Pharmacology for Pharmacy and the Health Sciences

A patient-centred approach

Michael Boarder
Professor of Pharmacology, Leicester School of Pharmacy, De Montfort University, UK

David Newby
Senior Lecturer in Clinical Pharmacology, School of Medicine and Public Health, University of Newcastle, Australia

Phyllis Navti
Divisional Lead Prescribing Advisor, Leicestershire County and Rutland Primary Care Trust NHS, and Senior Lecturer in Pharmacy Practice, Leicester School of Pharmacy, UK

OXFORD
UNIVERSITY PRESS

OXFORD
UNIVERSITY PRESS

Great Clarendon Street, Oxford OX2 6DP

Oxford University Press is a department of the University of Oxford.
It furthers the University's objective of excellence in research, scholarship,
and education by publishing worldwide in

Oxford New York

Auckland Cape Town Dar es Salaam Hong Kong Karachi
Kuala Lumpur Madrid Melbourne Mexico City Nairobi
New Delhi Shanghai Taipei Toronto

With offices in

Argentina Austria Brazil Chile Czech Republic France Greece
Guatemala Hungary Italy Japan Poland Portugal Singapore
South Korea Switzerland Thailand Turkey Ukraine Vietnam

Oxford is a registered trade mark of Oxford University Press
in the UK and in certain other countries

Published in the United States
by Oxford University Press Inc., New York

British Library Cataloguing in Publication Data

Data available

Library of Congress Cataloging in Publication Data

Data available

Typeset by MPS Limited, A Macmillan Company
Printed in Italy on acid-free paper by
L.E.G.O. S.p.A.

ISBN 978–0–19–955982–4

1 3 5 7 9 10 8 6 4 2

Abbreviations

5'-dFUrd	5'-deoxy-5'-fluorouridine
5-FU	5-Fluourouracil
6-MTG	6-methylthioguanine
6-TG	6-thioguanine
6-TGMP	6-thioguanine monophosphate
6-TGTP	6-thioguanine triphosphate
6-TIMP	6-thioinosine monophosphate
6-TUA	6-thiouric acid
6-TXMP	6-thioxanthosine monophosphate
5'-dFCyd	5'dexoy-5'fluorocytidine
5ASA	5-aminosalicylic acid
5-FU	5-fluorouracil
5-HT	5-hydroxytryptamine
5-HTT	serotonin (5-hydroxytryptamine) 5-HT transporter
6-MMP	6-methylmercaptopurine
6-MP	6-mercaptopurine
6-MP	6-mercaptopurine
6-MTIMP	6-methylthioinosine monophosphate
6-MTITP	6-methylthioinosine monophosphate
6-MTITP	6-methylthioinosine triphosphate
6-TGTP	6-thioguanine triphosphate
7-TM	7-transmembrane
A&E	Accident and Emergency
A2RAs	angiotensin II receptor antagonists
ABC	airway breathing circulation
AC	anthracycline, doxorubicin and cyclophosphamide
ACC	anterior cingulate cortex
ACE	angiotensin-converting enzyme
ACEI	angiotensin-converting enzyme inhibitors
ACh	acetylcholine
AChR	acetylcholine receptor
ACS	acute coronary syndrome
ACTH	adrenocorticotrophic hormone
ADCC	antibody dependent cellular cytotoxicity
ADH	antidiuretic hormone
ADME	absorption, distribution, metabolism, elimination
ADP	adenosine diphosphate
A&E	accident and emergency

AEDs	anti-epileptic drugs
AF	atrial fibrillation
AGEs	advanced glycosylation end products
AgRP	agouti-related protein
AIC	5-aminoimidazole-4-carboxamide
ALL	acute lymphoblastic leukaemia
AMI	acute myocardial infarct
AML	acute myeloid leukaemia
AMP	adenosine monophosphate
AMPA	α-amino-3-hydroxy-5-methyl-isoxazole
AMPK	AMP-activated protein kinase
α-MSH	α-melanocyte stimulating hormone
ANA	antinuclear antibody
ANS	autonomic nervous system
antiCCP	anticyclic citrullinated peptide
APC	antigen-presenting cell
aPTT	activated partial thromboplastin time
AR	allergic rhinitis
ARBs	angiotensin receptor blockers
ARC	arcuate nucleus
ASW	approved social worker
ATP	adenosine triphosphate
ATRA	all-trans retinoic acid
AV	atrioventricular
BCR	breakpoint cluster region
bFGF	basic fibroblast growth factor
BGL	blood glucose level
BMI	body mass index
BNF	brain-derived neurotrophic factor
BP	blood pressures
CAD	coronary artery disease
cAMP	cyclic adenosine monophosphate
CB_1	cannabinoid receptor
CB1	endogenous cannabinoid receptor
CCK	cholecystokinin
CCU	cardiac care unit
CD	cytidine deaminase
CD20	cluster of differentiation 20
CD52	cluster of differentiation 52
CDC	Centre for Disease Control and Prevention

CDC	complement-dependent cytotoxicity
CES	carboxylesterase
CHF	congestive heart failure
c-Kit	stem cell factor receptor
CL	corpus luteum
CLO	camplyobacter-like organism
CMF	cyclophospahmide, methotrexate and fluouracil
CML	chronic myeloid leukaemia
CMV	cytomegalovirus
CNS	central nervous system
CO	cardiac output
COC	combined oral contraceptive pills
COMT	catechol O-methyl transferase
COPD	chronic obstructive pulmonary disease
CORB	confusion, oxygen, respiratory rate, blood pressure
COX	cyclooxygenase
CRF	corticotrophin releasing factor
CRP	C-reactive protein
CSM	Committee on Safety of Medicines
CTPA	computer tomography pulmonary angiography
CTZ	chemoreceptor trigger zone
CV	cardiovascular
CVD	cardiovascular disease
DAG	diacylglycerol
dCMP	deoxycytidine monophosphate
dCTP	deoxycytidine triphosphate
DFR	dihydrofolate reductase
DHFR	dihydrofolate reductase
DKA	diabetic ketoacidosis
DM	diabetes mellitus
DMARDs	disease modifying antirheumatic drugs
DP	diphosphate
DPK	diphosphate kinase
DPP-4	dipeptidyl peptidase 4
DSM-IV-TR	Diagnostic and Statistical Manual of Mental Disorders
DTIC	dacarbazine
dTMP	2'-deoxythymidylate monophophosphate
dUMP	2'-deoxyuridylate monophosphate
DVT	deep vein thrombosis
EC50	Concentration giving 50% of maximum response
ECG	electrocardiogram
ECL	enterochromaffin-like
ECP	eosinophil cationic protein

EDN	eosinophil-derived neurotoxin
EDRF	endothelium-derived relaxing factor
EDV	end diastolic volume
EE	ethinyl oestradiol
EEGs	electroencephalograms
EGFR	epidermal growth factor receptor
EMBP	eosinophil major basic protein
ENS	enteric nervous system
EP	eosinophil peroxidase
ER	oestrogen receptor
ERCC1	excision repair cross-complementing protein
ERK	extracellular signal-regulated kinases
ESR	erythrocyte sedimentary rate
FBC	full blood count
FDA	Food and Drug Administration
FdUDP	fluorodeoxyuridylate diphosphate
FdUMP	fluorodeoxyuridylate monophosphate
FdUTP	fluorodeoxyuridylate triphosphate
FEV_1	forced expiratory volume
FSH	follicle stimulating hormone
FUDP	fluorouracil diphosphate
FUMP	fluorouracil monophosphate
FUTP	fluorouracil triphosphate
FVC	forced vital capacity
$GABA_A$	gamma-aminobutyric acid
GAD	generalized anxiety disorder
GARFT	5-phosphoribosylglycinamide formyltransferase
G-CSF	granulocyte colony-stimulating factors
GDP	guanine diphosphate
GDP	guanosine-5'-diphosphate
GERD	gastro esophageal reflux disease
GF	Graafian follicle
GI	gastrointestinal
GINA	Global Initiative for Asthma
GIP	glucose-dependent insulinotropic polypeptide, gastric inhibitory polypeptide
GLP-1	glucagon-like peptide-1
GLUT2	glucose transporter 2
GMP	guanine monophosphate
GMPS	guanosine monophosphate synthetase
GnRH	gonadotrophin-releasing hormone
GORD	gastro oesophageal reflux disease
GPCR	G-protein coupled receptors
GTI	gastrointestinal tract infection
GTN	glyceryl trinitrate

GTP	guanine triphosphate	LMWH	low-molecular weight heparin
GTP	guanosine-5′-triphosphate	LOS	lower oesophageal sphincter
H2Ras	histamine-2-receptor antagonists	LSD	lysergic acid diethylamide
Hb	haemoglobin	LVEF	left ventricular ejection fraction
HDL	high-density lipoproteins	MAC	mycobacterium avium complex
HEPA	high efficiency particulate air	mAChR	muscarinic acetylcholine receptor
HER1	human epidermal growth factor receptor 1	MAO-B	monoamine oxidase B
HER2	human epidermal growth factor receptor 2	MAOI	mono-amine oxidase inhibitor
		MAPK	mitogen-activated protein kinase
HF	chronic heart failure	MCV	mean cell volume
HFAs	hydrofluoroalkanes	MDIs	metered dose inhalers
HIF-1a	hypoxia-inducible factor-1a	MDT	multidisciplinary team
HIT	heparin-induced thrombocytopaenia	MHC	major histocompatibility complex
HMG	hydroxymethylglutaryl	MI	myocardial infarct
HPA	hypothalamic-pituitary-adrenal	MIC	minimum inhibitory concentration
HPC	history of presenting complaint	MLCK	myosin light chain kinase
HPRT	hypoxanthine phosphoribosyl transferase	mLDL	modified LDL
HR	heart rate	MMC	migratory motor complexes
HSD	hydroxysteroid dehydrogenase	MMP	matrix metalloproteinases
HSV	herpes simplex virus	MP	monophosphate
IBD	inflammatory bowel disease	MPK	monophosphate kinase
IBS	irritable bowel syndrome	MRI	magnetic resonance imaging
IBS-A	alternating diarrhoea and constipation	mRNA	messenger ribonucleic acid
IBS-C	constipation dominant	MRSA	methicillin resistant *Staphylococcus aureus*
IBS-D	diarrhoea dominant	MTIC	methyltriazenyl-imidazole-carboxamide
IBS-M	mixed diarrhoea and constipation	mTOR	mammalian target of rapamycin
ICAM-1	inter-cellular adhesion molecule 1	NA	noradrenaline, norepinephrine
ICD-10	International Statistical Classification of Diseases and Related Health Problems	nAChR	nicotinic aceylcholine receptor
		NADH	nicotinamide adenine dinucleotide
ICU	intensive care unit	NADPH	nicotinamide adenine dinucleotide phosphate
IFL	irinotecan, fluorouracil and leucovorin		
IGF-1	insulin-like growth factor 1	NAG	N-acetylglucosamine
IHD	ischaemic heart disease	NAM	N-acetylmuramic acid
IL-2	interleukin 2	NARI	selective noradrenaline reuptake inhibitor
IL-6	interleukin-6	NARTI	nucleoside analogue RTI
IMPDH	inosine monophosphate dehydrogenase	NaSSA	noardrenergic and specific serotoninergic antidepressant
INR	international normalized ratio		
IP_3	inositol triphosphate	NDP	nucleoside diphosphate
IPANs	intrinsic primary afferent neurones	NFAT	nuclear factor of activated T-cells
JAK	janus kinase	NF-κB	nuclear factor κB
K_D	Dissociation constant, a measure of affinity of a ligand for its receptor	NICE	National Institute of Clinical Excellence
		NK	natural killer
LDL	low-density lipoprotein	NK1	neurokinin
LFTs	liver function tests	NMDA	N-methyl-D-aspartate
LH	luteinizing hormone	NNRTIs	non-nucleoside reverse transcriptase inhibitors
LHA	lateral hypothalamic area		
LHRH	luteinizing hormone-releasing hormone	NO	nitric oxide

NOP	nociceptin/orphanin
NPY	neuropeptide Y
NSAIDs	non-steroidal anti-inflammatory drugs
NSTEMI	without ST-segment elevation
NtARTIs	Nucleotide analogue RTIs
ORS	oral rehydration solutions
OTC	over the counter
PABA	para-aminobenzoic acid
PAE	post-antibiotic effect
PAI1 and PAI2	plasminogen activator inhibitors 1 and 2
PARs	platelet thrombin receptors
PCA	patient controlled analgesia
PCI	percutaneous coronary intervention
PCP	phencyclidine
PD	Parkinson's disease
PDE	Phosphodiesterase
PDGFR	platelet derived growth factor receptor
PE	pulmonary embolism
PEF	peak expiratory flow
PEGs	polyethylene glycols
PET	positron emission tomography
PGE_1	prostaglandin E_1
PGE_2	prostaglandin E_2
PGI_2	prostacyclin
$PG\text{-}I_2$	prostaglandin I_2
PI3K	phosphoinositide 3-kinase
PIP_2	phosphatidylinositol bisphosphate
Pis	protease inhibitors
PK	pharmacokinetics
PLA_2	phospholipase A_2
PLC	phospholipase C
PMH	past medical history
PML	promyelocytic leukemia gene
POMC	pro-opiomelanocortin
POP	progestogen only pill
PP	pancreatic polypeptide
PPARγ	peroxisome proliferator activator receptor gamma
PPIs	proton pump inhibitors
PSI	pneumonia severity index
PUVA	psoralen + UVA treatment
PVN	paraventricular nucleus
QRS	QRS-complex on an electrocardiogram
QT	QT-segment on an electrocardiogram
RA	rheumatoid arthritis
RAAS	renin-aldosterone-angiotensin system

RANKL	receptor activator of nuclear factor κβ ligand
RBC	red blood cells
RF	rheumatoid factor
rRNA	ribosomal RNA
RSV	respiratory syncytial virus
RTA	road traffic accident
RTI	respiratory tract infection
RTIs	reverse transcriptase inhibitors
RXR	retinoid X receptor
SA	sinoatrial node
SERDs	selective estrogen receptor down-regulators
SERMs	selective estrogen receptor modulators
SERT	serotonin (5-hydroxytryptamine) 5-HT transporter
SERT	serotonin reuptake transporter
SHBG	sex hormone binding globulin
SIADH	syndrome of inappropriate antidiuretic hormone
SMAC	second mitochondria-derived activator of caspases
SNP	sodium nitroprusside
SNRI	serotonin and noradrenaline reuptake inhibitor
SSRIs	selective serotonin reuptake inhibitors
STAT	signal transducers and activators of transcription
STEMI	ST-segment elevation MI
STI	sexually transmitted infection
SV	stroke volume
T_3	triiodothyronine
TB	tuberculosis
TC	total plasma cholesterol
TCA	tricyclic antidepressants
TDM	therapeutic drug monitoring
TENS	transcutaneous electrical stimulation
TFTs	thyroid function tests
ThioTEPA	N,N'N'-triethylenethiophosphoramide
TNF	tumour necrosis factor
TNF-α	tumor necrosis factor-alpha
TNM	T, extent of the tumour; N, number of lymph nodes involved; M, presence of metastasis
TP	thymidine phosphorylase
TP	triphosphate
tPA	tissue plasminogen activator
TPR	total peripheral resistance
TR	thyroid receptor

TRH	thyrotropin-releasing hormone		VEGF	vascular endothelial growth factor
tRNA	transfer RNA		VEGF-A	vascular endothelial growth factor A
TS	thymidylate synthetase		VIP	vasoactive intestinal peptide
TSH	thyroid stimulating hormone		VLDL	very low density lipoproteins
TXA_2	thromboxane A_2		VMH	ventromedial hypothalamic nucleus
UDP	uridine diphosphate		VTE	venous thromboembolism
UGT	uridine diphosphate-glucuronyltransferase		WBC	white blood cells
UV	ultraviolet		WCC	white cell count
UTI	urinary tract infection		WHO	World Health Organization
UVA	ultraviolet A		TPMT	thiopurine S-methyl transferase
UVB	ultraviolet B		XO	xanthine oxidase
VCAM-1	vascular cell adhesion molecule-1			

Clinical clerking abbreviations

PC	Presenting complaint		DS	Drug sensitivities
HPC	History of presenting complaint		O/E	On examination
PMH	Past medical history		FH	Family history
SH	Social history		O/Q	On questioning
DH	Drug history		O/O	On observation

Acknowledgements

This book arises out of teaching experience in both the United Kingdom and Australia, so firstly we should thank the many students over the years who have participated in, tested and challenged our attempts to develop the teaching of patient-centred pharmacology. We are grateful to our colleagues in our institutions, and beyond, who have helped us develop our approach to teaching pharmacology and extended it beyond its original boundaries. In particular we would like to thank the following of our colleagues and collaborators who have generously given up their time to read and comment on parts of this book: David Lambert, Gary Willars, Geoff Hall, Sandra Hall, Tania Webb (with special thanks for material in the workbooks in chapters 12 & 13), Ben Gronier (with special thanks for material in the workbooks in chapters 14 & 15), Rasha Salama (with special thanks for material in the workbook in chapter 11), Tyra Zetterstrom, Martin Elliott, Jane Dixon, Rowena Jones, Andrew Casinader, Jennifer Schneider, Namit Kathoria, Carmel Davison, Zeibun Patel, Bhavisha Pattani, Helen Knight, Olajide Ajetunmobi, Patricia Shorrock and Lucy Holt. Finally we would like to thank Jonathan Crowe, our editor at Oxford University Press, who did everything right – helped us build the project from its origins, guided us in details and broad issues, provided common sense when that was lacking from the authors, and was always ready with encouragement.

Figure acknowledgements

We would like to extend our thanks to everyone who helped obtain figures for this book, to Simon Tegg for the illustrations

Figure 3.8 Adapted from: Birkett DJ Half-life. *Australian Prescriber* 1988; 11(3): 57–9.

Figure 3.9 Adapted from: Birkett DJ Bioavailability and First Pass Clearance. *Australian Prescriber* 1991; 14(1): 14–16.

S4.1 and Figure 9.1 From Pocock G, Richards C, *The Human Body*, 2009. By permission of Oxford University Press.

Figures 8.1a–8.1c, 8.2, 8.4, 21.10, and 21.16 Saxe N, Jessop S, Todd G, *Handbook of Dermatology for Primary Care, 2nd edn*, 2007. By permission of Oxford University Press Southern Africa.

Figure 8.1d © NZ DermNet.

Figure B8.3 By permission of Brendan Thomas.

Figure S5.2a © Tissuepix/Science Photo Library.

Figure 17.4 © CNRI/Science Photo Library.

Figure 18.4 Reprinted by permission from Macmillan Publishers Ltd: Seeman P, *et al.* Antipsychotic drug doses and neuroleptic/dopamine receptors. *Nature* 261:717, 1976**.**

Figure 21.20 Adapted from Clavel F, Hance AJ. HIV drug resistance. *N Engl J Med* 2004; 350(10): 1023–35.

Figure 22.9 Adapted from: Zaboikin M, *et al.* Gene therapy with drug resistance genes. *Cancer Gene Therapy* 2005; 13: 335–45.

Figure 22.10 Adapted from: Derijks LJJ, *et al.* Thiopurines in inflammatory bowel disease. *Alimentary Pharmacology & Therapeutics* 2006; 24: 715–29.

Figure 22.12 Adapted from: Jin Y, Zeruesenay D, Stearns V, *et al.* CYP2D6 genotype, antidepressant use, and tamoxifen metabolism during adjuvant breast cancer treatment. *Journal of the National Cancer Institute* 2005; 97: 30–9.

Contents at a glance

Contents in full

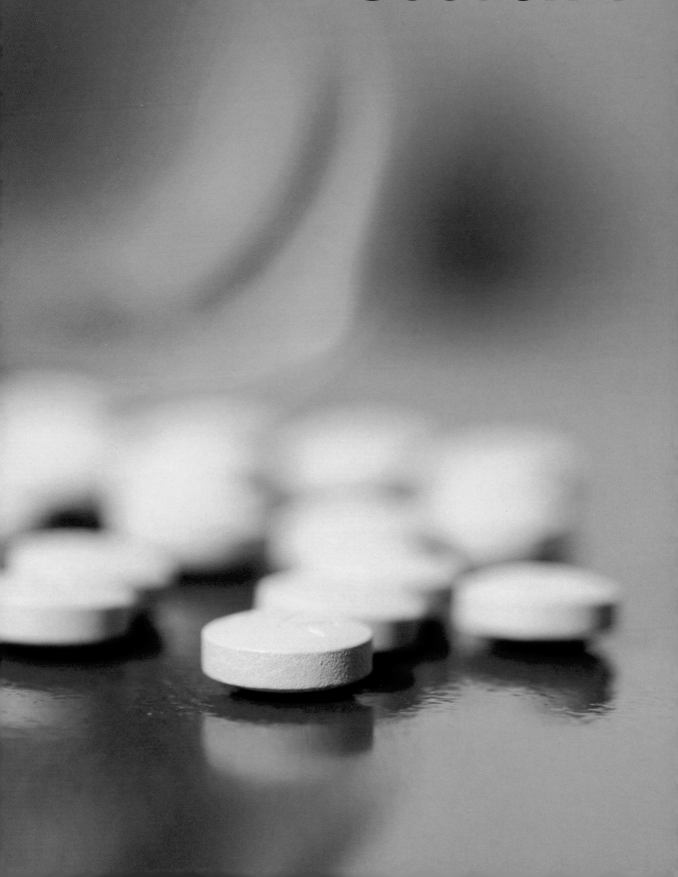

Section 1

Chapter 1
Drugs, patients, and this book

Pharmacology—*a **patient-centred** approach??* What does this mean? Let's start with a patient.

> It's morning. Gerald is in his own home, sitting hunched in his chair, talking in a quiet monotone, without movement of his mask-like face, his hands trembling, but otherwise still. He doesn't get up to greet you, doesn't reach out to shake your hand. It's not that he can't do these things, but they are difficult for him; sometimes he doesn't know whether he can do them or not. Two patches of cells have died in his brain, and this means his brain cannot plan movements and control his body. He takes his medication—it's not easy: his hands are shaking, swallowing is difficult. Half an hour later he stands, upright and confident, moves across the room normally, and now he reaches out to firmly shake your hand, smiling and chatting.[1]

We want you to be able to **understand** the various aspects of this situation:

1) What is wrong with the patient in the first place. **We need to understand this at the cellular and molecular level** if we are to understand the action of drugs.

2) The main drug treatments that are used to treat or manage the condition so that the patient benefits.

3) **How drugs work at the cellular and molecular level to benefit the patient**. This is where you really *understand* how drugs help people.

This book is written on the basis that understanding the patient's response to drugs and the cellular and molecular basis of drug treatment are the same thing.

When you look at our patient Gerald and see his initial disability, then watch the drugs change him, you should be able to picture in your mind what is happening in his brain, how the drug is entering his brain, and how his brain is being changed. As a result you will understand what the strengths and weaknesses of his treatment are, and what the future holds for him. You will also be in a good position to understand new drugs and new approaches to treatment as they come along in the future.

We introduce our patients as individuals. We tell stories around our patients so that you will think of them as individuals. They are people, like you and me, our mums and dads, our children. They *are* you and me. **Pharmacology is about people.**

1.1 How does this fit in with your career development in the changing world of healthcare delivery?

The need for this book stems from the likely nature of healthcare delivery in the future. Changes in this are under way, driven by governments, professional bodies, and the healthcare professionals themselves. Pharmacists are, in a number of countries, expected to play a greater role in

healthcare delivery in the future: pharmacists are expected to become more **patient-centred, with both** pharmacists and nurses playing a primary role in prescribing drugs in many healthcare settings.

As Patrick Vallance and Trevor Smart wrote in 2006:[2]

---

1. Gerald and his illness are explored in Chapter 17.

2. Vallance P. and Smart T. (2006) British Journal of Pharmacology, 147 (Suppl 1), S304–S307.

Prescribers are changing. Getting onto the register to practice as a doctor brings rather few specific rights. In fact just about the only one is the right to prescribe medicines. However, nurses and pharmacists are also gaining these rights and this trend seems unlikely to reverse. Indeed, it makes sense to broaden the range of prescribers, and the challenge will be to ensure an appropriate pharmacological underpinning to ensure safe and effective use of medicines.

This is a book to prepare you for these future challenges.

1.2 So, what is pharmacology?

Firstly, **pharmacology is a science**, so be prepared to learn a lot of science in this book. And be prepared to refer back to your basic biology, to refresh you memory about systems in the body—blood, heart and circulation, digestive system, the nervous system, etc. After all, it is these that go wrong when we get ill, so it is these that we will discuss as we go through medical conditions and their treatment.

In 1968, in a book called *Principles of Drug Action*, Avram Goldstein and colleagues defined pharmacology as follows:

> Pharmacology is the science of drugs, their chemical constitution, their biologic action, and their therapeutic application in man.

Pharmacology is a broad science, running from the chemistry of drugs, through their effect on physiology, to treatment of the sick.

Today, molecular and cell biology is at the heart of pharmacology—drugs are molecules, and they interact with other molecules inside us. This changes cells, organ systems, and eventually our bodies and our minds, for good or for bad.

The molecules with which drugs interact are often, but not always, proteins in our cells. The composition of the protein assemblies within our cells is initially defined by what we inherit from our parents—our genome. It's not surprising then that modern pharmacology is dependent on the understanding and techniques of molecular biology and genomics. This is where future advances, the nature of which we can only guess at, will have their beginnings. This is not an academic exercise—it is at the heart of the drug discovery of the pharmaceutical industry, and the treatment of the sick.

You will encounter a lot of science in this book, but you will not encounter much molecular biology. However, you should be aware that it is the molecular biology of life that lies beneath the efforts of pharmacologists to provide medical practice with improved drugs.

1.3 How to use this book

The chapters in this book are divided into six sections. The first section is this Introduction followed by Chapter 2 on how drugs change the body, and Chapter 3 on what happens to drugs when they enter the body. All of the other chapters are on clinical topics, starting with thromboembolic disorders, ending with cancers, and on the way dealing with such subjects as heart attacks, asthma, epilepsy, depression, and infections.

All of the chapters except the one you are reading now have **boxes** separated from the main text, which develop subjects and issues in greater detail. In some cases this is a more in-depth treatment of the science, in others it is a further exploration of clinical issues. It is anticipated that you can read the main text independent of the material in the boxes.

The main clinically oriented chapters, in Sections 2–6, have **workbooks** as the last part of each chapter. Here this book takes on an unusual aspect.

Fictional characters appear in a storyline in these workbooks; some of these characters get ill and are admitted to hospital. In hospital their details and clinical history are presented in a **clinical clerking** format. The medical staff treating them are introduced into the narrative, and the patient's diagnosis is made on the basis of the clinical clerking. A treatment plan is devised, and the workbook follows the progress of the fictional patients, mainly with respect to their medical condition, but also looking at the impact this has on their lives. The narratives are simple and intended to graphically illustrate the individual nature of patient care. The storyline in many cases uses the same, or overlapping, characters as they progress through different chapters.

From the point at which the diagnosis is made the workbooks have a further feature: questions and answers. Questions appear about the science underpinning the drugs and the drug treatments themselves. There are spaces in the workbook for you to write your own answers to these questions directly into the text. In this way you will not only have been taken through the subject in an interactive manner, probing and developing your understanding of the subject, but will also have created in the completed workbooks a learning resource for yourself.

The material to enable you to think through the answers to the questions in the workbooks is all provided in the main text (and boxes) in the relevant chapter. In this sense, each chapter is self contained, and the clinical subject each pursues may therefore be taken in any order. The only exception to this is that it is necessary first to understand fundamental aspects of drug action and drug use explained in Chapters 2 and 3. For example, you need

to understand the term 'antagonist', and to have a picture of how the body handles drugs introduced by different routes, in order to approach much of the material in the clinical chapters. If, however, you are confident in your basic pharmacology background then you may wish to read each of these clinical chapters independently of the rest of the book.

Asking students to write directly into their textbooks may seem odd. For those who do not wish to do this, or who wish to create separate collections of workbooks, or revise and review their answers, the workbooks are made available online as described below. They may then be completed independently of the bound text. In addition to the main text, boxes, and workbooks, you will find that each chapter has a **drug summary table**. This is a quick reference source for principle drugs in each clinical subject to which you can refer across and within chapters.

Further reading suggestions for each of the main chapters are provided at the end of the book, with examples exploring the basic science as well as the clinical application of pharmacology.

1.4 Comment for instructors

This book, with the feature of workbooks with narrative based around fictional characters, arose out of our experience of moving towards teaching patient-centred pharmacology to pharmacy students. The workbooks present in this text have their origin in those used in our teaching. The workbooks form the activity in small group teaching sessions, each of which is preceded by a series of lectures covering the subject of the workbook. Here we have replaced the lectures with illustrated text, and revised and extended the breadth of subjects covered in

the workbooks. In our strong emphasis on patients, we have strived to integrate the scientific basis of therapeutics with the clinical material. Our objective is that the science and the individual's therapeutic response are not seen as sequential (or, even worse, separate) material, but as a single, integrated subject. We hope you find this book interesting, but mostly we hope that it enthuses your students, motivating them to truly understand the pharmacological basis of therapeutics.

1.5 Online Resource Centre

Pharmacology for Pharmacy and the Health Sciences doesn't end with this printed book. Further materials are also available in the book's Online Resource Centre at www.oxfordtextbooks.co.uk/orc/boarder/.

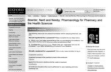

The Online Resource Centre includes the following material for registered adopters of the book:

- **figures from the book** in electronic format, ready to download
- all **workbooks** included in this book in pdf format, for use in teaching seminars, workshops, etc.
- **suggested answers** to the questions posed in the workbooks.

Chapter 2
How do drugs work?
An introduction

The drugs we are mainly interested in are those used to treat illnesses (therapeutic drugs). These are mainly (although not only) small molecules prepared by pharmaceutical companies, and our objective in this chapter is to provide an overview of how these drugs change bodily function. These principles of drug action will then be encountered again and again in the medical use of drugs that are discussed in the rest of this book. We discuss here the most commonly encountered forms of drug action—there are other modes of action of drugs used in the clinic that we do not discuss in this chapter, and some of these are explained later in this book.

To begin thinking about how drugs act we can note the following points:

1) **Most drugs act at cellular targets**, but some act outside cells. The simplest example is the treatment of acid indigestion with bicarbonate. The stomach contains hydrochloric acid, giving it a very low pH. When this causes discomfort, the bicarbonate will chemically neutralize part of the acid. This occurs in the lumen of the stomach outside any cells. A broader range of examples is found in drugs acting at proteins in the soluble part of the blood (the plasma). For example, in Chapter 4 we encounter drugs interacting with the enzymes in the plasma that are required for blood clotting. These enzymes (the clotting factors) may be inhibited by drugs such as heparin.

2) **The large majority of drug targets are proteins.** The plasma enzymes are an example of this, but are unusual in that most of these protein targets are cellular. The cellular target proteins may be at the surface of the cell or inside the cell (intracellular).

3) **The majority of protein targets are receptors.**[1] These are often cell surface receptors (e.g. the receptors for adrenaline (epinephrine) introduced in this chapter), but in many cases (e.g. steroid drugs) they are intracellular receptors.

4) **Apart from receptors** the most common protein targets are:

   a. **ion channels** (mainly cell surface, such as the blood pressure-lowering calcium channel blockers in Chapter 5)

   b. **enzymes** (mainly intracellular), such as enzyme substrates or inhibitors (e.g. L-dopa or the monoamine oxidase inhibitors used to treat Parkinson's disease in Chapter 17).

   c. **transport proteins** (mainly cell surface) such as the inhibitors of neurotransmitter uptake used to treat depression (e.g. Prozac-like drugs, Chapter 19).

---

1. The term 'receptor' is sometimes used to mean the molecule, or part of a molecule, that a drug interacts with to have its effect. This would mean that all molecular targets of drugs are receptors. This is not how the term is used in this book. Here a receptor is mostly taken to mean the molecule (usually a protein) that naturally-occuring biological mediators (e.g. neurotransmitter, hormones, local mediators) bind to to have their effect. This distinguishes receptors from other enzymes, ion channels, transporters, or other proteins, which are all the molecular targets for drug action, as set out in Box 2.1.

Box 2.1

First targets of drugs—they are mostly proteins.

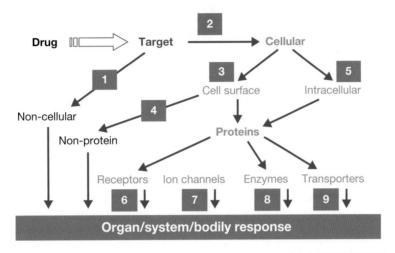

Figure a First drug targets.

When a drug is administered it will interact with an initial target. The main classes of drug target are numbered on the scheme.

1. A small minority of drugs interact with drug targets in the extracellular compartment.

2. The vast majority of drugs interact directly with molecules that are part of cells.

3. Some of these molecules are on the cell surface. This means that drugs that cannot enter cells (i.e. cannot pass thorough the lipid cell membrane because they are not lipid soluble) can bind to the membrane components and change the cells.

4. Some of the cell surface interactions are not in the first case with proteins, but with the lipid layer itself. This may contribute to the response to inhaled general anaesthetics, although the action of such drugs is increasingly described through the consequences for cell membrane proteins such as ion channels.

5. Most of the interactions of drugs are with proteins, which may be on the cell surface [3] or inside the cell [5]. If they are inside the cell then the drug must be able to pass through the cell membrane to reach the target protein.

6–8. Receptors are the most common type of protein drug target, either at the cell surface (usually intrinsic membrane proteins) or within the cell. Other common types of protein target are ion channels, enzymes, or transporter proteins.

In what follows we review the nature of drug action at these four main protein targets: receptors, ion channels, enzymes, and transport proteins.

2.1 Agonists and antagonists: drugs acting at receptors

Receptors have complex three-dimensional structures, within which pockets are formed that can be occupied by a small molecule: either by the neurotransmitters, hormones, etc. produced by the body, or by drugs. These small molecules may be collectively referred to as **ligands**. These ligands **bind** to specific sites on receptors.

When bound they are said to **occupy** the receptors. Some (nearly all the natural ligands and some of the drugs) then **activate** the receptor, changing the cell in which they are found. These ligands (natural and drugs) are called **agonists**. Some ligands, however, bind but do not activate the receptor. These are called **antagonists**. They have an

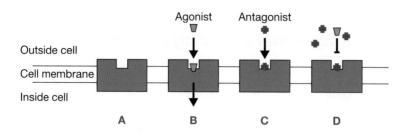

Figure 2.1 Agonists and antagonists at a cell surface receptor.

The cell membrane is shown, with the receptor in orange crossing the membrane from outside the cell to inside. In **A** there is no ligand (i.e. no agonist and no antagonist). In **B** an agonist (green symbol) is present in the extracellular compartment. This could be the naturally occurring hormone or neurotransmitter, or it could be a drug. It stimulates the receptor, sending signals into the cell which change cellular function. In **C** an antagonist is present (blue symbol) outside the cell—it binds to the same receptor site, but does not stimulate it. The cell's function is not changed. In **D** the agonist is again present as in **B**, but this time with antagonist molecules. The antagonist occupies the receptor, and so despite the presence of the agonist the receptor is not stimulated. The effect of the antagonist is seen by comparing **D** with **B**. Note that the effect of the antagonist is dependent on the presence of the agonist. A more complex illustration of these issues, emphasizing the equilibrium of bound and free drugs with populations of receptors, appears in Figure 2.5.

effect because, by occupying receptors, they reduce the binding of the natural agonist. The general situation is illustrated in Figure 2.1, considering events at a cell surface receptor in the presence of an agonist, an antagonist, or both.

2.1.1 Both agonists and antagonists are important in therapeutics

To help understand the principles of agonist and antagonist action we can consider adrenaline (epinephrine), a hormone from the adrenal medulla which stimulates its receptors in many cell types throughout the body. Adrenaline is an agonist at adrenoceptors, a family of cell surface receptors—the main members (that is those that are important for understanding commonly used drugs) are α_1-, α_2-, β_1-, and β_2-adrenoceptors.

Here is a clinical example of when an agonist drug at adrenoceptors is used.

Amritpal is a pharmacy student who has asthma. She gets up early for an 8 am lecture, rushes to catch the train to university, and then finds she is struggling to breathe, with wheezing and coughing. She finds her blue inhaler, takes two puffs, and within a few seconds she is breathing freely.

The inhaler contains a drug called salbutamol. When she inhales the salbutamol it reaches the small airways (the bronchioles) in her lungs. When she is having an asthmatic episode these small tubes, which have flexible walls, are too narrow. This is partly because they have smooth muscle wrapped around them that has contracted too much, squeezing the bronchioles and making the passage of air difficult.[2] These smooth muscle cells have β_2-adrenoceptors on their surface. The salbutamol *stimulates* these receptors, i.e. it is an *agonist* at β_2-adrenoceptors. The stimulated receptors send signals inside the cell that make the muscle relax, the airways open up, and breathing becomes easier.

Now consider another case, in which an antagonist drug is used:

Balrag is 60 years old, and has high blood pressure.[3] This means that his heart is pumping too much blood per minute against too high a resistance from the blood vessels around his body, so the pressure in the vessels carrying blood away from the heart (the arteries) is too high. Balrag's heart is stimulated by the hormone adrenaline, released from the adrenal medulla. His heart muscle cells have adrenoceptors on them, mainly β_1-adrenoceptors. His natural adrenaline

---

2. This is only one of several aspects of asthma. See Chapter 11 to learn about this condition and its treatment.
3. See Chapter 5.

stimulates the adrenoceptors (i.e. it is an agonist at these receptors) and this makes his heart beat more strongly, contributing to his high blood pressure. Many years ago he was prescribed a drug called atenolol, which he has taken as a pill every morning since. This drug is a β_1-adrenoceptor *antagonist*. When he takes atenolol it spreads around his body, including his heart, where it competes with the natural adrenaline at the β_1-adrenoceptors. It occupies these receptors but does not stimulate them, reducing the stimulation of the receptors by adrenaline (see Figure 2.1). As a result the receptors are stimulated less and his heart beats less strongly, contributing to a reduced blood pressure and a reduced risk of heart attack and stroke.

These two commonplace scenarios illustrate that both agonists and antagonists have a role to play in therapeutics.

2.1.2 The subdivision of receptors into types and subtypes is important for therapeutics

The examples above, of treatment of asthma with β_2-adrenoceptor agonists and treatment of high blood pressure with β_1-adrenoceptor antagonists also illustrates the importance of the study of receptor subtypes, their classification, and the development by pharmacologists and chemists of subtype-specific ligands (and potential drugs). The major adrenoceptors in airway smooth muscle cells are β_2-adrenoceptors, while those in the heart are principally β_1-adrenoceptors. This opened the way for the development of β_2-selective agonists in inhalers for asthma which were largely free of cardiac effects. In this case receptor classification has revolutionized life for millions of asthma sufferers the world over, and saved countless lives (Figure 2.2).

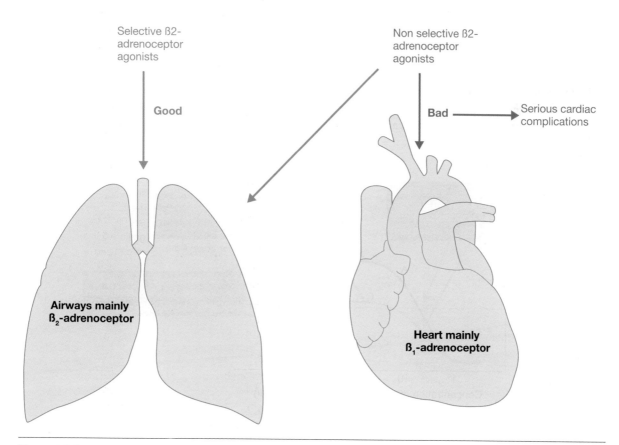

Figure 2.2 Importance of β-adrenoceptor subtypes in the treatment of asthma.

Both β_2-selective (β_2-adrenoceptors only) and non-selective (both β_1- and β_2-) agonists have beneficial effect at opening airways. However, the non-selective drug also gives significant cardiac effects, which means it cannot be used in the treatment of asthma. So, effective safe treatment of the symptoms of asthma was dependent on understanding β-adrenoceptor subtypes and their differing pharmacologies.

As mentioned above, the α-adrenoceptors (subdivided into α_1- and α_2-adrenoceptors) are also important for clinical pharmacology, as illustrated by the following example of the significance of receptor classification.

After a few years of taking his β_1-adrenoceptor antagonist, Balrag finds his blood pressure is not adequately controlled (see Chapter 5 for clarification) and he ends up taking several drugs. One of the drugs he takes is doxazosin, which is a selective α_1-adrenoceptor antagonist. α_1-adrenoceptors are found on the vascular smooth muscle cells, which are wrapped around the smaller blood vessels that the heart is pumping blood through. Stimulation of these receptors by naturally occurring adrenaline (and noradrenaline/norepinephrine) leads to constriction of the blood vessels and an increase in resistance to blood flow, resulting in an increased blood pressure. When doxazosin is present it will occupy the α_1-adrenoceptors, reduce binding of adrenaline and noradrenaline, reduce vasoconstriction, and therefore reduce blood pressure.

Note here that by paying attention to receptor subtypes we have a patient who is treating his high blood pressure at the two crucial locations, the pump (the heart) and the resistance to flow (small blood vessels; see also Chapter 5). We are able to target our drugs to a particular anatomical site, and a particular physiological function, and either increase the activity at the receptors (agonists) or reduce receptor activation (antagonists). The principal objective of treatment with any drug is to generate a highly specific effect in a particular region of the body. This can sometimes be achieved by localized administration of the drug (e.g. the use of antibiotic ointment to treat a skin infection). However, within the body this is generally accomplished by using drugs that are highly selective for particular receptor subtypes, such as in the examples given above.

2.1.3 Partial agonists show properties of both agonists and antagonists and offer flexible treatment options

Consider a strip of muscle tissue suspended in a bath of physiological fluid from both ends, so that any contraction of the muscle can be recorded and quantified. Then add an agonist (drug A) for a receptor you know is on the muscle cells and which stimulates contraction. If you add different concentrations of agonist then you will get different sized responses. This will give you data to plot as a concentration–response curve, i.e. the relationship between the concentration of drug and the response. A typical curve is shown in Figure 2.3, for drug A (blue line).

It can be seen that the response gets larger as more agonist is added, but only up to a point—beyond this the

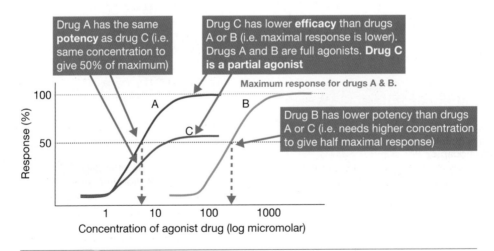

Figure 2.3 Concentration-response curves for three different agonists, all of which act on the same receptor to give the response.

Drugs A and B are both full agonists. Drug A is more potent than drug B. Drug C is a partial agonist. It has the same EC_{50} as drug A, so it has equal potency, but it can only give a fraction of the maximal response that drug A can give, i.e. drug C has a lower efficacy than drug A.

response remains the same despite more drug being added. A plateau is reached. This is because drug A can only generate a response when it is bound to the receptor—in effect when it **occupies** the receptor. So when there is no drug present then none of the receptors are occupied by drug A and the response size is 0. As the concentration of drug A around the receptors increases then more of the drug binds to the receptors so the size of the response increases. However, there must be a fixed number of receptors on this piece of tissue so if we continue to increase the concentration of drug A then eventually it will occupy all of the receptors. Increasing the concentration of drug A further will not increase the size of the response, since all the receptors are now fully stimulated so the response cannot get any bigger—a plateau is formed at the top of the concentration-response curve. The binding/occupation issues are further explored below (Figures 2.5 and 2.6).

Returning to our experimental situation, Figure 2.3 shows concentration-response curves for three different drugs (A, B, and C) added to the fluid bathing the strip of muscle. Note that these three drugs all act on the same receptor population. If we add drug B instead of drug A it gives the same maximum response as drug A, but this requires a higher concentration of drug. It is helpful to consider the concentration of drug which gives **half the maximal response** (the EC_{50}). Compared to drug A, drug B requires a higher concentration to give half the maximal response, so the EC_{50} for drug B is *higher* than the EC_{50} for drug A. We say that drug A has a higher **potency** than drug B because we can achieve 50% of the maximal response with a lower concentration.

Now look at drug C in Figure 2.3. The concentration-response curve for this drug also reaches a plateau, but this is lower than that for drug A. However much drug C we add we can never get as big a response as we can with drug A. And yet these two drugs have the same EC_{50}. (Note that the EC_{50} is the concentration giving half the maximal response for *that* drug). We make two observations:

1) The lower plateau for drug C is evidence that drug C has a lower **efficacy** than drug A. When it occupies the receptor it does not stimulate the receptor as strongly.

2) The two drugs have the same potency. We know this because the concentration to give half the maximal response (the EC_{50}) is the same.

So drug C can give a response. It binds to the same receptors as drug A and acts as an agonist, but cannot give a full response. It is a **partial agonist**, in contrast to drugs A and B, which are called full agonists.

This may be useful in itself. You may want a drug which has an effect but which is not as powerful as some other drugs.

Steve is a patient with moderate but quite troubling persistent abdominal pain. His position is stable, and he is at home, but he finds that ibuprofen does not adequately control his pain. His doctor wants to give him an opiate (i.e. morphine-like) drug, but knows that moderate pain does not warrant such a powerful drug with such addiction/abuse potential. A number of options are available,[4] but one he considers is a drug called buprenorphine. This acts at the same receptors as morphine, but it is a partial agonist so for this example, in Figure 2.3 morphine is drug A and buprenorphine is drug C, and the response is pain reduction. Buprenorphine gives less maximal pain relief, but it is sufficient for Steve's moderate pain and he becomes more comfortable.

Here a partial agonist was more appropriate than a full agonist. A partial agonist has another feature which follows from our experimental example, where both drug A and drug C are binding at the same receptor site.

Joe is a drug addict. He regularly takes heroin. Heroin is closely related to morphine, and acts on the same receptors as morphine. He has a sufficient supply of heroin to take frequently, to prevent the horrible effects of withdrawal (se Chapter 20). Sometimes he takes other drugs as well. On this day he takes a new drug that has recently been stolen from a clinic. He doesn't know it, but he takes buprenorphine. He immediately starts to become very ill—he is rapidly precipitated into partial withdrawal.

Buprenorphine binds very strongly to the same receptor as heroin, and so if heroin is present it will displace the heroin, and being only a partial agonist will produce a much lower level of response from the receptors, precipitating withdrawal. Buprenorphine is acting as an antagonist in the presence of heroin.

What this means is that a partial agonist can also act as an antagonist when given at the same time as a full agonist (Figures 2.1 and 2.5), binding to the receptor and reducing the response to a full agonist, as illustrated in Figure 2.4.

4. See Chapter 20, where the management of pain with drugs is explored.

12

Chapter 2 How do drugs work? An introduction

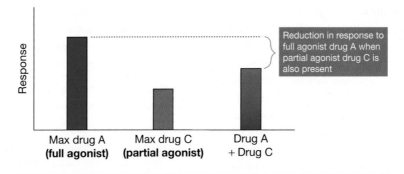

Figure 2.4 Drug C is a full agonist and drug C is a partial agonist at the same receptor.

Both are used at their maximally effective concentration (see Figure 2.3). When both drugs are added together some of the receptors will be occupied by drug A and some by drug C. The final response will be lower than that produced by drug A alone, meaning that drug C seems to be working like an antagonist.

From Figure 2.4 we can say that a drug like drug C acts partly as an agonist and partly as an antagonist, but that **it is not a pure antagonist** because it has some agonist activity.

2.1.4 What determines the potency of drugs: efficacy and affinity

Remember that we have already considered the term 'potency' when looking at the response curves to agonists in Figure 2.3. It is potency which determines the concentration of an agonist drug that is needed to give half its maximal response. Why is it that two similarly acting drugs may require very different doses to give a similar clinical response? It is likely that a major influence is potency, so it is important that we have some understanding of what determines this.

We have said that these drugs are ligands that bind to receptors and stimulate them to different degrees. Pure antagonists don't stimulate them at all; full agonists at maximally effective concentrations stimulate them to give the largest response possible. Above we have used the term **efficacy**[5] to describe this attribute—the ability of a drug, once bound to the receptor to stimulate it. Further aspects of efficacy and what they tell us about how drugs and receptors work are considered in Box 2.2.

A separate but equally important property of drugs is how *tightly* they bind to their receptors—some drugs bind more strongly than others. A drug that binds very strongly to its receptor is said to have a high **affinity**. From our example above, buprenorphine binds *very* strongly to the opiate (morphine) receptor (Chapter 20, section 20.3.1) and yet it cannot fully activate it. Many pure antagonists bind very strongly to their receptors, but they do not activate them at all. So binding and activation are two different things, which we need to comprehend if we are to understand how drugs work. We introduced the binding/occupation of drugs and receptors above (section 2.1.3), and we will now develop these ideas further. This is important when we consider how drugs work in the clinic, since we are so often dealing in clinical outcome with the competition between introduced drugs and native ligands at binding to the receptor.

The affinity of a drug for its receptor: binding is an equilibrium business

Pharmacologists have devised ways of measuring the binding of drugs to receptors. Given that receptors are specific cellular proteins, then there is a limited number of binding sites on any one cell, or in any given tissue. So if we expose our cells to increasing concentrations of drug (the ligand) then we will get more and more ligand bound, until we have saturated the receptors (i.e. they are all occupied).

There is a danger that this may give the impression that a ligand binds to and sticks to a receptor, making it

---

5. Strictly speaking we should use the term 'intrinsic efficacy' to describe the attribute of the drug which results in the size of the response at the level of the receptor, but here we will be satisfied with a simplified terminology. It is also worth noting that in a clinical setting the term 'efficacy' may be used in a much broader sense than here, i.e. to describe how effective a drug is at generating a desirable clinical outcome.

Box 2.2
Receptor reserve, efficacy and irreversible antagonists

For an agonist to give a response at a receptor it must occupy it. As explained in the text (section 2.1.4) this is an equilibrium binding, with the free agonist (i.e. that in solution) in equilibrium and constant exchange with the bound (attached to cell surface receptors) molecules.

We also know from the main text of this chapter that occupation is not enough to give a response—an antagonist may occupy exactly the same binding site but will give no response. The additional factor, what the agonist *does* to the receptor to turn it on, we are calling efficacy (see footnote 5, this chapter).

We can get an interesting insight into how agonist drugs work by comparing the binding of a drug, its occupation curve, to the concentration-response curve. This is done in Figure b. The striking thing is that the response curve is not the same as the occupancy curve – it lies to the left.

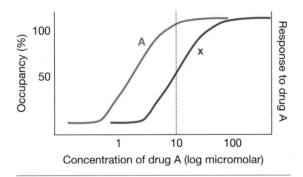

Figure b The occupation curve and the concentration-response curve for an agonist are often not the same.

The blue line (x) is the occupation curve for agonist drug A, and the red line (A) is the response curve for drug A. The dotted line shows 50% occupancy at 10 micromolar concentration of agonist A.

Examining this closely we can see that we get a full response with only 50% occupancy of the receptors. This occurs at a drug concentration of 10 micromolar. As we increase the concentration beyond this more receptors are occupied but there is no more response. This may seem curious: if we are occupying more receptors why does the response not get larger? Pharmacologists describe this as a 'receptor reserve' or they may say that there are 'spare receptors', which simply is a way of saying that there are more receptors than needed to give a full response—stimulating half the receptors at any moment in time is sufficient to give a full response.

So what would happen if we were to reduce the number of receptors? This should remove the spare receptors. If this is done precisely then it would mean that all receptors would need to be occupied to give a full response. If we have the right type of non-competitive antagonist then it is possible to effectively remove receptors from being able to generate a response. Remember from the main text in this chapter that most antagonists used in the clinic are competitive antagonists. A non-competitive antagonist will effectively knock out receptors. What would happen if we took the situation in Figure b and added increasing concentrations of a non-competitive antagonist? The result is shown in Figure c. As the concentration of non-competitive antagonist is increased the number of receptors available is decreased. The curve shifts to the right as the receptor reserve is removed. Eventually the response curve becomes identical to the occupation curve—to get full response all receptors must be stimulated. If we were to carry on increasing the concentration of the antagonist it would mean that there were not enough receptors, even when all were stimulated, to generate a full response, and so the maximum of the curve would reduce, and the curve would collapse, as shown in Figure c.

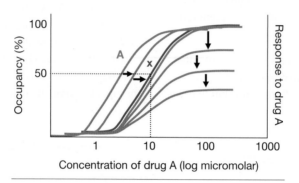

Figure c Effect of a non-competitive antagonist.

The blue line (x) is the occupation curve for drug A, and the far left red line (A) is the concentration-response curve for drug A. The other red curves are concentration response curves for drug A in the presence of increasing concentrations of a non-competitive antagonist.

Now let us consider a little further the significance of efficacy of our agonist. If we return to the situation in Figure b, but consider a second agonist drug B with the same *affinity* for the receptor as drug A, so it has the same occupation curve, but with a greater *efficacy*. The consequence is shown in Figure d. The drug with the higher efficacy does not give a bigger maximum response than the lower efficacy drug A (since both are full agonists) but it does generate this response at a lower concentration. This type of observation is of obvious clinical importance—drug B will be more *potent* than drug A.

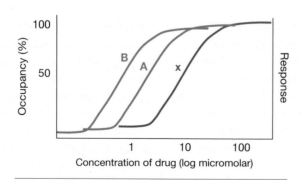

Figure d Comparison of drug A with a higher efficacy drug B.

It is assumed that the drugs have the same affinity for the receptor, and so the occupation curve in blue (x) is the same for both drugs. However, the efficacy of drug B is greater than that of drug A.

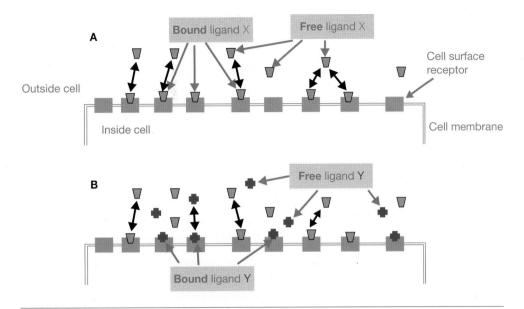

Figure 2.5 Free and bound ligands are in equilibrium and competition.

Free ligand is in solution in the extracellular space. This is like the drug bathing the cells. **Bound ligand** is temporally attached to the receptors at the membrane. The bound ligand goes on and off the membrane repeatedly, interchanging with the free ligand—there is an **equilibrium** between the bound and the free. There are only a limited number of receptors. In **panel A** the cell is bathed only by ligand (drug) X, shown as the **green** symbol. There is bound and free ligand, and not all receptors are occupied. In **panel B** the cell is bathed by two different ligands (drugs), both X and Y, with ligand Y shown as the **blue** symbol. When Y is added with X, then Y **competes** with X for occupation of receptors. The result is both Y and X occupy receptors. But Y acts by displacing some of X from binding so that there is less X bound. The action of drug Y is **competitive**: if the affinity of Y for the receptor was greater, then there would be even less binding of X. Note that if X is an agonist and Y is a pure antagonist then there will be less **response** to X when Y is added, and even less response if Y had a greater affinity than X.

unavailable for future binding. This is not the case, at least not for natural ligands (e.g. neurotransmitters and hormones), nor for the vast majority of drugs. When a ligand is added to the solution bathing the receptor it binds **reversibly**, so that individual molecules of the ligand bind then free themselves (dissociate) from the receptor. They are then available to bind again. This 'on–off' binding has well understood **kinetics**, which means the rate at which the molecule binds to, and the rate at which it dissociates from, the receptor. There is an **equilibrium** between the bound and the free ligand (illustrated in Figure 2.5).

The balance of this equilibrium will be different for different ligands. Some will have kinetics that shift the equilibrium in favour of more binding, but it is still an on–off process, so that the receptor is always available for different ligands to bind to it. Pharmacologists measure these processes, coming up with an index of how strongly ligands bind. In Figure 2.6 the blue line indicates the

amount of binding of drug A to the receptors as the concentration of the drug increases until it reaches a maximum, which is then denoted as 100% binding (meaning all the receptors are now occupied by the drug).

The position of the binding curve along the concentration axis (Figure 2.6) is an indication of the strength of binding. We can represent this numerically as the concentration giving 50% of the maximum binding (or 50% saturation). So a drug with an on–off equilibrium that gives strong binding will generate 50% saturation at a lower concentration than one that is only weakly bound. This is a measure of affinity, and is expressed as the dissociation constant, the K_D, as illustrated in Figure 2.6. A drug with a high affinity will reach 50% occupancy at a low concentration and so will have a low K_D value.

Returning to Figure 2.5, we see that if there is more than one ligand in the vicinity of the receptor then they will compete with each other in trying to bind onto the receptor. A ligand with a low K_D and therefore high affinity

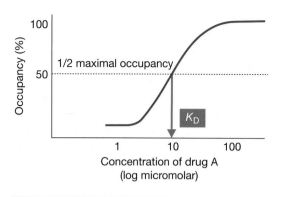

Figure 2.6 Occupancy of the receptor by a ligand is concentration dependent.

The concentration which gives half the maximum is a measure of how strongly the ligand binds to the receptor, and is designated the dissociation constant, or K_D. The K_D in our example here is 10 micromolar, or 10^{-5} M.

will bind more effectively against a ligand with a low affinity (high K_D). So for a drug to have a major effect at a low dose it needs to have a high affinity for its target receptor. It is no wonder that pharmaceutical companies attach considerable importance to the K_D of drugs under development, since most of them act at receptors in competition with the natural ligand (e.g. neurotransmitter or hormone).

Note that the consideration of affinity relates to drugs that are agonists and antagonists, whereas efficacy issues only

apply to drugs that are agonists (because a pure antagonist has, by definition, no efficacy).

2.1.5 Back to antagonists: competitive and non-competitive

We have said that antagonists reduce the effect of an agonist by **competing** for the same binding sites. This idea is illustrated in both Figure 2.1 and Figure 2.5. This is the way most clinically useful antagonists work—such drugs are called **competitive antagonists**. To explore this further consider a concentration-response curve to an agonist. What happens to this curve if we add a competitive antagonist in with the agonist?

The notable thing about Figure 2.7 is that the concentration–response curve for agonist A reaches the same maximum in the presence of the competitive agonist, but the curve is shifted to the right: the concentration of A required to reach the maximum is higher in the presence of the competitor drug. What this means is that a competitive antagonist will not reduce the response to a natural agonist that is at a very high concentration.

Clare suffers from hay fever. When the pollen count rises she takes antihistamines. She finds that many of her symptoms are reduced if she takes the antihistamines early enough, but the distressing scraping itchiness and swelling of the tissue around her eyes doesn't seem to be affected by the drug.

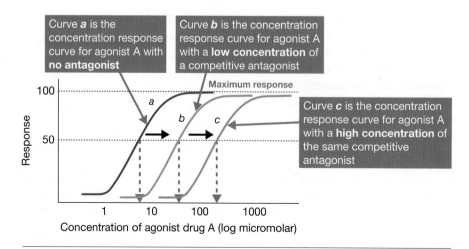

Figure 2.7 Three concentration-response curves to a single agonist A in the absence of an antagonist (a), in the presence of a **competitive** antagonist at low (b) or high concentration (c).

The antihistamines used to treat hayfever are competitive antagonists. Hayfever is caused in part by histamine released from cells called mast cells, which are concentrated in parts of the body exposed to the environment like the skin, and particularly the skin around the eyes. Mast cells release a large amount of histamine when stimulated by, for example, pollen, and it is likely that part of the reason Clare does not get relief from these symptoms is that the histamine concentration at the histamine receptors is so high that it out-competes the antihistamine drug—the drug can't bind, so it has no effect.

Since most clinical drugs are competitive antagonists, the ideas introduced here have a widespread influence on the effectiveness of drug-based therapies.

A non-competitive antagonist, while not very common as a therapeutic agent, has a more profound effect on the maximal response. If the agonist does not compete at the same site as the antagonist then the response will, under many circumstances, be lower, even at the highest concentration of agonist (Box 2.2).

2.2 How receptors change cells

Drugs that act at receptors either activate them (agonists such as salbutamol used in asthma) or prevent their activation (antagonists such as atenolol used in high blood pressure); if we want to understand therapeutics then we need to know how the receptors work.

The receptor, when activated by a native agonist such as a neurotransmitter or a hormone or by an agonist drug, must send a signal within the cell that changes the function of the cell in some way. There are a very large number of ways in which receptors do this, but here we will limit ourselves to a simple introduction to a few of those that are encountered in the clinical context of the rest of this book.

Receptors are located either on the surface of cells or inside the cells. Firstly, we will provide an overview of some of the many mechanisms activated by **cell surface** receptors.

2.2.1 Cell surface receptors: some examples with different effector mechanisms

There are many different types of cell surface receptors with widely different structures. One thing they all have in common is that they are intrinsic proteins of the cell membrane, which means they cross the cell membrane

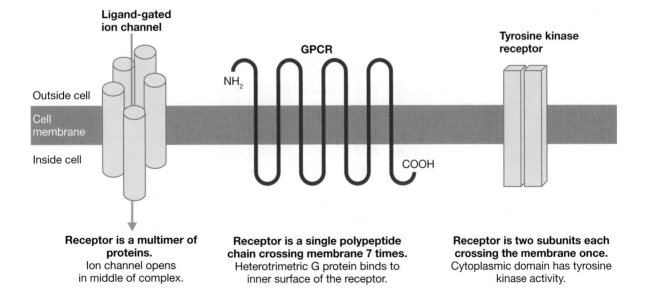

Ligand-gated ion channel

GPCR

Tyrosine kinase receptor

NH₂

Outside cell

Cell membrane

Inside cell

COOH

Receptor is a multimer of proteins.
Ion channel opens in middle of complex.

Receptor is a single polypeptide chain crossing membrane 7 times.
Heterotrimeric G protein binds to inner surface of the receptor.

Receptor is two subunits each crossing the membrane once.
Cytoplasmic domain has tyrosine kinase activity.

Figure 2.8 Three different types of cell surface receptor.
In each case the cartoon of the protein crossing the membrane (in orange) shows the presence of an extracellular domain poking out of the membrane into the extracellular space, a transmembrane domain, which may involve multiple crossings of the membrane by one or more polypeptide chains, and an intracellular domain. GPCR, G protein-coupled receptor.

and therefore have an extracellular domain, a transmembrane domain, and an intracellular domain. Figure 2.8 illustrates some of the common structures of the receptor proteins crossing the membrane.

Pharmacologists classify receptors in a number of different, overlapping, and not necessarily logically organized ways. Features which guide classification include the native agonist(s), the mechanism by which they operate, the relative affinity of other ligands, including antagonists, and structural relationships revealed by molecular biology. For example, receptors for acetylcholine (AChRs) include ligand-gated ion channels and G protein-coupled receptors (GPCRs). These two groups of AChR are, for historical reasons, named after the plant-derived drugs nicotine (from the tobacco plant) and muscarine (found in some mushrooms): the ligand-gated ion channel is called the **nicotinic aceylcholine receptor** (**nAChR**) and the GPCR is called the **muscarinic acetylcholine receptor** (**mAChR**).

Ligand-gated ion channels and GPCRs account for most of the cell surface receptors we encounter in clinical pharmacology. We will also consider here the mechanism of action of the insulin receptor, which operates in a manner used by classical growth factor receptors, collectively called tyrosine kinase receptors. In limiting the account in this section to these three mechanisms—ligand-gated, GPCR and tyrosine kinase receptors (Figure 2.8)—we will not forget that there are many other important mechanisms whereby cell surface receptors regulate cellular function.

2.2.2 Ligand-gated ion channel receptors

Ligand-gated ion channels are commonly found in excitable cells, which essentially means in muscle and nerve cells. One important characteristic is that they are the fastest class of receptors, so they are found where rapid responses (e.g. skeletal muscle) or fast information processing (e.g. in the brain) is required. Excitable cells have gradients of ions across the cell membrane at rest, and are often capable of firing action potentials. The receptor is composed of several subunits that cross the membrane, clustering together to form a pore or ion channel in the middle (Figure 2.8). On binding of the agonist to the extracellular domain of the receptor complex the ion channel opens. This is what **gating** means: the gate is opened when the agonist binds.

The channels also have **selectivity**, which means they are selective for the ions they let through. This might be Na^+, Ca^{2+}, K^+, or Cl^-. In each case ions only move when the channel opens if the concentration is higher on one side of the membrane than the other. For example, K^+ is higher inside the cell (the cytosol) than outside, so opening a K^+ channel will let the ion flow out of the cell. Figure 2.9 illustrates this for a ligand-gated channel that is selective for Na^+, which is at a higher concentration outside the cell than inside, so that when the ligand binds, the channel

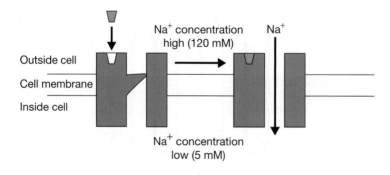

Figure 2.9 Ligand-gated ion channels.

The ion channel has a binding site for the agonist (green symbol). When this site is empty (left) the channel is closed, but when occupied by the agonist (right) the ion channel flips open. The open channel will have selectivity, e.g. for Na^+, Ca^{2+}, K^+, or Cl^-. The consequences of opening the ion channel will depend on which ion(s) the channel is selective for. In the example shown the channel is selective for Na+, which is higher outside the cell than inside. So when the agonist binds, the channel opens, and Na^+ flows into the cell, making the inside of the membrane more positive, i.e. the membrane depolarizes.

opens and Na⁺ flows in. Where there is a voltage difference across the membrane then this will also affect the flow of ions, for example with positively charged ions attracted to the negatively charged side of the membrane.

We will consider the nAChR as an example of a ligand-gated channel.

The nAChR is a ligand-gated channel for Na⁺, as shown in Figure 2.9. This means that aceylcholine acting at this receptor in a nerve or muscle cell will always be excitatory. This is because an excitable cell will always have more Na⁺ outside the cell than inside, so when the nAChR is operated, the inside of the cell will become less negative, stimulating the muscle to contract and the nerve cell to form action potentials. It is the nAChR at the neuromuscular junction that enables motor nerves, releasing acetylcholine onto muscle nAChR, to stimulate skeletal muscle contraction. It is the nAChR at the autonomic nervous system ganglion (both sympathetic and parasympathetic) that enables the acetylcholine released from the pre-ganglionic neuron onto postganglionic cell bodies to stimulate action potential in the post-ganglionic neuron. This results in the control of most aspects of bodily function as a result of the

consequent release from the terminals of post-ganglionic neurons of acetylcholine (mainly parasympathetic) and noradrenaline (most sympathetic) neurons (Figure 2.10).

Brain ligand-gated ion channel receptors: glutamate and GABA accelerators and brakes

There are also some nAChRs in the brain. Their role is poorly defined and they have no direct impact on our understanding of therapeutics, so they are not considered further here. However, the brain does depend on glutamate receptors, which are ligand-gated ion channels. These glutamate receptors, illustrated in Box 16.1 Figure b are excitatory (the channel selectivity is for Na⁺ and Ca²⁺), and it is this excitatory neurotransmission that underlies brain activity—without it our brains would shut down. Some of the fascinating complexities of brain glutamate and gamma-aminobutyric acid (GABA) ion channel receptors, and the possibilities for drug interaction, are introduced in later chapters in Section 5. The central importance in the brain of ligand-gated ion channels is not limited to glutamate receptors. If these are the accelerator pedal of the brain, then we need a brake pedal as well, and this is provided by the neurotransmitter GABA, acting on the ligand-gated ion channel GABA_A receptors (see Box 16.1 for more on

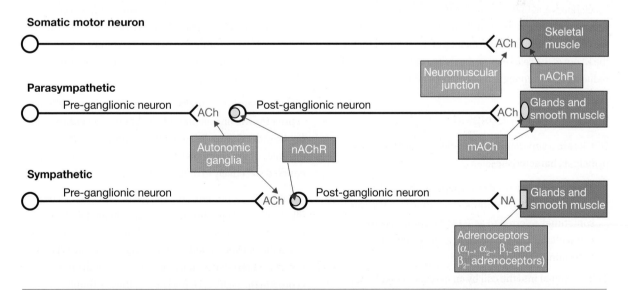

Figure 2.10 Receptors for acetylcholine and noradrenaline (norepinephrine) in tissues receiving neurons from the somatic motor system (to the skeletal muscle neuromuscular junction), at the sympathetic and autonomic ganglia and at the cells innervated by the sympathetic and parasympathetic postganglionic cells.

Note that the neuromuscular junction skeletal muscle cells and the postganglionic neurons of the autonomic system have **nicotinic** acetyl choline receptors. ACh, acetylcholine; nAChR, nicotinic aceylcholine receptor; mACh, muscarinic acetylcholine; NA, noradrenaline (noreplinephrine).

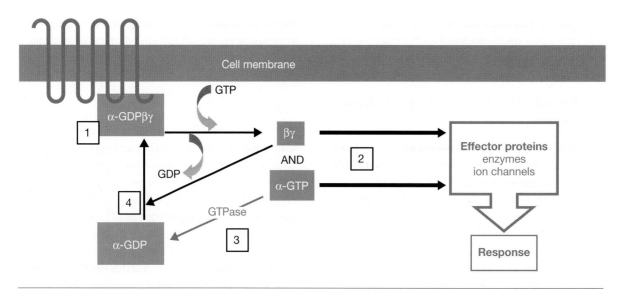

Figure 2.11 Heterotrimeric G protein function.

The blue symbols represent the G protein, initally as a heterotrimer of α_{GDP}, β, and γ subunits all associated with each other [1]. Following activation by an agonist-receptor complex the α-subunits lose their affinity for GDP and gain affinity for GTP. The GTP-bound α-subunits then dissociate from the βγ subunits—both α_{GTP} and βγ then interact with the enzymes and ion channels, which results in the response of the cell to the agonist [2]. The system turns itself off because the α subunit also has an enzyme activity that converts GTP to GDP (this is the GTPase activity [3]). When this happens the α_{GDP} once again associates with the βγ subunits [4], which are then available once more for activation by the agonist–receptor complex [1].

accelerators and brakes in the brain). Their selectivity is for K$^+$ ions, and since these are at higher concentration inside the cell than outside, GABA opening of the channel allows the K$^+$ out of the cell, keeping the resting potential low, and reducing or preventing action potential firing.

2.2.3 G protein-coupled receptors

GPCRs are a superfamily of receptors that have two principal characteristics:

1) They consist of a single polypeptide chain which crosses the cell membrane seven times (so they are sometimes referred to as 7-TM receptors), with an extracellular C-terminus and an intracellular N-terminal tail (Figure 2.8).

2) They signal into the cell by an agonist-controlled interaction with a heterotrimeric G protein at the inner face of the cell membrane.

Heterotrimeric G proteins

This is a family of G proteins, each of which comprises three different α, β, and γ subunits (hence 'heterotrimeric'). The heterotrimeric G protein acts as the interface

between the receptor and the enzymes and/or ion channels that are the usual targets of GPCRs. It is usually the activation or inhibition of these enzymes and ion channels which gives rise to the response to stimulation of GPCRs (Figure 2.11).

Heterotrimeric G proteins are not all the same: different G proteins will link on one side to different receptors and on the other side to different effector proteins (e.g. enzymes or ion channels). In this way different GPCRs are coupled selectively to different responses.

A G protein is a protein with a single pocket that can be filled with either guanosine-5'-diphosphate (GDP) or guanosine-5'-triphosphate (GTP). The protein is activated when the pocket is filled with the small molecule GTP, but inactive when GDP is attached. With a heterotrimeric G protein the GDP/GTP pocket is in the α-subunit. The agonist interaction with a GPCR leads to a change in the associated G protein. The result is that the GDP falls off the α-subunit and GTP becomes attached. With the GTP attached the α-subunit separates from the βγ-subunits (which remain stuck to each other). Both the GTP-α-subunit and the βγ-subunits may then regulate enzymes or ion channels (Figure 2.11).

This account of the manner in which GPCRs change cell function is the bare outline of what has become a vast and complex branch of pharmacology. The heterotrimeric G protein mechanism outlined in Figure 2.11 has many additional aspects to it, and the issue of GPCRs operating in a manner partly independent of the heterotrimeric G proteins has also been established. However, the central story told in Figure 2.11, when coupled with a discussion of the effector proteins (e.g. enzymes and ion channels), is sufficient for us to understand many aspects of drug use in the clinic.

2.2.4 Second messengers, protein phosphorylation, and cellular regulation by GPCRs

One of the ways that activation of cell surface receptors changes events within cells is by regulating enzymes that make small molecules called **second messengers**. These then act within the same cell to control other events. They are often water soluble and diffuse a short distance within the cytosol to reach target proteins, or they may be lipid based and stay within the membrane. Agonists (first messengers) therefore stimulate receptors at the cell surface, leading to the formation of second messengers, which act as signalling molecules, meaning that they carry signals into the cell.

Commonly the response of the cell is then mediated by enzymes called **protein kinases**. These enzymes phosphorylate proteins, changing their function and so changing cell and tissue functions such as muscle contraction and gland secretion.

Here we shall introduce two GPCR-regulated enzyme systems that control most cells in the body, and which we will frequently encounter in the clinical material that follows. These are (1) the systems which regulate **cyclic AMP** synthesis and (2) activation of an enzyme called **phospholipase C** and resultant effects on cytosolic

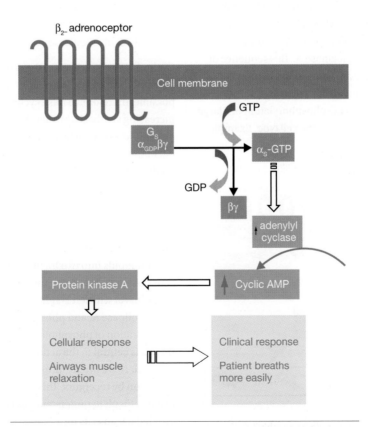

Figure 2.12 Stimulation of β_2-adrenoceptors in bronchiolar smooth muscle increases cyclic AMP synthesis.

β_2-adrenoceptors are an example of a GPCR coupled through a G protein called G_s. When activated by a receptor G_s dissociates, freeing the GTP-α_s-subunit, which activates adenylyl cyclase, the enzyme responsible for cyclic AMP synthesis. In the example given (smooth muscle cells of the small airways, the bronchioles) the physiological response to elevated cyclic AMP is relaxation.

calcium concentrations ($[Ca^{2+}]_c$) and protein phosphorylation.

GPCR control of cyclic AMP synthesis underlies much drug action

Let us consider our asthma patient Amritpal, whom we encountered earlier. When she inhaled salbutamol her asthma was quickly relieved. We mentioned above that the salbutamol stimulates the β_2-adrenoceptors on the surface of the smooth muscle wrapped around the small airways, and that stimulation of these receptors sends signals into the cell, causing the muscle to relax. The major signalling molecule involved here is cyclic AMP: stimulation of the receptor increases its synthesis, raising cyclic AMP levels in the cell, and resulting in muscle relaxation (Figure 2.12; see also Chapter 11).

There are a variety of types of heterotrimeric G proteins. The β_2-adrenoceptors are coupled to cyclic AMP synthesis by a G protein called G_s, and it is the freed GTP-α_s subunit that leads to increased cyclic AMP synthesis. Once its levels in the cytosol are raised, cyclic AMP stimulates a protein kinase called protein kinase A. This sequence of events is extremely common, being found in most cells. Protein kinase A is widespread in its distribution, and once activated it stimulates the phosphorylation of a large variety of proteins, depending on the cell type. Examples

include proteins associated with muscle contractile mechanisms and ion channels (e.g. those controlling entry of Ca^{2+} into cells). The result in the case of bronchiolar smooth muscle cells is relaxation, but it should be noted that the response in other muscles cells may be the opposite, as when contractility is increased in heart myocytes.

In this account agonists stimulate receptors which *raise* cyclic AMP synthesis. However, it should be noted that there are a large number of receptors that are coupled through a different G protein, called G_i, which results in the *inhibition* of adenylyl cyclase causing *lower* cyclic AMP levels (Figure 2.13).

Of particular note here is that both the increase or decease in cyclic AMP synthesis are due to **agonists** acting on their respective receptors—whether it goes up or down depends on the G protein (G_s or G_i) to which that receptor couples.

Drugs may also increase cyclic AMP levels by reducing its breakdown: phosphodiesterase inhibitors

Cyclic AMP is destroyed in the cytosol by enzymes called phosphodiesterases. When considering drugs it is possible, therefore, to raise cyclic AMP levels not only by increasing synthesis, but also by the use of **phosphodiesterase inhibitors**. This strategy is encountered, for example, when we cover cardiovascular medications in Section 2.

GPCR control of the phospholipase C pathway regulates the function of most cells and tissues

Phospholipases are a group of enzymes which split phospholipids into two fragments. A phospholipid general structure is illustrated later in Box 3.1 along with the points at which it is split by the enzymes phospholipase A_2 and phospholipase C (PLC). Further consideration of phospholipase A_2 is found in Section 3, since it is central to the action of many anti-inflammatory drugs. Here we briefly introduce the significance of PLC activation by receptors. This can seem a complex subject that is difficult to understand, but it should not be avoided because its importance to bodily function and drug action is enormous.

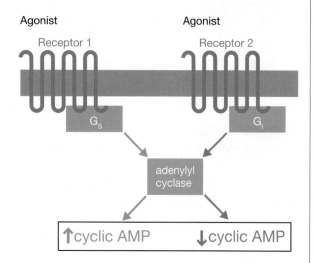

Figure 2.13 Receptors may couple to an inhibiton (through G_i) or stimulation (G_s) of cyclic AMP synthesis.

Note that the scheme shows two different receptors, one of which couples to G_s and one to G_i, and that both the increase and the decrease in cyclic AMP synthesis are caused by the actions of agonists acting at their respective receptors.

The phospholipids are found in the inner face of the cell membrane, with the lipid part stuck into the membrane and the water soluble part poking into the cytosol. This is illustrated for the inositol lipid called PIP_2 in Figure 2.14.

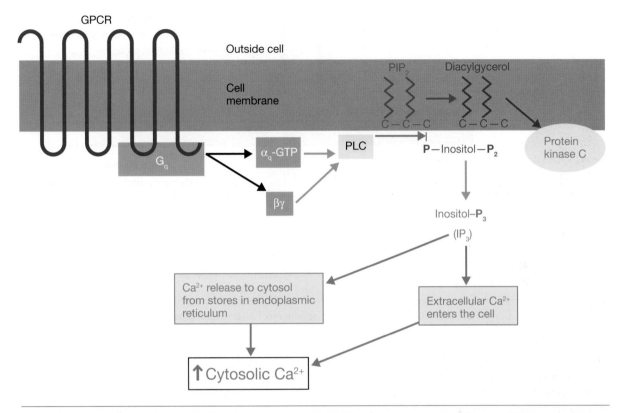

Figure 2.14 Receptor-regulated activation of phospholipase C (PLC) and formation of diacylgycerol (PIP$_2$) and inositol trisphosphate (IP$_3$).

The GPCR, on binding an agonist, acts through a heterotrimeric protein called G$_q$ to activate PLC. The substrate of PLC shown in blue is phosphatidylinositol-bisphosphate (PIP$_2$). This has a C–C–C glycerol backbone with carbon chains (indicated by the zig-zag lines) attached to two of these glycerol carbons. The third glycerol carbon is linked to a phosphate group, which is itself linked to an inositol sugar unit. The inositol has two more phosphates attached, making three phosphate groups in total. PLC cuts this molecule into two fragments in a position that leaves the three phosphates on the inositol, forming inositol trisphosphate (IP$_3$) and the lipid part, diacylgycerol. The IP$_3$ is water soluble, and so leaves the membrane to enter the cytosol, where it meets its protein targets. The diacylgycerol is a lipid, and stays in the membrane and so can only regulate membrane bound proteins, namely protein kinase C. GPCR, G protein-coupled receptor; GTP, guanosine-5´-triphosphate; PLC, phospholipase C; **P**. phosphate

Inositol is a sugar (like glucose) and it can have a variable number of phosphates attached to it at different positions. Its importance lies in the fact that when it is split by PLC it generates two fragments, inositol trisphosphate (IP$_3$) and diacylgycerol, both of which are second messengers that influence most aspects of bodily function (Figure 2.14):

1) The lipid-hating part of the sugar with phosphates attached is IP$_3$. This small molecule moves into the cytosol from where it controls **Ca^{2+} levels in the cell**, raising the cytosolic calcium ($[Ca^{2+}]_c$) from its basal level of around 100 nM in a fast and often highly localized way within the cell. Cytosolic calcium controls many aspects of cell and tissue function, from muscle contraction and gland secretion to cell division and cell death.

2) The remaining lipid fraction of PIP$_2$ (diacylgycerol) remains in the membrane, from where it activates a family of protein kinases called protein kinase C, which also regulate the function of most cells and tissues.

2.2.5 Tyrosine kinase receptors: the insulin receptor as an example

In Figure 2.8 the third major class of cell surface receptor illustrated is the superfamily of tyrosine kinase receptors. An example is the insulin receptor—a subject

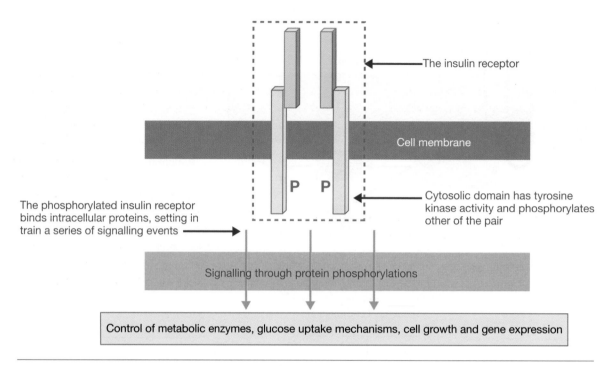

Figure 2.15 The insulin receptor as an example of a tyrosine kinase receptor.

The basic tyrosine kinase structure of two protein subunits crossing the cell membrane once is present, with the addition of two extracellular subunits to make up the insulin receptor. The binding of insulin to the extracellular domain leads to autophosphorylation in the intracellular domain, which means that the kinase activity of each chain phosphorylates the other chain. As a result the intracellular part of the receptor attracts proteins, which bind to it and the complex then activates signalling cascades.

of obvious importance in understanding a number of diseases and their treatment, particularly to do with the way the body handles glucose and the various forms of diabetes.

In Figure 2.8 we have shown these receptors as being two subunits, each crossing the membrane once. For many **growth factor receptors** this is true. For the **insulin receptor** each transmembrane subunit has an extracellular subunit attached, as shown in Figure 2.15.

The basic mechanism of all tyrosine kinase receptors is that the agonist binding to the extracellular face leads to the phosphorylation of the intracellular face, and this leads to the activation of complex signalling pathways. In the case of insulin this includes not only complex changes in glucose metabolism and uptake, but also signalling to the nucleus controlling gene expression and the cell cycle.

2.2.6 Intracellular receptors

We shall use as our main example here the actions of **steroids**, which are explored in their clinical drug context in Section 3.

Steroids change gene expression

An important difference between steroids and the other natural agonists, such as adrenaline and insulin, which we have discussed previously, is that they can enter the cells they are influencing. Adrenaline, insulin, and many of the other agonists we shall consider cannot cross the cell membrane because they are not lipid soluble. To influence the cell they must therefore bind to receptors that are accessible from outside the cell, and these receptors must then send signals across the membrane into the cell. Steroids, however, are lipid soluble and so pass through the cell membrane into the cell, where they bind to their intracellular protein receptor and the steroid/receptor complex enters the nucleus. Not surprisingly, several things can then happen, depending on which steroid, which receptor, and which cell is involved. However, a central part of the story is that gene expression is altered. In the case of the anti-inflammatory steroids that are so important in clinical practice, the result is the reduced expression of genes that cause and promote inflammation and an increase in expression of genes encoding anti-inflammatory proteins. It is because of this combined mechanism that anti-inflammatory steroids are so effective.

2.3 Ion channels as drug targets

Ion channels are intrinsic membrane protein complexes that cross the cell membrane. We have encountered one class of ion channel already in Figures 2.8 and 2.9: the ligand-gated ion channel, in which the receptor and the channel are the same. Ion channels are usually cell surface drug targets.

Voltage-gated channels

Channels can be open or closed. This is the gating of the channel. Ligand-gated ion channels are opened and closed (gated) by naturally occurring ligands (e.g. hormones or neurotransmitters). **Voltage-gated ion channels**, by contrast, are dependent on the voltage across the cell membrane to determine whether they are open or closed. Muscle cells and nerve cells (excitable cells) have an electrical charge across their cell membrane that at rest is negative to about –70 mV inside the cell compared to outside. Some of the ion channels we are interested in are closed under these conditions. If an action potential comes along that starts to depolarize the membrane, to, say, –40 mV inside, then voltage-sensitive Na^+ channels may open, allowing Na^+ into the cell from its higher concentration outside the cell. As the membrane becomes even less polarized, moving towards a positive charge inside, then voltage-sensitive Ca^{2+} channels (for example, L-type channels on smooth muscle cells) may open, and Ca^{2+} can

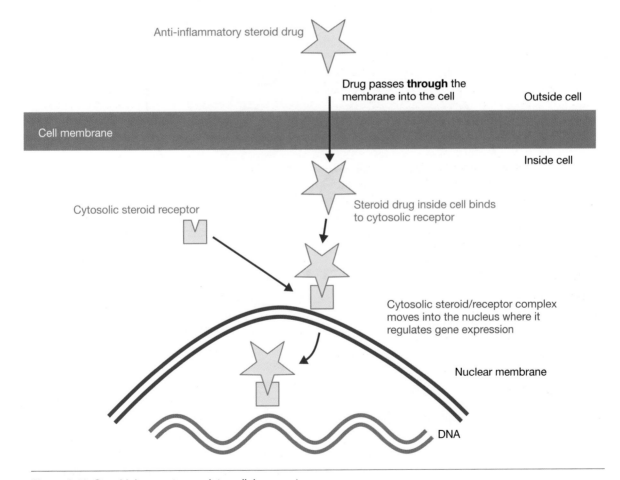

Figure 2.16 Steroid drugs act on an intracellular receptor.

The steroid molecule passes straight through the membrane, binds to a receptor inside the cell, this complex enters the nucleus and gene expression is changed. If the drug is an **anti-inflammatory** steroid then the gene expression changes in the direction of increased expression of genes for anti-inflammatory proteins (e.g. that for lipocortin) and decreased expression of genes for pro-inflammatory proteins (e.g. inflammatory cytokines), as discussed further in Section 3.

then flow into the cell (like Na⁺, Ca^{2+} is also at a higher concentration outside the cell). Under some circumstances the voltage-sensitive K⁺ channels may open—then K⁺ will flow from inside the cell to the outside (its concentration is higher *inside* the cell), tending to move the membrane back to being negatively charged inside.

We will encounter all these types of voltage-gated channels later in this book. We will encounter drugs that specifically block certain of these channels, such as the drug amlodipine, an example of an L-type Ca^{2+} channel blocker used in the treatment of hypertension. (There are also drugs that open

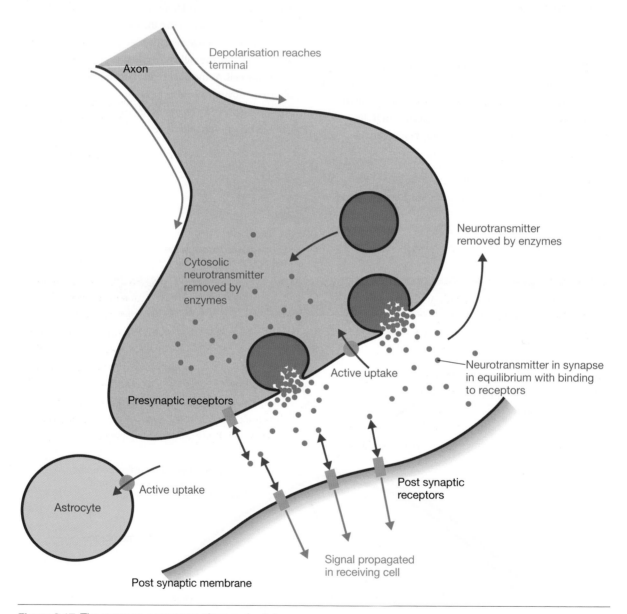

Figure 2.17 The synapse, neurotransmitter, and uptake.

The diagram shows a nerve terminal with neurotransmitter released into the synaptic space. While there the neurotransmitter molecules can stimulate the receptors (both postsynaptic, generating neurotransmission, and presynaptic, controlling further neurotransmitter release). The neurotransmitter is rapidly removed from the synaptic space—in the case of brain neurotransmitters (e.g. noradrenaline, dopamine, and serotonin) this is largely by active uptake by transporter proteins in the membranes of the nerve terminal or adjacent cells. Drugs that inhibit this reuptake (such as certain antidepressant drugs, Chapter 19) can be expected to increase the availability of neurotransmitter to stimulate its receptors.

channels, such as nicorandil increasing opening of a type of K$^+$ channel sensitive to intracellular ATP).

When a voltage-gated Na$^+$ channel in a nerve cell has opened allowing Na$^+$ into the cell, exciting it, the channel will rapidly close and for a very short time it will enter a state in which it *cannot* be opened. This is the refractory state. There are some drugs which bind to this refractory state. Because their effect is greater when cells are very active (i.e. lots of action potentials) these drugs are referred to as 'use dependent'. They provide a more sophisticated way in which to manipulate voltage-sensitive channels than simply blocking the channels, and such drugs have found clinical use in the treatment of cardiac arrythmias (Chapter 7) and epilepsy (Chapter 16). The principle of 'use dependence' is described more fully in Box 16.2.

2.4 Enzymes as drug targets

When an enzyme is a drug target we normally think of intracellular enzymes. We have noted above that this is not always the case, as when we inhibit the blood plasma enzymes necessary for blood clotting.

In the majority of cases therapeutic drugs acting at enzymes inhibit them. However, activity through an enzymic step may be *increased* by clinically used drugs, as when L-dopa is used to boost dopamine levels in the brain, in this case the supply of L-dopa to the decarboxylase enzyme is increased by its administration as a drug, and it is converted into dopamine (Chapter 17).

2.5 Transporter proteins as drug targets

The simplest example to use to illustrate this type of drug action is the antidepressants, which act as inhibitors of the uptake of specific types of neurotransmitter in the brain. The general situation here, with respect to a synapse in the brain, is illustrated in Figure 2.17.

Some of these antidepressants inhibit the uptake of noradrenaline (norepinephrine) and serotonin (5-hydroxytryptamine), for example. When a neurotransmitter is release in the brain it is in many cases removed by being drawn into local cells, across the cell membrane. This is achieved by specific uptake proteins capable of picking up the neurotransmitter and transporting it from the synapse, across the cell membrane, and into the cell, thus terminating its action. Drugs which bind and block these uptake proteins will increase the amount of neurotransmitter in the synapse, thus boosting its activity in the brain. This accounts for the action of some very well known antidepressant drugs such as fluoxetine and citalopram. The action of these drugs is more fully explored in Chapter 19.

Chapter 3
Pharmacokinetics

Pick up any monograph about a drug, and buried among information about the dosage, indications, precautions, and side effects will be something about the **pharmacokinetics** of the drug. The term 'pharmacokinetics' quite literally means drug (pharmaco) movement (kinetics), and is the science related to what happens to a drug when it gets into the body. Put simply, it can be thought of as what the body does to the drug. This is contrast to **pharmacodynamics**, which is about the action of drugs or, in other words, what the drug does to the body. The relationship of pharmacokinetics with pharmacodynamics is outlined in Figure 3.1.

This chapter will review the basics of pharmacokinetics (PK). The study of PK is a branch of pharmaceutical science in its own right, and this chapter is in no way meant to replace the more comprehensive resources on the subject. However, a basic understanding of the principles of PK is essential when considering the pharmacology of the drug. After all, pharmacology is literally the science of the interaction of a drug with the body, and the PK of a drug can dictate everything from the route of administration through to how long the effect will last, side effects, and precautions with its use.

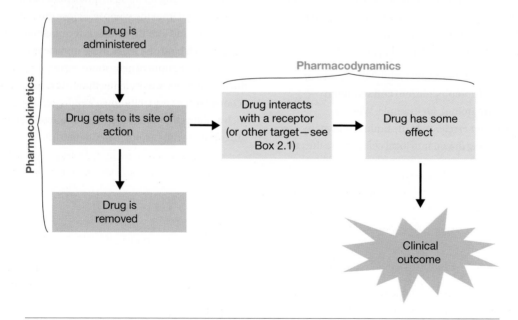

Figure 3.1 Pharmacokinetics versus pharmacodynamics.

3.1 The core principles of pharmacokinetics: ADME

When you read about the PK of a drug you will often come across the acronym **ADME**. This stands for:

- Absorption
- Distribution
- Metabolism
- Elimination

These four steps, which to differing extents are sequential, are the key aspects of the PK of a drug. However, to understand some of the concepts we will need to work backwards, starting with elimination (clearance) and finishing with absorption.

3.2 Drug elimination: clearance

Clearance is one of two fundamental concepts in understanding PK (the other is volume of distribution, which we will cover later). The clearance of a drug is the irreversible elimination of the drug from the body. The two main routes of elimination for most drugs are the kidneys and the liver. Drugs can be eliminated in their original form (unchanged) or they can be converted to other molecules (called metabolism). Unchanged drugs are eliminated primarily in the urine, but can also be excreted in the gut (faeces), sweat, breath, etc. Metabolism for most drugs occurs primarily in the liver, but many other cells have the capacity to convert drugs to other forms. Once converted, the metabolites are then eliminated through the same routes as unchanged drugs (e.g. urine, sweat, etc).

The clearance of a drug can be discussed in terms of routes of elimination (e.g. renal clearance) or as total clearance, which is the sum of the clearance by all routes. This is expressed as the volume of blood cleared of the drug per unit time. Conventionally this is presented as L/h or mL/min.

The total clearance of a drug is important because it determines the dosage rate required to maintain a certain concentration in the blood. As discussed in Chapter 2, for most drugs to work there usually needs to be a certain amount of them around to be able to interact with a receptor. The relationship between drug concentration and clearance is:

dosage rate = plasma concentration × clearance

It can be seen from this equation that if the clearance goes down, so must the dosage rate to maintain the same plasma concentration, and vice versa. The other way to think about this is that if the clearance goes down the plasma concentration will go up if you keep the same administration rate. As we will see later, this is important to consider when certain health states (e.g. renal disease) or drug interactions (e.g. blockers of liver enzymes) can cause the clearance to go down, resulting in increased blood levels that can cause toxicity. Here is an example:

> Steven has chronic obstructive airways disease[1] and is admitted to hospital. The decision is to give him some theophylline by intravenous infusion. The recommended blood level for theophylline is 10–20 mg/L. The total body clearance in an average adult (70 kg) is approximately 3 L/h. It was decided to try to aim for the upper **blood level** limit (20 mg/L). To maintain that concentration you would need to give 60 mg/h (20 mg/L × 3 L/h). However, Steven is a smoker, and in smokers the clearance can increase by as much as 50% because smoking causes the enzymes in the liver to *increase* in activity (more about this later), so in Steven the clearance could be 4.5 L/h, in which case he would need 90 mg/h **of theophylline** to keep the same concentration.

You can see from this example that the blood concentration and the clearance both have to be measured in the same volume (in this case in litres) so that they cancel out in the equation. Also, note in the example that we give the drug by intravenous infusion, which means we know that 100% will get into the bloodstream at a constant rate. If we looked at a graph of the blood levels, we would see something like Figure 3.2.

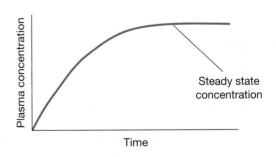

Figure 3.2 Plot of concentration versus time for a continuous intravenous infusion.

1. Airways disease and its treatment are discussed fully in Chapter 11.

It can be seen from Figure 3.2 that the concentration rises over time until it plateaus. Initially the drug is being cleared faster than it is being administered. However, as we continue to give the drug we eventually reach the plateau where the rate of administration is equal to the rate of clearance, and this is called the steady state concentration.

The situation is quite different if we give drugs orally as they need to be absorbed first to get into the bloodstream, and that may not be complete (more later) and is not immediate. Therefore, if we look at the concentration curve for oral medications we see something like Figure 3.3.

You can see that to start with the drug is absorbed faster than it is being eliminated. After some time, the rate of absorption equals the rate of elimination, which is the point at which the maximal concentration occurs (called C_{max}). The time at which C_{max} occurs is referred to as t_{max}. After this, the body starts to eliminate the drug faster than it is absorbing it, and the levels in the plasma decrease.

3.2.1 Drug clearance by the liver: metabolism

The liver plays a vital role in clearing drugs, and other molecules, from the body. The ultimate aim of hepatic metabolism is usually to make the drug more easily cleared by other routes, primarily the kidneys. It does this through what are broadly classified as phase I and phase II reactions. Phase I reactions include hydroxylation, oxidation, and dealkylation. The enzyme systems most often involved in these reactions are members of the cytochrome P450 family. The aim of phase I reactions is to prepare the molecule for phase II reactions. These include glucuronidation, acetylation, and conjugation. The phase II reactions usually result in making the molecule more polar and therefore more water soluble. This makes the molecule easier to remove by the kidney (more later). Phase II reactions usually, with a few exceptions such as morphine, result in inactive metabolites. Phase I reactions, on the other hand, can produce active metabolites, sometimes more active than the parent compound. For some drugs, hepatic metabolism is a requirement before the drug becomes active (e.g. thalidomide), in which case the parent drug is called a pro-drug.

Hepatic extraction ratio

All blood in the body passes at some time through the liver. It does this through the portal vein. Once a drug gets into the blood, therefore, it will eventually be presented to the liver for possible metabolism. However, generally only free (unbound) drug can be taken up by the liver cells and metabolized. Many drugs are 'carried' in the blood attached to proteins, the main one being albumin (Figure 3.4).

Once taken into the hepatocyte (the main cell type in the liver), the drug is metabolized by enzymes. How active these enzyme are is called the intrinsic clearance. There are therefore three factors that impact on hepatic clearance: liver blood flow, protein binding, and intrinsic clearance.

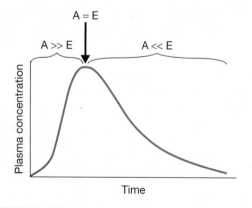

Figure 3.3 Plot of concentration versus time curve for an oral drug.

A, rate of absorption; E, rate of elimination.

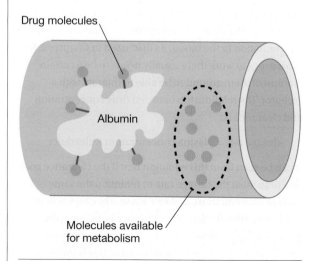

Figure 3.4 Example of drug binding to albumin.

If the liver has low enzyme activity (low intrinsic clearance) then the rate of hepatic clearance is related to the degree of protein binding and the enzyme activity, and does not depend on liver blood flow. In essence, the liver is so poor at removing the drug, it doesn't matter how fast or slow you present the drug to it (i.e. liver blood flow). If you want to visualize this, imagine the liver enzymes are a robotic arm taking golf balls off a conveyer belt, and the speed at which the conveyer belt moves is liver blood flow. If the robot arm is very slow at removing the golf balls, say only taking one off every hour, it doesn't matter how slow or fast the conveyer belt moves because it still only takes off very few of the golf balls!

If the liver has high levels of enzyme activity for a drug, then the main determinant of hepatic clearance is liver blood flow. Using the robot example above, the robotic arm is so efficient that it actually removes the golf balls faster than the conveyer belt can present them, therefore how many golf balls are removed will depend on how fast (or slow) you present them (i.e. if you only present one per hour, it can only remove one per hour, but if you present 100 per hour it will remove 100 per hour).

The term used to measure the extent of liver capacity for a drug is called the hepatic extraction ratio. This can range from 0 (no drug removed by the liver) to 1 (all of the drug removed the first time it passes through the liver). For example, if a drug has a hepatic extraction ratio of 0.7, it means that 70% of the drug is removed each time the blood passes through the liver. Given that the average liver blood flow is 1.5 L/h (the maximum hepatic clearance rate possible), this would mean that the hepatic clearance would be approximately 1 L/h (i.e. $0.7 \times 1.5 = 1.05$). Knowing whether the liver has high, or low, capacity for a drug helps predict what factors will impact on its clearance, as we can see in this example:

> Margaret is taking warfarin because of a long history of deep vein thrombosis,[2] and propranolol for her blood pressure.[3] She develops a chest infection and her GP decides to prescribe a macrolide antibiotic,[4] erythromycin. He decides he should check first whether there is likely to be any problems. He finds that erythromycin can increase the effect of warfarin, but has little effect on propranolol, even though both are metabolized by the liver. It turns out that warfarin has low clearance by the liver (hepatic extraction ratio of <0.3), whereas propranolol has a high clearance (extraction ratio ~0.7). The interaction with warfarin is because erythromycin is an inhibitor of hepatic enzymes, which causes a decrease in its clearance and therefore an increase in the warfarin levels. It does not affect propranolol because the liver has such great capacity to metabolize it, it is not affected by having some of the enzymes blocked by erythromycin.

3.2.2 Elimination by the kidney

The kidney is a complex organ that is the second major site of drug elimination. The key parts of the kidney are outlined in Figure 3.5.

Drugs are cleared by the kidney through one of three processes: filtration; secretion, or reabsorption. The kidney filters drugs and other substances through the glomerulus (an intertwined mass of semi-permeable blood vessels that sit inside the Bowman's capsule) and clears approximately 10% of the blood as it passes though at a rate of about 1200 mL/min. Thus, the glomerular filtration rate is about 120 mL/min. The process of filtration is passive and, just like the liver, only unbound drugs can be cleared by filtration.

The kidney also has several active transport systems that occur in the proximal tubule. The two main systems affect acidic drugs (e.g. penicillin) and basic drugs (e.g. procainamide). These 'pump' drugs from the bloodstream into the proximal tubule. Drugs that compete for these secretion methods (e.g. cimetidine and procainamide) can lead to decreased clearance and potential toxicity. However, this competition is used therapeutically when probenecid is given with penicillins to reduce their clearance, increasing their blood levels and effectiveness.

Starting in the proximal tubules drugs can be reabsorbed from the Loop of Henle, the distal tubules, and the collecting ducts. This occurs because nearly 99% of the water that is filtered in the glomerulus is reabsorbed in these parts of the kidney, leaving only about 1–2 mL from the original 120 mL filtered from the blood each minute at the end as the urine. Thus, drugs that are only filtered would increase in concentration nearly 100 fold as they pass through (e.g. if there was 1 mg of drug in the 120 mL of water originally filtered, by the time it got to the collecting ducts the 1 mg would be in 1–2 mL). This increased concentration as the drug passes along the tubules encourages passive reabsorption. Several things influence the reabsorption. First, only unionized (non-charged) molecules can pass the membranes, therefore drugs that are weak acids and weak bases will change their state (ionized versus unionized) depending on the pH of the urine. It is possible to increase the pH using urinary alkalinisers (e.g. sodium bicarbonate) and decrease the

---

2. Chapter 4.
3. Chapter 5.
4. Chapter 21.

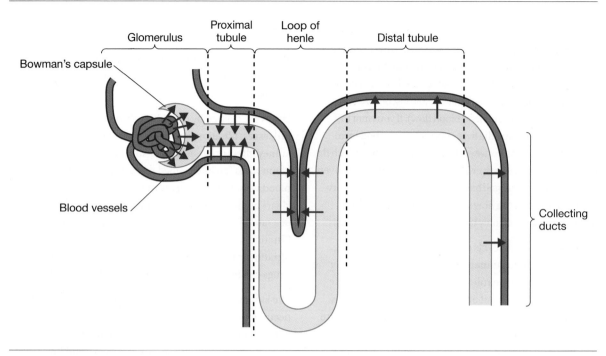

Figure 3.5 Major elements of the kidney.
Arrows indicate the directions in which drugs can travel.

pH with agents such as ascorbic acid. The other influence on drug reabsorption is urine flow rate. If someone drinks large amounts of water, the kidney will increase the filtration of water and produce urine that is more dilute. This would decrease the concentration gradient for any drugs in the urine and decrease the reabsorption. These two influences, particularly urinary pH, can cause interactions with some drugs (increasing their toxicity) but can also be useful as we can see in this example:

> Simon is receiving methotrexate, a folate antagonist anticancer drug,[5] as part of his treatment for lymphoma. While he is receiving the methotrexate, he is given plenty of fluid and a urinary alkaliniser (e.g. sodium citrate + sodium bicarbonate). This is done to enhance the renal clearance of methotrexate by first increasing the dilution of the methotrexate in the urine, making it less likely to be reabsorbed. Second, methotrexate is a weak acid (pKa = 4.3) and therefore is ionized in alkaline urine, reducing its ability to cross membranes. This interaction is used to reduce the toxicity of methotrexate to the kidneys by increasing its removal.

Why is renal clearance important?

Understanding the factors that can influence renal excretion helps predict drug interactions (as above) as

well as the effect of disease states. The most important factor is the effect of renal dysfunction because, irrespective of whether a drug is actively secreted or reabsorbed, the most important determinant of renal elimination is filtration. We measure renal filtration (or glomerular filtration) rate using creatinine clearance. Creatinine is a by-product of the breakdown of creatine phosphate in the muscle. It is primarily filtered with little or no secretion or reabsorption. Using serum creatinine levels, and adjusting for age, weight, and gender, it is possible to calculate the glomerular filtration rate:

$$\text{creatine clearance} = \frac{(140 - \text{age}) \times (\text{weight in kg})}{814 \times \text{serum creatinine (mmol/L)}}$$
$$[\times 0.85 \text{ for females}]$$

As a rule, for most drugs adjustment for reduced renal filtration is only required if creatinine clearance has decreased by 50% or more (i.e. <60 mL/min). If required, the dosage adjustment is usually proportional to the degree of renal clearance reduction. However, you must adjust for the contribution of renal clearance to the total clearance of the drug. If a drug is entirely removed by the kidney, then generally if the renal function is decreased by 50%, the dose needs to be reduced by 50%. However, if, say, only 50% of total elimination is due to the kidneys, and the renal function is reduced to 50%, then only a 25%

---

5. Cancer drug therapy is discussed in Chapter 22.

reduction in dose is required (e.g. 50% hepatic + 50% renal and a 50% reduction in renal function means the total will be 50%(hepatic) + 25% ($0.5 \times 0.5 = 0.25 = 25\%$ renal) = 75% of normal = 25% reduction). However, when deciding the need to reduce doses in renal failure two things must be considered. First, does the drug have what is called a 'low therapeutic index', meaning that the difference between toxic levels and therapeutic levels is small? In this case, the need for reductions in doses in renal failure may be more important. Second, you must consider whether the drug has active metabolites that are also cleared by the kidneys.

3.2.3 Protein binding

We have seen that with both renal clearance and hepatic clearance, only free or unbound drug is removed from the blood. In addition, only unbound drug is available to interact with receptors to give a pharmacological effect. As mentioned above, drugs can be bound to proteins in the plasma, and these include albumin, α_1-acid glycoprotein, and lipoproteins. Albumin is one of the major proteins and has several binding sites, which can carry drugs or endogenous substances such as bilirubin. α_1-acid glycoprotein is an acute phase protein that increases in concentration in response to systemic tissue injury and inflammation, and contains a single binding site.

Protein binding is similar to competitive receptor binding (see Chapter 2) in that free and bound drugs exist in equilibrium:

free drug + protein $\leftrightarrows$ drug–protein complex

The degree of protein binding is determined by the physicochemical properties of the drug and its affinity for the protein, the amount of free drug around, and the amount of protein available. Examples of highly protein bound drugs include warfarin, propranolol, phenytoin, and diazepam. The degree of protein binding can change

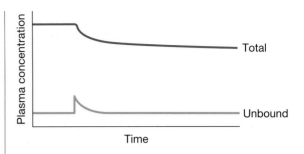

Figure 3.6 Comparison of total and unbound drug concentrations if protein displacement occurs.

due to displacement (e.g. another drug or an endogenous molecule 'pushing' the bound molecule off the albumin) or reduced levels of proteins (e.g. in hepatic failure, as the liver is the major producer of albumin).

As you would expect, changes in protein binding affect primarily drugs that are highly protein bound. If the protein binding decreases for these drugs, there is an effect on the free and total concentrations of the drug. The free levels initially rise. However, because there is more unbound drug available, more of the drug is cleared, therefore the free levels return to the starting level. However, the total drug levels will go down because more of the drug has been eliminated. The net effect is a reduction in total drug, but little change in free levels (Figure 3.6)

Because free levels are unaltered, and it is free drug that exerts the pharmacological effect, changes in protein binding do not usually alter the effect of the drug. However, it is important to consider protein binding changes when interpreting blood levels when undertaking therapeutic drug monitoring, as the blood levels used are often the total drug levels (i.e. the total levels may go down, which would usually be a sign to increase the dose, but the free drug level, and therefore the therapeutic effectiveness, is unchanged).

3.3 Volume of distribution

This is the second of the two fundamental concepts of PK. The volume of distribution (Vd) relates the amount of drug measured in the blood to the amount that is given. It is a 'virtual' volume and is usually called the 'apparent volume of distribution'. The Vd reflects the extent to which the drug distributes into tissues, and binds to proteins and other structures in the body. The formula to determine Vd is:

$$Vd = \frac{\text{total amount in the body}}{\text{concentration in blood/plasma}}$$

If a drug is highly distributed/bound to structures outside the blood the Vd is large because the apparent free concentration in blood will be small (Box 3.1), whereas if tissue binding is very low (e.g. warfarin), the Vd approximates blood volume. The degree of binding is

Box 3.1
Illustration of volume of distribution

1 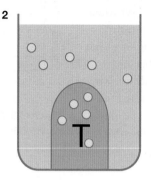 **2** **3**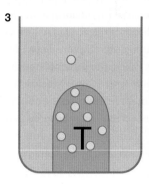

Figure a

1. In this example, there is very little binding, with only 1 mg of drug attached to tissue. If we measured the concentration we would find it to be 9 mg/L. The Vd would be 10 mg/9 mg per litre = 1.11 L. It can be seen that if binding is very low, then the Vd approximates the total volume. For a drug in the body this would approximate blood volume (~8 L).

2. In this example, there is modest tissue binding with about half of the drug bound. The concentration in the liquid is 5 mg/L, and the Vd is 10 mg/5 mg per litre = 2 L.

3. In this case the binding is very high, with 9 mg of drug attached to tissue. The concentration in the liquid is 1 mg/L. The Vd is 10 mg/1 mg per litre = 10 L.

Figure a shows three beakers, each representing the body. The grey liquid represents blood and the yellow mass represents tissues (T). For simplicity, let us assume each beaker contains 1 L of liquid. In each beaker, imagine we have added 10 mg of drug (each red dot represents 1 mg). The volume of distribution is calculated as:

$$Vd = \frac{\text{total amount in the body}}{\text{concentration in blood/plasma}}$$

Table 3.1 Apparent volumes of distribution for common drugs

Drug	Apparent Vd (L)
Warfarin	8
Theophylline	30
Diazepam	80
Imipramine	>700
Chloroquine	>7000

determined by the physicochemical properties of the drug, including the size of the molecule, solubility, and the state of ionization. Examples of the Vd for some drugs are given in Table 3.1. You can see that highly lipid-soluble drugs like imipramine and chloroquine have large Vd because they are bound to fat stores in the body.

3.3.1 When is knowing the Vd helpful?

The Vd is used to calculate the loading dose of a drug. A loading dose is a higher than normal dose used when you want to get the blood levels to steady state quicker (see Figure 3.1). As we saw in the example above with Steven, who was given theophylline by continuous infusion, it took some time to reach steady state (the plateau concentration). If we rearrange the equation above, you can see that if we know the Vd and concentration required, we can calculate the loading dose:

If we want to get the blood levels of the theophylline for Steven (who had chronic obstructive pulmonary disease) to the desired level (20 mg/L) quickly, we can calculate the required dose as Vd × concentration required. For Steven this would be 30 L × 20 mg/L = 600 mg.

3.4 Half-life of a drug

The plasma half-life of a drug is the time it takes for the blood levels to drop by half. If we gave someone a single bolus injection of a drug and measured the blood levels over time we would see something like Figure 3.7.

In Figure 3.7 we can see it takes 2 hours for the blood level of the drug to drop from 100 mg/L to 50 mg/L, and another 2 hours for the level to halve again to 25 mg/L, therefore the half-life for this drug is 2 hours.

The half-life ($t_{1/2}$) is related to the two key parameters already discussed, Vd and clearance, by the following formula:

$$t_{1/2} = \frac{0.693 \times Vd}{clearance}$$

What this tells us is that changes in Vd and clearance have opposite effects on the half-life. If the Vd decreases (e.g. if binding to tissues changes) the half-life decreases

because more is available for elimination, whereas if the clearance decreases (e.g. in renal or hepatic disease) the half-life increases because less of the drug is being eliminated.

3.4.1 Why is knowing the half-life useful?

First, as we saw in Figure 3.7, the half-life can help predict how long it will take drug levels to fall, and this can help to predict the duration of action after a single dose of drug as there is usually a minimum concentration of a drug required in the plasma for it to have an effect. If we use the example in Figure 3.7, and say the minimum amount is 20 mg/L to have an effect, then after a single dose the effect will stop after just over 4 hours. Because the decline in blood levels is exponential, not linear (as Figure 3.7 shows), it also tells us that doubling the dose does not double the duration of action (in the example in Figure 3.7, if we gave twice the dose so the initial concentration was 200 mg/L, the time until the levels dropped to below 20 mg/L would be just over 6 hours, not 8 hours).

Second, the half-life helps to determine the fluctuations in plasma levels of drug between dosing. Taking the example of theophylline again (Figure 3.8).

Theophylline has a plasma half-life of approximately 4 hours. Figure 3.8 shows two dosing regimens in a 20 kg child. In both dosing regimens we are giving a total of 600 mg per 24 hours. However, if we give 300 mg every 12 hours we get a peak level of about 35 mg/L, and what we call a trough level (the lowest level before the next does) of about 4.5 mg/L. For

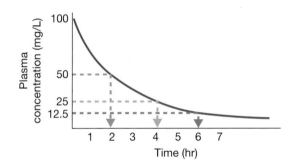

Figure 3.7 Concentration versus time curve for a hypothetical drug.

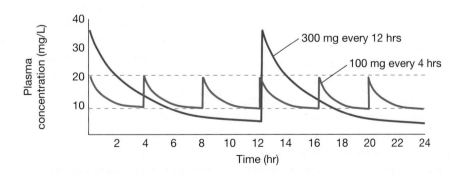

Figure 3.8 Example of two dosing regimens with theophylline.

Adapted from: Birkett D.J. Half-life. *Australian Prescriber* 1988; **11**(3): 57–9.

theophylline, levels above 20 mg/L can cause toxicity (e.g. cardiac arrhythmias and neurological side effects), while levels below 10 mg/L are ineffective. If we give 300 mg every 12 hours the drug is only between 10 mg/L and 20 mg/L (called the therapeutic range) for about 4 hours. However, if we give 100 mg every 4 hours, then the fluctuations in the levels of the drug remain within the therapeutic range for the entire period.

For most drugs with half-lives of up to 24 hours, giving doses every half-life is appropriate. However, if a drug has a very short half-life, it means that the dosing will be so frequent that patients may find it difficult to keep taking the medicine, leading to non-compliance. The solution to this is to develop a sustained-release version that releases the drug more slowly over time.

The third aspect of drug dosing that the half-life determines is the time to reach steady state (see Figure 3.2). With chronic oral dosing, or continuous intravenous infusions, it takes about five half-lives to reach steady state. Knowing this will help to determine how long it will take to get to a therapeutic level. Here is an example of why this is important:

> Julia is rushed into the emergency department with an episode of status epilepticus,[6] a very severe and potentially life-threatening form of epilepsy. One of the drugs used for this is phenytoin, which has a half-life of about 24 hours. It is obviously not possible to wait 5 days for the levels of phenytoin to get high enough in Julia to start having an effect, therefore the emergency physician gives her a loading dose (a higher than normal dose) to get the levels up quickly. However, once under control, Julia's epilepsy is maintained with once-daily dosing of phenytoin.

3.5 Absorption and bioavailability

The first step when giving a drug systemically involves absorption. The vast majority of drugs are given orally, therefore we will focus on this route in this chapter. However, drugs can be given by many other routes for a systemic effect. These include parenterally, topically, and rectally. The parenteral route, that is by injection, is arguably the most invasive, and least liked by most people. However, giving a drug intravenously (IV) by injection has the advantage that absorption is 100%.

When a drug is given orally, several things have to happen. First, it is swallowed and delivered to the stomach, and from there it passes into the intestines, where the majority of drugs are absorbed. Before it can be absorbed, the tablet or capsule has to break apart and dissolve, usually in the stomach. The solution of drug then has to get through the gut wall. All drugs absorbed in the gut enter the portal circulation first. This comprises the capillary beds that surround the gut and drain into the liver. Once it has passed through the liver, the drug is into the systemic circulation. The term 'absorption' is used to describe the fraction of drug that is given that makes it into the portal circulation. Bioavailability is the fraction of total dose that gets absorbed and then passes through the liver. Many things influence the first step, absorption, as outlined in Figure 3.9.

Once the drug is absorbed it is exposed to possible hepatic metabolism. If the extraction ratio of a drug is very high, then little or no drug may enter the systemic circulation. In this case the bioavailability is low and the drug is said to have a high first-pass metabolism (or there is a high first-pass effect). Examples of drugs with high first-pass effects include verapamil, propranolol, lignocaine, and glyceryl trinitrate. For some drugs, such as glyceryl trinitrate (GTN, a vasodilator used for angina) and buprenorphine (an opioid analgesic used for pain), the extraction ratio is so high that oral bioavailability is nearly 0%. This means alternative routes of administration must be used. Both GTN and buprenorphine are given as a topical patch, so the drug is absorbed through the skin. They are also given sublingually (under the tongue), as the blood supply here does not drain into the liver first. Drugs are sometimes given rectally to avoid the first pass. However, it should be noted that the blood supply from the rectum does drain in part into the liver, and so some first-pass effects are possible.

As discussed above, for drugs with high hepatic extraction ratios, changing enzyme activity has little effect on systemic clearance. However, it has a dramatic effect on the bioavailability. For example, if a drug has an extraction ratio of 90% (0.9) and it goes down to 85% (0.85) because of enzyme inhibition, the bioavailability increases from 10 to 15%, a 50% relative increase.

---

6. The subject of epilepsy is introduced in Chapter 16.

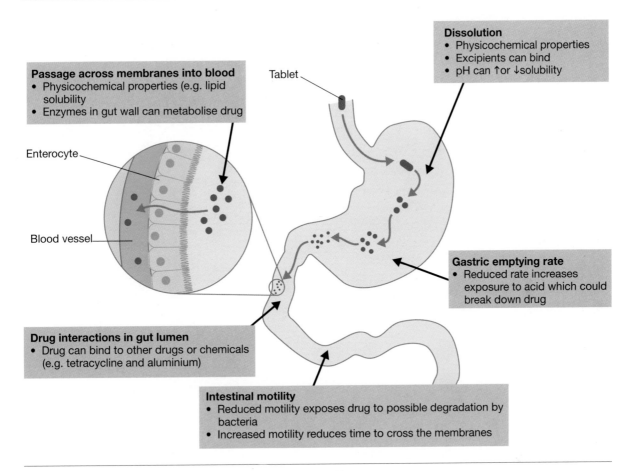

Dissolution
- Physicochemical properties
- Excipients can bind
- pH can ↑or ↓solubility

Tablet

Passage across membranes into blood
- Physicochemical properties (e.g. lipid solubility
- Enzymes in gut wall can metabolise drug

Enterocyte

Blood vessel

Gastric emptying rate
- Reduced rate increases exposure to acid which could break down drug

Drug interactions in gut lumen
- Drug can bind to other drugs or chemicals (e.g. tetracycline and aluminium)

Intestinal motility
- Reduced motility exposes drug to possible degradation by bacteria
- Increased motility reduces time to cross the membranes

Figure 3.9 Factors influencing the absorption of a drug from a tablet.

Adapted from: Birkett, DJ. Bioavailability and first pass clearance. Australian Prescriber 1991; **14**(1): 14–16.

Section 2
The cardiovascular system

In this book we mostly focus on common disorders: those most often encountered in doctors surgeries, general hospitals, and pharmacies throughout the world. Frequently these conditions are not life threatening, but remain serious, for example skin disorders (Chapter 8) or most manifestations of depression (Chapter 19). By contrast, in this section we will mainly be considering a set of conditions caused by disease of the heart or blood vessels (the cardiovascular system) that are both common and life threatening. What will most of us die of? Well, the answer is very clear: most of us will die from cardiovascular disease or from cancer. Taken together cardiovascular diseases will kill more of us than any other set of conditions. As we discuss in Chapter 6, in the USA alone approximately one person every minute dies as a result of diseased blood vessels in the heart.

For a large percentage of these people death will be sudden and unexpected. The most common cause of these sudden deaths is heart attacks—the blood supply to part of the heart is reduced by clogged up vessels, oxygen supply to the heart is inadequate, and as a result part of the heart tissue dies.

However, we are not helpless to reduce the likelihood of this happening. We can eat well, exercise, and avoid cigarette smoke and stress. Taken together these measures can have a profound effect on cardiovascular risk reduction. Here we are concerned with understanding how we can use drugs as therapeutic agents to reduce patients' risk of establishing diseases of the heart or blood vessels, and how we can modify the course of such illnesses when they occur. The objective is to improve longevity and the quality of life.

In this section we will encounter a number of patients who develop a range of common and serious cardiovascular conditions. Monique has developed a blood clot in a leg vein following a long-haul flight (Workbook 1). For her this creates discomfort, but also a risk of more serious and potentially life-threatening consequences—the risk of these occurring is reduced by the drugs she takes. Once her illness is resolved there is no reason to think her long-term risk is increased. Andreas (Workbook 2) has high blood pressure (hypertension), a condition in which, typically, the patient feels perfectly well. Despite the absence of symptoms, Andreas will have to take antihypertensive drugs for the rest of his life—the long-term reduction in blood pressure will substantially reduce Andreas' risk of developing serious cardiovascular conditions such as heart attacks and stroke. Contrasting with this, poor Brian in Workbook 3 has already developed clogged-up coronary arteries—we need to reduce his long-term risk with drugs that modify his blood lipid profile, but in his case it is too late to prevent a heart attack. In Workbooks 3 and 4 we will explore the pathology and blood treatment of patients with other common types of heart diseases (arrhythmias and heart failure). In every case we will describe the physiological basis of these illnesses, and set out to understand how the action of the drugs at a cellular and molecular level changes the physiology of the heart and blood vessels, and why this results in a therapeutic outcome.

Chapter 4
Haemostasis and thromboembolic disorders

What happens when you cut yourself and bleed? Eventually the flow of blood from the wound reduces and a clot forms. The underlying mechanism behind this arrest of blood loss from a damaged vessel is called **haemostasis**. Here, formation of a clot is beneficial. In Workbook 1, our fictional patient Monique experiences pain in her leg and it is concluded that a blood clot has formed on the inner face of an intact vein.

- A clot on the inside of the wall of an intact blood vessel is called a **thrombus**, and in this patient has led to a condition called deep vein thrombosis (DVT); the thrombus may block (occlude) or reduce blood flow at its site of formation.

- Furthermore, part of the thrombus may break away from the vessel wall, forming an **embolus**, which may block a smaller vessel upstream.

In this chapter, we will explore thrombus formation and removal, and the serious and common illnesses to which thrombus formation contributes. We will then look at the cellular and molecular basis of action of the drugs used to manage these pathologies, and the way this helps us to understand the pattern of use of these drugs in the clinic. We will concentrate on the most commonly used drugs, such as **heparin**, **aspirin**, and **warfarin**, but will also introduce some less well-known drugs that are useful in clinical practice.

In Monique's case, the clot (thrombus) causing the blockage dislodged and moved to her lungs, occluding blood vessels there. This creates a further dangerous condition called pulmonary embolism (PE). The process by which blood clots occur and travel through the veins is commonly known as venous thromboembolism (VTE), a collective term for DVT and PE. These common and potentially serious conditions associated with blood vessel occlusion by thrombi and emboli are also known as **thromboembolic disorders**. Included in such disorders are DVTs, PEs (which were complications for this patient), stroke, angina, and myocardial infarct (MI; heart attack). These disorders are summarized in Table 4.1. In Workbook 1 in this chapter, we consider Monique as a patient with DVT leading to a PE. Patients with other conditions in which thrombus formation plays a role are discussed in Chapters 6 and 7.

Table 4.1 Thromboembolic disorders

	Thromboembolic disorder	Site of clot
1	Deep vein thrombosis	Deep veins
2	Pulmonary embolism	Lung arterial vessels
3	Stroke	Brain arterial vessels
4	Myocardial infarct	Heart arterial vessels

4.1 How thrombi are formed and destroyed: the targets for drug action

Numerous drugs are available to modify the processes of haemostasis, which underlies thromboembolic disorders. These are mainly **antithrombotic drugs**. However, under some conditions, agents that *increase* thrombus formation or stability (haemostatic or antifibrinolytic drugs) are clinically useful. To understand the clinical use of these drugs you must develop a working picture of how thrombi are formed and removed. The mechanisms discussed below are those that underlie the occurrence of thromboembolic disorders. From a clinical perspective

Table 4.2 Risk factors for thromboembolism

Abnormality of blood flow (e.g. pooling of blood)	Abnormality of surface in contact with blood	Abnormality relating to clotting proteins
Immobilization (e.g. long plane flights)	Heart valve disease/replacement	Estrogen therapy (oral contraceptives)
Bed rest	Acute myocardial infarct	Pregnancy
Paralysis	Indwelling catheters	Malignancy
Atrial fibrillation	Previous DVT/PE	Thrombocytosis
Venous obstruction from obesity, pregnancy, tumour	Fractures	Protein C and S deficiency
Myocardial infarct	Tumour invasion	Antithrombin-III and activated protein C deficiency

these are the events stimulated in different ways by the risk factors set out in Table 4.2.

4.1.1 Platelet activation and coagulation in thrombus formation

One event contributing to haemostasis when you cut yourself is **vascular spasm**: the contraction of smooth muscle in the wall of pre-capillary arterioles supplying blood to the damaged area reduces blood flow and loss. This is fast and important in resolving a wound. The remaining events form the blood coagulation/platelet processes that lead to a clot, which blocks blood loss. So haemostasis, the arrest of blood flow from a broken blood vessel, has three components:

1) vascular spasm

2) coagulation cascade

3) platelet activation and plug formation.

The last two of these clotting processes also occur in an intact vessel in thrombus formation. **It is these coagulation/platelet events that are targeted by the antithrombotic drugs**.

While they are part of the same process, we will introduce the elements of the coagulation cascade and platelet recruitment separately.

1) **Coagulation.** This is the solidification of blood into a gel. Coagulation occurs via two convergent coagulation cascades, the intrinsic and the extrinsic cascade, as set out in Box 4.1. Each cascade comprises a series of clotting factors. These factors are proteins, which are synthesized in the liver and released into the bloodstream as inactive precursors. Specifically, each

protein is a proteolytic enzyme: an enzyme that catalyses the breakdown of other proteins. As such, each member of the cascade cleaves and activates the next member of the cascade. The signal being transmitted by the cascade is amplified at each step since each active factor formed can activate a very large number of molecules in the next step.

For example, Box 4.1 shows how the inactive factor X is activated to factor Xa, which then cleaves inactive factor II (also known as prothrombin) to form the active enzyme factor IIa (thrombin). Fibrinogen is another soluble protein, which is made in the liver and circulates in the blood. When thrombin is activated, fibrinogen is cleaved to form insoluble fibrin. This is stabilized and cross-linked by local factor XIIIa, forming the fibrin mesh, which is the scaffold for a thrombus. The coagulation cascades and their initiation are described in Box 4.1.

2) **Platelet recruitment**. This is characterized by **platelet adhesion** to the vessel wall, **platelet activation** with a change in shape and release of active chemical mediators, and **platelet aggregation**, in which platelets clump together (Box 4.2). Three important themes for understanding drug action are:

 • the two-way communication between platelets and local vascular endothelial cells (Box 4.3)

 • the role played by the biosynthesis, and release from platelets, of thromboxane A_2 (TXA_2), adenosine diphosphate (ADP), and other chemical mediators (Box 4.2)

 • the control of expression of certain receptors on the surface of platelets, notably the central role of glycoprotein receptors GPIIb/IIIa (Box 4.2).

Box 4.1

The coagulation pathways are integrated with the platelet aggregation process

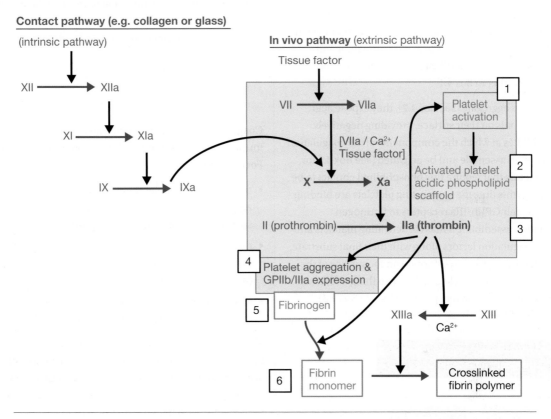

Figure a Interaction between coagulation cascades and platelet activation as the coagulation factors assemble on the surface of the activated platelets.

The pink shaded areas indicate events occurring on the surface of activating platelets. The scheme shows changes in structure (e.g. to activated form of factor) in blue arrows, and stimulating influences on these reactions in black arrows. The numbered steps are referred to in the text.

Setting the stage The coagulation cascades are conventionally described as the 'intrinsic pathway' (or more usefully the 'contact pathway') and the 'extrinsic pathway' (described here as the '*in vivo* pathway'), which converge at the level of factor Xa activation and have in common the sequence of events following this activation. Therefore, the pathway from Xa activation to the formation of the cross-linked fibrin polymer may be described as the 'common pathway'. The role of platelet activation/aggregation in thrombus formation cannot be separated from the coagulation cascades—they are part of an integrated process from initiation of a cascade to the formation of a thrombus.

Role of platelets The involvement of platelets is shown in Figure a in the form of **1**, platelet activation leading to the exposure of the acidic phospholipids; **2**, these act as scaffolds for the assembly of complexes leading to thrombin formation; **3**, the enhanced thrombin availability itself stimulates (via platelet thrombin receptors) more platelet activation, and expression of platelet GPIIb/IIIa receptors (**4**), with binding of fibrinogen to the complex (**5**) and its conversion to fibrin (**6**). In this way the platelet/thrombotic cascade forms a functional unit for the formation of a thrombus.

4.1.2 Coagulation and platelet recruitment are part of the same process, leading to platelet-fibrin plug formation

While they are often presented as separate processes, blood coagulation and platelet recruitment occur together as a series of simultaneous and interconnected events leading to platelet–fibrin plug formation and thrombus formation, as illustrated in Figure 4.1 and explored further in Box 4.1.

As platelets aggregate (see Box 4.2), they expose acid phospholipids on their surface, providing negatively charged sites at which the components of the coagulation cascade can assemble and be activated (see Box 4.1 for those factors that require this phospholipid contact to be active). At this time the aggregating platelets are binding through their GPIIb/IIIa receptors to fibrinogen molecules, assembling a mass of activating platelets and active coagulation factors along with their final substrate, fibrinogen. As thrombin is formed on the surface of the fibrinogen-bound platelets, it does two things: (1) it acts on protease-activated receptors (PARs; see Box 4.3),

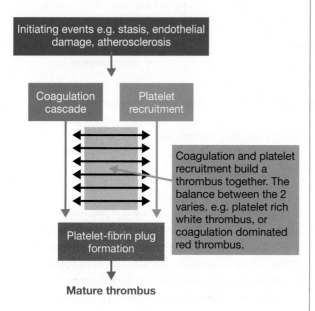

Figure 4.1 Elements of thrombus formation.

Thrombus formation involves the concerted activation of the coagulation cascade and activation of platelets: they occur together, the coagulation cascade is typically assembled on the surface of activating platelets. In this way platelet stimulation activates coagulation. Similarly, products of coagulation, e.g. thrombin, directly stimulate platelets. See also Box 4.1.

activating platelets and recruiting more into the thrombus-forming process, and (2) it converts fibrinogen to insoluble fibrin, forming the mesh of fibrin with platelets attached. This is the **platelet–fibrin plug**. As the thrombus matures, the fibrin becomes cross-linked to form a tighter mesh, and platelets (which are packed with actin/myosin) contract, compressing and strengthening the thrombus.

There is a further crosstalk between mechanisms of haemostasis

Coagulation and platelet involvement in thrombus formation involves many additional points of interaction. For example:

- the activating platelets being drawn into the aggregating mass release vasoconstrictor substances such as TXA_2, causing vascular spasm
- thrombin formed in the coagulation cascade can promote both platelet activation and vasoconstriction (acting through PARs, see Box 4.3)
- activating platelets can attenuate the anticoagulant influences of locally produced heparin (see below).

This crosstalk has important implications for understanding drug action. It means, for example, that antiplatelet drugs may be expected to modulate all three mechanisms of haemostasis. This being the case, when we consider Workbook 1 it may lead us to the question of whether Monique should have been advised to take aspirin as part of her therapy, and if not why not?

Further features of thrombus formation affect our understanding of drug use

The processes of coagulation and platelet plug formation are major targets for the action of antithrombotic drugs, and in Monique's case we will see how knowledge of drugs modifying the thrombotic process allows us to plan and understand her drug treatment. In addition, drugs which promote thrombus dissolution ('clot-busters') have an important clinical role. Before discussing the action and use of these drugs, there are some interesting topics to consider that will improve our ability to manage the clinical conditions presented by Monique and other patients we will encounter later.

Maturation of coagulation factors requires reduced vitamin K The coagulation factors II, VII, IX, and X set out in Box 4.1 are proteins in which the amino acid chain has been chemically modified after it has been

Box 4.2
Platelets: their role in the haemostatic process

Setting the stage Platelet activation is a key event in most heart attacks (Chapter 6) and strokes (Chapter 17), and so the role of platelets is clearly of importance to us. Platelets are non-nucleated components of blood. They have a life-span of 5–9 days. They release a variety of chemical mediators when activated, both those that are pre-stored in granules and those released as they are synthesized. These mediators act on neighbouring platelets (and local endothelial cells), recruiting them into the formation of a thrombus. Platelets also become 'sticky' on activation, when they will clump together and adhere to the vessel wall. The activated platelets also expose surfaces, which promotes the coagulation cascade, so that platelet plug formation and coagulation occur together (platelet–fibrin plug formation) in the development of a platelet-rich thrombus (see also Box 4.1). The process of recruiting platelets into haemostasis, leading to platelet plug formation, may be divided into three steps: adhesion, activation, and aggregation.

Role of thrombin Thrombin is the main active product of the coagulation cascade. It is also a potent activator of platelets. It is a major way in which the coagulation cascade activates platelets (see also Box 4.1). Thrombin acts upon a family of receptors

called protease-activated receptors (PARs). Platelets stimulated by thrombin will expose acid phospholipids on their surface, which become the sites of thrombin formation by the coagulation cascade, forming a positive feedback system for thrombin formation (see Box 4.1).

Platelet adhesion Platelet adhesion describes the sticking of platelets to the inner face (luminal aspect) of the blood vessel. In a healthy blood vessel, there is an active communication between platelets and endothelial cells, which means platelets pass freely over the inner face of blood vessels (see Box 4.3). However, when endothelial function is compromised, by disease (e.g. atherosclerosis; Chapter 6) or trauma, the antiplatelet influence is reduced and thrombotic influences such as von Willebrand factor takes over.

Von Willebrand factor

- A large protein, which plays a role in the coagulation cascade as well as platelet recruitment.

- It is released from endothelial cells and damaged blood vessel walls.

- Its main function is to bind other proteins. For example, it binds to subendothelial collagen

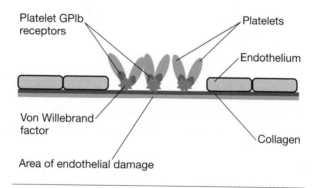

Platelet GPIb receptors

Platelets

Endothelium

Von Willebrand factor

Collagen

Area of endothelial damage

Figure b Von Willebrand protein acts as a bridge between collagen exposed in damaged blood vessels and the GP1b receptors on platelets.

This leads to the platelets adhering to the vessel wall at the site of damage.

Box 4.2 **Platelets: their role in the haemostatic process**

exposed as a result of endothelial damage, and to receptor proteins on the surface of platelets (e.g. GPIb receptors), **thus causing platelets to adhere to the blood vessel wall**.

Platelet activation Two components to platelet activation can be identified: shape change and release of active chemical mediators.

Shape change Platelets are normally discoid in shape with a smooth surface, but on activation, e.g. by binding to collagen, they become irregular in shape with a somewhat spiky surface.

Release of mediators Numerous highly potent chemical mediators are released from activating platelets. These can be classified into two groups:

1. **Substances pre-stored in the granules and released by exocytosis.** Here we are concerned with adenosine diphosphate (**ADP**), which is released from its stores to act on local platelets via their $P2Y_{12}$ receptors. However, we also note that platelets release other stored substances, such as adrenaline (epinephrine) and 5-hydroxytryptamine (serotonin).

2. **Substances which are lipid soluble, not stored, and leave the cell by passing through cell membranes as they are synthesized.** For this group it is the rate of synthesis that determines the rate of release from platelets, and not surprisingly therefore the enzymes responsible for synthesis are prime drug targets (see also Figure 4.6 and discussions elsewhere of steroidal

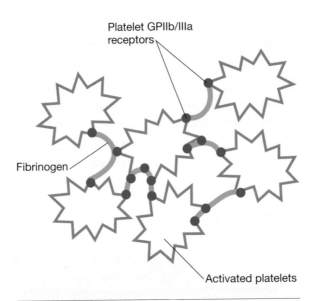

Figure c Activated platelets express GPIIb/IIIa receptors—fibrinogen binds to these, pulling the platelets together.

The fibrinogen is converted to insoluble fibrin strands by thrombin produced on the surface of the platelets (Box 4.1), and the platelets themselves contract, forming a solid thrombus. Notably, as the activated platelets bind to fibrinogen they are also attaching to the inner face of the blood vessel (Figure b above), explaining why the thrombus grows attached to the blood vessel.

and non-steroidal anti-inflammatory drugs). The significant example here is thromboxane A_2 (**TXA_2**).

Key role of GPIIb/IIIa receptors in platelet–fibrin plug formation The significance of ADP and TXA_2 is that, along with thrombin formed as part of the parallel coagulation cascade, they stimulate platelets to express glycoprotein receptors **GPIIb/IIIa**. These receptors are essential for platelet aggregation (see below). Not surprisingly, therefore, they have been the target of drug development programmes, leading to the antiplatelet drugs abciximab, eptifibatide, and tirofiban.

Platelet aggregation Platelet aggregation refers to the process of activated platelets sticking with fibrin/fibrinogen together to form aggregates. GPIIb/IIIa receptors expressed on the surface of platelets exposed to thrombin, ADP, and TXA_2 bind to fibrinogen, which pulls the platelets together in aggregate (Figure c). This fibrinogen is then a substrate for the local thrombin being formed by the coagulation cascades, which converts it to insoluble fibrin. These fibrin strands become cross-linked (under the influence of factor XIIIa) and stabilize to form a mesh that, with the attached platelets, is the platelet–fibrin plug, which is the basis of a platelet-rich thrombus.

---

synthesized. This takes the form of modification of some of the glutamic acid residues, which are part of the protein structure. The alteration in these glutamic acid residues is called γ-carboxylation. Without this modification these factors are not active and coagulation cannot take place. The γ-carboxylation of these coagulation factors requires reduced vitamin K; during carboxylation the reduced vitamin K is converted to its oxidized form. The enzyme vitamin K reductase restores the vitamin to its reduced form for another round of γ-carboxylation of coagulation factors (Figure 4.2).

A deficit in vitamin K, such as may be a risk in the newborn, will result in a potentially serious bleeding disorder. This risk is avoided by the post-partum administration of vitamin K. A more routine encounter with the requirement for reduced vitamin K is seen in the use of warfarin as an anticoagulant (Figure 4.2 and below), and indeed this manipulation of clotting factor, γ-carboxylation by warfarin, plays a major role in the management of patients such as Monique.

Arterial and venous thrombi are not the same Arterial and venous thrombi differ as a result of a different relative contribution of the platelet and coagulation elements leading to thrombus formation.

Understanding the difference between venous and arterial thrombi helps us understand why different drugs are used in their management. Arterial thrombi, or **white thrombi**, are mainly platelets in a mesh of fibrin and cell debris. They are formed when an atherosclerotic plaque becomes thrombogenic and accumulates activating platelets on its surface (see Chapter 5). This platelet colony then recruits the coagulation cascade by the mechanisms indicated above, leading to a fibrin cross-linked structure with few red blood cells. Venous thrombi, by contrast, are commonly associated with pooled static blood (e.g. DVT), leading to coagulation cascade activation with relatively little platelet involvement. This is what is thought to have happened to Monique. These thrombi have a red colour derived from the high number of red blood cells trapped within the fibrin mesh, and a low contribution from platelets. Not surprisingly, antiplatelet therapy (which reduces the recruitment of platelets into thrombi, as set out below) is more effective in the management of arterial white thrombi than venous red thrombi.

Endogenous brakes prevent uncontrolled coagulation The accelerating amplification of the coagulation cascade might seem likely to lead to the uncontrolled spread of coagulation. Such a disastrous

Box 4.3

Two examples of endothelial–platelet interactions

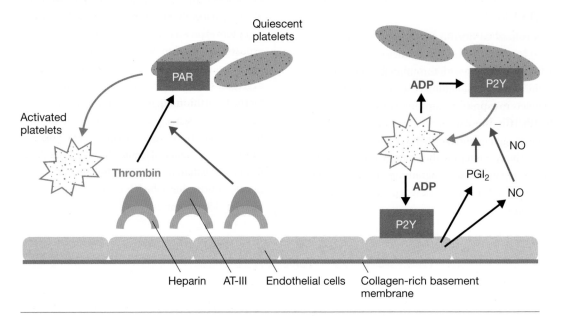

Figure d Two examples of the communication between platelets and endothelial cells.

Figure d illustrates how endothelial cells drive platelets away from activation and adhesion, stopping platelets from sticking to the inside of the blood vessel and consequently preventing thrombus formation and maintaining blood flow.

On the left the activation of platelets by thrombin is illustrated. Activation of platelets by thrombin is considered to be one of the most potent mechanisms for platelet recruitment into thrombus formation. This activation then exposes further acidic surfaces on the platelets, which promote the coagulation cascade to produce more thrombin (Box 4.1). If this process progresses unchecked, there will be accelerating fibrin formation and platelet–fibrin plug development. However, in a healthy blood vessel this sequence will be blocked by the binding of antithrombin-III (AT-III) binding to heparin. The AT-III-heparin complex inhibits thrombin, therefore preventing the PAR-mediated activation of platelets. The heparin in the figure is the native heparin, produced by endothelial cells as in one of the ways they inhibit coagulation in healthy blood vessels. When **heparin** is administered as a drug this can supplement the native heparin, which is particularly important when damaged endothelium results in lowered heparin production.

On the right the role of ADP in prostacyclin (PGI2) and nitric oxide (NO) production is illustrated. As platelets activate they release a range of mediators, including ADP (see Box 4.2). ADP acts on platelets via $P2Y_1$ and $P2Y_{12}$ receptors, contributing to progression towards platelet adhesion to blood vessel walls. However, in a healthy blood vessel this is prevented by ADP released from platelets also stimulating the endothelial cells, where ADP acts on $P2Y_1$ receptors to enhance synthesis and release of PGI_2 and nitric oxide (NO). These then act directly on platelets to (1) prevent progression towards adhesion and aggregation, (2) prevent release of further platelet-stimulating mediators, and (3) prevent recruitment of other platelets.

Many other mechanisms operate in healthy blood vessels. Activating platelets release other local mediators (Box 4.2). Notable for our purposes is the release of TXA_2, a potent stimulator of platelets whose synthesis and release is effectively inhibited by **aspirin**.

In disease states the balance of communication is disturbed. Disruption of endothelial function can have many consequences. For example:

1) endothelial cells act as a barrier between platelets and the collagen of the basement membrane (see Figure c for an illustration of the consequences of removal of this barrier)

2) endothelial cells provide a barrier preventing mediators released from platelets reaching underlying vascular smooth muscle cells. When this barrier is removed, platelets activate and release mediators such as ADP and TXA_2, which stimulate these muscle cells to contract and **proliferate, contributing to reduced blood flow as a result of vascular spasm and atherosclerosis (Chapter 6)**

3) the growth of an atherosclerotic plaque removes the local influence of endothelial cells and can, when mature and rupturing, present a focus for platelet activation unrestrained by the presence of adjacent endothelial cells (see Chapter 6).

---

outcome is prevented because the activation of cascades also leads to their inhibition; it is a self-regulating system. These inhibitory mechanisms are central to the action of anticoagulant drugs, as illustrated by the following three examples:

- Antithrombin-III (AT-III) is a plasma protein, which combines with heparin to inhibit thrombin and other coagulation factors, including factor Xa, which is responsible for the formation of thrombin from its prothrombin precursor (see Box 4.1).

- The heparins are an endogenous group of mucopolysaccharides of varying molecular weight that come from the vascular endothelium, mast cells, and basophils. Endothelial-derived heparin binds with AT-III to give a powerful local anticoagulant effect.

- Protein C is another plasma protein. It is activated by thrombin, inhibiting factor Va and factor VIIIa.

Clots and thrombi must be removed—incorporating the seeds of destruction To avoid the accumulation of clots and thrombi during a lifetime, it is necessary that a mechanism for removal exists, and it is therefore not surprising that as a thrombus forms it incorporates the mechanism for its own destruction. This clot-dissolving process is called **fibrinolysis**, and is achieved by the breakdown of the fibrin by plasmin, a proteolytic enzyme that can also degrade other proteins, including fibrinogen and factors II, V, and VIII. Several mechanisms ensure that plasmin activity is restricted to within clots, and does not circulate throughout the body.

Plasmin comes from its inactive precursor plasminogen, a plasma protein, which accumulates on fibrin as it is formed by the coagulation cascade. This fibrin-bound plasminogen is a good substrate for tissue plasminogen activator (tPA), which is released from damaged blood vessels and also binds to the fibrin, where it cleaves plasminogen into active plasmin (Figure 4.3). This locally formed plasmin then breaks the fibrin into soluble

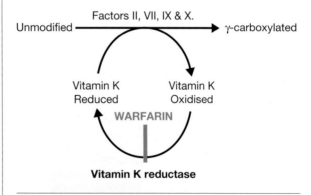

Figure 4.2 Role of vitamin K in clotting factor maturation.

Reduced vitamin K is necessary for the γ-carboxylation of the clotting factors. Without this the clotting factors cannot later be activated and participate in the coagulation cascade. The reduction of vitamin K is prevented by warfarin, preventing the synthesis of mature clotting factors and eventually leading to the loss of these factors in the blood.

fragments, causing the clot to dissolve. The fibrin-dependent nature of tPA action prevents formation of plasmin from circulating plasminogen. Plasminogen activator inhibitors 1 and 2 (PAI1 and PAI2) further attenuate any plasmin activity outside of the thrombus.

In Monique's case, all of these mechanisms will have been set in place as her VTE became established. The drugs she was prescribed reduced the thrombogenic processes in her leg and lungs, leaving removal of the original thrombus to the endogenous mechanisms just described.

4.2 Drugs used in the treatment of thromboembolic disorders

While we understand the involvement of platelets and coagulation as a single process in thrombus formation, it is conventional to classify clinically useful antithrombotic agents as drugs interfering with the coagulation cascades (anticoagulant drugs), those that reduce platelet activation (antiplatelet drugs), and those which promote clot dissolution (fibrinolytic drugs, also called thrombolytics). This is a valuable approach because it relates clearly to their clinical patterns of use. In each case, if you understand the mechanism of action of the drugs, and their pharmacokinetics, then you will be able to understand how they are used to benefit patients. The workbooks (both in this chapter and later) provide a way of developing your understanding of the relationship between the mechanisms of drug action and the treatment of individual patients.

4.2.1 Anticoagulant drugs

The clinical use of drugs that attenuate coagulation cascades is dominated by the heparin group of preparations and warfarin. Their mechanisms of action and resulting clinical use are explored below. In addition, some other related drugs used in anticoagulant therapy are introduced.

Heparins

Heparin sulphate is secreted by endothelial cells, providing an anticoagulant surface to blood vessel linings. Along with the antiplatelet mediators released by endothelial cells (Box 4.3) endothelial-derived heparin contributes to the free flow of blood through healthy vessels.

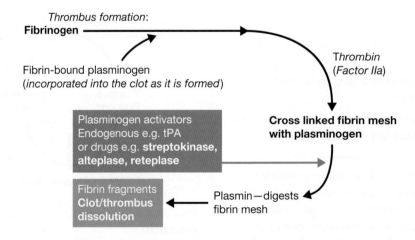

Figure 4.3 Clots/thrombi remove themselves by digestion from within.

As the thrombus (clot) is formed, fibrinogen is converted to fibrin. Plasminogen binds to the fibrin so that it is brought into the thrombus. The plasminogen activators can then convert this fibrin-bound plasminogen into plasmin, which is a proteolytic enzyme capable of breaking the fibrin up, leading to the thrombus falling apart.

Heparin is a polymer of sugars that is extracted from animal tissues to be used as a drug. In clinical preparations it comes in two size ranges. The activity of **unfractionated heparin** depends on larger forms of 18 saccharide (sugar) units or longer, while the preparation of smaller **low-molecular weight heparin (LMWH)** requires a minimum pentasaccharide (five units) size for its clinical effect. An example of LMWH is **enoxaparin**.

In Workbook 1, Monique develops VTE. Her clotting factors have been activated as part of the process, generating abnormally large quantities of thrombin. Since this leaves her at risk of complications, it is important that antithrombotic therapy works very quickly. Although an LMWH would be used first line in most DVT patients, unfractionated heparin was used in Monique's case because she developed multiple PEs and became haemodynamically unstable (see Workbook 1). When unfractionated heparin is used, a large initial dose is administered intravenously for a rapid response by quickly achieving therapeutic levels.

Mechanism of action of the heparin preparations

Both clinically available forms of heparin depend for their action on stimulating the AT-III action, one of the natural anticoagulant mechanisms introduced above. Understanding the pattern of clinical use of unfractionated heparin and LMWH depends on understanding their different manner of binding to AT-III as well as the way the pharmacokinetics of the two preparations varies. Binding to AT-III is illustrated in Figure 4.4.

Heparin acts as a cofactor for AT-III, increasing its ability to inhibit coagulation factors. Unfractionated heparin can bind directly to both AT-III and thrombin; this is necessary for the inhibition of thrombin by AT-III. Factors IXa–XIIa are effectively inhibited by the AT-III/heparin complex in the absence of direct binding of heparin to the clotting factors. As a result both unfractionated and LMWH can inhibit factor Xa, but LMWH cannot inhibit thrombin.

Several points of therapeutic significance follow from this account of the mechanisms of action of heparins:

- Considering that factor Xa is required for thrombin (factor IIa) production, and that the AT-III/heparin dimer is a very effective inhibitor of factor Xa, it is not surprising that both are very effective as anticoagulants.

- Furthermore, the mechanism of action ensures that both types of heparin act quickly: AT-III is already in the plasma and inhibits clotting factor activity immediately the heparin levels in the blood are raised. The speed of inhibition depends on the route of administration. Neither drug can be given orally: subcutaneous injection will take about 30 minutes for effective action, while an IV injection will have an essentially immediate effect. However, clinical trials have shown that subcutaneous LMWH are as effective and safer than unfractionated heparin.

- Both heparins can have an antiplatelet effect. This is not unwelcome and is because, as mentioned above, thrombin activates platelets directly.

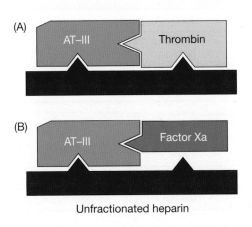

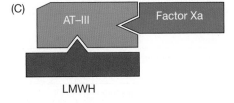

Figure 4.4 Action of heparins at AT-III and clotting factors.

This figure shows both short (C) (fractionated) and long (B) (unfractionated) heparin molecules (in brown) binding to AT-III (green), creating an effective inhibitor of factor Xa (dark blue). However, only long heparin can also bind thrombin (A) (light blue), necessary for inhibition by AT-III.

Pharmacokinetics of heparin

Most **unfractionated heparin** binds to AT-III. However, a significant remainder (about a third) binds to other sites such as plasma proteins and endothelial cells, contributing to its dose-dependent pharmacokinetic profile and reducing its bioavailability.

Other properties affected are detailed in Table 4.3.

Almost all bound LMWH is complexed with AT-III. There is little or no binding to plasma proteins, endothelial cells, etc., leading to improved bioavailability, predictable dose response, and a more sustained clinical effect.

How is unfractionated heparin used in hospital?

Heparins are given intravenously or by subcutaneous injection. The clinical use of unfractionated heparin is more complicated than that of many drugs. The complexities arise for a number of reasons, including unpredictable pharmacokinetics and a variable antithrombotic response from one patient to the next. It is important that the anticoagulant response is sufficient to protect the patient, but not so over-effective that the patient is left vulnerable to severe bleeding. Working out the correct dose for the continuous infusion is guided by testing each patient's blood by measurement of the activated partial thromboplastin time (aPTT), which reflects the alterations by heparin of the clotting cascade.

Adverse effects of heparin

Haemorrhage (bleeding) is the most common side effect of unfractionated heparin. Factors that influence this are length of therapy, advanced age of patient, comorbidity (patient has other disease states), concomitant antiplatelet treatment (e.g. aspirin), and dose of heparin too high (raised aPTT).

Bleeding as a result of heparin use should be managed by:

- discontinuing heparin
- fluid infusion to maintain volume if bleeding
- blood/plasma/clotting factor infusion
- **protamine** may be administered intravenously to neutralize heparin by forming an inactive protamine–heparin complex. Protamine has a rapid onset of action and its effect lasts 2 hours.

Thrombocytopaenia (low-platelet count in the blood) can be caused by heparin. This is known as heparin-induced thrombocytopaenia (HIT), the two types of which are:

- type I HIT, which occurs as a direct result of the effect of heparin on platelet function, resulting in platelet clumping and significant reduction in platelet count. It is reversible, patients remain asymptomatic, and platelet counts return to normal even if heparin is continued.

Table 4.3 Comparison of unfractionated heparin and low molecular weight heparin

	Unfractionated heparin	Low molecular weight heparin
Molecular weight	3000–30,000	1000–10,000
Fraction bound to AT-III	2/3 (++)	Almost all (+++)
Fraction bound to plasma protein	1/3 of molecule (+++)	Almost none (+)
Inhibition of platelet function	++++	++
Increases vascular permeability	Yes	No
Bioavailability	++	++++
Dose-dependent clearance	Yes	No
Elimination half-life	30–150 minutes	60–750 minutes
Endothelial cell binding	++++	–
Primary route of elimination	Saturable binding processes Renal	Renal
Activated partial thromboplastin time monitoring required	Yes (complex binds to thrombin)	No (complex does not bind to thrombin)

• type II HIT, which occurs when prolonged use of thrombin (5 to 14 days after start of heparin treatment) generates antiplatelet antibodies. Heparin then binds to these antiplatelet antibodies to form a heparin–antibody complex that binds to the surface of platelets, resulting in platelet aggregation despite the thrombocytopaenia. Type II HIT is a more severe condition than type I, with a greater fall in platelet count. Monique, our patient in Workbook 1, only received heparin for 5 days and therefore was at minimal risk.

Type II HIT can result in limb thrombosis, requiring amputation in 25% of cases. Stroke, MI, skin necrosis, and thrombosis of other major organs can also occur.

In cases of thrombocytopaenia, heparin must be discontinued. Because LMWH are less likely to activate platelets, the risk of thrombocytopaenia is reduced. However, if antibodies to the heparin complex have been formed, it is possible for LMWH to also cause the type II HIT; cross-reactivity has been reported to be as high as 90%. **Danaparoid** is an LMWH-related preparation with a greater affinity for Xa, which has a role in patients with immune heparin-induced thrombocytopaenia. In such patients requiring parenteral antithrombotics there are also alternatives derived from hirudin (see section below on other anticoagulants).

Warfarin

Warfarin is the most commonly prescribed anticoagulant. In Monique's case the Workbook 1 treatment began with heparins. It then moved to both heparins and warfarin before maintaining the warfarin and discontinuing the heparin. Why was this done? Heparins have a very rapid anticoagulant action (minutes). Warfarin is an anticoagulant with a very slow onset of action (days). Heparins are given by injection, while warfarin is by oral administration. These differences define the clinical use of these two compounds. Typically, as in the case of Monique, heparins are used to rapidly establish an antithrombotic state. Warfarin therapy is normally started on the same day, so for some days, from the outset of therapy, both drugs are given. This avoids harm from a pro-coagulant effect that warfarin may have when first used, which comes from its effect on protein C, a vitamin K dependent factor (see below). Overlap of this nature therefore ensures that heparin secures the antithrombotic status of the patient during the few days it takes before warfarin has its anticoagulant effect. When warfarin is effective, heparin is discontinued. Many patients will continue to take warfarin for years, facilitated by its oral administration.

Why is onset of warfarin action so slow?

Warfarin acts by preventing the maturation of clotting factors. The mature factors are already present in the blood in the form of a circulating pool of inactive precursor factors (e.g. factors II, VII, IX, and X) ready to be converted on activation of the coagulation cascade into the active (e.g. factor IIa, etc.) form. The anticoagulant effects of warfarin are only seen when these precursor factors are cleared from the circulation and this takes a few days. This is why Monique's warfarin and heparin were overlapped for several days.

Figure 4.5 shows the relationship between the maturation and activation of clotting factors, and illustrates the point of action of warfarin and heparin in these processes.

How can the effect of warfarin be reduced by vitamin K administration?

Warfarin competes directly with vitamin K at its binding site on the vitamin K reductase enzyme (Figure 4.2). This means that it prevents vitamin K having access to the reductase enzyme, resulting in the depletion of

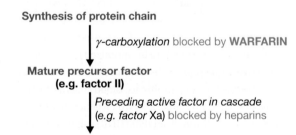

Figure 4.5 Sequential maturation and activation of clotting factors.

The sequence starts with the synthesis of the protein chain of the factor protein, which is the clotting factor. This then must be γ-carboxylated (see also Figure 4.2), resulting in the mature factors, which normally circulate. This process is inhibited by warfarin. These mature precursor factors (inactive) have to be cleared from the body before warfarin administration results in an antithrombotic effect. The heparin preparations block the proteolytic activity of the activated factors (Figure 4.4), which is required during the coagulation cascade, as the clot/thrombus is forming.

reduced vitamin K and the consequent loss of γ-carboxylation. Eventually, over several days, this leads to a loss of mature clotting factors in the blood. Being a competitive antagonist, the binding of warfarin to the reductase enzyme can be effectively overcome by an elevated vitamin K concentration. This explains why warfarin overdose is effectively treated by intravenous vitamin K.

Pharmacokinetics of warfarin

Warfarin is 99% bound to albumin. It is metabolized in the liver by cytochrome P450 enzymes, with the subsequent production of inactive metabolites that are excreted in the urine and stool. Some drugs increase this metabolism of warfarin, while some inhibit it. Drug interactions can therefore have an important effect on the correct dosage for the individual patient. Drugs which inhibit warfarin breakdown include macrolide antibiotics, azole antifungal agents, and cimetidine. Metabolism may be increased by drugs such as phenytoin, phenobarbitone, and rifampicin. The mean plasma half-life of warfarin is approximately 36 hours.

How is warfarin used in the clinic?

Warfarin is taken orally, facilitating its use for long-term maintenance therapy at home. This enhances the need for good patient education (see below). However, even with prolonged home use, warfarin therapy needs to be monitored to ensure the best dose is used. As with heparin, the dose needs to be optimized to provide effective protection against thrombus formation while minimizing bleeding problems. Blood coagulation is measured using a simple test, which generates an International Normalized Ratio (INR) value. A high INR means the blood clots quickly. The INR is used to adjust the patient's dosage. In a patient such as Monique an INR of 2–3 is required. Administration and dosage of warfarin are further explored in Box 4.4.

Adverse effects of warfarin

The most common adverse effects of warfarin include bleeding and skin necrosis.

There are several factors that influence the risk of bleeding. Bleeding mostly occurs in the nose, pharynx, gastrointestinal tract, and urinary tract. Bleeding tends to be dose-dependent. Withdrawal or suspension of warfarin therapy and/or vitamin K administration are used to control the bleed. Bleeding occurred in Monique's

case because of the interaction of warfarin with her antibiotics.

Other anticoagulants

There is interest in clinically useful anticoagulants that directly inhibit thrombin or other factors, independent of AT-III. Some derive from **hirudin**, which medicinal leaches use to ensure a free flow of blood. **Lepirudin** is a recombinant mimic of hirudin, which may be given by intravenous injection or infusion in patients requiring anticoagulation who have heparin-induced thrombocytopaenia (see above). **Fondaparinux** is another synthetic drug, an inhibitor of factor Xa, available for use in the management of VTEs, administered by intravenous or subcutaneous injection. **Ximelagatran** was the first of the class of direct thrombin inhibitors, which acts by the sole inhibition of the action of thrombin. It was an oral drug with a fixed dose and would have resolved the problem of dosing, interaction, and monitoring with warfarin, but had to be withdrawn in 2006 after reports of hepatotoxicity. Recently **dabigatran** has been introduced as an acceptable direct thrombin inhibitor. Acting higher up the coagulation cascade is **rivaroxaban**, a direct factor Xa inhibitor. These types of drugs may be the oral anticoagulants of the future, displacing warfarin in many clinical settings, reducing the burden of regular attendance at anticoagulant clinics and of bleeding/thrombotic complications.

Summary of clinical uses of anticoagulants

Warfarin is used in a wide range of clinical conditions that predispose to thrombin-rich clots (red clots). Warfarin is used in patients who have suffered a DVT or PE for a period of 3–6 months after their first clot and lifelong if there is a second clot. Warfarin is also used to prevent a stroke in patients with chronic atrial fibrillation because clots that could form in a fibrillating heart could dislodge and cause a blockage in the brain (see also Chapter 7).

Patients with artificial implants, e.g. valves, pacemakers, and defibrillators, may in some cases be put on warfarin for 3 months to lifelong, depending on the type of implant and any concurrent risk factors.

4.2.2 Antiplatelet drugs

The inhibition of platelet activation will reduce platelet plug formation, but will also indirectly attenuate activation of the coagulation cascade by reducing the assembly of coagulation factors at the surface of the

Box 4.4
How heparins and warfarin are used in the clinic

When wishing to anti-coagulate a patient it is commonplace for heparin to be used first for its fast onset, followed by long-term treatment with warfarin, with an overlap of several days in which both are given, because of the long delay before warfarin is effective. Heparin is administered i.v. in clinic or subcutaneously, while warfarin, being orally available, is suitable for long-term home use.

HEPARIN

Heparin is aviable as unfractioned (UH) or a purified low molecular weight preparation (LMWH). Differences between these preparations are set out in Table 4.3 and Figure 4.4.

Heparin administration, aPTT tests and dosage. Three modes of administration of heparins are available.

1. **Loading dose followed by continuous infusion.** In patients with acute PE and who are compromised haemodynamicaly, such as Monique, it is also important that effective anticoagulant levels are reached very quickly. UH should be used because the efficacy of LMWH in this situation is unknown. To achieve this it is common to give an initial high dose (loading dose) followed by continuous infusion (intravenous) to maintain the desired anticoagulant effect. A loading dose is usually required in an emergency such as haemodynamicaly compromised PE because it provides rapid achievement of therapeutic levels, and because while there are ongoing clotting processes there is resistance to anticoagulation within the thrombus. So the concentration required to shut the thrombotic process down is higher than that required to prevent it starting up again (inhibition of the effects of heparin by activating platelets is mentioned above).

    Working out the correct dose for the continuous infusion is then guided by measurement of the activated partial prothrombin time (aPTT) which reflects the alterations in the intrinsic pathway of the clotting cascade. Using a heparin dose which prolongs the aPTT to 1.5 to 2.5 times the mean normal value has been considered adequate to prevent extension of the thrombus.

2. **Subcutaneous unfractionated heparin.** Twice daily subcutaneous injection of heparin has been shown to be as safe and as efficacious as the continuous infusion for the initial period of treatment of DVT. It has some advantages over the infusion technique

    *   Alternative in patients without IV access
    *   More mobility for patients as not hooked up continuously to infusion
    *   Less nursing time
    *   More easily reversible than LMWH.
    *   cheaper

    This could have been an alternative for Monique if she had been more stable. Note that aPPT measurement is still required for dosing (contrast with subcutaneous LMWH below).

3. **Subcutaneous LMWH.** These have been shown to be as safe and effective as unfractionated heparin.

    Advantages of LMWH are

    *   No aPPT monitoring required
    *   Easy calculation of correct dose based on the weight of the patient.
    *   Can be used at home.
    *   Although the drug cost of these are usually higher, the overall cost turns to be lower.

LMWH preparations. Monique was treated with a LMWH. Examples of LMWH used in the treatment of VTE are **dalteparin**, **enoxaparin** and **tinzaparin**. There are significant differences in their molecular weight, pharmacokinetic and pharmacodynamic characteristics. Dalteparin was chosen for Monique because it was the first line LMWH for VTE on the formulary in Monique's hospital.

WARFARIN THERAPY AT HOME AND IN THE CLINIC. There are two main methods of initiating warfarin therapy.

a) **The average daily dosing method** which is based on the principle that although patient's warfarin dosing requirements vary significantly, an average dosing requirement in mg per day of warfarin to maintain an INR of 2–3 is chosen. Patients are generally started on this dose, which is adjusted if required until the desired INR is attained. INR is evaluated within 3–5 days of warfarin initiation. Patients with increased sensitivity to warfarin are started on a lower dose. Factors that increase sensitivity are : age > 70, congestive heart failure, malignancy, renal and hepatic disease, malignancy and concurrent use of interacting medication.

b) **The flexible warfarin initiation method** evaluates the rate of increase in INR and daily adjustments are made according to the rate of increase in INR. The aim is to determine a maintenance dose. below. The flexible dosing method offers an approach tailored to the individual patient.

---

activated platelets. Antiplatelet drugs may be mechanistically divided into two classes: (1) those acting at an intracellular location to inhibit enzymes, for example aspirin and dipyradimole, and (2) those acting at platelet-surface receptors, such as clopidogrel and abciximab.

Aspirin

Aspirin is a drug with a single mode of action at the molecular level (it is a cyclooxygenase (COX) inhibitor, see below) but with diverse significant applications. The actions and applications of aspirin therefore occur at a number of different locations in this book.

In Workbook 3, we discuss another fictional patient, Brian, who takes aspirin in connection with his angina. We will encounter aspirin in a variety of other clinical contexts, and in particular will discuss aspirin and related drugs as anti-inflammatory and analgesic agents. Here we will consider aspirin as an example of an antiplatelet drug.

In Box 4.3, various aspects of platelet and endothelial interactions are discussed, and a simplified account given of the pathway leading to prostacyclin and TXA_2 synthesis. The diagrams in Box 4.3 and Figure 4.6 show how synthesis of both these compounds is dependent on COX. After the COX-catalysed step, the pathway diverges, either to prostacyclin in endothelial cells or to TXA_2 in platelets. Box 4.3 illustrates how this affects platelet function: prostacyclin is antiplatelet, and contributes to the antithrombotic influence of endothelial cells, while TXA_2 promotes platelet aggregation. Figure 4.6 illustrates the inhibition of COX by aspirin.

The illustration shows how aspirin, acting on both endothelial cells and platelets, could produce both an increase and a decrease in platelet recruitment. In fact, the effect of low-dose aspirin (e.g. 75 mg per day) is predominantly on platelets, leaving the endothelial prostacyclin pathway intact, with the result that aspirin is antiplatelet and antithrombotic. The reason for this is in part that the COX enzyme is permanently knocked out by aspirin. Individual platelets cannot recover from this since they have no nucleus and therefore cannot make new enzyme. Recovery of platelet activity in the patient depends therefore on the natural turnover of platelets (7–10 days). The endothelial cells by contrast continually make more COX protein, and so, with low-dose aspirin, reach an equilibrium, which preserves prostacyclin production.

Another reason why low-dose aspirin has a greater effect on platelets than endothelial cells is that it is subject to considerable first-pass metabolism, which means that

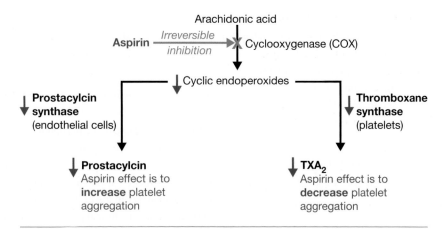

Figure 4.6 Aspirin has different effects on platelets and endothelial cells.

Aspirin acts on the same molecular target in the two cell types, but the consequences are very different. This is because the enzyme cyclooxygenase, which aspirin inhibits, leads to prostacyclin in the endothelial cells but thromboxane in the platelets.

while it influences the blood as it passes the intestines and liver circulation, its distribution around most of the tissues of the body is limited.

Clinical use of aspirin as an antiplatelet drug

Clinical use of aspirin is essentially summarized by noting that it is most effective at preventing or limiting arterial occlusions, in which platelet involvement is high and where anticoagulants have a limited effect. This contrasts with the VTEs, where anticoagulants are most effective. This explains why Monique is not treated with aspirin in Workbook 1, while Brian, with his arterial occlusion, is treated with aspirin. In these cases, it is common to prescribe an initial dose of 150–300 mg immediately following the ischaemic event, followed by the low maintenance dose of 75 mg per day to prevent further events. Aspirin may also be used following heart surgery and in the management of atrial dysrhythmias (Chapter 7).

Adverse effects of aspirin are discussed elsewhere (section 9.3.1), however, it is important to note here that aspirin should not usually be used in patients with a wide variety of bleeding disorders, or those under the age of 16 due to association with Reye's syndrome; a potentially fatal condition that affects many organs of the body.

Other antiplatelet drugs

While other COX inhibitors have been produced for clinical use by the pharmaceutical industry, aspirin

remains the only one used for its antiplatelet effect. Other antiplatelet drugs therefore act by separate mechanisms.

Clopidogrel is a prodrug, which means that it acts after conversion within the body to an active metabolite, which reduces the stimulation of platelets by ADP. The release of ADP from platelets, and its action on platelet $P2Y_{12}$ receptors to enhance aggregation, is set out in Box 4.2. The clopidogrel metabolite is an antagonist at these $P2Y_{12}$ receptors. Like aspirin, it is useful in the prevention of reoccurrence of arterial ischaemic disease and in most cases of acute coronary syndrome. It is also used in patients who have received coronary stents. Because it acts in a manner entirely separate from aspirin it is not surprising that its effects may be additive, and in some cases this is seen as an improved clinical outcome when both drugs are administered together.

Following evidence from clinical trials, it is used in acute coronary syndrome in combination with aspirin to reduce risk of further events.

Dipyradimole acts to increase the level of cyclic AMP in platelets by inhibition of phosphodiesterase (see section 2.2.4), stabilizing platelets and reducing activation. In patients with a history of occlusion of blood vessels in the brain (cerebral ischaemic events such as stroke), it may be useful to prevent further events. It is routinely used with aspirin.

Abciximab is a preparation of an antibody fragment, which binds to the GPIIb/IIIa receptors expressed on platelets as a central mechanism in platelet recruitment, as explained in Box 4.2. **Eptifibatide** and **tirofiban** act as antagonists at the GPIIb/IIIa receptors. These drugs, administered intravenously in hospital, are useful for certain patients undergoing coronary angioplasty or stenting—procedures to secure blood flow through arteries supplying the heart—and in some cases of acute coronary syndrome.

Not surprisingly, these antiplatelet drugs all carry a risk of bleeding disorders; this risk must be weighed against the benefits.

4.2.3 Fibrinolytics (thrombolytics)

In Workbook 3, our patient Brian has a heart attack (MI). One possibility for immediate treatment is that the patient is 'thrombolyzed', which means that a drug is given that will lead to the breakdown of the clot that has blocked an artery serving part of his heart. Such a drug will encourage the digestion of the fibrin mesh of the clot, and so is called a **fibrinolytic** or a thrombolytic. Figure 4.2 illustrates the native fibrinolytic system, whereby clots are broken down and removed. As also indicated in this figure, fibrinolytic drugs promote the conversion of fibrin-bound plasminogen to the proteolytic enzyme plasmin, which cuts the fibrin mesh into pieces.

Streptokinase is a bacterial protein that is administered by intravenous infusion. Because the patient develops antibodies, which bind and inactivate the streptokinase, at least a year must elapse before it may be used again.

The other fibrinolytic drugs available are all synthetic (recombinant) versions of the endogenous tPA, such as **alteplase**, **reteplase**, and **tenecteplase**. Again given by intravenous infusion, they are selective for their action on the plasminogen bound to fibrin within clots.

Fibrinolytics play a central role in saving lives when used immediately (at least within a few hours) following an MI (see also Chapter 6). They unblock the affected coronary artery, securing improved perfusion of blood and restored oxygen delivery to the working muscle of the heart. In addition, in some patients they have a role in the management of DVT, ischaemic stroke (where there is a block of an artery in the brain), and in preventing shunts and tubes used in clinical procedures from becoming blocked by clots.

4.2.4 Antifibrinolytic drugs and haemostatics

Treatments that inhibit fibrinolysis will stabilize clots and promote haemostasis. Let us consider two examples with interesting modes of action.

Tranexamic acid binds to plasminogen. As a result the action of tPA leads to the formation of a plasmin–tranexamate conjugate that is inactive. Tranexamic acid is available for oral administration or intravenous infusion. Its main use is severe menorrhagia and overdose of streptokinase or plasminogen activator fibrinolytics.

Aprotinin is a wide spectrum protease inhibitor with diverse effects, including inhibition of plasmin activity, and conversely inhibition of components of the coagulation cascade and thrombin activation of platelets. Clinically, the antifibrinolytic activity dominates, leading to its use to reduce blood loss with certain major surgical procedures.

SUMMARY OF DRUGS USED FOR HAEMOSTASIS AND THROMBOEMBOLIC DISORDERS

Therapeutic class	Drugs	Mechanism of action	Common clinical uses	Comments	Examples of adverse drug reactions
Heparins	Unfractionated heparin Heparin	Indirectly binds to AT-III and factor Xa to form complexes that inactivate thrombin and coagulation factors	VTE treatment and prophylaxis Acute coronary syndromes	Extremely short half-life Extensive protein binding, leading to dose-dependent response	Haemorrhage Thrombocytopenia Bruising and pain at injection site
	Low molecular weight heparin Examples: dalteparin enoxaparin tinzaparin	Binds to factor Xa to form complex that inactivates thrombin and coagulation factors		Longer half-life than unfractionated heparin Minimum protein binding, leading to predictable dose response profile	
	Heparinoid Danaparoid	Contains a specific pentasaccharide that activates AT-III, resulting in inactivation of factor Xa and sometimes factor IIa	Prophylaxis of VTE Heparin-induced thrombocytopenia		Haemorrhage Bruising and pain at injection site
Vitamin K antagonist	Warfarin	Inhibits epoxide reductase and subsequently vitamin K-dependent synthesis of activated factors II, VII, IX, and X, proteins C and S	VTE treatment and prophylaxis Stroke prophylaxis	Approximately 2 days required for effect Metabolized by cytochrome P450, leading to interactions Very long half-life of 1 week	Bleeding Skin necrosis Hepatic dysfunction
	Phenindione			Used less commonly because of side effects Shorter time to effect and duration Many interactions	Liver and kidney damage Rash Myocarditis Blood dyscrasia
Other anticoagulants	Fondaparinux	AT-III-mediated selective inhibition of factor Xa.	VTE prophylaxis	Elimination half-life of 17–21 hours	Bleeding Anaemia Thrombocytopenia
	Dabigatran	Inhibits free thrombin, fibrin-bound thrombin, and thrombin-induced platelet aggregation	VTE prophylaxis	Taken orally and although theoretically could be substitute for warfarin, more evidence required Elimination half-life of 12–14 hours	Bleeding Anaemia Bruising
	Rivaroxaban	Selectively inhibits factor Xa directly	VTE prophylaxis	Taken orally and although theoretically could be substitute for warfarin, more evidence required Partially metabolized by hepatic cytochrome P450 Elimination half-life of 7–11 hours	Bleeding Anaemia Bruising
	Bivaluridin	Reversibly inhibits thrombin directly	Percutaneous coronary intervention Acute coronary syndrome	Clearance reduced in renal impairment	Nausea Bleeding
	Lepirudin	Directly inhibits thrombin	Acute heparin-induced thrombocytopenia type 2		Bleeding Cough Bronchospasm

Therapeutic class	Drugs	Mechanism of action	Common clinical uses	Comments	Examples of adverse drug reactions
Oral antiplatelets	Aspirin	Irreversibly inhibits COX and thereby reduces thromboxane and prostaglandines production	Ischaemic cardiovascular and cerebrovascular disease	Low dose required for antiplatelet effect (higher dose for analgesic effect) Very long-lasting effect	Gastric ulcer Bronchospasm
	Clopidogrel	Selectively inhibits ADP binding to platelet receptor, and ADP-mediated activation of the GPIIb/IIIa complex, inhibiting platelet aggregation		Metabolized by hepatic cytochrome P450	Bleeding Diarrhoea Rash
	Dipyridamole	Increase the level of cyclic AMP in platelets by inhibition of phosphodiesterase		Used in combination with aspirin	Bleeding Headache Tachycardia
	Ticlopidine	Irreversibly changes function of platelet membranes by preventing ADP stimulation of platelet-fibrinogen binding and subsequent interactions between platelets	Second–third line ischaemic cardiovascular and cerebrovascular disease	Limited use due to risk of neutropenia	Haemorrhage and neutropenia
Other antiplatelet drugs: glycoprotein inhibitors	Abciximab Tirofiban Eptafibatide	Occupies glycoprotein IIb/IIIa receptor, thereby preventing binding of fibrinogen to platelet and blocking platelet aggregation	Acute coronary syndrome Percutaneous coronary intervention	Administered intravenously Used in combination with heparin	Bleeding Thrombocytopenia Allergic reactions (abciximab: development of antibodies)
Fibrinolytics (thrombolytics)	Non-synthetic Streptokinase Urokinase	Activates plasminogen and catalyses the cleavage of endogenous plasminogen to generate plasmin	Acute MI Stroke PE (survival rate increases if drug given within 1 hour of symptoms)	Body produces antibodies to streptokinase (patients not to have for second time for minimum 1 year later)	Bleeding Hypotension Allergic reactions
	Synthetic recombinant TPA Alteplase Reteplase Tenecteplase			Reteplase and tenecteplase can be given by injection, which could ensure patients receive drug faster	
Antifibrinolytics	Tranexamic acid	(1) Competitively inhibits activation of plasminogen, → reduced conversion of plasminogen to plasmin (fibrinolysin) (2) Directly inhibits plasmin activity	Prevention or treatment of haemorrhage associated with excessive fibrinolysis, e.g. menorrhagia	Given both orally or intravenously	Nausea Vomiting Diarrhoea
	Aprotinin	Inhibits proteinase	Prevention of perioperative haemorrhage	Elimination half-life of 10 hours	Anaphylaxis MI Gastrointestinal

AT-III, antithrombin-III; VTE, venous thromboembolism; COX, cyclooxegenase; ADP, adenosine diphosphate; AMP,TPA, ;MI, myocardial infarct; PE, pulmonary embolism

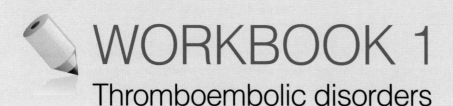

WORKBOOK 1
Thromboembolic disorders

Introducing Monique, a patient with deep vein thrombosis and pulmonary embolism

The patient: a simplified case history

On Sunday morning Monique awoke with a headache, but as she crawled out of bed to get a glass of water and some paracetamol she also found she had a sharp pain in her right leg. The headache was probably due to the wine that she and her closest friend had drunk last night. However, she could not explain the distressing pain in her leg.

When Monique described the leg pain on Sunday morning, Sunita, who is a final-year pharmacy student, convinced her that they should go to Accident and Emergency (A&E) at the local University Hospital. On their way, Monique got more and more breathless, and Sunita had to pull over and call an ambulance, which arrived in 5 minutes. Monique is seen by the doctor as soon as she arrives in hospital.

While examining Monique, the doctor asks her detailed questions about herself, which are relevant to her symptoms.

A table of clinical clerking abbreviations is given on page xi.

CLINICAL CLERKING FOR MONIQUE RICHARDS AT A&E DEPARTMENT

PC: Pain in leg and chest, shortness of breath, sweating, lightheadedness, haemoptysis

Haemoptysis: Monique is coughing up blood.

HPC: Pain in leg spreading to chest, worse on exertion; shortness of breath progressing

PMH: Nil significant

This means Monique currently suffers or has suffered from no major or significant medical conditions.

SH: Secretary who sits at a cramped desk all day. Recently returned from Australia on a 26-hour flight. Drinks about 40 UK units of alcohol at irregular intervals every week.

1 Monique sits cramped at a little desk all day long. Altered blood flow resulting from cramped long sitting could increase the risk of deep vein thrombosis (DVT).

2 Cramped sitting on a long journey could alter blood flow and increase the risk of thrombosis.

One unit (UK) is 8 g or 10 ml of pure alcohol. High alcohol intake could influence certain metabolic enzymes in the liver. Irregular alcohol intake could make this effect erratic. Oral anticoagulants are metabolized by the liver. Any profound effect on these metabolic enzymes would therefore indirectly influence the effect of oral anticoagulants. This would need to be considered if Monique is prescribed an oral anticoagulant later. She should be told of the maximum recommended units of alcohol per week and what the long-term effect of going above this recommendation is.

DH: Nil

This means Monique is not currently taking any regular medication.

O/E:

1) Pulse = 120/minute

   Monique's pulse is very elevated.

2) Dyspnoea, tachypnoea and ⇓ oxygen saturations

   Dyspnoea: shortness of breath.

   Tachypnoea: rapid breathing.

   ⇓ oxygen saturations.

   Monique is finding it difficult to breathe, which could be due to a blockage in her lungs or a heart attack.

3) Calf circumference: right leg = 39 cm, left leg = 37 cm

   Note the difference of 2 cm between left and right legs. A difference of >2 cm is used to diagnose DVT.

4) Blood pressure = 90/50 mm Hg

   Monique's blood pressure (BP) is below normal and a cause for concern (more about BP in the next case study).

5) Cyanosis

   Monique's lips and fingers are coloured blue.

6) Weight = 90 kg

   Monique is overweight and her weight could increase her risk of DVT, heart problems, and diabetes.

Biochemistry:

INR 1.1 (2–3)

(Note this for question regarding warfarin later)

Simplified, the International Normalized Ratio (INR) is the ratio of the time taken before a clot is formed in a patient blood sample compared to a standard blood sample. It is used to monitor the effect of oral anticoagulants. Normally, people have an INR between 0.8 and 1. Patients like Monique, with risk factors of clot formation, are required to have higher values within a set range. This is called the target range. The target range varies with risk of thrombosis. The current range for treatment of venous thromboembolism (VTE) in Monique and patients like her is between 2 and 3. This range is attained with the help of anticoagulant medication. The medication makes their blood take longer to form clots. If they cut themselves, they bleed for longer.

Investigations:

1) Doppler scan for DVT

The Doppler scan obtains information about the movement of blood flowing in vessels. It provides information about vascular disease and is commonly used to diagnose thrombi in veins.

2) Assessment for symptoms of pulmonary embolism

Pulmonary embolism (PE) refers to blockages in the blood vessels of the lung. Clot fragments from the vein may break and travel to the lung and cause a block called PE. All patients diagnosed with DVT are therefore assessed for symptoms of a PE. If there are no symptoms, no further testing is performed.

The following symptoms were investigated and found in Monique:

- chest pain
- breathlessness
- hypotension
- low oxygen saturations
- haemoptysis

3) D-dimers: elevated

D-dimers are fragments of cross-linked fibrin formed as plasmin degrades clots (see Figure 4.3). Levels become elevated following thrombus formation. Testing is usually reserved when the suspicion of PE is low to moderate. In Monique's case it was high and so it was not really required.

4) Computer tomography pulmonary angiography

Computer tomography pulmonary angiography (CTPA) is increasingly used as the gold standard for PE diagnosis. It is non-invasive imaging of the lungs. Advantages include the possibility of picking up other lung disorders from the differential diagnosis in case there is no pulmonary embolism.

Diagnosis: DVT; multiple PE with haemodynamic instability

Plan:

Oxygen

Analgesia

Commence heparin infusion

Note: Thrombosis is a major cause of death and disability. It is divided into:

1 arterial block:

- *mainly caused by damage to the endothelial wall*
- *has a large platelet component therefore aspirin is most effective to prevent and treat these blocks*
- *leads to myocardial infarct, stroke, and peripheral ischaemia*

2 venous block:

- *mainly caused by stasis, i.e. pooled, non-flowing blood*
- *has a large fibrin component and a small platelet component, therefore aspirin is not as effective*
- *leads to DVT and pulmonary embolism (venous thromboembolism, or VTE).*

Dr Carter Brown tells Monique, who can barely breathe, that she has VTE, i.e. DVT and multiple PEs. He prescribes intravenous heparin.

The nurse sets up the heparin using a vein in Monique's hand.

Carter explains to Monique that she has a clot (thrombus) as a result of thrombosis in a vein in her right leg as well as several in her lung.

EXPLORING MONIQUE'S CONDITION

1a) What is haemostasis?

....

....

....

1b) What is this thing called thrombosis that occurred in the vein in Monique's right leg?

....

....

....

Carter explains that unfortunately Monique 's DVT had led to PEs.

2) A PE is a *pulmonary embolism*. What type of embolism is this? Where does it occur?

....

....

....

Sunita asks Carter if emboli can travel to other parts of the body. He agrees that they could.

He asks them to imagine that Monique had an embolus that travels with her blood through her aorta into the arteries supplying her heart and her brain. He says there are several life-threatening conditions that could result from the blockage of these arteries with emboli.

3) List at least two of these life-threatening conditions. Explain what these are.

....

....

....

Carter explains to Monique that the main factors contributing to venous thrombosis fall into four main groups:

a) pooled static blood (stasis), e.g. caused by immobilization of legs or venous obstruction
b) pregnancy
c) clotting contents abnormality. e.g. with oral contraceptives, malignancy
d) blood in contact with surface abnormality, e.g. fractures.

4a) Which of these factors probably contributed to Monique's DVT?

Refer back to the A&E investigations and clerking.

4b) List three factors that could cause thromboembolism as a result of abnormality of the surface in contact with blood (see Table 4.2).

Monique asks Carter how the swelling suddenly appeared in her leg. Before he can explain, Sunita, to impress him, starts talking about coagulation.

She says the swelling in Monique's right leg (DVT) was caused by inappropriate coagulation in the affected veins in her leg and lungs. Sunita explains how the different drugs on Monique's prescription chart target different elements of what she and Carter refer to as 'thrombus formation'.

5) What are the two main elements of thrombus formation that are targeted by antithrombotic drugs?

6a) What is coagulation?

6b) What are the two clotting cascades called? (Give traditional names as well as more recent descriptive names.)

....

....

....

7) What is the first of the three main steps which platelets undergo during haemostasis? Will this lead to activation of the clotting cascade?

....

....

....

8a) List three chemical mediators involved in platelet recruitment during thrombos formation?

....

....

....

8b) What is the name of the receptor on the platelets that plays the most prominent and final role in platelet aggregation?

....

....

....

9a) What are the main differences in formation and content between arterial and venous thrombi?

....

....

....

9b) What are the consequences for this for choosing first-line drugs to treat thromboembolic disorders?

....

....

....

Sunita and Carter also mention thrombin and antithrombin.

10) Identify and list the four roles that are played by thrombin (factor IIa) in the coagulation cascade, during the coagulation, leading to the DVT formation that Sunita mentioned.

The pharmacist on call is asked to supply some more heparin for the heparin infusion. She introduces herself as Jo.

Jo talks to Monique about the infusion called heparin, which she is currently receiving.

She tells Monique that her body actually produces some heparin to prevent uncontrolled clotting.

11a) List three chemicals in Monique's blood that are involved in preventing uncontrolled coagulation.

11b) Describe how they interact to prevent uncontrolled coagulation.

When Monique asks how heparin works, the nurse tries to explain.

She uses strange words like thrombin, which confuses Monique.

12) What two substances in Monique's blood does heparin interact with in order to be effective (Figure 4.4)? How does this reduce coagulation?

Monique is moved to ward 17. This is awkward, involving the movement of the drip stand down the winding corridor.

Monique asks Sunita why heparin was not given to her in tablet form or as a quick injection.

13a) Why has Monique been given heparin as a continuous infusion and not as an intravenous injection or a subcutaneous (sc) injection (section 4.2.1)?

> *Note:*
>
> *Intravenous infusion = a solution of a drug is administered directly into a vein, continuously over more than 8–10 minutes.*
>
> *Intravenous injection = a solution of a drug is administered into a vein by injection over a short period.*
>
> *Subcutaneous injection = a solution of a drug is administered under the skin.*
>
> *Hint: What is half-life, and how long after subcutaneous injection is the effect of heparin evident?*

13b) Could Monique have been given heparin orally? Explain your answer.

> Monique is also fed up because every 6 hours the nurse comes round and takes blood from her to check what they refer to as her aPTT.

14) What does aPTT stand for and what does it measure?

After Monique becomes stable and does not require oxygen, Jo suggests that the unfractionated heparin be changed to an LMWH.

> The doctor agrees to do this, and an LMWH is started as a subcutaneous injection to be given once a day only.
>
> The following questions explore the reasons for the suggestions.

15) In terms of clotting cascades what is the difference in site of action of unfractionated heparin and LMWH?

16) Why is the pharmacokinetic profile of unfractionated heparin less predictable than that of LMWH?

17) List two advantages of LMWH over unfractionated heparin.

Monique could actually name one!!

18) List one advantage of heparin over LMWH.

What drug is used to reverse bleeding with heparin?

19) Why was heparin given first, rather than administering LMWH from the outset?

Much later, the consultant on call stops to see Monique during his rounds. He requests that warfarin be commenced for Monique. He chastises the junior doctor for not having prescribed it at the same time as heparin.

He insists that warfarin and the LMWH should be given simultaneously for at least 6 days, until Monique's target INR has been maintained in the therapeutic range for 2 days.

The next day Monique is surprised when Andreas, her boss, comes to visit her in hospital. Andreas is a quality control pharmacist for a pharmaceutical company in a nearby town. She had a crush on him 2 years ago, when she met him through his secretary, but kept it secret because he always had a string of dates. She still finds him attractive but that is her most closely guarded secret.

They chat about work and then Monique's illness.

Andreas says his dad has been taking warfarin since he was diagnosed with pulmonary embolism after a second DVT 2 years ago. He and Sunita continue discussing warfarin and clotting factors.

They explain to Monique that clotting factors II, VII, IX, and X are involved in the way warfarin works.

20) Explain how these factors are involved in the mechanism of action of warfarin. Refer in particular to the role of vitamin K.

Jo, the pharmacist, drops by and explains why the consultant had insisted that Monique should still be given LMWH injections during the first few days of taking warfarin tablets.

21) What does Jo say is the reason for giving LMWH and warfarin simultaneously?
How long does it take before the effect of each dose of warfarin is experienced?
What is warfarin's effect on protein C?

22) If LMWH action ultimately depends on preventing formation of factor IIa (thrombin), then it cannot be clinically effective until the existing circulating factor IIa has been lost from the blood. Why then does it work so much faster than warfarin?

23) What is the name of the test used to monitor warfarin? Explain what this test measures.

Refer back to biochemistry section of clinical clerking.

Sunita has started seeing Carter regularly.

Sunita and Monique wonder why Andreas is so concerned about Monique. When he is out of earshot, Sunita makes jokes to Monique about Monique and Andreas getting together.

Because Monique blushes each time, the jokes get more and more outrageous. Sunita is already planning their wedding and kids' names.

On day 5 post-admission, Monique's INR is 2.5 and has been between 2 and 3 for 2 days therefore the LMWH is discontinued and it is decided to discharge her in 2 days if her INR is maintained between 2 and 3.

She develops a chest infection and because she is allergic to penicillin antibiotics, she is commenced on the non-penicillin antibiotic called erythromycin, 500 mg tablets.

Her INR result 2 days later is 8 and she has several nosebleeds. Vitamin K is given orally.

25a) What could have caused Monique to bleed?

Many drugs or clinical conditions such as a damaged liver could influence the effect of warfarin.

This is because warfarin is metabolized by a liver enzyme that is affected by these drugs, and therefore increases or decreases the effect of warfarin. Vitamin K, which is found in some vegetables, will counteract the effect of warfarin.

25b) How will the vitamin K that Monique was given influence her INR? Explain the mechanism.

26a) List four other drugs that could increase the activity of warfarin. (See for example, warfarin in Appendix 1 of the BNF.)

Andreas wonders if aspirin could be an option to treat Monique's DVT.

He had been told warfarin was better than aspirin for his dad, but wonders if aspirin could be used for Monique. He asks Jo, the pharmacist, when she comes around.

26b) Which of the two drugs do you think Jo would recommend for Monique's DVT?

Andreas tells Monique that his father was told that certain foods and drinks could affect his warfarin. He asks her if anyone has talked to her about this.

27) Referring back to Monique's history on page 2, i.e. social history, what do you think Jo will tell her when she counsels her about warfarin and her social life?

Monique's INR normalizes after 5 days and it is decided that she can be discharged.

She is told that she should continue to take warfarin for 6 months. She will have to attend a clinic regularly for blood tests, after which her dose of warfarin could be altered.

She is given a warfarin booklet with more information about warfarin. Jo explains the content and recommends that she carries the booklet around with her and also that she always tells every healthcare professional attending to her that she takes warfarin.

28) List six other things which patients on warfarin must be educated about.

Andreas insists on taking her home.

Before they leave, Monique wants to stop by and say goodbye to Mrs Goodfellow, whom she had become quite close to while on the ward.

Mrs Goodfellow, who had been in the bed next to Monique's for 2 days, had been moved to intensive care after she had a nasty reaction to heparin. The nurses told Monique that the name of the reaction was HIT II.

29a) What does HIT mean? How does it manifest itself?

29b) What is the difference between HIT I and HIT II in terms of mechanism and severity?

Monique is pleased to see an improvement in Mrs Goodfellow, who is waiting to be transferred back to the ward. She tells Monique that her heparin was replaced with a drug called lepirudin.

30a) What is lepirudin and how does it differ from heparin?

30b) Why was Mrs Goodfellow not given an low-molecular weight heparin instead of lepirudin?

Monique promises Mrs Goodfellow she will come back and visit her in a couple of days.

Monique has read a lot about anticoagulation and antiplatelet drugs while bored on the ward and she asks Andreas about the difference between aspirin, clopidogrel, and tirofiban, which other patients on the ward were taking.

31) What are the differences between aspirin, clopidogrel, and tirofiban?

Monique also asks Andreas about drugs working in the opposite way to thrombolytics but cannot remember their names.

32) List two antifibrinolytic drugs and their clinical uses.

Monique completes her 6-month course of warfarin with no problems.

Chapter 5
Hypertension

Imagine if you feel perfectly well, go to your doctor for a routine check, and are told you must start taking drugs every day for the rest of your life for a condition with no symptoms. Furthermore, you may be told as time goes by that you must increase the number of different drugs you take, perhaps to four a day, despite no perceptible increase in your wellbeing. Of course, many do not need to imagine this, for they will be among the millions worldwide who have already experienced this situation, having been diagnosed as hypertensive. If the physician is asked by the patient about the criteria used to decide to treat in this manner, then the physician may, in the spirit of openness, advance the view that the dividing line between who is and who is not to be treated for hypertension is arbitrary.

Given this commonplace scenario, it is clear that patient education is paramount. This can only be effective if prescribers have a solid understanding of the biological basis of hypertension and its consequences, and the way in which both of these are modified by the profusion of drugs available.

The consequences of hypertension are profound (e.g. Table 5.1), offering, if left untreated, a greater probability of major cardiovascular disease and disaster, and consequently a shorter lifespan. The potentially disastrous cardiovascular events referred to are familiar to patients; they include atherosclerotic disease (clogged up arteries, Chapter 6), ischaemic heart disease in the form of angina and myocardial infarcts (heart attacks, Chapter 6), arrhythmias, and heart failure (Chapter 7). The *benefits* of blood pressure treatment can therefore be explained as a reduction in the risk of getting conditions such as strokes and heart attacks.

There are a very large number of different drugs available to treat hypertension. The objective of this chapter is to provide the healthcare professional with a secure

Table 5.1 Hypertension is a risk factor for various conditions

Primary condition	Secondary consequence
Atherosclerosis of coronary arteries	Angina
	Myocardial infarct
	Stroke (ischaemic or haemorrhagic)
Myocardial infarct	Heart failure
	Arrythmias
Kidney disease[a]	Hypertension[a]
Hypertension[a]	Kidney disease[a]
Retinal disease	
Diabetes	

[a] Kidney disease is a cause of hypertension, and hypertension may cause kidney disease.

foundation in the mechanisms of drug action that gives the therapeutic response, and to help understand and devise individualized therapeutic strategies, and advise patients on their own drug usage.

Hypertension is a common condition, with a prevalence rate of about 25% of total population and a higher prevalence in black (African origin) people. Other risk factors include family history, ageing, lifestyle (e.g. stress, diet, alcohol), and obesity. In the vast majority of cases, the cause is unknown (so-called essential hypertension), while in other rare cases there is an identifiable cause (secondary hypertension), such as renal disease or a tumour of the adrenal medulla catecholamine secreting cells (phaeochromocytoma). Blood pressure is measured in the aortic side of the vasculature, and while hypertension of the pulmonary circulation is a recognized condition, here we are concerned only with hypertension of the systemic circulation.

Table 5.2 Three different schemes for designating blood pressure ranges (note their different uses in different parts of the world)

A. Version 1. Used in UK

	Systolic (mm Hg)	Diastolic (mm Hg)
Optimal	<120	<80
Normal	<130	<85
High-normal	130–139	85–89
Hypertension	>140	>90

B. Version 2. Used in USA

	Systolic (mm Hg)	Diastolic (mm Hg)
Normal	<120	<80
Prehypertension	121–139	80–89
Stage I	140–159	90–99
Stage II	>159	>99

C. Version 3. Used in Europe (excluding UK)

	Systolic (mm Hg)	Diastolic (mm Hg)
Optimal	<120	<80
Normal	121–129	80–84
High normal	130–139	85–89
Hypertension Grade 1	140–159	90–99
Hypertension Grade 2	160–179	100–109
Hypertension Grade 3	>179	>110

The clinical definition of hypertension is based on data relating elevated blood pressures to increased risk of cardiovascular disease (CVD). For example, a non-smoking man of 55 years old with normal blood lipids (see Chapter 6) has a 1 in 10 chance of CVD within 10 years if his systolic blood pressure is 120 mm Hg; however, this risk rises to over 1 in 5 if his systolic blood pressure is over 160 mm Hg. Table 5.2 sets out three schemes for defining optimal-to-high blood pressure readings; each indicating that sustained blood pressures over 140 systolic and 90 mm Hg diastolic are diagnostic of hypertension and should be considered for drug treatment. In practice, the decision to treat is based not only on these blood pressure schemes, but also on other factors, e.g. co-existing conditions, and potential benefit from lifestyle changes.

In addition, patients with extremely high blood pressures may be classified as having a **hypertensive crisis**, requiring a more urgent and separate approach to treatment (see also Workbook 2).

Later in this chapter and Workbook 2 we will consider how this leads to decisions and choices in the drug treatment of individual patients. Before that, however, we must review the mechanisms generating and controlling arterial blood pressure, and then review the fundamental mechanisms by which antihypertensive drugs act on these mechanisms to reduce blood pressure.

5.1 The physiological control of arterial blood pressure

Antihypertensive drugs can only be understood by reference to the mechanisms that regulate and set our blood pressures. These lie in the blood vessels and heart, and the way these are influenced by both the nervous system (this means the brain acting via the sympathetic and parasympathetic branches of the autonomic nervous system) and the endocrine system (acting via the release of hormones in the blood). Drugs in common use act at all these levels of control.

5.1.1 What determines our blood pressure: heart and blood vessels

Arterial blood pressure is largely determined by only two factors, cardiac output and total peripheral resistance. The first is located in the heart and the second in the blood vessels.

Cardiac output. The central question about cardiac function is how much blood is being pumped per minute. This is the cardiac output (CO); it is determined by the **heart rate** (HR; the number of beats per minute) × **stroke volume** (SV; the volume per heart beat).

$$CO = HR \times SV \qquad (5.1)$$

Arterial blood pressure = cardiac output × **total peripheral resistance** (TPR), which is the resistance to flow offered by the blood vessels. It is determined by the degree of contraction of the smooth muscle in the walls of the precapillary arterioles.

$$BP = CO \times TPR \qquad (5.2)$$

Substituting eq. 5.1 into eq. 5.2, we see that arterial blood pressure is determined by three factors—heart rate, stroke volume, and total peripheral resistance:

$$BP = HR \times SV \times TPR \qquad (5.3)$$

We shall consider those aspects of these three parameters, which help us devise an individual drug treatment plan for a patient with hypertension.

5.1.2 What determines the heart rate?

In a healthy heart, the electrical excitation of each heart beat has its origin at the top right-hand side of the heart, in a patch of tissue at the upper segment of the right atrium called the sinoatrial node (SA node). From here the excitation spreads through the atria. It is then held up for a moment by the barrier formed between the atria and ventricles before it gathers at the atrioventricular node to pass down specialized conduction cells to rapidly spread throughout the ventricles (Figure 5.1).

The cells of the SA node fire action potentials on their own. That is, they do not require a neuronal input to tell them when to fire—they show automaticity. It is the frequency with which they fire action potentials that determines your heart rate. In Figure 5.2 action potentials of the SA node are shown; it is apparent that the frequency of the heart rate is determined by the steepness

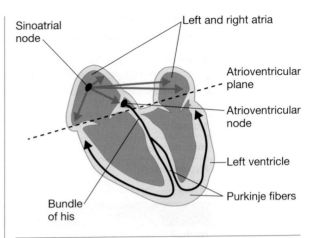

Figure 5.1 The origin and spread of excitation in the heart.

In a healthy heart, the excitation arises spontaneously as depolarizations in the sinoatrial (SA) node. A wave of depolarizations spreads through the muscle cells of the atria. The atrioventricular plane is impermeable to depolarizations, except at the atrioventricular (AV) node–bundle of His path, through which the excitation travels to reach the Purkinje fibres, then spreads rapidly throughout the ventricles. See also Box 7.1.

of the *pacemaker* slope of the SA node action potentials; if the slope is steep it takes less time to reach threshold, and action potentials fire more frequently, resulting in an increase in heart rate. This is illustrated in Figure 5.2.

The steepness of the slope is determined by a set of ion channels; it is these proteins localized in the membrane of the SA node cells that are the molecular target of drugs that regulate the heart rate. The physiological determinants of heart rate, such as the activity in the sympathetic and parasympathetic branches of the autonomic nervous system, also act at these SA node molecular targets. In summary, the release of acetylcholine from the parasympathetic system will decrease the steepness of the slope, and decrease heart rate (**negative chronotropic effect**); the release of noradrenaline from the sympathetic nerve terminals (or adrenaline from adrenal medulla via the bloodstream) will increase the steepness of the slope and increase heart rate (**positive chronotropic effect**).

While the parasympathetic mAChR influence on the pacemaker slope is profound (and unopposed can cause a very substantial lowering of heart rate), it is noteworthy that it is the β-adrenoceptors that are a more significant target for therapeutic agents, such as the antihypertensive β-adrenoceptor antagonists described later.

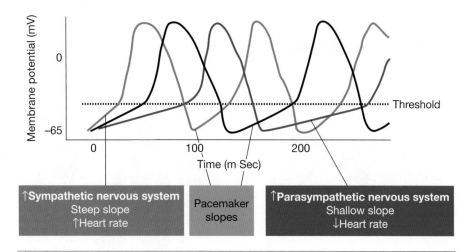

Figure 5.2 The sinoatrial node action potential.

The action potentials are characterized by the pacemaker slope, which controls the heart rate. The slope may be increased by stimulation from the sympathetic nervous system (red lines)—it reaches threshold more quickly, the heart rate rises—or it may be shallow, e.g. parasympathetic stimulation dominates when the heart rate falls. The pacemaker slope is formed by the action of several channels, including the current labelled I_f (f for 'funny'), which carries Na^+ and Ca^{2+} into the cell and is the target of the anti-angina drug ivabradine (Chapter 6).

Receptors for noradrenaline and adrenaline in the SA node cells are mainly of the $β_1$-*adrenoceptor* subtype (although other subtypes are also to be found). Cellular responses include a stimulation of cyclic AMP synthesis (which will affect the ion channels by increasing their phosphorylation) and various effects on ion channels, all of which will collude to steepen the pacemaker slope (Box 5.1).

5.1.3 What determines stroke volume?

The determinants of stroke volume are complex, and here we will only cover those issues necessary to understand the action of therapeutic agents. We will divide the influences on stroke volume into two groups: those directly influencing the ventricular myocytes and those which influence cardiac function by acting via the blood vessels.

Direct influences on cardiac myocytes are mainly changes to the action potentials. These determine the strength of the stimulus, which drives the contraction of those cells. This can be understood by considering the effect of noradrenaline or adrenaline on the ventricular action potential. The ventricular action potential in a healthy heart is characterized by no pacemaker slope (its depolarization is dependent on action potentials passing down from the atria) and a plateau (Figure 5.3).

These ventricular cells have a large number of voltage-dependent Ca^{2+} channels—when the upsweep of the action potential occurs they open and Ca^{2+} can then flow into the cell. This maintains the depolarization (hence the plateau) and provides the raised intracellular Ca^{2+}, which stimulates the muscle contractile mechanism. An increase in the rate of Ca^{2+} influx will raise the plateau and increase the force of contraction (*positive ionotropic effect*). This will result in an increased stroke volume.

Receptors for noradrenaline or adrenaline in the ventricles are β-adrenoceptors; clinically they are mainly considered to be $β_1$-adrenoceptors (although $β_2$ subtypes are also found and may become more important in certain pathologies, e.g. heart failure). They are again coupled to a stimulation of cyclic AMP synthesis—this leads to an enhanced phosphorylation of the voltage-dependent Ca^{2+} channels, which results in an increased probability of opening and an enhanced height of the Ca^{2+} plateau. Other channel influences mean that the duration of the action potential is shortened. This means there can be a simultaneous increased rate of action potential firing as a result of the concurrent influence on the SA node. The consequence is greater influx of Ca^{2+} and increased stroke volume. The cardiac β receptors are a major target for drug action.

Box 5.1
The renin-aldosterone-angiotensin system

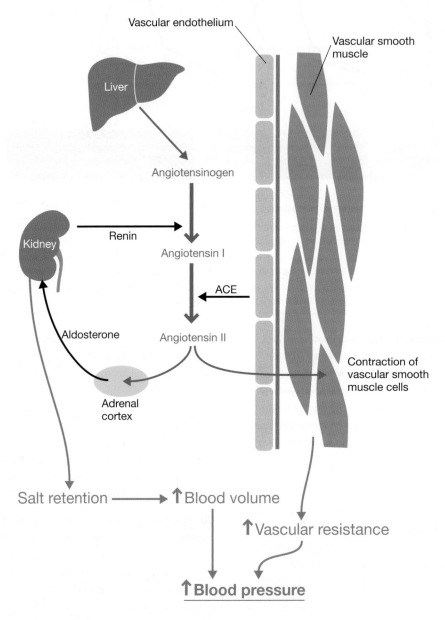

Vascular endothelium

Vascular smooth muscle

Liver

Angiotensinogen

Kidney

Renin

Angiotensin I

ACE

Aldosterone

Angiotensin II

Adrenal cortex

Contraction of vascular smooth muscle cells

Salt retention → ↑Blood volume

↑Vascular resistance

↑Blood pressure

Aspects of the renin-aldosterone-angiotensin system (RAAS) and the control of arterial blood pressure. Figure a illustrates the relationship between the various tissues of the body and the main features of the **renin-aldosterone-angiotensin system** (RAAS). Angiotensinogen is constitutively released from the liver and circulates in the blood. Renin is a proteolytic enzyme. Its release from the juxtaglomerular cells of the kidney is under the control of the sympathetic nervous system. Stimulation of β-adrenoceptors by noradrenaline increases renin release; conversely, the presence of β-adrenoceptor antagonists will reduce renin release. Renin then meets angiotensinogen in the blood, converting it to angiotensin I. This is then converted to angiotensin II by angiotensin converting enzyme (ACE). Angiotensin II has the effect of raising blood pressure by acting on its

Receptors for acetylcholine in the SA node are **muscarinic acetylcholine receptors (mAChR)** of the M_2 subtype. Principle cellular responses include a reduction in cyclic AMP synthesis (which will affect the ion channels by reducing their phosphorylation), inhibition of Ca^{2+} channels, and enhancement of K^+ channels. These types of mechanisms will combine to reduce the pacemaker slope (see Figure 5.2).

Other mechanisms may increase cyclic AMP and intracellular Ca^{2+}, leading to increased force of contraction. For example caffeine may inhibit the breakdown of cyclic AMP by phosphodiesterases, leading to increased force (and rate) of contraction. Agents which activate other receptors coupled to enhanced cyclic AMP synthesis include histamine acting at H_2-receptors, explaining a direct effect of histamine on cardiac output. Digoxin is a clinically useful drug (see Chapter 7), which includes in its action an increase in Ca^{2+} that is independent of cyclic AMP, with a consequent increased force of contraction.

Receptors for acetylcholine in the ventricles are again M_2 mAChR, coupled to a decrease in cyclic AMP and reduced force of contraction. However, the direct influence of the parasympathetic/mAChR system on ventricular function is weak—the main effect on ventricular stroke volume may be due to decreased contraction of the atria.

Indirect influences on stroke volume are mainly due to changes in blood vessels. These affect the heart in a number of ways—two of them are explored here, dividing them into changes to the venous side, or the arterial side, of the circulation.

Changes to the venous side: the importance of venous return, preload and end diastolic volume

The sympathetic influence on the large capacitance vessels will be to cause contraction of smooth muscle, leading to vasoconstriction. The valves in the large veins mean that the blood is forced in one direction only—back to the heart, giving an increased **venous return** and an increased **central venous pressure** (the pressure in the large veins and the atria at the end of the filling phase). As a result, just before the contraction starts, the walls of the atria will be more stretched (sometimes referred to as an increase in **preload**) and the volume of blood in the atria (**end diastolic volume**) will be increased (Figure 5.4). This has an effect on stroke volume because of Starling's law. When a muscle is stretched *before* it begins to contract, the force of the subsequent contraction will be increased.

So we can sum up the situation by:

> **sympathetic stimulation of large veins** = ↑ **venous return**, = ↑ **end-diastolic volume**, = ↑ **stretching of the atria walls**, = ↑ **force of contraction**, = ↑ **increased stroke volume**

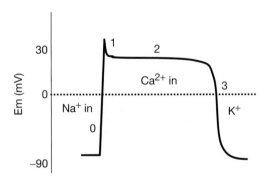

Figure 5.3 The action potential of a ventricular myocyte. This is a plot of the voltage (mV) across the cell membrane (designated Em) against time. A negative Em indicates that the cell is electrically negative inside the membrane compared to outside. The notable points are the absence of a pacemaker slope, the rapid rise caused by opening of fast Na^+ voltage sensitive sodium channels, giving a rapid depolarizing influx of Na^+, the Ca^{2+} plateau in which depolarization is maintained by a sustained influx of Ca^{2+}, and the eventual return to a negative potential when the inward Na^+ and Ca^{2+} currents have both been shut down and there is an increase in K^+ permeability, enabling K^+ ions to leave the cell, returning the membrane to the resting potential.

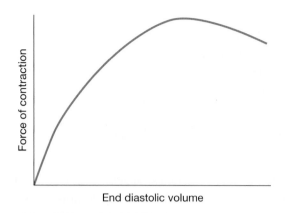

Figure 5.4 Ventricular function curve.

The relationship between end diastolic volume and the force of the next contraction. When the end diastolic volume is increased, the walls of the ventricle are more stretched *before the contraction begins*, and so the muscle will then contract with greater force.

The preload will also be augmented by an increase in blood volume, providing some insight into the role of the kidney and salt-retaining hormones such as aldosterone in healthy physiological regulation. This effect of blood volume is important for us since it shows how drugs such as the thiazide diuretics act in a patient such as Andreas. The enhanced elimination of water and sodium by diuretics decreases blood volume, with a consequent reduction in preload and stroke volume, contributing to the management of hypertension in many patients.

However, note that thiazides in addition have an unrelated vasodilatory effect that contributes to their blood pressure-lowering activity (see below).

Changes to the arterial side: the importance of arterial blood pressure and afterload

When your left ventricle begins to contract, the left ventricular pressure rises rapidly. At first this is below the aortic pressure, and so your aortic valve is closed. This means there is a short delay between the beginning of systole (muscle begins to contract) and the beginning of ejection of blood into the aorta. This is the period when the pressure inside the ventricles rises fast. Within a few milliseconds it reaches aortic pressure, your aortic valve flips opens, and blood flow begins. If the arterial blood pressure is increased, your ventricular pressure will have to reach a higher level for blood flow to begin (Figure 5.5). This may be referred to as an increase in **afterload**. Similarly, as the contraction phase passes, its peak and the blood flow begin to fall; the aortic valve will close earlier if the arterial blood pressure is higher. Both changes will shorten the ventricular ejection phase (when blood is being pumped out) and so for a given force of contraction there will be a reduced volume of blood ejected, i.e. there will be a reduced stroke volume.

Taken together these determinants of stroke volume are summarized in Figure 5.6. They show that if you have a healthy cardiovascular system your heart will respond to

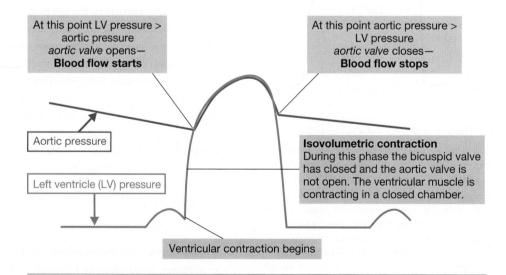

Figure 5.5 Changes in ventricular and aortic pressures.

Note that blood can only be ejected from the heart when the red line (pressure in the left ventricle) exceeds the pressure in the aorta (blue line). LV, left ventricle. See also Box 7.1.

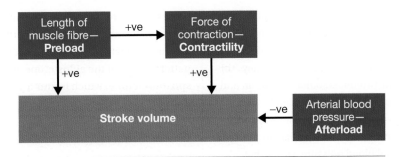

Figure 5.6 Summary of regulation of stroke volume.

an increased arterial pressure by reducing cardiac output and thus bringing arterial pressure down, and respond to an increase in central venous pressure by an increased cardiac output, thus preventing a build-up of pressure on the venous side.

What we must consider is what happens when this adaptive system breaks down and there is a chronic rise in arterial pressure (hypertension) or central venous pressure (heart failure, Chapter 7). To understand these conditions further, we must consider the regulation of total peripheral resistance by the autonomic nervous system and the renin-angiotensin-aldosterone system (RAAS).

5.1.4 What determines our peripheral resistance?

Peripheral resistance lies at the level of the precapillary arterioles, with their small lumen regulated by contraction of their smooth muscle cells. The presence of a suitable resistance to flow at the arteriolar level is essential for the maintenance of normal blood pressure and perfusion of tissues. This can be graphically seen in a patient with, for example, anaphylactic shock, who may have a very high cardiac output but a blood pressure too low to effectively perfuse the tissues because there is no resistance to flow. In such a case it is essential to rapidly cause contraction of the arteriolar vascular smooth muscle to re-establish pressure, for example with intramuscular adrenaline/epinephrine (see below). So there is normally a degree of tonic contraction of the arterioles, offering sufficient resistance to flow to generate the systolic and diastolic blood pressures. This is important since it explains how we can have drugs that *increase* or *decrease* peripheral resistance.

Receptors for noradrenaline or adrenaline in the arterioles are both α_1-adrenoceptors (which stimulate

contraction of smooth muscle) and β_2-adrenoceptors (which stimulate relaxation). Both are significant, but the effect of the α_1-adrenoceptors, which increases peripheral resistance, dominates. This explains the increase in peripheral resistance that is part of the clinical response to administration of adrenaline/epinephrine or noradrenaline/norepinephrine, which will stimulate both these types of adrenoceptors. The expression of α_1-adrenoceptors receptors in vascular smooth muscle cells is widespread, controlling resistance in such major vascular beds as mesenteric and skin. The response is mediated by receptor coupling through G-proteins to the phospholipase C system, leading to raised intracellular Ca^{2+}, which stimulates the contractile mechanism. The expression of vascular β_2-adrenoceptors is much more restricted, being present mainly in skeletal and cardiac arterioles. This relaxation response is in common with β_2-adrenoceptors found in airways smooth muscle, which also cause relaxation—in this case the response is directly targeted by anti-asthma drugs (Chapter 11), while the vascular β_2-adrenoceptor response is not intentionally manipulated in therapeutics.

Note that this apparently perplexing conflict in action between α_1- and β_2-adrenoceptors makes sense when considering the classical fight-or-flight scenario, in which an urgent necessity for physical response is accompanied by an increase in adrenaline (adrenal medulla) and noradrenaline (sympathetic nervous system) release— blood supply to the skin and viscera are reduced, while the supply of oxygen to skeletal muscle and heart are increased.

The role of the RAAS in controlling peripheral resistance is essentially due to the action of the potent vasoconstrictor angiotensin II. Go to Box 5.1 for a review of the organization of the RAAS. As a central target of antihypertensive drugs, it is important to note that both angiotensin II and aldosterone are physiologically active products of the RAAS, the latter acting as a hormone, which increases sodium reabsorption from the distal convoluted tubule and collecting duct of the kidney. This means that aldosterone promotes sodium retention and increases blood volume, so both angiotensin II, via a direct effect on increasing peripheral resistance, and aldosterone, via an indirect effect on cardiac output, lead to an increase in arterial blood pressure. Drugs that modify these influences are now amongst the most widely prescribed in the clinical management of cardiovascular conditions, and so it is not surprising that they have been prescribed to our fictional patient Andreas (Workbook 2). The key to the pharmacological control of the system is to note from Box 5.1 and Figure 5.7 that angiotensin II acts not only to regulate peripheral resistance at the arterioles, but also to control the secretion of aldosterone from adrenal cortex cells. In both cases this is via AT-1 receptors. Figure 5.7 shows that the physiological control of the system lies upstream, at the juxtaglomerular cells of the kidney, with renin secretion.

The role of aldosterone at the kidney distal tubule is not limited to sodium retention: it also enhances potassium secretion in the urine. High plasma potassium has a direct effect on the aldosterone secreting cells of the adrenal cortex, stimulating

potassium secretion. Interestingly, this provides renin/angiotensin-independent control of aldosterone. This action of aldosterone has a direct effect on the clinical pattern of use of the aldosterone antagonist **spironolactone**, which is thus a potassium-sparing diuretic.

Ethnicity correlates with the role of renin in hypertension

We may note from this scheme that kidney and renin secretion are central to the control of blood pressure, particularly when challenged with the high sodium intake characteristic of modern diets. There is individual variation in the manner in which we respond to these challenges, and some of this correlates with race. This includes renin responses, explaining why the recommendations for initial antihypertensive drug treatment may depend on ethnicity (e.g. Figure 5.10).

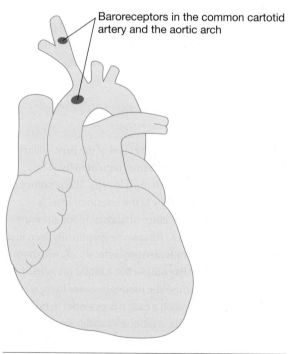

Figure 5.8 Location of arterial baroreceptors.
Baroreceptors are stretch receptors—when stretched they increase the rate of firing of their sensory neurons. Placed in the strategic locations shown they stretch as arterial blood pressure is increased. The rate of neuronal firing from baroreceptors constantly sends information concerning blood pressure to the central nervous system, resulting in a modification of the autonomic (sympathetic and parasympathetic) control of the cardiovascular system.

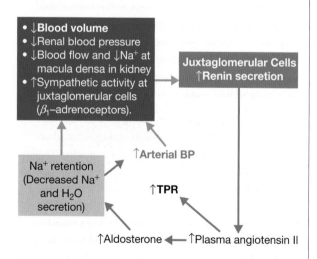

Figure 5.7 The central role of renin.
Renin secretion is highly regulated, as indicated by the items in the blue box. This includes control by the sympathetic nervous system, influencing peripheral resistance and cardiac output (through Na^+ retention and blood volume). BP, blood pressure; TPR, total peripheral resistance.

5.1.5 The role of baroreceptors in controlling blood pressure

Baroreceptors in blood vessels are stretch receptors: they increase their firing when the walls of the vessels are stretched by increased blood pressure. Two examples of baroreceptors in major arteries are indicated in Figure 5.8. These form a feedback loop regulating the autonomic nervous system via the brain.

Baroreceptors are also found in other strategic locations. For example, we have already encountered the juxtaglomerular cells of the kidney—these are baroreceptors, which when stretched decrease their renin secretion, providing a short feedback loop that is independent of the autonomic nervous system.

These types of feedback loop explain some of the complexities in the clinical control of blood pressure, and why it is not possible to simply titrate blood pressure down using a drug that reduces peripheral resistance. For example, if arterial blood pressure falls in response to a vasodilator drug, this is detected by the baroreceptors, sympathetic activity is increased, cardiac output and peripheral resistance will increase, and blood pressure will be raised. The successful long-term management of hypertension (and we are talking about life-long drug taking) often requires the manipulation by drugs of several of the regulatory mechanisms described.

5.2 Antihypertensive drugs

At the beginning of this chapter we described the blood pressure measurements that define clinical hypertension and form the basis for criteria for treatment. In practice, treatment is guided by sets of recommendations, as we describe below. These guidelines derive from clinical trials and past experience. It is also apparent that some guidance is not based on rock-solid evidence. The recommendations also include considerable choice by the prescriber. This can be seen when we consider the UK 2006 recommendations below—firstly they are a strategy only for newly diagnosed hypertensives, and secondly they provide **options** for the prescriber, e.g. for patients of 55 or over of a calcium channel inhibitor or a diuretic as the first drug. There is, however, considerable scope for effective prescribing to be informed by an understanding of how the drugs work, as well as clinical experience. With no greater knowledge of the cardiovascular system than is set out above, you can interpret the clinical response of the patient in terms of the cellular changes brought about by the drug, and can understand how different combinations of drugs may work to achieve the best clinical outcome. Here we will first set out the mode of action of the most widely used classes of antihypertensive agents, and will then discuss therapeutic strategies using these which provide for most patients. Following that, we will briefly overview other less commonly used antihypertensive drugs.

5.2.1 Drugs that act on the RAAS

The outline of the RAAS set out in this chapter is modified by three main classes of clinically useful drugs: angiotensin converting enzyme (ACE) inhibitors,

angiotensin II receptor antagonists, and aldosterone antagonists. Of these, only the first two are used in the management of hypertension. In addition, a new class of antihypertensive agent, which inhibits renin, has been developed.

ACE inhibitors

In Box 5.1 the outline of the RAAS shows how renin converts the liver-derived plasma protein angiotensinogen into angiotensin I. This 10-aminoacid peptide has the last two amino acid residues clipped off by ACE to form the 8-amino acid peptide angiotensin II. This occurs within the circulation, particularly at the surface of endothelial cells. Angiotensin II then acts at AT-1 receptors, stimulating vasoconstriction and aldosterone release. ACE inhibitors will reduce both the vasoconstrictor and Na^+ retention effects of the RAAS, explaining their antihypertensive action. They are commonly prescribed and effective antihypertensives, which are generally well tolerated. Issues of particular note for prescribers are:

- ACE is not the only enzyme capable of converting plasma angiotensin I into angiotensin II, hence there is a theoretical reason for thinking that AT-1 antagonists (see below) may be more effective.

- ACE also acts on bradykinin, in this case to break it down, therefore ACE inhibitors lead to accumulation of bradykinin. This is important because it is probably the cause of dry cough seen with some patients taking these drugs. This is the most common adverse effect of these drugs; the cough can be intolerable, requiring an alternative drug choice, such as an AT-1 antagonist.

- There is a potentially serious interaction between ACE inhibitors, diuretics, and NSAIDs such as ibuprofen (sometimes called the 'triple whammy'), leading to renal failure. This interaction is particularly important given NSAIDs are available as non-prescription drugs, and combination ACE inhibitors and diuretics are increasingly prescribed together.

Examples of ACE inhibitors in use are **lisinopril**, **enalapril**, **ramipril**, **captopril**, and **perindopril**. Factors indicating the choice of drug here will include coexisting conditions. For example, if the patient has liver impairment then the choice will be a drug eliminated exclusively by the kidney (e.g. lisinopril or ramipril) and not one with substantial liver metabolism (e.g. perindopril). Additionally, choosing a long-acting, once-daily preparation has advantages in terms of concordance/compliance/adherence.

Angiotensin II antagonists (ARBs, A2RAs)

Angiotensin II antagonists may also be referred to as AT-1 antagonists, ARBs (angiotensin receptor blockers), sartans, and A2RAs (angiotensin 2 receptor antagonists). They are prescribed for patients unable to tolerate ACE inhibitors due to the cough mentioned above. Other adverse effects of ACE inhibitors, which may be of concern in certain classes of patients, may also be seen with ARBs. In some patients ARBs may be more effective than ACE inhibitors, as predicted from the alternative routes for angiotensin II formation mentioned above. Like ACE inhibitors, ARBs make their antihypertensive effects by down-regulating both the vasoconstrictor and aldosterone limbs of the RAAS. Examples of ARBs are **candesartan**, **eprosartan**, **irbesartan**, **losartan**, **olmesartan**, **telmisartan**, and **valsartan**.

Aldosterone antagonists

Aldosterone antagonists (**spironolactone** and **eplerenone**) are not routinely used as antihypertensives, but may be useful in heart failure (see Chapter 7). They are the third class of drugs that directly modify the RAAS. While downregulating the action of aldosterone in Na^+ retention and K^+ excretion, they do not inhibit the vasoconstrictor effects of angiotensin II. They are potassium-sparing diuretics.

Renin inhibitors

Inhibition of renin makes sense as a strategy to control hypertension, alongside ACE inhibitors and ARBs. One renin-inhibiting drug, **aliskiren**, has become available for use as an alternative fourth- or fifth-line drug. Reported to give a good blood pressure response even in combination with ACE inhibitors and ARBs, this may prove to be a useful class of drug in the management of hypertension. It may develop a role for those patients unable to tolerate ACE inhibitors due to cough, as an alternative to ARBs.

It is interesting to note that ACE inhibitors give a compensatory increase in renin secretion, increasing angiotensin I synthesis. We noted above that the conversion of angiotensin I to angiotensin II can occur independently of ACE, so elevated renin limits the effectiveness of ACE inhibitors. Compensatory increases of renin release should have less impact on the effectiveness of aliskiren.

5.2.2 Diuretics

Stimulating natriuresis (sodium excretion) is an important mechanism by which thiazide diuretics have their antihypertensive effects. Thiazides act on the distal tubule—they directly inhibit the mechanism for transport of Na^+ from the tubule lumen into the cells of the tubule wall, and hence enhance the amount of Na^+ lost in the urine. The consequences for blood volume and cardiac output can be deduced from the information presented above, from which it may also be predicted that the reduced blood volume will lead to increased renin output and increased angiotensin II activity, counteracting the effect of the diuretic (Figure 5.9). This provides another example of the complexity of antihypertensive therapy, leading to the scientific rationale behind the treatment with drugs of more than one class.

Thiazides are weaker diuretics than loop diuretics, less likely to cause adverse effects, and are routinely used in the management of commonly presenting hypertension. The most widely used thiazide diuretics are **bendroflumethiazide** and, with a slightly longer duration of action, the thiazide-like drug **chlorthalidone**. Another thiazide-like drug favoured in some parts of the world is **indapamide**.

It should be noted that while thiazides are correctly classified as diuretics, they also have a direct vasodilatory effect; this is believed to have an important role in sustaining their antihypertensive actions by counteracting the effects of enhanced angiotensin II activity mentioned above. The vasodilatory effect may

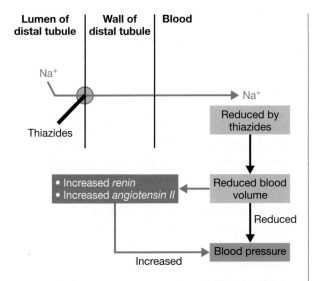

Figure 5.9 Thiazide action as a diuretic will lead to a compensatory increase in renin output.

Thiazide diuretics act at the distal tubule to increase the amount of Na⁺ lost in the urine. This results in a reduced blood volume, which contributes to lowering blood pressure. However, the reduced blood volume will be detected at the renin-secreting cells of the kidney, resulting in an increased release of renin, increased formation of angiotensin, and an increase in blood pressure. Thiazide antihypertensive drugs also have an entirely separate vasodilating effect, and this may explain why the overall response is a reduction in blood pressure.

prove to be the major mechanism for sustained blood pressure lowering in the clinical context.

5.2.3 Calcium channel blockers

Calcium channel blockers in clinical use can be initially classified according to the type of calcium channel they maintain in a closed state. In the case of those used to treat hypertension, the drugs target the L-type calcium channels, which are found in both heart and vascular muscle cells. Binding to these channels they reduce calcium influx. This can have its effect at three locations:

- the conducting system of the heart—the drugs slow the conductance of cardiac excitation
- the contractile cardiac myocytes—the drugs reduce the force of contraction
- the vascular smooth muscle cells—the drugs vasodilate, seen in a wide manner across arterial beds. This is predominantly on the arterial side, including the resistance precapillary arterioles, leading to a reduction in peripheral resistance.

There are three types of L-type calcium channel blockers in common clinical use: dihydropyridines, verapamil, and diltiazem. The choice between them is by various criteria, including whether they act on the heart as well as the blood vessels. They also vary in their pharmacokinetics, e.g. amlodipine is long lasting and so can be given once a day, whereas nifedipine, diltiazem, and verapamil are more rapidly eliminated and so are prescribed for multiple daily dosage or in slow-release preparations.

Dihydropyridines

This is a class of drugs defined by their chemical structure. They have preferential action on the vasculature, acting as vasodilators, accounting for their widespread use in the management of hypertension. They have little or no action on heart contractile strength, making it possible to consider some of these drugs (e.g. amlodipine) for patients with heart failure (see Chapter 7). In the management of hypertension, the lowering of blood pressure caused by drugs such as these results in a predictable reflex increase in cardiac output (e.g. via baroreceptors and increased sympathetic activity at the heart). Dihydropyridines are the most common choice of calcium channel drugs in the treatment of hypertension.

There are a large number of dihydropyridines available, including **amlodipine**, **nifedipine**, **felodipine**, **lercanidipine**, and **nisoldipine**. The choice of dihydropyridine is influenced by additional conditions (e.g. avoid all except amlodipine in heart failure). As well as hypertension, the dihydropyridines are useful for angina (particularly when associated with coronary artery spasm, see Chapter 6).

Verapamil

This is a single drug with distinct cardiac effects, including prolonging the refractory period within the sinoatrial and atrioventricular nodes.

Verapamil reduces:

- heart rate
- conduction of the excitation from atria to ventricles
- calcium influx in the ventricular action potential plateau (reducing force of contraction)
- calcium influx in the vasculature, giving generalized arterial vasodilation.

The combined cardiac and vascular effects explain the antihypertensive action. The cardiac effects of verapamil make it unsuitable for patients with heart failure, but explain its usefulness in the treatment of arrhythmias (see Chapter 7). In hypertension it may be particularly useful in heart attack or angina patients who cannot be prescribed β-blockers, for example because they are asthmatic.

Diltiazem

Diltiazem is available for antihypertensive treatment, particularly in the slow release form. It has less effect on heart rate than verapamil, but it does extend the action potential and refractory period within the sinoatrial and atrioventricular nodes, which, combined with peripheral vasodilation, reduces the work load, and therefore the oxygen demand, of the heart. This explains its use in the management of angina (Chapter 6).

5.2.4 α_1-Adrenoceptor antagonists

α_1-Adrenoceptors are widespread at vascular smooth muscle cells (section 5.1.4); stimulation by noradrenaline and adrenaline at these receptors leads to vasoconstriction, generating the vascular tone that maintains peripheral resistance. There is normally background stimulation (sympathetic tone) at these receptors, maintaining the peripheral resistance necessary for an arterial blood pressure that can effectively perfuse our tissues. In addition, the noradrenaline release from the local sympathetic terminals varies rapidly in response to demand. For example, when standing up from a lying position peripheral resistance in the viscera is increased, maintaining blood flow to the brain. Not surprisingly then, drugs that act as competitive antagonists at these α_1-adrenoceptors reduce peripheral resistance and have a place in the treatment of hypertension.

Two issues are relevant to understanding the usefulness, and limitations, of these drugs as antihypertensive agents.

- A reduction in blood pressure in response to reduced peripheral resistance will be detected by baroreceptors (Figure 5.8), leading to a compensatory increase in sympathetic release of noradrenaline, with effects on β-adrenoceptors in the heart and increased competition for vascular α_1-adrenoceptors (reducing the effectiveness of the competitive antagonist). This will tend to a reflex restoration of the blood pressure,

explaining why a patient with hypertension cannot simply have their blood pressure titrated down with an α_1-adrenoceptor antagonist. The outcome is that these drugs are normally taken in combination with other antihypertensives (see below).

- The α_1-adrenoceptor antagonists do not act at α_2-adrenoceptors that are located at the noradrenaline-releasing nerve terminal. This means that the released noradrenaline can still stimulate these presynaptic receptors, which will reduce further release of noradrenaline. Non-selective α-adrenoceptor antagonists, acting on both α_1 and α_2 subtypes, will block this presynaptic inhibition, leading to more noradrenaline release. The α_1-adrenoceptor selective agents are therefore generally preferred for the treatment of commonly presenting hypertension.

α_1-Adrenoceptor antagonists used for hypertension include **doxazosin**, **prazosin**, **terazosin**, and **indoramin**. The very potent non-selective (α_1 and α_2) antagonists **phenoxybenzamine** and **phentolamine** are used in the treatment of the very rare cases of hypertension caused by adrenal medulla tumours (phaeochromocytoma). A common unwanted effect of all these drugs is postural hypotension (leading to dizziness on standing).

5.2.5 β-adrenoceptor antagonists

Commonly referred to as β-blockers, this class of drugs has been very widely used as a mainstay of antihypertensive therapy in the past. However, in some parts of the world they are now not routinely prescribed to newly presenting hypertensives (see strategy set out below). While they may no longer be part of the main scheme of recommended prescribing for most new patients, there is such a large number of those doing well on β-adrenoreceptor antagonists, and others for whom there is a particular case for using them, that these drugs will remain common for hypertension for a considerable time. In addition they are important medication for patients with other conditions, notably angina, myocardial infarction, arrhythmias and heart failure (see later chapters).

Mode of action

Previously in this chapter we have mentioned the prevalence of β_1-adrenoceptors in the heart, stimulation of which leads to increased heart rate and force of contraction, increasing cardiac output and blood pressure. At first sight, therefore, it seems that the antihypertensive action of β-antagonists is simple—a reduction in cardiac output. However, baroreceptor-mediated feedback will lead to increased sympathetic activity, increasing the amount of noradrenaline competing with the competitive antagonists and combining with other feedback mechanisms to restore blood pressure. It seems that we must have a broader explanation for the antihypertensive action of these drugs:

- at the heart to reduce cardiac output
- at the kidney to reduce renin release (by action at the β-receptors of the juxtaglomerular cells—section 5.1.4 and Box 5.1)
- at the brain, where the effect is to reduce the activity of the sympathetic nervous system, reducing the release of noradrenaline at the β-receptors.

It is notable that the major effects of β-adrenoceptor antagonists are seen when sympathetic activity is high (physical activity, stress) and understandable therefore that the argument for using these drugs is greatest in patients where excess sympathetic activity contributes most to their hypertension.

Not all β-adrenoceptor antagonists are the same There are a large number of β-adrenoceptor antagonists from which a prescriber must choose the most appropriate for each individual. Significant differences are to be found in selectivity between β-adrenoceptor subtypes, selectively between α- and β-adrenoceptors, and partial agonism.

β_1–β_2-subtype selectivity of β-adrenoceptor antagonists The early β-adrenoceptor antagonist propranolol is equally effective at both β_1- and β_2-subtypes. This is of particular clinical importance since β_2-adrenoceptors found in bronchiolar smooth muscle help keep airways open—in asthmatic patients antagonists at these β_2-receptors may precipitate a significant increase in airways resistance (see Chapter 11). As a result β-adrenoceptor antagonists are generally not to be prescribed to asthmatics. Not surprisingly, there has been considerable interest in developing β_1-adrenoceptor-selective antagonists. The following drugs are described as selective for β_1- over β_2-adrenoceptors: **bisoprolol, atenolol, metoprolol,** and **nebivolol.** Importantly, none are devoid of β_2-adrenoceptor antagonism, and so even these are generally not recommended for asthmatics.

Partial agonists such as **oxprenolol** will occupy the β-adrenoceptors and weakly stimulate them while antagonising the stronger stimulation by noradrenaline or adrenaline. They may be expected, therefore, to smooth out the peaks and troughs of activity at these receptors.

Selectivity between α- and β-adrenoceptors Given the significance of α_1-adrenoceptors in maintaining peripheral resistance, it seems that a combined α_1- and β-adrenoceptor antagonist would be desirable. **Carvedilol** and **labetalol** are two examples of such a drug.

5.2.6 Other drugs available to treat hypertension

The drugs and guidelines set out above describe the tools that provide a satisfactory blood pressure control for the majority of patients presenting with uncomplicated hypertension. However, a number of other drugs are available that may be used on patients with unusual hypertensive issues. These patients may present with extremely high pressures (e.g. 220/120 mm Hg systolic/diastolic), with blood pressures resistant to the mainstream strategy, or with other relevant conditions such as heart failure or arrhythmias.

Vasodilators

This group, in addition to the widely employed α_1-adrenoceptor antagonists mentioned above, includes the following less commonly used drugs.

Sodium nitroprusside In Workbook 2 Andreas presents with a blood pressure of 210/135 mm Hg, requiring immediate treatment. While in most cases this may be treated with prompt oral β-adrenoceptor antagonists or calcium channel blockers, in Workbook 2 the possibility of using sodium nitroprusside (SNP) is introduced. Sodium nitroprusside acts as a nitric oxide (NO) donor—the NO enters the vascular smooth muscle cells, stimulating the synthesis of cyclic GMP, causing a rapid and profound vasodilatation (Box 5.2). Sodium nitroprusside has a very short half-life and so must be given as an intravenous perfusion. This generally gives a rapid reduction in blood pressure, after which SNP is discontinued and a long-term blood pressure management strategy based on the information above is pursued. Sodium nitroprusside is only used for short-term therapy, and has two major disadvantages:

Box 5.2
The vascular nitric oxide system

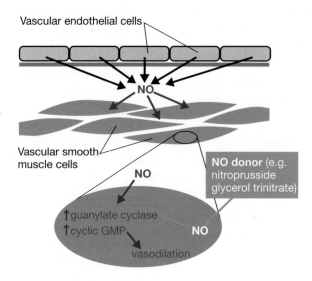

Nitric oxide (NO) release from vascular endothelial cells and its effect on vascular smooth muscle cells. Endothelial cells in green/orange and smooth muscle cells in blue/yellow.

Nitric oxide (NO) is a major endothelium-derived relaxing factor (EDRF), and is released from endothelial cells in response to many vasodilating influences (e.g. shear stress and pressure from the blood passing over the endothelium, stimulation of bradykinin or acetylcholine receptors). This is a very small molecule—once synthesized it passes through membranes and drifts out of the cells—and its rate of release is therefore determined by its rate of synthesis. NO is unstable once released, so only influences local cells, and does not survive to circulate in the blood. The NO released from endothelial cells can also act in the luminal direction, where it exerts a local anti-platelet effect. Various drugs interact with the NO system. These include NO donors such as sodium nitroprusside and glycerol trinitrate, which enter the smooth muscle cells, interact with intracellular protein SH groups, and form NO inside the target cells, causing vasodilation.

- Very rapid blood pressure reduction is not usually desirable and can have serious adverse consequences.
- A product of SNP decomposition is cyanide, and so patients must be monitored for cyanosis (see Workbook 2).

For these reasons SNP's use in hypertensive crises is in decline.

Minoxidil is a potassium channel activator, which means it will keep the membrane potential low, reducing vascular smooth muscle contraction. It is reserved for severe drug-resistant hypertension. **Diazoxide** is another potassium channel activator available (by intravenous injection) in cases of hypertensive emergency. **Hydralazine** is a vasodilator mainly on the arterial side, acting in a poorly understood manner to interfere with mechanisms of Ca^{2+} elevation.

Centrally acting sympatholytics

A sympatholytic is a drug that reduces the influence of the sympathetic system. A centrally acting sympatholytic acts in the brain to reduce the amount of activity in the sympathetic system, which means it will reduce noradrenaline release from nerve terminals in the cardiovascular system and elsewhere.

Methyldopa is metabolised into α-methyl noradrenaline, which is an agonist at brain α_2-adrenoceptors This accumulates in the vesicles of noradrenergic terminals and is released instead of noradrenaline. Stimulation of

α_2-adrenoceptors, in the brain and elsewhere, has a powerful noradrenaline release-inhibiting effect. **Clonidine** is a direct α_2-adrenoceptor agonist that similarly inhibits noradrenaline release, principally by its action in the brain. **Moxonidine** is an antihypertensive agent, which also reduces sympathetic outflow by a central mechanism.

5.3 Strategies for the drug treatment of hypertension

With respect to decisions about drug treatment, we can consider five questions:

1) What **co-morbidities** (other known illnesses or conditions) are there?

2) Have **non-drug measures** been attempted.

3) What is the **threshold** for treatment?

4) How **urgent** is treatment?

5) What are the **target** blood pressures the treatment is aimed at achieving?

With respect to the first point, the coexistence of other medical conditions will influence the outcome of the 'threshold' question—who to treat? If there is evidence of cardiovascular complications, end-organ damage (e.g. kidney or retina), diabetes, or a 10-year risk of over 20% (e.g. with concurrent dyslipidaemias, see Chapter 6), then thresholds may be lowered and there should be a greater urgency to drug treatment in the mid-hypertensive range.

'Non-drug measures' means lifestyle changes, such as stress reduction, smoking cessation, exercise regimes, etc. These should be pursued in all patients with hypertension. They may be the only interventions necessary in some patients, particularly those with mild hypertension and low risk.

Thresholds and urgency With respect to the first two of these, the following may act as a guide:

- Sustained (repeated measurements over months) blood pressures between 140 and 159 systolic or 90 and 99 diastolic (mm Hg) are treated with lifestyle guidance and, if this is not sufficient, with drugs, with the target of bringing readings down to below 140/90.

- A patient recording pressures of 160–179 mm Hg systolic or 100–109 mm Hg diastolic should be reassessed weekly on four or more occasions and if readings are consistent despite lifestyle advice drug therapy should be initiated.

- Patients with pressures of 180–219 mm Hg systolic or 110–119 mm Hg diastolic maintained over 1–2 weeks should be prescribed drugs without delay.

- Pressures of 220 mm Hg systolic or 120 mm Hg diastolic or above indicate a hypertensive crisis that should be treated immediately.

Target blood pressures With respect to target blood pressures that treatments are aiming at, unless there are complications, this is likely to be <140/90 (systolic/diastolic mm Hg). Issues which modify this include diabetes and chronic kidney disease, when lower targets (typically <130/80 (systolic/diastolic mm Hg) are likely to be set.

Dangers of 'overtreating' hypertension and the 'J curve' There are two commonly encountered situations when concerns may be raised about drug treatments that bring down hypertension too far or too quickly.

6) The use of intravenous vasodilators to treat hypertensive crisis, where concerns about a very rapid reduction from a very high level have made intravenous drug administration less popular (see Workbook 2).

7) The management of a standard hypertensive patient— is there a danger in setting the target too low (sometimes described as the 'J curve')? There is some evidence that excessive pharmacological reduction of diastolic blood pressure (e.g. below 80 mm Hg) may reduce cardiac perfusion during diastole, increasing the risk of an myocardial infarct (MI) in certain patients (e.g. those with a history of coronary artery disease).

We have described hypertension as a symptom-less disease, but in Workbook 2 we encounter Andreas, whose hypertension has caused symptoms of a persistent headache and an acute attack of dizziness and confusion. Andreas, presenting with pressures of 220/140 (systolic/diastolic mm Hg), is treated as a case of **hypertensive crisis** and he illustrates that hypertension at the upper end may not be symptom-free. These very high blood pressures should be treated with urgency. They are associated with end organ damage (e.g. damage to kidney or retina) and much enhanced risk of major cardiovascular accidents such as MI or stroke.

Andreas is a patient who illustrates two other aspects of hypertension treatment.

- Only one measurement, his diastolic pressure of 140 mm Hg, fell within the highest category in the scheme set out above, and yet this was sufficient to include him. The categories are defined by the highest indicated by *either* systolic *or* diastolic pressures; both do not need to be above the cut off to meet the definition.

- He has previously been diagnosed as hypertensive and prescribed drugs, but has not maintained his drug therapy—poor compliance is understandably commonplace, whereas in the vast majority of hypertension cases there are no symptoms. Andreas' crisis is contributed to poor compliance.

Strategy in the treatment of hypertension

Combining the clinical pharmacology and the outcome of trials and clinical experience to create a strategy for the treatment of hypertension across the population is complex. It is not surprising therefore that strategies vary across countries, and are subject to change. The differences in recommendations between countries or regions may be seen in the recommendation for the first class of drug prescribed. However, as the majority of patients will require more than one drug type, regardless of which is administered first, this may not be the most significant issue. Despite this, substantive differences do exist. In the UK there has, over a number of years, been a downgrading of the recommended role for β-adrenoceptor antagonists; firstly removing it as the recommended drug for first-line treatment, and most recently relegating it to possible use as a fourth-line drug. In Europe (excluding UK) and the USA there has been no such substantial change—rather other drugs have risen in profile to compete with β-blockers as mainstream therapy. It should always be remembered that the actual choice of drugs will depend on the individual patient, most notably what other clinical conditions coexist. For example, asthmatic patients, diabetic patients, or those with high risk of diabetes: in such patients β-adrenoceptor antagonists should not be prescribed, and in particular, where diabetes is an issue, in combination with thiazide diuretics.

In the UK, the recommended drug-choice strategy for uncomplicated hypertension, typically presenting repeatedly with pressures in the region of 140–179 mm Hg systolic and 90–109 mm Hg diastolic, is defined by the plan set out in Figure 5.10.

- The scheme is divided, in terms of *initial* treatment, into those on the left, expected to have a high RAAS contribution (high renin), and those on the right, expected to have less RAAS involvement in their hypertension and therefore less likely to respond well to ACE inhibitors.

- Reaching blood pressure targets with a single drug should always be the first objective of drug treatment.

- However, as most patients will not respond sufficiently to their initial drug, the distinction between the two groups of patients in the scheme above disappears as more drugs are added.

- Note also that ACE inhibitors can be replaced by ARBs as necessary, e.g. as discussed above for those patients with unacceptable cough.

- Importantly, the scheme relegates the β-adrenoceptor antagonists to a possible role as fourth-line treatment—in reality many patients will be prescribed α-adrenoceptor antagonists instead.

The scheme is only intended as a guide for newly diagnosed patients. It differs from previous recommendations: as mentioned above, it reduces the role for β-adrenoceptor antagonists, and also removes thiazide diuretics as first-line treatment for under 55 non-black patients. The scheme does not direct prescribers to change the medication for these established patients to fit into this scheme.

In the USA recommendations are:

> Stage 1 hypertension (see Table 5.2B): a thiazide diuretic for most patients, with the alternatives of ACE inhibitor, ARB, calcium channel blocker or β-blocker.

> Stage 2 hypertension (Table 5.2B): use the same variety of drugs but with the expectation of using a two-drug combination.

Use of additional drugs until target blood pressure is achieved.

In Europe (excluding UK) recommendations are for choice of drugs from the same five classes (thiazide diuretic, ACE inhibitor, ARB, calcium channel blocker, and β-blocker) at initiation and maintenance, alone or in

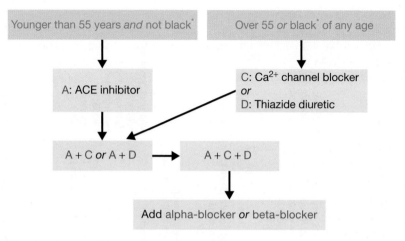

*Black is defined as of African or Afro-Caribbean origin.

Figure 5.10

A scheme in used in the UK for prescribing to newly diagnosed hypertensive patients. *Black is defined as of African or Afro-Caribbean origin.

combination, with clinical judgement determining the drugs used, depending on the individual patient.

In Australia the National Prescribing Service recommends low-dose thiazides as a start for most patients, ACE inhibitors in patients with diabetes, and calcium channel blockers/β-blockers in patients with angina.

The information given above outlining the physiological control of blood pressure enables the prescriber to understand, up to a point, why certain drug combinations

are optimal. For example, diuretic effects on blood volume and cardiac output complement a dihydropyridine calcium channel drug, which mainly affects the vasculature and peripheral resistance. From a mechanistic point of view it can then be predicted that adding an ACE inhibitor, with its independent effects on cardiac output and vasculature by attenuating the kidney/renin influence, has additional effects beyond those of diuretics and calcium channel blockers. In this way it is possible to understand the pharmacological basis of strategies for drug treatment of hypertension.

SUMMARY OF DRUGS USED FOR HYPERTENSION

Therapeutic class	Drugs	Mechanism of action	Common clinical uses	Comments	Examples of adverse drug reactions
ACE inhibitors	Lisinopril Enalapril Ramipril Captopril Perindopril Trandolapril Fosinopril Quinalapril	Inhibits ACE, preventing conversion of angiotensin I to angiotensin II, leading to: a) reduced peripheral arterial resistance b) aldosterone secretion c) accumulation of bradykinin	Hypertension Ischaemic heart disease Heart failure Diabetic nephropathy	Pharmacokinetics vary widely Captopril has shortest time to peak and duration Bradykinin could cause dry cough	Hypotension Persistent angioedema Rash Dry cough
Angiotensin II receptor blockers (ARBs, A2RAs)	Candesartan Losartan Irbesartan Valsartan Olmesartan Telmisartan Eprosartan	Antagonist at angiotensin II receptor, leading to: a) reduced peripheral arterial resistance b) aldosterone secretion	Hypertension Ischaemic heart disease Heart failure Diabetic nephropathy	Pharmacokinetics vary widely Usually reserved for second line use in patients who cannot tolerate ACE inhibitors due to cost and sometimes evidence	Hypotension Persistent angioedema Hyperkalaemia
Renin inhibitors	Aliskiren	Directly inhibits renin, which decreases plasma renin activity and inhibits conversion of angiotensinogen to angiotensin I	Hypertension	Metabolized by hepatic CYPA4, leading to interactions Very long half-life Relatively new class/drug Usually reserved for third line use	Diarrhoea Rash
Loop diuretics	Furosemide	Blocks the reabsorption of sodium and chloride in kidney tubules (proximal and distal tubules and loop of Henle), causing a profound increase in urine output	Resistant hypertension Heart failure Oedema	Quick onset of action	Mild gastrointestinal effects Hypokalaemia Hyperglycaemia Headache Dizziness
Thiazide diuretics	Bendroflumethiazide Chlortalidone Indapamide	Directly inhibits the mechanism for transport of Na+ from the tubule lumen into the cells of the tubule wall, and hence enhance the amount of Na+ lost in the urine	Heart failure Hypertension Oedema	Slower onset of action and longer duration	
Calcium channel blockers	Dihydropyridines: amlodipine nifedipine felodipine lercanidipine nisoldipine Non-dihydropyridines: verapamil diltiazem	Antagonist at calcium channel blocks the influx of calcium ions via calcium channel into cardiac and vascular smooth muscles	Hypertension Angina	Dihydropyridines act predominatly on vascular smooth muscle Verapamil acts on heart whilst diltiazem is intermediate Diltiazem and verapamil metabolized by hepatic cytochrome P450 system	Abdominal pain Nausea Palpitations Oedema

Class	Drugs	Mechanism	Indications	Notes	Side effects
Selective α_1-adrenoceptor antagonists	Doxazosin Prazosin Indoramin	1) Selectively inhibits the post synaptic α_1 and α_{1a} adrenergic receptors, causing arterial and venous dilation 2) Binds highly to α_{1c} adrenoceptor subtype predominant in the prostate	Hypertension BPH	Have little effect on presynaptic α_2 receptors and are therefore less likely to cause reflex tachycardia than the non-selective α-blockers. Useful for patients with both BPH and hypertension	Orthostatic hypotension Nasal congestion Urinary urgency Dizziness Headache
Non-selective α_1 and α_2 antagonists	Phenoxybenzamine phentolamine	Blocks the effect of adrenaline and noradrenaline at α_1 and α_2 receptors both pre and post synaptically, leading to arterial and venous vasodilation and inhibition of catecholamine-mediated vasoconstriction	Hypertensive crises caused by phaechromocytoma	Blockade of presynaptic α_2 receptors results in increased noradrenaline release and enhances reflex tachycardia	Reflex tachycardia Dizziness Drowsiness Fatigue
β-adrenoceptor antagonists	Propranolol Bisoprolol Atenolol Metoprolol Nebivolol Carvedilol Labetalol	Competitively block β-receptors in heart, peripheral vasculature, bronchi, pancreas, uterus, kidney, brain, and liver, resulting in reduced cardiac output and antihypertensive effect	Hypertension Ischaemic heart disease Heart failure (not all)	Selectivity and specificity vary widely Pharmacokinetics vary widely	Bronchospasm Dyspnoea Cold extremities
Vasodilators	Sodium nitroprusside	A pro-drug that releases nitric oxide, a potent vasodilator that increases cGMP levels, leading to phosphorylation of protein kinase, which causes relaxation of vascular smooth muscles	Hypertensive emergency Controlled hypotension during surgery to reduce bleeding Acute heart failure	Degraded to thiocyanate, which could accumulate and cause toxicity Infusion should be protected from light Rarely used because of thiocyanate toxicity	(usually resulting from thiocyanate toxicity) Nausea Vomiting Sweating Headache Palpitations Abdominal pain
	Minoxidil Hydralazine Diazoxide	Causes direct relaxation of vascular smooth muscle, leading to vasodilation in the periphery	Resistant hypertension Alopecia (minoxidil)		Flushing Headache Dizziness
Centrally acting sympatholytics	Methyldopa clonidine	Directly stimulates α_2-receptor in the vasomotor centre of the medulla, leading to reduced sympathetic outflow from the brain	Hypertension	Methyldopa can be used in pregnancy Clonidine also used for menopausal flushing	Headache Dizziness Drymouth Bradycadia
	Moxonidine	Agonist at central imidazoline-l-1 and α_2 receptor	Hypertension	Not to be used in renal impairment	Weight gain Tachycardia

ACE, angiotensin converting enzyme; MI, myocardial infarction; PE, pulmonary embolism; BPH, benign prostate hypertrophy

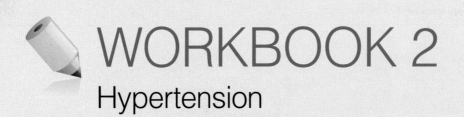

WORKBOOK 2
Hypertension

Andreas, a non-compliant patient. A case of hypertensive crisis followed by long-term management

The patient: a simplified case history

The day of Monique and Andreas' wedding has finally arrived. Andreas has arrived at the registry office 30 minutes early, anxious for nothing to go wrong. He sits and waits with his father Brian and his brother Eoin, who is also his best man. Eoin is a world-renowned Formula 1 driver who has missed a championship to attend this wedding.

Suddenly Andreas feels dizzy and wobbly; the headache he has had for the last few days has got worse. He wonders if this has anything to do with his high blood pressure. His doctor keeps trying to get him to take the treatment for this seriously. Eoin notices his pallor but before he can say anything, Andreas says he needs to lie down on the waiting bench. Eoin rings for an ambulance.

While in the ambulance, Eoin has to do all the talking because Andreas is too confused to be coherent. He tells the paramedics that although Andreas' family doctor prescribed tablets for his blood pressure 6 months ago, Andreas only took them for 2 days and threw the rest away. The paramedics take his blood pressure; it is extremely high, requiring urgent hospitalization.

And so instead of getting married Monique rushes to the local hospital. She meets Dr Lucy Knight, a young doctor who talks with them and confirms Andreas' details, which were compiled with Eoin's help.

A table of clinical clerking abbreviations is given on page xi.

CLINICAL CLERKING FOR ANDREAS KAISER

Age: 35 years

PMH: Moderate hypertension, poorly controlled

SH: Lives with fiancée and twin daughters. Smokes 20 cigarettes a day. Weight 95 kg (overweight).

> *1) Smoking, like hypertension, also increases his risk of having a stroke or heart attack, although there is little evidence that long-term smoking leads to increased blood pressure.*

> *2) Weight reduction will contribute to reducing his blood pressure.*

DH:

1) Bendroflumethiazide

2) Lisinopril

Note: In some parts of the world bendroflumethiazide has been called bendrofluazide.

Poor control of hypertension by drugs may be due to poor compliance (i.e. patient not taking drugs as prescribed). This may even be true of those educated in drug treatment. Andreas (who is an industry pharmacist, see Workbook 1) openly admits to not taking the medication prescribed.

O/E:

1) Blood pressure = 220/140 mm Hg (<140/90 mm Hg)

Less than 140/90 mm Hg is the recommended value. Andreas' blood pressure (BP) is extremely elevated. Blood pressures this high represents a medical emergency because of the high risk of renal damage, retinopathy, stroke, encephalopathy or myocardial infarct (heart attack).

2) Pulse = 60/minute (normal)

Biochemistry:

1) Sodium = 142 mmol/L (135–145)

2) Potassium = 4.2 mmol/L (3.5–5.5)

These are both within recommended range.

Diagnosis: Hypertensive crisis

Plan:

Scenario 1: Start sodium nitroprusside infusion

Scenario 2: Start oral labetalol

Lucy explains to Andreas that his headache and dizziness were all brought about by his very high BP. She says a BP of 210/135 mm Hg is a medical emergency and could lead to permanent damage or death.

PART 1: EXPLORING ANDREAS' CONDITION

1) Andreas' BP was extremely elevated at 220/140 mm Hg.

1a) What is the meaning of the two numbers? Use the terms 'systolic' and 'diastolic' in your answer.

....

....

....

1b) What are considered normal pressures? How do you assess urgency of treatment on the basis of blood pressure readings?

....

....

....

2a) What is systole and what is diastole?

2b) Explain the meaning of the following statement: 'When left ventricular systole starts pressure inside the ventricles rises immediately, but there is a short delay before the ejection of blood into the aorta (ejection phase) begins' (refer to Figure 5.5).

2c) Andreas' diastolic BP is very high (his afterload is high). Will this increase or decrease the delay between onset of left ventricular systole and the beginning of the ejection phase? What effect would this have on stroke volume?

See section 5.1.3.

3) Do you think the activity of the sinoatrial (SA) node is a problem in Andreas' case? Is his pacemaker slope appropriate? Should we think in his case of using drugs intended to target the SA node pacemaker slope?

Clue: Consider his pulse. Also refer to section 5.1.2 and Figure 5.2.

4) Considering that blood pressure = HR x SV x TPR (section 5.1.1) which of these three determinants of BP should be the target of drug therapy for Andreas?

5) If we wish to target total peripheral resistance (TPR) using a vasodilatory drug, suggest two types of drug, one type acting directly as a vasodilator and one type acting at defined receptor subtypes. Give examples.

6) If we wish to directly target stroke volume (SV) with drugs acting at the heart cells, suggest a receptor target and indicate how drugs acting at this receptor may influence SV.

....

....

....

Immediate treatments for Andreas' hypertension

For this imaginary patient with hypertensive crisis we provide two alternative approaches to immediate drug treatment once the patient has been admitted to hospital. In the first the patient has been treated with an intravenous antihypertensive drug to rapidly reduce BP. However, it is recognized that a very rapid drop in BP may promote the very conditions which the treatment is intended to avoid, i.e. heart, brain, retina, and kidney pathologies. Because of this the intravenous vasodilator approach (Scenario 1) has fallen out of favour. Nevertheless very high BP (e.g. 140 mm Hg diastolic or above) does require urgent hospital treatment, but clinical judgement may favour oral labetalol, atenolol, or amlodipine, with the intention of bringing the diastolic pressure to around 100 mm Hg over 24 hours, followed by a long-term strategy aimed at the lower than 140/90 mm Hg systolic/diastolic target.

To explore these alternative strategies, two scenarios are presented below for Andreas once he arrives at hospital. The first is to use the intravenous vasodilator sodium nitroprusside and the second, now more likely, is to use oral labetalol.

Scenario 1: Intravenous vasodilator

Lucy explains that the drug sodium nitroprusside (SNP) will be administered to quickly bring down Andreas' BP. This is because if his BP was not reduced immediately, it could lead to damage to the retina, heart attack, stroke, or kidney failure. The drug has a very short half-life so must be given by intravenous infusion, which in itself adds to a rapid onset of action.

Once introduced into the bloodstream, SNP rapidly distributes itself around the body, including the vascular smooth muscle cells (arterial and venous), where it interacts with sulphydryl groups and generates nitric oxide (NO) within the cells, causing widespread vasodilatation. For more on NO, see Box 5.5.

7) In normal vascular physiology endothelial cells regulate local vasodilatation by synthesis and release of NO, which then acts on the adjacent vascular smooth muscle cells. Draw a simple diagram showing how this works (see Box 5.2) and add the manner in which SNP interacts with this system.

....

....

....

8a) What effect will SNP have on peripheral resistance?

....

....

8b) How does this affect:

- afterload
- blood pressures
- stroke volume?

8c) What effect will SNP have on central venous pressure and how will this lead to changes in:

- preload
- end diastolic volume
- force of contraction (of the ventricles).

Note the widespread vasodilator action of the drug, and use the knowledge you have gained of the cardiovascular system to work out the consequences for heart function.

Andreas' BP is checked every 5 minutes after commencing the SNP infusion. Fifteen minutes later it has dropped to an acceptable level and the SNP can be discontinued.

Investigations 15 minutes after infusion: BP = 170/95 mm Hg (<145/95).

This is still elevated, but he can be considered as being over the 'crisis'. His current BP can now slowly be reduced with oral medication.

Monique is amazed at how quickly this drug has worked.

Sodium nitroprusside is mainly used for a fast effect, although it may be given intravenously over a large number of hours if necessary. However, in the body SNP is broken down to produce a toxic thiocyanate product. For longer term (e.g. 48 hours) administration, the patient is monitored for thiocyanate toxicity, as a result of which SNP treatment would be stopped. In such a case intravenous labetalol might be an alternative (see below).

Scenario 2: Oral labetalol

Lucy explains that a strategy of bringing down Andreas' BP over 24 hours will be used. This is considered the safest option and Andreas will be kept in hospital during this time.

Andreas is started on oral labetalol, with regular checks on his BP.

After 24 hours his BP is down to 175/100 mm Hg.

Labetalol can also be administered intravenously short term (e.g. 15 minutes) for a rapid response.

9) What is the mechanism of action of labetalol? What makes it different from other widely used β-adrenoceptor antagonists?

Note: What receptor subtype(s) does it act on? Is it an agonist or antagonist?

Long-term treatments for Andreas' hypertension

By the next day Andreas is feeling well, and talks with Lucy about his condition and its treatment. He is embarrassed that he failed to take his earlier medication for hypertension—after all he is a pharmacist! —and he recognizes that this means he was partly responsible for his crisis the day before. He wants to discuss his treatment.

10) List three illnesses which Andreas' hypertension could cause if it is left untreated.

The doctor explains to Andreas that the choice of antihypertensive is based on the following:

- cost
- tolerability in individual patients
- concomitant disorders and contraindications (e.g. patients with heart failure should use ACE inhibitors, patients with gout should not be given diuretics)
- race and age

It is decided not to prescribe bendroflumethiazide.

11) Why has Andreas been taken off bendroflumethiazide? Consider the treatment algorithm for newly diagnosed hypertensives (Figure 5.10 and section 5.3). How do you think this should be applied to Andreas, who is a young white male?

12) Bendroflumethiazide is still commonly prescribed to control hypertension. When is it likely to be appropriate to do this?

13a) To which class of drugs does bendroflumethiazide belong?

....

....

13b) Where is the site of action of bendroflumethiazide?

....

....

13c) What is the mechanism of action by which bendroflumethiazide reduces Andreas' BP (section 5.2.2)?

....

....

13d) Is there reason to consider that the antihypertensive effect of bendroflumethiazide may NOT be solely due to its diuretic action (Figure 5.9)?

....

....

Lucy explains that Andreas' BP had probably risen gradually over a long period.

Andreas sheepishly admitted that he had often experienced strange headaches and dizzy spells, but had dismissed them as minor.

He admitted that he had intentionally refused treatment with bendroflumethiazide for his hypertension. This was because after taking the tablets for a week, he had realized that he had to urinate more often, particularly at night. He said the hypertension had only been diagnosed during a physical examination requested by his insurance company and that he had no symptoms or effects on his life, and so quite quickly stopped taking both types of tablets.

14) To minimize non-compliance Andreas should have been advised to take bendroflumethiazide in the morning. Explain this.

Bendroflumethiazide is also called a 'water tablet' because it makes patients urinate more often.

....

....

15) What first-line treatment should be considered for Andreas once his hypertensive crisis is over?

Jo, the pharmacist, discusses Andreas' case with the doctor and they agree that using an angiotensin converting enzyme (ACE) inhibitor is the best treatment for Andreas, and so he is prescribed lisinopril. This is the same drug he had been prescribed previously, but now without the bendroflumethiazide. Andreas agrees that from now on he will take his medication every day without fail.

16) Do you think the ACE inhibitor alone is likely to be sufficient to control Andreas' BP in the long run? Explain.

17) Which octapeptide's formation will be blocked by ACE inhibitors when Andreas starts taking it to reduce his BP? What is the whole system called?

18) Referring back to question 4, which of the three determinants of BP (stroke volume, heart rate or peripheral resistance) will be most directly modified by the ACE inhibitor?

19) The ACE inhibitor will also be expected to have an indirect effect on kidney function, through aldosterone. Explain this effect.

When Andreas was training he was taught that β-adrenoceptor antagonists (β-blockers) were commonly prescribed for the long-term treatment of hypertension. He mentions this to Lucy, and asks why they have not considered β-blockers for him. Lucy asks the pharmacist Jo to join them, and they discuss the situation regarding β-blockers.

20) Why were β-blockers not prescribed for Andreas?

> *β-blocker prescribing has changed over the last few years. These drugs are more formally called β-adrenoceptor antagonists. They have a long history as major antihypertensive drugs, and are still used for hypertension and other indications (see labetalol use above, and later). Students must therefore understand the types and mode of action of β adrenoceptor antagonists. However, in some countries these drugs are no longer recommended as first-line antihypertensive therapy for most newly diagnosed patients.*

21) Following recommendations, when might it be appropriate for a patient to be taking β-blockers to control hypertension?

22a) If Andreas is put on a β-blocker, what is the molecular mechanism by which it will influence his BP?

Which receptors are influenced and where are they found (see section 5.2.5)?

22b) How does activity at this receptor change cardiac function?

> *Clue: Draw a ventricular myocyte action potential and illustrate the effect of (i) stimulating β-adrenoceptors and (ii) a β-adrenoceptor antagonist on the calcium plateau. Describe what will be the effect on cardiac function (i.e. force of contraction, stroke volume, cardiac output).*

22c) Is the effect on the calcium channel seen as an effect mainly at stroke volume or heart rate? Are effects of β-blockers also expected at sinoatrial node action potentials?

> Jo and the registrar talk about choosing the right β-adrenoceptor antagonists (β-blockers). They use words like cardioselective and nonselective.

23a) Indicate some possible unwanted effects of using β-blockers.

23b) Why might a drug that is selective for β_1 receptors over β_2 receptors be of clinical interest? How would this relate to the notion of a cardioselective drug?

23c) Are there β-blockers that we can freely prescribe to asthmatics?

Jo and Lucy discuss with Andreas that the current guidelines do not recommend β-blockers for a young non-black patient, and also that because of some of the side effects of β-blockers they may not be the most suitable drugs for Andreas. The side effects she mentions are impotence and the risks associated with sudden discontinuation when Andreas' compliance history is taken into consideration.

Andreas is determined to try and remember his cardiovascular pharmacology from his college days, and asks why he has not been prescribed calcium channel blockers. He also mentions that his line manager at work was newly diagnosed as hypertensive and was given amlopidine. Lucy asks whether he is black, and it turns out he is African.

Jo points out that initial prescribing for hypertension is related to race, and that black patients, expected to have a less satisfactory response to ACE inhibitors as a first-line drug, are likely to be prescribed a diuretic or calcium channel drug.

24a) What is the effect of a calcium antagonist on calcium channels?

What type of calcium channels are blocked by therapeutically significant calcium channel blockers?

24b) What effect does the administration of calcium channel blockers have on blood vessels?

Andreas knows the dihydropyridine calcium channel blockers but cannot remember the names of the non-dihydropyridines. Lucy tells him.

25) List the two non-dihydropyridine calcium channel blockers Lucy mentions.

Which one is cardioselective?

- *A cardioselective non-dihydropyridine reduces BP by directly acting on the heart.*
- *The dihydropyridine Nifedipine only affects calcium channels in the periphery and has no action on the heart*
- *When the BP is rapidly dropped by nifedipine the heart compensates by beating faster and this is called reflex tachycardia.*
- *A cardioselective non-dihydropyridine does not cause this because it directly slows the cardiac pacemaker. A cardioselective non-dihydropyridine reduces BP by directly acting on the heart pacemaker.*

Andreas was discharged from hospital and took his lisinopril regularly. He was asked to attend the local hypertension clinic frequently to check his BP.

Treating Andreas with the ACE inhibitor was not successful because he quickly developed a horrible dry cough. The ACE inhibitors not only reduce synthesis of angiotensin II, they also prevent bradykinin breakdown, causing the accumulation of this peptide in the upper respiratory tract. This bradykinin is thought to be the reason for the cough.

In place of ACE inhibitors Andreas was prescribed losartan, an angiotensin II receptor antagonist (or ARB: angiotensin receptor blocker, also known as 'sartans').

26a) What is the mechanism of action of angiotensin II receptor antagonists? At which receptor are they antagonists? How does this lead to reduced blood pressure?

See section 5.2.1 and Box 5.1.

26b) List three physiological functions controlled by angiotensin II acting on this receptor.

27) Why are angiotensin II receptor antagonists less likely to cause a cough?

Andreas took his losartan as instructed and the cough disappeared. However, this treatment was also unsatisfactory since on repeated measurements in the hypertension clinic his BP was around 170/105 mm Hg, a long way from the target of 140/90 mm Hg or less, substantially increasing (by more than twice) his chances of having a major cardiovascular event. The doctor mentions that eventually bendroflumethiazide could be prescribed again, assuming that this time Andreas would take his medication regularly, but that he also wants to consider other drugs.

28a) Multiple drug prescribing is commonly required to reach target BP. What are the three main drug types used in hypertension, one or more of which are likely to be added to Andreas' treatment?

Clue: A, C, D.

28b) Which of these would you prescribe as a second drug for Andreas to take with his losartan? Explain your answer, not just in terms of the guidelines indicated in Figure 5.10, but also in terms of the complementary mechanisms of action of the drugs.

29) Other drugs are also available if targets are not reached with two drugs. Set out a long-term strategy for treating Andreas, making the assumption that first three drugs, then four drugs are prescribed in an attempt to reach target. Along with the A, C and D drugs also consider using drugs that act at α-adrenoceptors and at β-adrenoceptors.

Chapter 6
Atherosclerosis and ischaemic heart disease

If a man of 20 develops acute and uncomfortable chest pains, he is likely to put it down as indigestion and wait for it to go away. If this happens to a 60-year-old man the response may be quite different, with the recognition that the pain may come from heart disease, and fear of a heart attack. Of course the large majority of such patients recover quickly, but this patient's fear is not without foundation, and so the condition requires prompt clinical investigation. Such a situation is explored in the case of our imaginary patient Brian in Workbook 3 at the end of this chapter. In general, a patient's chest pain may be unrelated to heart disease, or it may be caused by partial blockage of coronary arteries serving the heart, leading to myocardial ischaemia or **ischaemic heart disease**. This can result in either chest pain without permanent damage to the heart (**angina pectoris**) or chest pain with the death of heart tissue (a heart attack, also called **myocardial infarction** (MI)). Angina pectoris refers to the symptom of chest pain, often radiating to arm and jaw. Commonly, but not always, there is underlying **coronary artery disease** caused by the development of **atherosclerosis** over the years preceding the onset of chest pain. Angina may be taken as a warning that coronary artery disease exists, enabling interventions to reduce the risk of a later MI. (More rarely, myocardial ischaemia can occur in the absence of chest pain). There are lifestyle changes and drugs that can have a major impact on the development of atherosclerotic disease, and of course there are a variety of drugs available which modify the course of angina or a heart attack. These drugs may profoundly affect the well-being, and perhaps chances of survival, of the patient. In this chapter, we will study the underlying process of atherosclerosis and the events associated with angina and heart attack so that we can understand how these drugs work, and how they may be best employed in the treatment of individual patients.

Coronary artery disease is the most common cause of death in the developed world. In the USA alone over 6 million people suffer from angina, with coronary artery disease causing approximately one death per minute. In the majority of these fatal cases there is no long-term record of heart disease. Faced with such observations the need to improve prevention and treatment is clear. While the greatest prospects for prevention lie with lifestyle changes, there is potential for improved use of drugs already available, and the development of better pharmacological tools, which will come from a more profound understanding of the cellular and molecular events underlying coronary artery disease.

Coronary arteries, heart muscle, and oxygen supply and demand

The heart is mainly a muscle, which contracts about once per second throughout a person's life. The frequency and force of contraction varies according to the activities of the individual, and it is this that determines the work done by the heart and the resulting demand for oxygen. Blood, and therefore oxygen, is supplied to the heart by the coronary arteries. These course along the surface of the heart (Figure 6.1), sending arterioles deep into the muscle tissue.

In healthy people the supply of oxygen to the heart increases when demand increases. This is by dilation of the coronary arterioles, leading to increased blood flow and oxygen supply to the heart. In coronary artery disease, the internal surface of the artery wall becomes lined with a growth, which reduces the maximum lumen

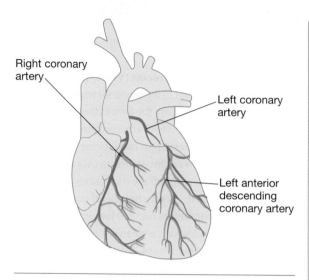

Figure 6.1 The major vessels that are subject to blockage by coronary artery disease are found on the surface of the heart.

In addition to those shown here, the left circumflex coronary artery is also often blocked in coronary artery disease. Arterioles of diminishing size then descend into the muscle walls of the ventricles. Partial blockage of the major vessels reduces the maximum flow that fully dilated arterioles can deliver to the muscle tissue.

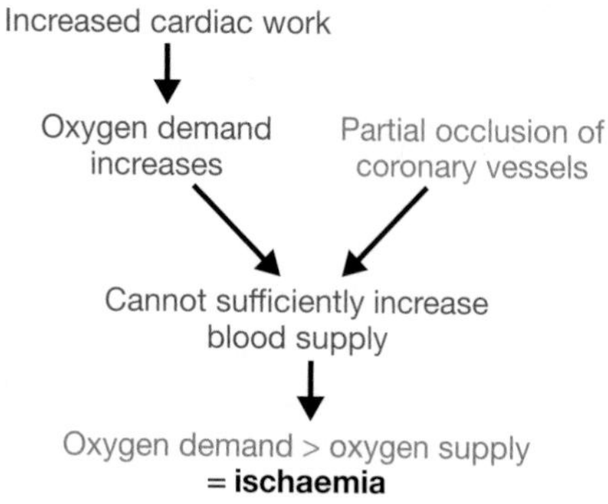

Increased cardiac work

↓

Oxygen demand increases   Partial occlusion of coronary vessels

Cannot sufficiently increase blood supply

↓

Oxygen demand > oxygen supply
= **ischaemia**

Figure 6.2 Cardiac ischaemia occurs when the coronary vessels cannot deliver enough blood for the oxygen supply to meet the oxygen demand.

of the vessel through which the blood can flow. This *partial occlusion* of the coronary arteries may mean that the maximum blood flow is not sufficient for oxygen supply to meet oxygen demand (e.g. when the heart works harder and oxygen demand increases), leading to ischaemia and angina (Figure 6.2).

The partial occlusion of the coronary arteries can come about in three ways:

1) due to atherosclerotic plaque growth from the vessel wall, producing a stable partial block

2) block by thrombus/embolus, which may develop rapidly and be unstable, and may occur as a consequence of long-term atherosclerosis

3) contraction (spasm) of coronary arterial smooth muscle.

These different causes of ischaemia relate to the different clinical categories of angina discussed below. Atherogenesis (the generation of an atheroma or atherosclerotic plaque) is the principle long-term pathological process contributing to ischaemic heart disease, and so we shall now consider atherosclerosis and the way in which its development may be modified by drugs.

6.1 Atherosclerosis

Atherosclerosis results in a growth on the inner face of a blood vessel wall, partly blocking the vessel; clearly if this happens in a blood vessel serving the heart (a coronary vessel) it is a serious situation—this is coronary artery disease.

The essential features of atherosclerosis are:

1) a focal disease of the arterial tree that affects the tunica intima (i.e. the inner lining) of large- and middle-sized arteries

2) the formation of a fibrous plaque (atheroma), which gives ↓ lumen size and ↓ blood flow

3) the danger that a ruptured plaque may act as a focus for thrombus formation.

Essential features of atheroma formation are a compromised endothelial layer, the accumulation within the intima of cholesterol/lipids, vascular smooth muscle cells, and cellular debris, occurring with local vascular inflammation, forming a plaque, which develops a calcified surface as it matures. The process is intimately affected by the levels and nature of circulating cholesterol, a subject we must review before looking at the initiation and maturation of an atheroma in more detail.

6.1.1 Cholesterol, triglycerides, and lipoproteins are found in the circulation

Cholesterol is an essential part of all cells within our bodies, forming part of the cell membranes. Its supply from the blood is required for cell growth and viability. It also has more specialized roles, such as the precursor for steroid hormone synthesis and a central component of bile. It is transported around the body in the blood, both towards and away from tissues, bound to lipoproteins.

Triglycerides are produced in liver from the metabolism of carbohydrates, alcohol, sugar, fats, and cholesterol. They are a transportable energy source, again moved in the blood bound to lipoproteins.

Lipoproteins serve to solubilize lipids and to target the lipids to specific cell types. Lipoproteins circulate in distinct forms, and these target different categories of cells, meaning that different types of lipoprotein transport their lipid cargoes in different directions between specific tissues. To understand the role of lipoproteins and the clinical use of drugs aimed at modifying them, we must consider these different types.

Types of lipoproteins: good and bad?

Lipoproteins are, as the name suggests, made up of one or more protein components (the *apo*lipoproteins), which combine in diverse ways with specific combinations of cholesterol and triglycerides to produce particles of different size and density. A high triglyceride content gives them a low density—as the triglycerides are delivered to the tissues the cholesterol remains in higher density particles, which are cleared by the liver. We can identify four main types of lipoprotein. Note that in clinical investigations the level of these different lipoproteins in the blood will play a central role in defining a therapeutic strategy, as illustrated in Workbook 3.

1 **Chylomicrons** are large low-density particles with a very high triglyceride content that transport dietary lipids away from the intestines to deliver them to muscle and other tissues for use as energy sources. As chylomicrons pass through the vascular beds, the triglycerides are freed by the action of **lipoprotein lipase**, leaving behind cholesterol-containing chylomicron remnants, which are cleared from the blood by uptake into the liver. In this way lipoprotein lipase activity contributes to the lowering of blood total cholesterol. In part this explains why drugs that increase lipoprotein lipase (section 6.2.4) can lower blood cholesterol.

2 **Very low density lipoproteins (VLDL)** provide the transport mechanism in the blood for triglyceride and cholesterol exported from the liver to the tissues. The major drugs used to prevent atherosclerosis (the statins, see below) act in part by reducing this traffic of VLDL from the liver. Once in the tissues the capillary lipoprotein lipase strips off the triglycerides. This increases the density of the cholesterol-containing remains, which therefore become low density lipoprotein (LDL), which is cleared from the blood by the liver and other tissues. This explains why drug-induced increases in lipoprotein lipase (section 6.2.4) facilitate the clearance of VLDL from the plasma.

3 **Low density lipoprotein (LDL)** accounts for most of the cholesterol found in the blood. It is this that provides for delivery of essential cholesterol to the tissues, where it is taken into cells by binding to cell surface LDL receptors followed by endocytosis. Following internalization, the cholesterol is released from the LDL complex to supply the cells' needs. In familial hypercholesterolaemia (where there is an inherited deficit in LDL receptors), this system of LDL uptake fails, circulating LDL-cholesterol levels may be very high, and there is a high risk of atherosclerosis. Where levels are high, LDL will be deposited in various tissue, and it is here that we see the link with atherosclerotic disease – it is excessive uptake of LDL cholesterol from the blood into the intima of the blood vessel that pays a central role in turning a healthy blood vessel into a dangerously diseased one. This is why high levels of LDL cholesterol are bad. Liver uptake of LDLs occurs by binding to specific LDL receptors. An increase in the number of these liver LDL receptors, and thus an increase in clearance by the liver of circulating LDL cholesterol, follows a number of lipid-lowering drug treatments (see below).

4 **High density lipoproteins (HDL)** by contrast scavenge cholesterol in the tissues, e.g. those originating from VLDL and LDL mentioned above. This cholesterol is then retuned to the liver. This movement of cholesterol away from the tissues explains why plasma HDL is seen as beneficial in maintaining a non-atherogenic balance of cholesterol transport.

Some of the relationships between the different forms of cholesterol circulating between liver, intestines, and other tissues are summarized in Figure 6.3.

In the light of these observations it is understandable that high total plasma cholesterol (TC) and high LDL cholesterol are undesirable. Lifestyle changes and drugs are aimed at bringing down high levels of TC and LDL cholesterol while maintaining HDL cholesterol levels, as explained below. In the example provided in Workbook 6, the normal levels of TC, LDL cholesterol, HDL cholesterol, and triglycerides are set out. The patient Brian's levels are compared to these and this is used to aid diagnosis and the setting of a treatment plan.

6.1.2 Sources of circulating cholesterol and the significance of bile

There are two sources of cholesterol. One is dietary, absorbed from the intestines and transported in chylomicrons to eventually arrive in the liver. The other is *de novo* synthesis in the liver.

Diet and bile

Bile is made in the liver and passed via the bile duct to the intestines. Bile is a mixture of detergents, which solubilize the dietary lipids, facilitating their absorbance. Importantly, the detergents are themselves a derivative of cholesterol. Cholesterol from the liver is therefore incorporated into bile, passed into the intestines, and reabsorbed into the bloodstream along with the dietary fats (Figure 6.3). Inhibition of bile reabsorption would therefore be expected to reduce cholesterol from both the diet and synthesis in the liver.

Cholesterol and synthesis in the liver

Cholesterol biosynthesis in the liver can be summarized as:

acetyl CoA → hydroxymethylglutaryl (HMG)-CoA $\overset{[1]}{\rightarrow}$ mevalonic acid → cholesterol

Step [1], the rate-limiting step in the synthesis of cholesterol, is dependent on the enzyme HMG–CoA reductase. If this enzyme is inhibited (see below) then the

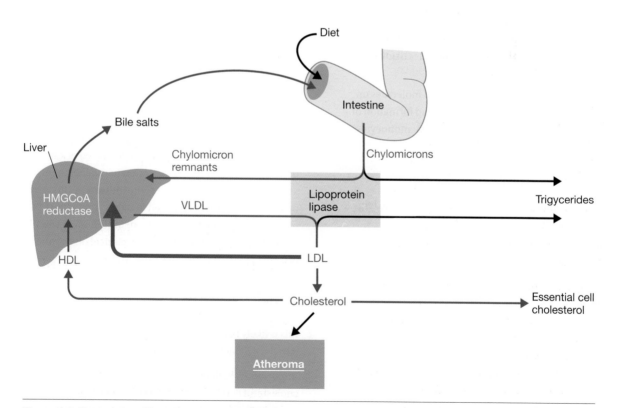

Figure 6.3 Transport and inter-conversion of cholesterol.

In this simplified scheme, a central role is given to lipoprotein lipase, acting on the lipids as they pass through the vascular beds. See section 6.1.1 for further explanation of events in this figure.

liver will reduce its output of cholesterol in the form of VLDL and will increase its uptake of LDL cholesterol.

Steps in atherosclerosis

The slow process of generating an atheroma in the inner face of a blood vessel wall begins with compromised endothelial function, progressing with the incorporation of cholesterol and infiltration of white blood cells, establishing a chronic inflammatory condition of the vessel wall.

Not all medium-sized arteries are equally susceptible to atherosclerosis. For example, the internal mammary artery is normally free of pathology in a patient with coronary artery disease, and so this vessel can be utilized as the donor artery by a surgeon performing bypass surgery. This difference between arterial vessels is likely to be due in part to different pressures, turbulence, and shear forces, all exacerbated by hypertension, which damage endothelium.

The main steps are conventionally described as follows.

1) Injury to endothelial lining (e.g. pressures, high LDL cholesterols, smoking-derived toxins) disrupting endothelial cell functions such as NO production.

2) LDL cholesterol crosses endothelial barrier, accumulates within the intima and is oxidized → modified LDL (mLDL).

3) Expression of monocyte adhesion molecules on dysfunctional endothelial cells, and formation of mLDL attracts monocytes to intima; monocytes become macrophages.

4) Macrophages and injured endothelial cells generate free radicals that further oxidize LDL.

5) Macrophages scavenge mLDL and become large foam cells which form fatty streaks.

6) T lymphocytes and other inflammatory cells infiltrate the diseased wall, establishing a chronic inflammatory condition, releasing proinflammatory cytokines, growth factors, and markers of inflammation such as C-reactive protein (CRP), promoting further LDL cholesterol uptake and white cell infiltration.

7) The plaque grows and matures, with proliferation of smooth muscle cells and extracellular matrix protein deposition, calcium accumulation, and a fibrous calcified surface (cap).

The development of a calcified cap to the plaque in step 7 is particularly ominous, since it is often here that a catastrophic sequence of events can rapidly escalate. The atheroma takes years to grow, and may remain unknown to the individual concerned until the calcified surface cracks, the plaque ruptures, and a thrombogenic surface is exposed at which platelets begin to activate and accumulate (see Chapter 4).

Calcification of fibrous plaque

⇒ ↑ rigidity and fragility ⇒ susceptible to rupture
⇒ exposure of thrombogenic material to circulating blood → foci for thrombus formation
⇒ fragmentation → emboli

Thrombus formation may quickly follow, leading to a rapid occlusion of the blood vessel or the breaking free of the thrombus (forming emboli) to block a further vessel upstream. These are the events that underlie the onset of unstable angina and MI.

Atherosclerosis as an inflammatory disease

Inflammation (see the introduction to Section 3) has been established as part of the atherosclerotic process. The standard anti-inflammatory drugs described elsewhere in this book have no role in prevention or management of atherosclerosis, but there are some indications that some of the drug treatments referred to below may accrue part of their therapeutic benefit from an inhibition of vascular inflammation, e.g. as evidenced by clinical observations of a fall in plasma C-reactive protein (CRP).

6.2 Preventing atherosclerosis? Lipid-lowering drugs

6.2.1 Thresholds and targets depend on the patient

Patients with high cholesterol are at increased risk of cardiovascular disease. In such individuals long-term lifestyle considerations must always be placed first, since they have the greatest potential benefit. Where this approach is inadequate and drug treatment is initiated, this is likely to be long term, and should always be in parallel with advice on lifestyle changes.

Importantly, high LDL cholesterol and low HDL cholesterol correlate with high risk, since LDL cholesterol accounts for the majority of circulating cholesterol; this means that such patients have a high total cholesterol (TC). In practice, the most common objective of preventative drug treatment is to lower TC and LDL cholesterol. There is also recognition that raised HDL cholesterol is desirable and that triglycerides may be targeted by certain drugs (see below).

When considering drug treatment what are the thresholds (e.g. what level of TC and LDL cholesterol have to be reached) for drug treatment to be started and what are the target levels of blood lipids aimed at? Thresholds and targets will vary greatly according to the individual patient. Does the patient have a prior history of ischaemic heart disease or co-morbidities such as hypertension or diabetes? What is the smoking history, sex, age, and race? Help is conveniently provided by rapidly collating such information into an integrated risk factor using algorithms such as that provided in many prescribing guides.

While thresholds and targets are variable, it is always the case that the objective is to lower circulating levels of TC and LDL cholesterol. As a starting guide we note that patients with TC > 4 mmol/L will be considered for treatment. In the case of Brian (Workbook 3), we see from his clinical clerking that he has a TC of 9.2 mmol/L and an LDL cholesterol of over 8 mmol/L (this should be less than 3 mmol/L), with a history of vascular disease (stroke, in his case). So we can imagine, from the account of blood lipids in atherosclerosis given above, the way these circulating cholesterols have been interacting with and damaging his coronary artery walls over the preceding years, leading to his heart disease. The decision is made to proceed with aggressive drug therapy to lower Brian's TC and LDL cholesterol. As a further general guide we might consider a target for a patient such as Brian of less than 4 mmol/L for TC and 2 mmol/L for LDL cholesterol.

Patients at risk may be prescribed lipid-lowering drugs in the absence of high blood lipids. This may include those with established cardiovascular disease (e.g. a history of angina) or type 2 diabetes patients; guidelines may recommend treatment of all such patients with lipid-lowering drugs, regardless of starting lipid levels. Where TC is over 4 mmol/L or LDL-cholesterol over 2 mmol/L, more aggressive treatment may be required.

It is worth noting that there is some variation in targets and guidelines between countries.

Four different pharmacological approaches to controlling blood lipids with drugs can be classified according to major mechanisms of action thought to contribute to their therapeutic effect.

1) inhibition of cholesterol biosynthesis
2) reduction of absorption of cholesterol from the intestines
3) elevation of lipoprotein lipase activity
4) elevation of circulating HDL.

Commonly prescribed drugs are found in each approach. It is important to consider the mechanism of action of these drugs to understand their clinical use and why some combinations may be beneficial in some patients.

6.2.2 Inhibition of cholesterol synthesis: the statins

Statins, the first choice in the control of plasma lipids, inhibit the enzyme HMG-CoA reductase, the rate-limiting step in cholesterol synthesis (section 6.1.2). If hepatic synthesis is effectively inhibited then uptake of LDL-cholesterol from the blood is increased. The statins may therefore be said to reduce circulating cholesterol by increasing its clearance.

Now best-selling drugs, statins include **simvastatin**, pravastatin, and those with longer half-lives: **atorvastatin** and **rosuvastatin**. They are generally effective as monotherapy (e.g. LDL cholesterol may be reduced by about 40% by high-dose simvastatin and by over 50% by atorvastatin). In some patients where response is not adequate, greater reductions may be sought by using statins in combination with other drugs acting by different mechanisms, such as ezetimibe (see below). However, importantly, statins alone are the first option treatment to lower cholesterol in the majority of patients.

Simvastatin has its greatest effect at night because it is then that liver cholesterol synthesis is highest and therefore, being a relatively short-lived drug, it is most effective taken in the evening. A drug such as atorvastatin is effective for much longer and so can be taken at any time.

Statins are now believed to have a number of other potentially therapeutic actions. These can be generally understood from the recognition that the HMG-CoA pathway is involved in regulating events beyond cholesterol metabolism. Many postulated benefits do relate to the vasculature, such as improvements in endothelial function, antiplatelet outcomes, attenuated inflammatory processes, etc. No doubt as our understanding of these non-cholesterol effects develops it will extend the future clinical use of statins.

Statins also have some unwanted effects. The pathway they inhibit is believed to play a role in development, and so statins are not used during pregnancy. The major side effect is myositis (inflammation of the muscles), usually resolved by withdrawing the drug. Myositis with tissue breakdown can (rarely) be serious. Curiously, the risk is enhanced if a patient takes grapefruit juice with the statin. The explanation turns out to be straightforward: grapefruit juice contains inhibitors of liver enzymes that break down simvastatin, resulting in higher levels of the drug in the body.

6.2.3 Reduce absorption of cholesterol from the gut: resins and ezetimibe

Intestinal cholesterol comes from both diet and synthesis in the liver (deposited in the intestines in the form of bile, Figure 6.3). Inhibiting gut absorption therefore increases elimination of both these sources of cholesterol. In order to meet its needs the liver will then increase its absorption of LDL-cholesterol, further contributing to lowering high circulating cholesterol. We will consider two types of agents: one is an old remedy acting as a bulk absorber in the intestines and the other is a newer molecularly targeted drug.

Anion exchange resins in clinical use include **cholestyramine** and **colestipol**. These bind cholesterol in the gut and are eliminated in the faeces. They are consumed in bulk, are unpalatable, may cause digestive problems, and interfere with the absorption of some drugs, including digoxin and warfarin. However, they have a proven history of long-term reduction in coronary artery disease. Also, since they are not absorbed into the body, they play a role, for example in pregnancy, when other treatments may be advised against.

Ezetimibe is a more recent small molecular weight inhibitor specifically targeted at a protein required for processing and uptake of cholesterol in the gut wall. It is a potent drug taken once a day which, combined with dietary advice, has assumed an important role in the management of high blood cholesterols under two circumstances:

1) as an adjunct to statin therapy (see below) when the response is inadequate

2) as an alternative when statins are not tolerated.

Its effectiveness in reducing high LDL cholesterol is proven, its proper place in treatment still unsettled. It is currently not recommended as the first option for either primary or secondary prevention of coronary artery disease. Despite this, in 2006 in the USA there were 34 million prescriptions for ezetimibe.

6.2.4 Elevation of lipoprotein lipase activity: the fibrates

Fibrates are a class of drugs with complex effects on circulating lipids that are only partly understood. Here they have been given a special class of 'lipoprotein lipase elevators' (from Figure 6.3 we can see the central role that lipoprotein lipase has in cellular cholesterol traffic). This reflects their action as enhancers of the expression of the lipoprotein lipase gene. They do this by increasing the action of a protein within the nucleus of cells, which acts as a transcription factor—a type of protein in the nucleus that controls gene expression. This increases the expression of the gene for lipoprotein lipase, increasing the amount of this enzyme within the cell.

Figure 6.4 explains a major clinical observation that fibrates reduce blood VLDL cholesterol, since increased lipoprotein lipase will increase the stripping of triglycerides from VLDL. This moves triglycerides from the plasma into the tissues, thus reducing their plasma levels. Additionally contributing to these changes, fibrates have an effect on liver cells, which reduce VLDL release into the blood. The second major observation is that there is an increase in circulating HDL, collecting cholesterol from the tissues and returning it for reprocessing in the liver. There is, as a consequence of long-term remodelling of the cholesterol traffic, also a reduction in LDL cholesterol. It seems reasonable to suggest that the benefit of fibrates to patients comes from the combined effect on VLDL:LDL:HDL ratios.

While this central action (on lipoprotein lipase) has been used to classify fibrates here, it is important to realize that the expression of other genes is also altered, and so it is not surprising that all the clinical observations cannot be simply explained as a consequence of the increase in lipoprotein lipase expression.

It was mentioned above that there is an inflammatory aspect to atherosclerosis. The fibrates decrease vascular inflammation by further selective anti-inflammatory changes in gene expression, presumably contributing to the therapeutic effect.

The fibrates are generally well tolerated, but do have a rare and potentially serious myositis effect, with muscle pain associated with inflammation and muscle cell

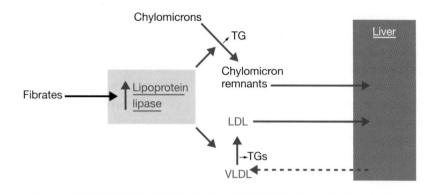

Figure 6.4 Fibrates as lipoprotein–lipase elevating drugs.
Increasing lipoprotein lipase within the vascular beds changes the balance of lipid trafficking between the liver and the circulation. Solid arrows indicate an increase, dotted arrow a decrease.

breakdown. Since this is also the case with statins, these two drugs are seldom used together, and then only with great caution.

Elevation of circulating HDL: nicotinic acid-receptor agonists

Nicotinic acid has long been known for two reasons: firstly, it is an essential vitamin and secondly, in high doses it has a major beneficial impact on circulating lipids. While it does reduce VLDL and LDL cholesterol, its main interest has come from its ability, more than the other drugs we have mentioned, to raise HDL. Its mechanism of action, which has been obscure, was clarified with the recent discovery of a receptor for nicotinic acid, which will illuminate at least some of its clinical effects. This raises the real prospect of new clinical agents acting as agonists at this receptor, targeting an

increase in circulating HDL. However, currently the only drug in this class is nicotinic acid.

Nicotinic acid has been shown to reduce the progression of coronary artery disease and consequent mortality. Nicotinic acid is available as an alternative for those who cannot tolerate statins, and as a partner to statins. The combination of the most effective LDL lowering agent with the most effective HDL elevating agent seems a marriage made in heaven. We look forward to the further exploitation of this with the advent of new nicotinic acid-targeting drugs.

Nicotinic acid has the common side effect of profound cutaneous vasodilatation with flushing—currently it is reported that the modified release preparations increase tolerance. It is hoped that future nicotinic acid-receptor agonist drugs will be free of this complication.

6.3 Ischaemic heart disease: angina

When you run up a set of stairs your heart does more work, and so the demand for oxygen increases. In a healthy heart this increased demand is met by increased supply: vasodilatation on the arterial side provides greater perfusion of the blood. If the coronary arteries are partially occluded then this increase in supply will be restrained, resulting in supply not meeting demand. This is ischaemic heart disease (Figure 6.2), resulting in angina or MI.

The severity of the ischaemic event will depend on:

1) the *extent* of the ↓ blood flow

2) the *duration* of ischaemia

3) the *rate* at which the blood flow is reduced.

6.3.1 Coronary blood flow during systole and diastole

Here we shall first consider the nature of perfusion of the heart during the cardiac cycle. (Some of these issues have already been introduced in Chapter 5 when we considered hypertension.) Remember that during systole, the left ventricle contracts and pressure with the ventricle rises until it exceeds pressure within the aorta—only then does the aortic valve flip open and blood flow from the heart (Figure 5.5). At the peak of systole, pressure in the coronary arteries is not greater than the pressure within the ventricular tissue—coronary blood flow falls during systole. Paradoxically, coronary blood flow is greatest during diastole, when aortic pressure is lowest. This pattern of events is illustrated in Figure 6.5, and explains why a cornerstone of treatment for angina is reducing heart rate.

By reviewing the comments on cardiac blood flow in Chapter 5 we can consider the consequences of changes in preload and afterload. This is done in Box 6.1. Understanding these relationships enables us to recognize what contributes to angina—for example, we can see that stress with sympathetic overactivity, or hypertension, exacerbate the situation—but importantly also helps us to further understand drug treatment of angina.

6.3.2 Types of angina

The three types of angina can be directly related to the processes underlying partial occlusion of the coronary arteries set out in the introduction to this chapter.

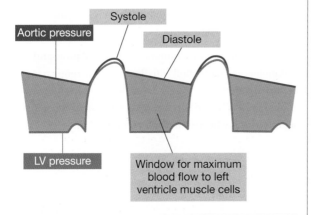

Figure 6.5 Why slowing the heart rate increases oxygen supply to the heart.

During ventricular systole the rise in pressure within the ventricle wall compresses the blood vessels within it, reducing blood flow. This effect is greatest in the *left* ventricle (LV) and in the tissue closest to the inside of the ventricle (the subendocardial layer). The result is that maximum blood flow to the muscle cells in the ventricle wall is during diastole. Consequently, slowing the heart rate, increasing the duration of diastole, increases coronary blood flow and oxygen supply to the working myocardium.

Stable angina is the most common form, and is due to a stable atheroma reducing the maximal capacity of a coronary artery. Stable does not mean that the ischaemia/pain is always there. It means that it does not occur at random, it occurs in response to specific precipitants, such as running up stairs or stress, and so might be better referred to as predictable angina. The predictable precipitants can be understood in terms of upsetting the oxygen supply/demand relationship discussed above.

Unstable angina presents as predictable accelerations of symptoms, often with rapid progression. It is caused by rupture of the surface of an atherosclerotic plaque, with platelet plug formation rapidly reducing blood flow. The platelet plug may dissipate, restoring flow only for the process to be repeated, or a more stable thrombus may form. This requires urgent treatment, partly because of the discomfort caused but mostly because a complete occlusion or breaking away of the thrombus to block vessels upstream may lead to progression to MI.

Variant angina (also called Prinzmetal's angina) is a transient reduction of blood flow caused by coronary artery spasm—this may occur in association with or independent of atherosclerotic disease.

6.3.3 Drug treatments and angina

Long-term preventative drug treatment is almost exclusively aimed at reducing the progression of atherosclerosis, covered above. Here we are concerned with drugs used to relieve the pain of angina or to avert the onset of angina in a patient with a history of this condition.

Most of the drugs described below act to reduce the workload of the heart or increase coronary perfusion. These drugs therefore do not modify the progression of the underlying disease—they treat and prevent symptoms, and with some uses may reduce the probability of progression to MI. Here we have divided the drugs into those where the therapeutic effect is largely due to a direct action on the heart and those (more commonly) where benefit is mainly due to action at the peripheral vasculature. In addition, the role of antiplatelet drugs in the management of angina is mentioned.

6.3.4 Action mainly at the heart

β-**adrenoceptor antagonists** are the main class of drugs in this group. We have encountered these before—they are perhaps best known as antihypertensive agents, and

Box 6.1

How arterial and venous vasoconstriction affect coronary blood flow

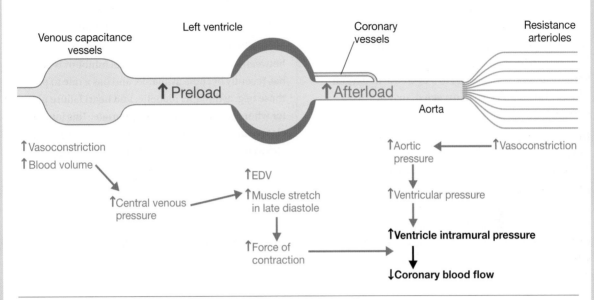

Figure a Relationship between venous and arterial vasoconstriction and coronary blood flow.

The consequences for drug therapy of angina

Venous vasoconstriction and an increase in blood volume will result in increased central venous pressure, increased *preload* and end diastolic volume (EDV). As a result of this the muscle cells will be more stretched and they will contract with greater force (Figure 5.4), generating greater pressures within the ventricle wall (intramural pressure).

Arterial vasoconstriction raises arterial blood pressures, increasing *afterload* and resulting in the raised ventricular pressures necessary to achieve a given ejection of blood, again leading to increased pressures within the tissue of the ventricle walls.

In both cases (Figure a) the consequence is increased compression of coronary arterioles and reduced blood flow to the myocardium. In both cases this restriction in oxygen supply is occurring, since the increased force of contraction increases oxygen demand, leading towards supply not meeting demand (ischaemia).

Increased sympathetic activity (e.g. as seen with exercise and stress) will lead to vasoconstriction on both venous and arterial side.

Drugs used to treat angina include those that reduce venous and/or arterial blood pressures, thereby reversing the effects described above. This will facilitate blood flow to the myocardium (as well as reducing work), helping to restore oxygen supply sufficiently to meet oxygen demand. Drugs used to treat angina by reducing vasoconstriction include **organic nitrates, calcium channel blockers** and **potassium channel activators**. In addition, drugs such as **ACE inhibitors** can be used in long-term management of angina patients, as a result of their ability to reduce vasoconstriction.

their cardiovascular actions have been reviewed in that context in Chapter 5. In Chapter 5 we saw how increased release of noradrenaline from the sympathetic system acting on the peripheral blood vessels changes heart function. Here we are concerned with the direct action of noradrenaline (and adrenaline) on the heart, essentially by actions at the β_1-adrenoceptors, which leads to a decrease in oxygen supply and an increase in oxygen demand. This is summarized in Figure 6.6.

If a patient who has partial block of coronary arteries is subject to stress or exercise, then the β_1-adrenoceptor-mediated changes in oxygen supply and demand illustrated in Figure 6.6 may lead to ischaemia and angina. (In reality, of course, the changes illustrated in heart function in Figure 6.6 and in vascular function in Box 6.1 will be occurring together.) The events set out in Figure 6.6 will be reduced by β-adrenoceptor antagonists and the onset of angina may be averted or its intensity reduced.

I_f **current inhibitors:** a reduction in heart rate will result in lengthened diastole, increasing the time during which heart muscle can be perfused, improving oxygen supply. Reduction in heart rate may be seen as a cornerstone in the treatment of angina, and the second class of

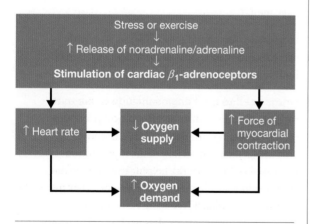

Figure 6.6 Effect of sympathetic stimulation of the heart on oxygen balance.

Note that increased heart rate reduces oxygen supply by reducing the time between the peaks of systole. This reduces the time in a given cardiac cycle such that blood can flow freely from the coronary vessels to the muscle of the heart. Similarly, an increased force of contraction means the reduction in blood flow in the peak of systole is more profound. Both therefore reduce oxygen supply at the same time when they are increasing the work of the heart muscle, thus increasing oxygen demand. β-adrenoceptor antagonists will reduce both these effects, increasing oxygen supply and decreasing oxygen demand.

anti-angina drugs that primarily act at the heart, **the I_f current inhibitors**, and directly target heart rate. The current carried by the sinoatrial I_f channels contributes to the sinoatrial node pacemaker slope, which is the sole determinant of heart rate (Box 5.3). Inhibiting this channel will reduce this slope, increasing the time between heart beats. The I_f channel inhibitor **ivabradine** has recently become available, and has a role to play in those (e.g. asthmatic, diabetic, and heart failure patients) for whom β-blockers are inappropriate. This interesting class of drug reduces heart rate while contractility and atrioventricular conduction remain unaffected.

Ranolazine is a recent antianginal drug of unclear mechanism of action involving attenuated late cardiac Na^+ entry, reduced Ca^{2+} and modulation of ventricular repolarisation and contractility. It is available for patients with chronic stable angina who are inadequately controlled by first-line drugs.

6.3.5 Action mainly at the peripheral vasculature

Drugs placed in this section are not necessarily free of a direct effect on heart, but have a major contribution from action at the vasculature. They have in common the effect of reducing vasoconstriction on the arterial and venous side. Box 6.1 explains how this leads to increased coronary blood flow (oxygen supply). Lowering blood pressure on the arterial side will also reduce the workload of the heart, reducing oxygen demand. Not surprisingly, we have met many of these drugs before in the treatment of hypertension (Chapter 5).

Organic nitrates

The main therapeutic effect of these drugs is caused by peripheral vasodilation; there is in addition a contribution from relaxing coronary arteries. Benefit derives chiefly from dilation of systemic veins, with reduction of preload (Box 6.1). There is, in addition, an arterial relaxation effect that will lead to some reduction in afterload. It might seem at first sight that coronary artery dilation should explain the effectiveness of nitrates, but in reality this may mainly increase perfusion by non-occluded vessels, and so this is thought in most cases not to be the main therapeutic event. However, in variant angina the nitrates may have a major role in reducing arterial spasm.

The nitrates act by entering vascular smooth muscle (and other) cells and there being converted to NO, to activate the cyclic GMP-based intracellular vasodilatation mechanism set out in Box 5.2. Nitrogen oxide from administered organic nitrates also has antiplatelet and anti-atherosclerotic effects, which may be beneficial.

The NO generated in the cells is very rapidly broken down, so the duration of the therapeutic effect is dependent on the kinetics of the organic nitrate chosen. **Glyceryl trinitrate** is used for fast short-term relief, given sublingually, providing absorption without first-pass metabolism (unlike the gut, the circulation from the mouth does not pass directly to the liver). It is rapidly distributed around the body; used during an angina attack pain relief may be rapid and effective or about 30 minutes. Extended action may be achieved with a transdermal patch.

Longer acting versions of organic nitrates are available to prevent an attack. **Isorbide mononitrate** lasts for about 4 hours, taken as a tablet.

Tolerance to organic nitrates is rapid and profound, and must be considered when using longer acting versions such as isorbide mononitrate. The generation of NO from the parent drug depends on the presence of –SH groups on the proteins. These become exhausted with exposure to nitrates, but are rapidly restored when the drug is removed. Longer term treatment with isorbide mononitrate must include a drug-free period in every 24 hours in order to maintain effectiveness.

Calcium channel blockers

The anti-angina effects of **calcium channel blockers** occur at both vasculature and heart. In each case they reduce calcium entry into muscle cells, giving less muscle contraction. The drugs are described more fully in the context of their antihypertensive action in Chapter 5.

Vascular effects are a reduction in calcium entry into the smooth muscle cells, leading to reduced arterial blood pressures and afterload, reduced cardiac work, and reduced oxygen demand.

Cardiac effects are:

a. reduced calcium entry at the sinoatrial node, reducing pacemaker slope and heart rate

b. reduced calcium entry into ventricular myocytes, reducing force of contraction, with a net effect of reduced oxygen demand.

Dihydropyridines (Chapter 5) act primarily on the vasculature. Examples indicated for prevention of angina include **nifedipine** (in long-acting modified release preparations), **nisoldipine**, **amlodipine**, and **felodipine**.

Verapamil is very effective in lowering heart rate, and both verapamil and **diltiazem** reduce cardiac contractility and coronary artery spasm.

Potassium channel activator

The only **potassium channel activator** in clinical use is **nicorandil**. Acting both to increase permeability of K^+ channels and as a nitric oxide (NO) donor, it causes vasodilation on both the venous and arterial side, including coronary vessels.

6.3.6 Anti-platelet drugs in the management of patients with angina

These drugs are discussed in Chapter 4. Acting to reduce the activation and recruitment of platelets, a daily low dose of **aspirin** has been shown to reduce the chance of ischaemic events in patients with evidence of coronary artery disease. **Clopidogrel**, another anti-platelet drug (Chapter 4), is slightly more effective than aspirin at reducing events in such patients. Given that a precipitating event in the onset of unstable angina and MI is platelet activation at a mature atherosclerotic plaque, it is understandable that this process is diminished by aspirin and clopidogrel. Aspirin and clopidogrel are used in combination in patients at moderate to high risk of having an MI.

6.4 Ischaemic heart disease: myocardial infarction

An MI (also called acute MI or AMI), or heart attack, is caused by a thrombotic event in a diseased coronary artery (see above). This may have a rapid onset and progression, leading to the death of working myocytes and causing a disruption of contraction and disordered transmission of the electrical impulse around the heart (arrhythmias, Chapter 7). This may lead to a catastrophic failure of orderly contraction of the heart and a collapse of cardiac output,

leading to sudden death (Figure 6.7). A significant number of patients die within a short time of having an MI.

The distinction between angina and MI is the death of myocardial tissue, and the resulting release of troponin into the blood and change in electrocardiograpgy (see Chapter 7) can therefore be used to distinguish between angina and MI in a patient presenting with chest pain.

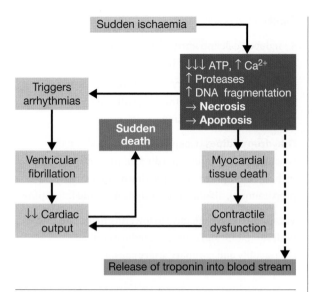

Figure 6.7 Sudden profound ischaemia leads to cell death, myocardial infarct, and risk of sudden or delayed death of the individual.

The ischaemic event normally occurs when rapid platelet plug formation on a fragmenting coronary artery atheroma leads to a thrombus-based sudden occlusion of the artery, shutting off the oxygen supply to contracting heart muscles. Intracellular events in these muscle cells (box in blue) leads to cell death and the subsequent life-threatening series of events. In addition, the dead cells release intracellular contents, such as the muscle-specific protein troponin, into the blood, providing a marker for the prior occurrence of an MI.

Survivors of heart attacks have a patch of dead muscle in their heart, and are liable to long-term heart failure and arrhythmias (Chapter 7) as a result and following the long-term formation of scar tissue. Importantly, MI survivors are at increased risk of further heart attack (secondary). In such patients preventative treatment is a more aggressive application of the drug therapy described above for prevention and treatment of angina.

Acute MI is a medical emergency best treated within cardiac care units, with the intention of increasing immediate and long-term survival of the patient. The acute management of such patients is a medical speciality and with respect to drugs includes thrombolysis with fibrinolytics, anti-platelet drugs (Chapter 4), and ACE inhibitors/β-adrenoceptor antagonists (Chapter 5) to reduce cardiac work and the dysrhythmic effects of excessive cardiac sympathetic stimulation. The immediate treatment of a patient admitted with an MI may be determined by the characteristics of the electrocardiogram, which records the pattern of electrical activity in the heart (Chapter 7). The distinction between patients with ST-segment elevation MI (STEMI) requiring immediate thrombolysis and/or surgical intervention and those without ST-segment elevation (NSTEMI) is further explored in Workbook 3.

SUMMARY OF DRUGS USED FOR ISCHAEMIC HEART DISEASE

Therapeutic class	Drugs	Mechanism of action	Common clinical uses	Comments	Common adverse drug reactions
Nitrates	Isosorbide mononitrate Isosorbide dinitrate	Releases nitric oxide, a potent vasodilator that increases cGMP levels, leading to phosphorylation of protein kinase, which causes relaxation of vascular smooth muscles	Angina Prophylaxis Heart failure	Nitrate-free period required to prevent tolerance	Headache Hypotension Flushing palpitations Orthostatic hypotension
	Glyceryl trinitrate		Treatment of acute angina attacks Treatment of heart failure	Tablets used sublingually or bucally (between upper lip and gum) Tablets expire 6 weeks after opening	
Potassium channel activator	Nicorandil	Increases potassium influx through ATP-sensitive sarcolemmal potassium channels, leading to hyperpolarization of the cell membrane and subsequent decrease in levels of cytoplasmic calcium (and dilation of arterial resistance)	Angina	Treatment commenced with low dose to reduce risk of headaches	Luminous blurred vision Bradycardia Ventricular extrasystoles Atrioventricular block Headache Dizziness
If channel blockers	Ivabradine	Selective and specific inhibition of the cardiac pacemaker I_f current that controls spontaneous diastolic depolarization in sinus node and regulates heart rate	Angina	Metabolized by hepatic Cyp3A4, leading to interactions	Bradycardia First-degree heart block Headache Dizziness Visual disturbances
ACE inhibitors	Examples: lisinopril ramipril captopril perindopril		See Drug summary table in Chapter 5		
Angiotensin II antagonists (ARBs, A2RAs)	Losartan Valsartan Candesartan				
Calcium channel blockers	Dihydropyridines: amlodipine nifedipine felodipine Non-dihydropyridines: verapamil diltiazem				

Therapeutic class	Drugs	Mechanism of action	Common clinical uses	Comments	Common adverse drug reactions
β-adrenoceptor antagonists	β₁-β₂-adrenoceptor antagonist: propranolol β₁-over-β₂-adrenoceptor antagonist: bisoprolol atenolol metoprolol nebivolol α1- and β-adrenoceptor antagonists: carvedilol labetalol		See Drug summary table in Chapter 5		
3-hydroxy-3-methylglutaryl coenzyme A inhibitor	Simvastatin Atorvastatin Rosuvastatin Pravastatin Fluvastatin lovastatin	Competitively inhibits 3-hydroxy-3-methylglutaryl coenzyme A reductase (HMG-CoA reductase), resulting in lowering of plasma cholesterol by inhibiting the body's synthesis of cholesterol to a small extent, and increasing the number of LDL receptors present on hepatic and extra-hepatic tissues	Hyperlipidaemia Primary and secondary CHD prevention	Simvastatin atorvastatin and rosuvastatin metabolized by hepatic P450 CYP 3A4 enzymes leading to interactions	Myalgia Mild transient gastrointestinal symptoms Headache Insomnia Dizziness Elevated transaminase concentrations
Anion exchange resin	Cholestyramine colestipol	Binds with bile acids in the intestine, preventing their reabsorption and producing an insoluble complex that is excreted in the faeces	Hyperlipidaemia	1 month required to peak effect	Constipation Diarrhoea Nausea Vomiting
Other cholesterol-lowering medication	Ezetimibe	Inhibits passage of dietary and biliary cholesterol across the brush border of the small intestine	Hyperlipidaemia	Very long half-life of 19–30 h	Gastrointestinal Headache Fatigue Myalgia
Fibrates	Bezafibrate Ciprofibrate Fenofibrate	Stimulates activity of lipoprotein and hepatic lipase, reduces synthesis of VLDL and enhances rate of receptor-mediated clearance of LDL from plasma	Hyperlipidaemia	Very short half-life and time to peak	Anorexia
Nicotinic acid group	Nicotinic acid Acipimox	May reduce esterification of hepatic triglycerides, decrease release of free fatty acids from adipose tissue and increase activity of lipoprotein lipase, which enhances the removal of chylomicron triglyceride from the plasma Increases HDL and reduces triglycerides, total cholesterol and LDL	Hyperlipidaemia	Very long elimination half-life	Diarrhoea Nausea Vomiting

ATP, adenosine triphosphate; ACE, angiotensin converting enzymes; LDL, low density lipoprotein; CHD, coronary heart disease; VLDL, very low density lipoprotein; HDL, high density lipoprotein.

WORKBOOK 3
Atherosclerosis, lipid-lowering drugs, and ischaemic heart diseases

The patient: a simplified case history

Their family and friends who are gathered in the church clap spontaneously, as the vicar announces that Andreas and Monique are now husband and wife. Everyone is relieved because the couple's last wedding was cancelled last minute after Andreas was rushed into hospital.

Andreas was diagnosed with a hypertensive crises and admitted into hospital for several days during which the right combination of medication for his hypertension was sorted.

Two hours later, whilst they are all gathered in the reception venue and laughing at a joke the best man has made, when suddenly, Andreas' dad, Brian collapses to the floor clutching his chest.

Dr. Carter Brown who is at the wedding as Sunita's date (Monique's best friend) is quick to take control. First he instructs Eoin to ring for an ambulance and then he sits Brian up against the wall and guides him to use a glyceryl trinitrate (GTN) spray and aspirin tablets. Ten minutes later, after using the spray the second time, Brian's pain subsides.

Brian is rushed into hospital and admitted onto the coronary care unit (CCU).

On CCU, the registrar proceeds to treat Brian, whose wife is accompanying him.

A table of clinical clerking abbreviations is given on page xi.

CLINICAL CLERKING FOR BRIAN KAISER

Age: 65 years

Weight: 70 kg

PC: Chest pain and nausea at rest

> *This means the chest pain did not start as a result of, or following, any form of exercise. Note this for later.*

HPC: Sudden onset of chest pain during reception of son's wedding. Started in his chest and radiated to his left arm and shoulder.

PMH:

1) Stroke in 1999

2) Dyslipidaemia diagnosed in 2000

3) Hypertension

> 1 Brian has had a previous stroke.
>
> 2 He also suffers from dyslipidaemia, which means his lipoprotein levels are above the recommended value.
>
> 3 He was diagnosed with hypertension in 1999 following his stroke.

SH: Retired and lives with wife. Smokes 20 cigarettes a day.

DH:

1) Asasantin retard

2) Gemfibrozil twice daily

3) Felodipine

4) Bendroflumethiazide

> Asasantin retard contains both dipyridamole (a vasodilator and antiplatelet drug) and aspirin (anti-platelet) to help prevent a further stroke.
>
> Gemfibrozil to reduce his cholesterol level. Elevated cholesterol increases his risk of having a heart attack.
>
> Felodipine and bendroflumethiazide for his hypertension.

O/E:

1) Blood pressure = 179/95 mm Hg (<140/90 mm Hg)

> His blood pressure is quite elevated and needs to be reduced.

2) Pulse = 60/minute (normal)

> Smoking, dyslipidaemia, his age and his sex all combine to increase his risk of having angina or a heart attack.

Biochemistry:

1) Electrolytes

  - Sodium = 143 mmol/L (reference 135–145)
  - Potassium = 4.1 mmol/L (reference 3.5–5.5)

> These are both within the recommended range.

2) Others

  - Total cholesterol = 9.2 (ideal < 4 mmol/L)
  - LDL cholesterol = 8.25 (ideal < 3 mmol/L)
  - HDL cholesterol = 2.0 (ideal > 0.84 mmol/L)
  - Triglycerides = 1.09 (0.8–1.7 mmol/L)
  - Troponin = 0.05 (<0.1 mcg/L)
  - Blood glucose level < 7 (normal)

> His total cholesterol, low density lipoprotein (LDL), and high density lipoprotein (HDL) and triglycerides are all indicators of dyslipidaemia.
>
> Troponin measurement is used to determine whether he has suffered from a heart attack. He has not.
>
> His blood glucose level is normal so they can rule out diabetes (one more risk factor of ischaemic heart disease).

3) Electrocardiogram: normal

> *Electrocardiography measures the electrical activity within the heart. An electrocardiogram (ECG) reading usually changes in the presence of a heart attack. It is used, along with troponin, to diagnose a heart attack.*

Diagnosis: Unstable angina

Plan:

Admit

Change gemfibrozil to simvastatin

Commence isosorbide mononitrate, clopidogrel, atenolol

> The doctor explains to Brian that he has suffered an attack of unstable angina. Brian's symptoms of severe left-sided chest pain accompanied by nausea are all classic symptoms of angina.
>
> Brian has heard of angina attacks before but has never heard of unstable angina. He asks the doctor, who explains that the heart, in order to function, requires a steady supply of oxygen carried in blood via blood vessels, and how in unstable angina the flow of blood can be interrupted in an unpredictable manner—he clearly indicates that this does need immediate hospital treatment.

EXPLORING BRIAN'S ANGINA AND ITS DRUG TREATMENT

1a) What is angina?

1b) List three types of angina

1c) What is the difference between stable and unstable angina in terms of:

i) the experience of the patient?

ii) events inside the coronary vessels?

_____

_____

_____

1d) Why is unstable angina considered so much more dangerous than stable angina?

_____

_____

_____

The doctor explains that angina and heart attacks (myocardial infarction, MI) are all presentations of what is generally called ischaemic heart disease.

He tells Brian that angina could eventually lead to a heart attack, with increased blockage of the blood vessels supplying the heart with blood.

Ischaemic heart disease (IHD): damage to the cardiac tissue resulting from reduced blood flow (ischaemia). The severity of symptoms depends on:

- _extent of ischaemia_
- _rate of ischaemia_
- _duration of ischaemia._

Brian's wife would like to know how this unstable angina can be managed.

The doctor explains that the key to management is prevention. Part of this involves reducing or avoiding factors that contribute to ischaemic heart disease. These are called risk factors.

He tells Brian that his blood tests showed that one of the risk factors he has is dyslipidaemia.

Dyslipidaemia: This is a term used to describe increased plasma concentrations of lipids (like cholesterol) as well as triglycerides.

2a) What are lipoproteins?

_____

_____

_____

2b) List their roles in the transportation of cholesterol and the quantity of cholesterol transported by each of them.

_____

_____

_____

3) List the two types of plasma lipoprotein that, when elevated, increase the risk of coronary artery disease.

The doctor tells Brian that the drug called gemfibrozil, which he has been using to treat his dyslipidaemia, does not appear to be effective. He can tell this because his blood lipids are still not satisfactory.

4) What evidence is this conclusion based on? (Go back and look at Brian's notes to see why the doctor has concluded this.)

Brian mentions that initially he had been told to alter his diet to treat his dyslipidaemia. This had been difficult but although he had lost weight, his levels had still been high and that is why the gemfibrozil had been commenced.

The doctor tells Brian that the change in diet combined with drug treatment has not been sufficient to bring down his lipids and halt the progression of the atherosclerosis in his heart's arteries.

5) What is atherosclerosis?

6) What are the seven main steps involved in atherogenesis (pathogenesis of atherosclerosis)?

7) Endothelial cells and LDL interact in atherogenesis. Explain.

8) List the names of the main classes of drugs used in management of dyslipidaemia. Which group does gemfibrozil belong to?

9a) The mechanism of action of fibrates involves an effect on lipoprotein lipase. What is the effect?

9b) Explain how this effect is beneficial.

10) What is the most common side effect of fibrates?

The doctor decides to change the gemfibrozil to simvastatin. Brian would like to know why he cannot use both drugs together, so that his levels will drop quickly.

11) Why were both drugs not used together?

Clue: Do statins cause myositis?

12) What is the mechanism of action of statins? Explain in your answer how statins affect the uptake and release of different forms of cholesterol by the liver.

The pharmacists tells Brian that the simvastatin has to be taken at night. She also advises that Brian should avoid grapefruit juice.

13a) Why should the simvastatin be taken at night?

13b) Why should Brian avoid grapefruit juice?

Brian is very worried he might forget to take his tablet if he must take it at night. He prefers to take all his tablets in the morning and get them out of the way.

The pharmacist, on reviewing Brian's notes, is alarmed at how high his cholesterol levels are. She discusses this with the doctor and together they agree to alter his simvastatin to atorvastatin.

13c) Why was atorvastatin chosen over simvastatin?

> Clue: In section 6.2.2 we saw that atorvastatin has a long duration of action and that it is more effective at lowering LDL than simvastatin.

Andreas and Monique both come to visit Brian. They look happy, as newly weds should. They ask Brian about what the doctors have said. Brian says he has been told to reduce his 'risk factors', to prevent a heart attack.

Andreas, who has just suffered a hypertensive crises, says he has been told to do exactly the same.

14a) Explain why hypertension is a risk factor for the development of coronary artery disease (CAD).

14b) Explain why, in a patient with established CAD, reducing hypertension is likely to reduce ischaemic events such as those giving rise to angina.

14c) Explain how β-adrenoceptor antagonist action at both arteries and veins may help to reduce ischaemic events in the heart. Use the terms 'preload' and 'afterload' in your explanation.

Reminder: Brian was put on atenolol, isosorbide mononitrate, and clopidogrel. These three drugs have very different effects, each contributing to a beneficial outcome.

15) Altering the balance between oxygen supply and demand is very important in the treatment of angina. List two ways of achieving this.

Think of one class of drug that could increase the size of blood vessels.

Which class of drug could reduce the heart rate and thereby the amount of work performed by the heart?

The doctor said Brian should be taking his isosorbide mononitrate tablets twice a day. The pharmacist tells Brian to take the isosorbide mononitrate tablets at 8am and at 2pm that is, at *irregular* intervals. She insists that he should take the second dose 6 to 8 hours after the first dose. This gives a large gap before the next dose, so that blood concentrations of the drugs are low for 4-8 hours every day.

16a) Explain the mechanism by which organic nitrates cause vasodilation of Brian's blood vessels (Chapter 5).

Clue: The mechanism includes cyclic GMP (Chapter 5).

16b) Why should nitrates be taken at irregular intervals (Chapter 5)?

Constant nitrate in the body leads to saturation of SH groups. What is the consequence of this and how can it be avoided?

Brian complains of indigestion pain to the pharmacist when she comes round and she explains that it is possibly due to gastric irritation brought about by the combination of aspirin, dipyridamole, and clopidogrel (Chapter 4).

Note: Aspirin and dipyridamole were originally prescribed (as the combined asasantin retard) because of Brian's earlier stroke, not because of his heart problems.

At the pharmacist's recommendation, the Asasantin retard is replaced with aspirin 75 mg and lansoprazole is prescribed to protect his stomach (lansoprazole is an anti-ulcer drug, see Chapter 12).

The pharmacist also tells him to take his aspirin and clopidogrel after food.

Brian wants to know how clopidogrel works. The pharmacist explains that it prevents the platelets from sticking together and blocking the heart vessels.

17) Explain in more detail the mechanism of action of clopidogrel (Chapter 4).

Brian, Andreas, and Monique talk about Sunita and Eoin when the newly weds come to visit again. Monique tells Brian how Sunita had found out that Dr. Brown had actually gotten married whilst they were dating. Sunita had been really heart broken, but was getting over him with Eoin's help. They wonder if the two could now get together because Eoin has always been secretly attracted to Sunita. Monique plans to play matchmaker.

Brian is told he will be kept in hospital for a couple of days.

PROGRESSION TO A HEART ATTACK (MI)

Overnight Brian complains of severe chest pain and the doctors are called immediately.

Blood tests are repeated and his ECG reading interpreted.

1) Electrocardiogram: ST segment is not elevated; however, there is ST depression in two leads.

> *The abnormal ECG with elevated troponin is diagnostic of an MI; because the ECG does not show an elevated ST segment this means it will be designated as a non-ST elevation myocardial infarction (NSTEMI).*

2) Troponin 6 hours after attack = 4.1 (<0.1 mcg/L)

> *Troponin is a protein produced when heart muscle is damaged following ischaemia.*

3) Blood pressure = 195/95 mm Hg

Diagnosis: Non-ST elevation myocardial infarction

Plan:

Change isosorbide mononitrate tablets to glyceryl trinitrate infusion

Commence tirofiban infusions for 72 hours minimum

Commence metoprolol intravenously

Commence subcutaneous enoxaparin (a low-molecular weight heparin, see section 4.2.1)

The doctor explains to Brian that while he previously had unstable angina, during the night he had an NSTEMI. Brian overhears the doctor telling the junior doctor that the NSTEMI was probably caused by a ruptured plaque, which is a common consequence of atherosclerosis. They also talk about him suffering from acute coronary syndrome (ACS).

Brian asks the doctor to help him understand whether his diagnosis is ACS or NSTEMI. The doctor explains to him that ACS is an umbrella term, which encompasses unstable angina, NSTEMI, and <u>ST</u>-<u>e</u>levation <u>m</u>yocardial <u>i</u>nfarct (STEMI). He tells Brian he initially had unstable angina and now he has suffered a NSTEMI, which is like a mini heart attack. However, the treatment has to be aggressive to prevent a STEMI, which is a full-blown heart attack.

The doctor explains to Brian that one of the infusions he is receiving called glyceryl trinitrate will reduce his heart work and improve the flow of blood to his heart and prevent angina.

---

18) Why is this helpful for patients recovering from an MI? Bring preload and afterload into your answer when you explain the consequences of GTN infusion for cardiac function.

Once Brian is considered stable his nitrate (GTN) infusion is discontinued and he can return to oral nitrates in the form of the isosorbide mononitrate tablets that he was taking earlier.

19) Name one side effect of nitrates that most patients complain about.

The pharmacist tells Brian that if he gets a headache he should ask for some paracetamol tablets. She explains that this is a common side effect of nitrates, caused by increased blood flow to the brain as well as to the heart.

She tells him that this usually gets better with time, but he should report to his GP if it is persistent.

Brian asks the pharmacist why he is getting injections under his skin, and what the other infusion, called tirofiban, is for.

She explains that they both work to prevent further blockage of the vessels supplying his heart with blood. The injections under the skin (subcutaneous) are of a heparin drug (in this case a LMWH called enoxaparin, see Chapter 4). Brian has heard of heparin. The combination of tirofiban and heparin provides an antiplatelet and anti-thrombotic effect, respectively.

20a) Explain exactly how tirofiban prevents platelet aggregation.

Clue: Cast your mind back to glycoprotein IIb/IIIa receptors (Chapter 4).

20b) Set out how this mechanism of action helps stabilize Brian, preventing further coronary artery occlusion.

The next day, Brian is told that he will also have to take a drug called nicorandil.

21a) To what class of drugs does nicorandil belong?

21b) What is the mechanism of action of this class of drugs?

....

....

....

Andreas and Monique come to visit Brian and meets Eoin who is also visiting.

As they chat, Brian suddenly clutches his chests and gasps for air. His ECG monitor starts beeping. Andreas calls the nurse, who runs to Brian and presses a red button at the top of his bed.

An alarm goes off, the curtains are pulled round, and about six doctors and nurses come running. Andreas and Monique are told to wait outside.

Later on Andreas is told that Brian has suffered a STEMI. They suspect a blockage in one of the main arteries.

Andreas wants to know if Brian was 'thrombolysed with streptokinase' (see Chapter 4). He tells the doctor that this should have been done when he was first diagnosed with NSTEMI. The doctor defends his position, saying that the patient was not thrombolysed because his blood pressure was too high and he had suffered a previous stroke. He explains that blood pressures above 200 mm Hg systolic/100 mm Hg diastolic are a clear contraindication for thrombolysis. With the history of stroke these would put Brian at a higher risk of bleeding if thrombolysed.

22) Looking back on Brian's clinical history do you think he should have been thrombolysed? Explain your answer.

....

....

....

Andreas says that since stroke can be a blockage (due to thromboembolism—ischaemic) or bleeding (haemorrhagic), only the haemorrhagic stroke is a good reason for not thrombolysing. (Stroke is discussed in Chapter 17).

23) Why would Andreas make this argument? Does it make sense to regard all stroke as a contraindication for thrombolysis?

....

....

....

The doctor again defends his position, saying that in fact under these conditions all types of stroke are contraindications to thrombolytics.

24a) What does 'thrombolysed with streptokinase' mean? (thrombolysis is a synonym for fibrinolysis)

What is the aim of giving a fibrinolytic drug to a patient having a myocardial infarction?

24b) What is the mechanism of action of fibrinolytics?

24c) If a patient has previously been given streptokinase within a year then this drug cannot be used. Why is this?

24d) In such a patient, what alternatives exist for thrombolysis?

Andreas suggests angrily that the right decisions, which might have prevented worsening of Brian's progression to a STEMI, were not taken.

25) Do you think that Andreas' attitude is justified? Were wrong decisions taken and did Brian's situation worsened because of this? What would you have done?

Brian is, however, given the following drugs in addition to his other medication:

- oxygen
- diamorphine (for pain relief)
- atenolol, a β-adrenoceptor antagonists (β-blocker), by intravenous injection.

24) What is the effect of β-blockers on cardiac work?

The doctor tells Brian that his felodipine tablets will be discontinued and the dose of his β-blocker increased. Brian is worried that his blood pressure will rise without the felodipine. The doctor and pharmacist explain that the β-blocker is also an antihypertensive and will treat his hypertension. He will also be started on ramipril, an ACE inhibitor (Chapter 5), which is used for both hypertension and after a heart attack.

25) What is the mechanism of action of ACE inhibitors? How does this explain a beneficial effect in Brian's case?

An echocardiogram is ordered and it shows that Brian now has left ventricular dysfunction and signs of heart failure.

He is started on a drug called eplerenone, which clinical trials have shown could improve outcomes in patients who have left ventricular dysfunction and evidence of heart failure following a heart attack.

26) To what class of drug does eplerenone belong (see Chapters 5 and 7)?

The doctors would also like to do a percutaneous coronary intervention (PCI) since thrombolytics are contraindicated.

Percutaneous coronary intervention (PCI), is used to describe a variety of procedures used to widen coronary arteries that have been narrowed by atherosclerosis. These procedures include angioplasty and stent insertion. PCI is usually performed by an invasive cardiologist. PCI can be performed to reduce or eliminate the symptoms of coronary artery disease, e.g. angina, or to abort an acute myocardial infarction.

During the PCI, the cardiologist realizes that two more of Brian's coronary arteries are blocked to varying degrees.

They perform balloon angioplasty using balloons fed via catheter through his femoral artery to the blockages, and inflated and supported by deploying two stents (metal scaffolding used during PCIs to keep blocked (stenosed) arteries open). Brian is told to take the clopidogrel for 1 year to prevent the platelets from aggregating round the stents and blocking the arteries.

After 2 weeks in hospital, Brian is discharged home on the following medication:

- aspirin tablets
- clopidogrel tablets
- isosorbide mononitrate tablets
- nicorandil tablets
- atenolol tablets
- eplerenone tablets
- ramipril tablets
- atorvastatin tablets
- lansoprazole tablets.

A letter is written to his GP advising that:
- his lipid levels should be monitored
- his ACE inhibitor dose should be increased as tolerated,
- his clopidogrel should be continued for 1 year
- his aspirin should be continued for life.

When Brian gets home, he is surprised to see Sunita and Eoin, who seem very happy and excited but nervous. They tell him they have some news for him. They tell him that they have decided to get married in 1 month's time. They would like to have the wedding in Trinidad, where Sunita's parents are and where Eoin's next competition is scheduled in 3 weeks' time.

Chapter 7
Arrhythmias and heart failure

If you get the feeling that 'your heart has missed a beat' or you feel palpitations (an uncomfortable fluttering), then you have probably experienced an irregularity in your heartbeat. If it is not seriously disturbing and not recurrent then you will probably forget about it, with no further consequences. However, if it is long-lasting or recurrent you may take your own pulse and find it to be irregular; a visit to your physician is then called for.

Further investigation, recording an **electrocardiogram (ECG)**, may reveal that the normally rhythmic pattern of activity in your heart is not always orderly. This means you have an **arrhythmia** (also called **dysrhythmia**). Most likely this will be uncoordinated electrical activity in the atria, which may lead to a variety of diagnoses, the most common of which is **atrial fibrillation (AF)**. This is a condition that can be responded to with a somewhat bewildering variety of possible drug interventions, as well as non-drug treatments designed to restore normal rhythm to your heart. With clinical management, it is seldom life-threatening; in some people it is resolved by treatment and others live satisfactorily with continuing atrial fibrillation.

In Workbook 4, we encounter Den, a patient whose onset of atrial fibrillation occurs after years of **heart failure**. In heart failure, a satisfactory cardiac output cannot be maintained—the patient is compromised. In Den's case, the combination of heart failure and arrhythmia leads to distressing symptoms at the onset of his atrial fibrillation. This combination is not uncommon in elderly patients, and Den provides us with an example of how we may use our understanding of pharmacology to help such people.

Before considering Den's case, we will look at the causes and varieties of arrhythmias, noting that in addition to those originating at the top of the heart (atria), which are not usually a medical emergency, less common ventricular arrhythmias such as **ventricular fibrillation** may be catastrophic and the cause of sudden death. We shall, however, concentrate most on the cellular and molecular basis of action of drugs used in the treatment of the most common of arrhythmias, atrial fibrillation. We will then outline the nature of heart failure, and the way in which drugs act to alleviate the effects of this condition.

7.1 Arrhythmias

A definition of arrhythmia is: an abnormality in the normal pattern of rhythmic excitation of the heart.

In Chapter 5 we introduced the normal pattern of origin and conductance of electrical excitation of the heart (Figure 5.1). We noted that depolarization of cells starts at the top right-hand part of the heart, with spontaneous rhythmic activity in the sinoatrial (SA) node as a result of the pacemaker slope (Figure 5.2). Excitation then spreads through the atria walls to reach

the atrio-ventricular boundary. Here, while the atria remains depolarized and contracted, the excitation reaches the atrio-ventricular node (AV node) and then passes very rapidly through specialized conduction fibres to depolarize the ventricles, causing contraction and ejection of blood. In Box 7.1 this conduction of excitation in the heart is illustrated in a simplified version of the cardiac cycle, from diastole to systole.

Box 7.1

The cardiac cycle, conduction pathways, and the ECG

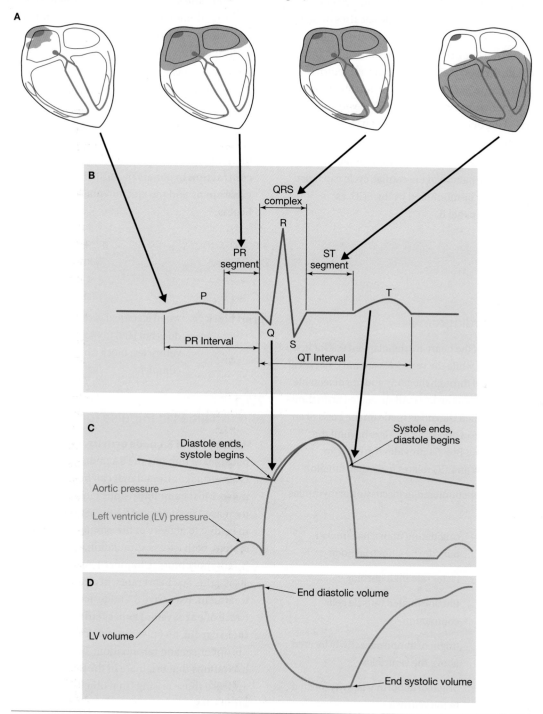

Figure a Panel A illustrates the origin (SA node) and spread of excitation through the atrial muscle walls, collecting at the atrioventricular (AV) node, and rapid excitation of ventricles through the specialized conducting fibres (bundle of His and Purkinje fibres).

The arrows indicate other events occurring at the same time. B, A typical electrocardiogram (ECG); C, Changes in left ventricular pressure and aortic pressure. D, Changes in volume of left ventricle. The following points are notable:

1) **Your pulse is created** when the ventricles contract and the pressure in your left ventricle rises until it reaches the pressure in the aorta (panel C, blue line reaches red line); the aortic valve flips open, and a volume of blood is ejected from the left ventricle into the aorta, sending a pulse of pressure through your arteries. You will note that when you are relaxed the duration of the pulse you feel is shorter than the spaces in-between.

2) Apart from taking your pulse and your blood pressure, the pattern of the cardiac cycle can most conveniently be monitored by the ECG, as illustrated in panel B.

3) **Diastolic and systolic blood pressures** are created by the rhythmic contractions of the left ventricle, and correspond to low and high points in the blue aortic pressure curve, panel C.

4) When the left ventricle begins to contract there is a short delay before the ventricle pressure reaches the pressure in the aorta. During this time no blood can flow out of the ventricle—the volume of the ventricle therefore remains the same (**isovolumetric contraction** in panel D)—until the aortic valve opens and the ejection phase begins.

The electrocardiogram

As different parts of the heart are depolarized (e.g. at first the top of the heart while the ventricles are not), electrical currents are carried through the body and are detectable by surface electrodes as an ECG. All suspected arrhythmia patients will have their diagnosis made on the basis of an ECG. Interpretation of abnormal ECGs is beyond the scope of this text, but Box 7.1 provides the basis for understanding how an ECG relates to cardiac function.

Terms commonly encountered in discussing arrhythmias include:

ectopic beats	originating from a pacemaker outside the sinoatrial node
tachycardia	faster rate than normal
fibrillation	uncoordinated muscle cell contraction
supraventricular	origin of abnormal activity located above the ventricles
ventricular	origin of abnormal activity located in the ventricles
sinus rhythm	orderly rhythmic activity originating in the SA node
rhythm control	restoring sinus rhythm
rate control	restoring ventricular depolarizations to a satisfactory rate
heart block	when electrical excitation in the atria does not lead to excitation of the ventricles; block can be partial or complete

7.1.1 Arrhythmias arising from abnormalities in impulse formation

1. **Modulation of SA node activity.** This is where the pacemaker remains the SA node, but its rate of firing is abnormal or irregular. It can be detected as a fast pulse. Most commonly sinus tachycardia, i.e. increased frequency of SA node firing. This is likely to be due to activity of the sympathetic nervous system, with excess stimulation of SA node β_1-adrenoceptors (Chapter 5). Associated with stress, this fast heart rate will often not require drug treatment. Excessive SA node activity may be a cause of **paroxysmal supraventricular tachycardia**, an episodic tachycardia exhibiting abrupt onset and termination. The term covers excitations that originate in the SA node, and also those arising from other atrial sites.

2. **Ectopic pacemaker.** Severe stress and excess stimulation by noradrenaline of contracting myocytes can change their action potential to create a pacemaker slope (Figure 7.1), resulting in excitation originating in cells outside of the SA node, disrupting normal function.

Normal action potential of a non-automatic working myocyte

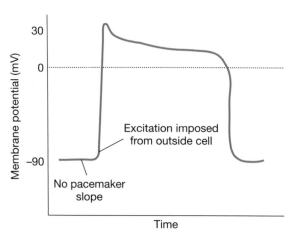

With cardiac injury, ischaemic or severe stress (excess catecholamines) the myocyte may develop a pacemaker slope

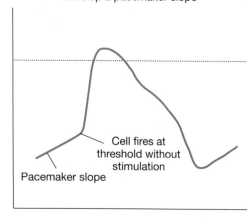

Figure 7.1 Generation of a pacemaker slope in heart muscle cells may lead to ectopic pacemaker activity.

The left panel shows the action potential of a normal contracting ventricular myocyte. The initial segment is flat—this means the cell will not fire spontaneously. Depolarization spreading from adjacent muscle cells will raise the membrane potential to threshold—this is when the voltage sensitive Na^+ channels will open, Na^+ flows into the cell down its gradient and the membrane potential rises to a positive value, an action potential is fired. However, if the muscle cell is damaged or changed, by, for example, ischaemia or excessive stimulation of its β-adrenoceptors, then it may develop a pacemaker slope (right hand panel), with a spontaneous rise in membrane potential to threshold and consequently fire and action potential in the absence of excitation from outside the cell. This cell is said to have developed 'automaticity' and has become a pacemaker, able to set abnormal excitations spreading in the cardiac tissue.

7.1.2 Arrhythmias arising from abnormalities in impulse conduction

1. **Re-entrant arrhythmias**. Damage to a group of cells in the wall of the heart can result in activity circulating round the damage and re-exciting itself. This can set up a self-perpetuating excitation, which can then spread out from the area around the damage, disrupting normal function. The original damage may be caused by ischaemia and is one way in which a myocardial infarction (MI) leads to arrhythmias. A diagrammatic representation of how patches of damaged tissue may give rise to one type of re-entrant arrhythmia is provided in Figure 7.2.

2. **Heart block.** In a normally functioning heart each action potential from the SA node passes through the atria and then excites the ventricles. Ischaemic damage or certain drugs may mean that some atrial excitations are 'lost'. This block occurs to different degrees: partial block when only a proportion of atrial beats reach the ventricles or complete block when no atrial excitations lead to ventricular activity. In some cases (e.g. when atrial excitations are very fast) it may be desirable to introduce a partial block with drugs (see below).

7.1.3 Atrial fibrillation—a supraventricular arrhythmia

There are a number of arrhythmias arising from the atrial tissues and they include abnormalities in impulse formation (e.g. atrial paroxysmal tachycardia) and in conductance (atrial fibrillation). Atrial fibrillation is the most common of arrhythmias, affecting around 1% of the population. It is uncoordinated electrical activity in the atria arising from multiple re-entry waves of depolarization. Atrial activity is very irregular and at a very high rate (e.g. 350–600 impulses/minutes). As a result there is uncoordinated ineffectual atrial contraction. Atrial fibrillation approximately doubles the mortality rate, mainly as a result of raised incidence of ischaemic stroke (to a rate of about 5% per year) as a result of cardiac thromboembolism (see below). Electrical cardioversion is the application of defibrillating current to the chest to restore normal function. This is the most common non-pharmacological treatment of atrial fibrillation. The pharmacological approaches to therapy are discussed below.

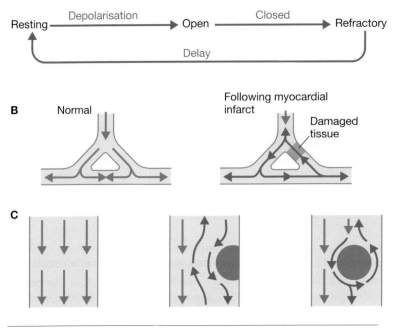

A   Action potentials carried by voltage dependent sodium channels

Figure 7.2 Damaged tissue (e.g. following MI) may lead to re-entrant arrhythmias.

Excitations (action potentials) are dependent on the opening of voltage-dependent sodium channels on the muscle cell surface. When opened by a change in the membrane potential (to less negative inside, depolarization) they allow Na^+ to enter the cell, carrying the action potential forward. Then they rapidly close, and for a moment cannot be opened (they are refractory, panel A). This ensures the orderly passage of an action potential in one direction down the walls of the heart—it cannot go backwards (panels B and C, left-hand illustrations). However, if a patch of tissue is damaged and carries the action potential with a delay (panel B) or via a diversion round dead tissue (panel C), then it may return to its origin after the refractory period is over, when it can re-excite the same tissue, setting up self-perpetuating excitations. If this is in the left ventricle wall then this may disrupt orderly contraction, resulting in a dangerous collapse of cardiac output.

The following points are notable:

a. The uncoordinated contractile activity characteristic of atrial fibrillation results in inefficient ejection of blood from the atria, with pooling of blood. A static volume of blood within the atria itself is potentially dangerous since static blood is prone to form a thrombus, which may be ejected as an embolus liable to block cerebral blood flow, leading to a stroke (see Chapter 17). Patients with atrial fibrillation have about a 5-fold risk of stroke—this is managed with antithrombotic therapy (see below).

b. Ventricular filling is not dependent on effective atrial contraction. This is because in ventricular diastole the pressure in the ventricles is lower than that in the atria even in the absence of atrial contraction. This explains why atrial fibrillation, in which effective contraction of the atria is lost, is not usually immediately life-threatening.

c. However, ventricular filling is dependent on a suitably long ventricular filling phase (i.e. ventricular diastole). Clearly if all these very fast atrial excitations were to reach the ventricles then there would be no efficient filling phase, contractions would be uncoordinated and ineffective, and the patient would be at immediate risk. This does not happen because the AV cannot conduct at this rate, so the ventricular rate is much lower than the atrial rate (only some atrial excitations reach the ventricles), and a life-sustaining cardiac output is maintained.

Recurrent atrial fibrillation may be usefully divided into three categories, dependent on the duration and persistence of the arrhythmia:

paroxysmal   repeated episodes, normally lasting no more than a few days, terminating spontaneously

persistent   recurrent episodes lasting over 7 days which do not terminate spontaneously, but do terminate with drug or electroshock (electrical cardioversion)

permanent   no spontaneous or induced termination

These categories affect the approach to treatment, as set out in Box 7.2. It should be recalled that atrial fibrillation may be treated by both drug and non-drug approaches.

7.1.4 Ventricular fibrillation

While atrial fibrillation is the most common arrhythmia and dominates prescribing for these types of conditions, the rarer ventricular arrhythmia is important as a cause of sudden death. Ventricular arrhythmia is the most common arrhythmia associated with cardiac arrest following MI (heart attack). Ventricular rate is too fast to allow adequate filling, and/or the uncoordinated contractions are ineffectual at ejecting blood, the cardiac output collapses, and death may occur within minutes. Management requires specialist care (see Chapter 6, section 6.4, and Workbook 3)—**lignocaine** is likely to feature in the immediate drug treatment.

7.2 Anti-arrhythmic drugs

We shall concentrate here on drugs used to manage atrial fibrillation, since it is the most common of arrhythmias and illustrates the mode of action of most anti-arrhythmic drugs. We will divide the drugs up according to the cellular basis of their action; following this we will consider their use in the treatment of atrial fibrillation in a case such as our fictional patient Den.

Classification by mechanism of action leads to four main classes plus two other drugs described as 'atypical':

Class I	Na⁺ channel blockers
Class II	β-adrenoceptor antagonists
Class III	drugs that delay repolarization
Class IV	Ca²⁺ channel blockers
'Atypical'	adenosine and digoxin

7.2.1 Class I: Use-dependent Na⁺ channel blockers

Taking a potent non-selective Na²⁺ channel blocker is likely to kill you (an example is the puffer fish poison, tetrodotoxin). However, a drug that binds selectively to the refractory (see Figure 7.3) state of the Na⁺ channel will result in a reduction in activity, which is greatest in cells excited with a high frequency. (In atrial fibrillation the frequency may be up to 600 excitations per minute—see below). **Here the term 'use-dependent' means a**

selective action at channels opening with high frequencies.

From panel A in Figure 7.2 you will see that the resting state is when the channels are available for opening, and in Figure 7.3 we can see the preferential binding means that there is a greater accumulation of channels in the

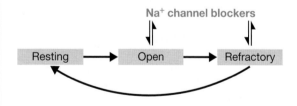

Figure 7.3 Use dependency in Class I anti-arrhythmic drugs.

The voltage-dependent Na⁺ channels on which conductance of cardiac excitation depends exist as an equilibrium between the three states shown in Figure 7.2A and here. The only one of these available for opening is the resting state. If a drug binds selectively to other states (notably the refractory state) then there will be a depletion of channels available for opening. There will be a greater drug effect in highly active channels. This is 'use dependency'. Cells firing slowly will be less affected than those firing with high frequency—activity in the latter will be selectively reduced.

Box 7.2
Classification of atrial fibrillation (AF) and drug therapy—an introduction

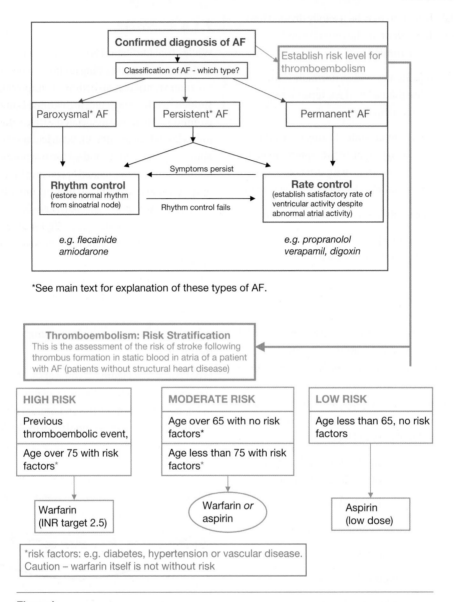

Figure b

Classification of the AF as paroxysmal, persistent or permanent will be overlaid with assessment of risk to inform the decision over the strategy of AF management (i.e. rate control vs rhythm control) and nature of antithrombotic drug treatment.

refractory state, with fewer available for opening. The use-dependent drug does not bind to, and so does not block, resting channels, but does delay the return of refractory channels to the resting state. So a second excitation following very rapidly from a first will find more Na^+ channels unavailable. The effect of this is:

a. Slow conduction velocity

b. reduced spontaneous firing of cells (i.e. reduced automaticity and ectopic pacemakers)

c. reduced high frequency of depolarizations.

The Class I drugs are subdivided into three groups:

1A The oldest of these drugs. Produce a moderate degree of Na^+ channel block, intermediate between Classes 1B and C below. Also notably these drugs prolong repolarization (see Class III above). Examples are **disopyramide**, **quinidine,** and **procainamide.**

1B Strong preference for refractory channels. Dissociation from the channel sufficiently rapid to allow normal rates of firing (e.g. around 1 per second) but not much faster rates, when there will be an accumulation of channels in the refractory state. Main example is **lignocaine**, which has important use in the prevention of arrhythmias following MI.

1C The slow association and dissociation of these drugs from Na^+ channels, and limited selectivity for refractory channels means they reduce all excitations, not just the high frequency (reduced heart rate, negative inotropy). They also slow conductance of excitation through the ventricles. Main example is **flecainide**, which is useful to prevent onset of atrial fibrillation and some ventricular arrhythmias, and suppress ectopic pacemakers. Not used for post-MI or heart failure patients.

7.2.2 Class II: β-adrenoceptor antagonists

These drugs mainly reduce sympathetic nervous system-induced enhancement of pacemaker activity and conductivity. Excessive sympathetic activity, including following a heart attack, contribute to ventricular tachycardias: β_1-adrenoceptor-dependent increase in pacemaker slope activity in ventricular myocytes (see Figure 7.1) will be countered by β-adrenoceptor antagonists. Conductance from atria through ventricles is enhanced by β_1-adrenoceptor stimulation, and so β-adrenoceptor antagonists will increase atrioventricular delay. An example is **propranolol**. **Sotalol** is a β-adrenoceptor antagonist that also has Class III activity (see below). It is of interest to note that when β-adrenoceptor antagonists are developed for many uses, e.g. as antihypertensives, a long duration of action is beneficial. This is not always the case for other indications, and **esmolol** is an example: a β-blocker with a short duration of action used intravenously for the short-term control of arrhythmias. As described elsewhere, β-adrenoceptor antagonists are avoided for asthmatic and diabetic patients.

7.2.3 Class III: Repolarization-delaying drugs

During an action potential the cell moves from negative inside (polarized) to positive inside (depolarized), and it must be repolarized (returned to negative) before another action potential can occur. A drug that prolongs the action potential will delay this repolarization, and increase the gap between action potentials; this will reduce frequency of firing. This may occur, for example, if the potassium channels that normally open and cause the membrane potential to fall back below zero are partially blocked. There are two significant repolarization-delaying anti-arrhythmic drugs, **amiodarone** and **sotalol**. Amiodarone is a powerful tool to counter arrhythmias, but is limited by serious side effects and a very long half-life, so is used under careful supervision. Sotalol combines both K^+-channel blocking (repolarization-delaying) and β-adrenoceptor antagonist activity and, like amiodarone, is useful in both ventricular and supraventricular arrhythmias.

7.2.4 Class IV: Calcium channel blocking drugs

We have previously encountered three types of L-type calcium channel blockers: dihydropyridines (e.g. nifedipine), **verapamil,** and **diltiazem**. In other uses, for example as antihypertensives (Chapter 5), the dihydropyridines are the main drugs. As anti-arrhythmias, verapamil is the main Class IV drug—it acts to decrease the rate of action potential generation in the SA node and to slow atrioventricular conduction, with additional negative inotropic and marked vasodilating effects. The main anti-arrhythmic use of verapamil is in the *prevention* of supraventricular tachycardia (adenosine—see below—is used to *terminate* existing supraventricular tachycardia) and in rate control for atrial fibrillation. It has little effect on ventricular arrhythmias.

7.2.5 Atypical anti-arrhythmic drugs

Adenosine is an agonist at A_1-adenosine receptors, which are coupled to K^+ channel opening, causing hyperpolarization and reduction in pacemaker slopes. A_1–K^+ channel coupling is present in the SA and AV nodes and the atria (but not in the ventricles).

This means adenosine reduces firing of SA and AV nodes, resulting in reduced heart rate and AV conductance. In addition, a hyperpolarization of atria cells reduces excess excitations. Overall the result is supraventricular anti-arrhythmic activity. Adenosine is administered by intravenous injection, with rapid onset and very short half-life (seconds). It is used for rapid and short-term control of paroxysmal supraventricular tachycardias, with an inhibition of re-entry excitations and a slowing of ventricular rate. Adenosine stimulates bronchospasm, and so is not advised for asthma patients.

Digoxin, the most commonly used among the group of drugs called cardiac glycosides, has clinical use in heart failure as well as arrhythmias, and so is discussed further below. Digoxin has two main mechanisms of action:

a. it inhibits the Na^+/K^+ pump in heart cells (see use in heart failure below)

b. it slows AV conduction as a result of increased parasympathetic (vagal) activity, accounting for its anti-arrhythmic activity.

Slowing AV conduction makes digoxin effective in **rate control** (see below) in the management of atrial fibrillation by reducing the ventricular rate despite a continuing atrial arrhythmia. Digoxin is therefore used to control persistent atrial fibrillation, but not to terminate paroxysmal atrial fibrillations.

7.3 Drugs and atrial fibrillation

Drug treatment in the management of atrial fibrillation has the objective of rate control or rhythm control, with prevention of thromboembolism.

7.3.1 Rhythm control

Drugs are used to restore the atria to control an orderly excitation from the sino-atrial node (restoration of sinus rhythm) by reducing excitability within the atria.

Class IA	(e.g. quinidine) and
Class IC	(e.g. flecainide)
	Na^+ channel drugs,
	i.e. membrane stabilizers
Class III	repolarization-delaying drugs (e.g. amiodarone)

7.3.2 Rate control

This strategy leaves the atrial fibrillations but keeps the number of ventricular excitations down by partially blocking transmission of excitation from the atria to the ventricles. Remember that, while you can keep going even if your atria are not effectively pumping, if the rate of firing of your left ventricle is too high it will not be able to fill and eject blood. This presents a danger of cardiovascular collapse. Rate control aims to achieve an effective ventricular rate in the face of continuing atrial fibrillation. AV node blocking agents:

Class II	β-adrenoceptor antagonists (e.g. propranolol)
Class IV	calcium channel blockers (e.g. verapamil).
Digoxin	AV delay

Estimation of the degree of risk of thromboembolism (risk stratification) is used to determine appropriate antithrombotic therapy. This is introduced in Box 7.2. In summary most or all patients with atrial fibrillation will be offered some antithrombotic therapy, most commonly in the form of daily aspirin or, where risk is greater, warfarin.

7.3.3 'Pill-in-the-pocket' approach

As an alternative or in addition to maintenance or routine daily drug use, the 'pill-in-the-pocket' approach provides for a drug to be carried and taken as needed at the onset of fibrillations. This approach has been used by some prescribers for the management of sporadic atrial fibrillations in the absence of structural heart disease, with, for example, flecainide.

7.4 Heart failure

Symptoms of breathlessness and fatigue and signs of fluid retention resulting in oedema[1] alert doctors to the possibility of heart failure. While many conditions we discuss in this book are under diagnosed, it is likely that heart failure is over diagnosed in the elderly. This is

---

1. Oedema (edema in US English): the accumulation of fluid in the interstitial spaces often producing a swelling, sometimes (e.g. pulmonary oedema in some heart failure patients) with serous consequences. In heart failure the leakage of water from blood vessels to the interstitial spaces is due to a raised pressure within the vasculature, especially in lower limbs (e.g. ankles). This is called *hydrostatic oedema*, distinguishing it from the oedema caused by a change in leakiness of blood vessels to protein seen in inflammation (Section 3).

because there are many other possible causes for the symptom cluster associated with heart failure, and these should be eliminated first. Useful confirming observations come from taking a chest X-ray and echocardiogram. An enlarged heart in the absence of other possible causes, and reduced ventricular function with an ejection fraction of less than 35%, is consistent with a diagnosis of heart failure. The symptoms are a direct consequence of the failure to maintain an adequate cardiac output.

Heart failure is one of the main causes of poor quality of life. Its effects can be disastrous. It is also a major cause of mortality. At any one time about 1–2% of the population suffer from heart failure, with a high prevalence in the elderly.

A definition of heart failure[2] **is**: a state where the heart is unable to maintain an adequate circulation for the needs of the body *despite* an adequate venous filling pressure.

In heart failure there is characteristically a raised central venous pressure. In other words there is an increased preload. In a healthy heart, an increased preload will mean an increased end-diastolic volume, resulting in an increased force of contraction and elevation of cardiac output (see Chapter 6). However, it is a cardinal feature of heart failure that an increased central venous pressure cannot result in increased cardiac output because *the left ventricle can no longer contract strongly enough.*

The increased venous pressure in the absence of increased cardiac output means blood accumulates in the venous system (this is the congestion referred to when the term 'congestive heart failure' is used).

The cause of the loss of contractile function in the left ventricle is commonly:

a. coronary artery disease

b. MI

c. arrhythmias

d. primary malfunction of the cardiac muscle cells.

The inadequate cardiac output elicits a compensatory increase in sympathetic stimulation which, because of the loss of contractile function, sets in place a futile cycle (Figure 7.5).

The role of the renin–angiotensin–aldosterone system. The diminished cardiac output also leads to a decreased blood flow to the kidneys and increased sympathetic activity at the juxtaglomerular apparatus—both of these lead to increased renin release.

2. Here we are discussing only systolic, left ventricular heart failure.

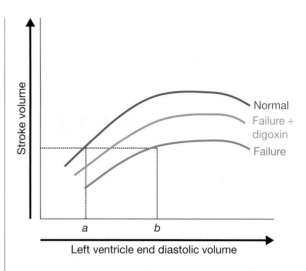

Figure 7.4 Ventricular function curve in the failing heart.

A ventricular function curve was first presented in Figure 5.4, and has been extended here to show the lowered response in the failing heart and the partial restoration of function, which may be achieved with digoxin. In a resting individual a healthy heart with an adequate stroke volume (dotted line) may have an end-diastolic volume 'a'. In a failing heart with raised central venous pressure, generating the same stroke volume requires a much greater end-diastolic volume 'b'. Digoxin is an inotropic drug (increases force of contraction) and partially restores function—note that the target stroke volume can be achieved with an end-diastolic volume between 'a' and 'b'.

The responses to reduced cardiac output set out in Figure 7.6 then contribute to the long-term progressive deterioration in heart function. Included in the structural deterioration of the heart is the diagnostic sign of cardiac hypertrophy (enlarged heart).

The cause of the enlarged heart is a consequence of increased stimulation, increasing stretch of ventricles

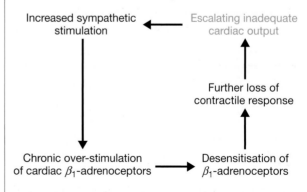

Figure 7.5

Chronic sympathetic over-stimulation of the failing heart cannot restore adequate cardiac output. Instead, occuring over months and years, it contributes to the long-term decline in function.

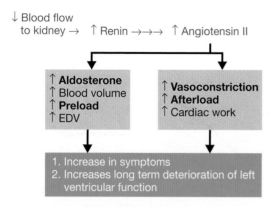

Figure 7.6 Changes in the renin–aldosterone–angiotensin system following the onset of heart failure.

The increase in afterload that follows from arterial vasoconstriction by angiotensin II will increase the work the heart must do to achieve the same cardiac output—the failing heart cannot increase its force of contraction, and so cardiac output falls further. The aldosterone-mediated increase in salt and water retention in the kidney leads to increased blood volume and further increases central venous pressure.

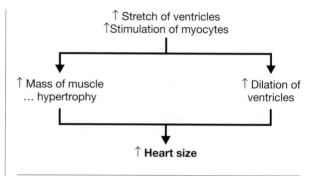

Figure 7.7 Cardiac hypertrophy in the failing heart.

The processes illustrated here start with an increased stretch of ventricles (see discussion of increased central venous pressure and end-diastolic volume above) and increased stimulation of the muscle cells (for example as a result of the chronic increased sympathetic nervous system activity of a heart failure patient). The resulting increase in heart size is then a result of both the increased size of the chambers of the heart and the increased thickness of the muscle walls.

(end-diastolic volume) and leading to both increased muscle mass (i.e. increased thickness of ventricle walls) and dilation of the ventricles (Figure 7.7).

7.5 Drugs used in heart failure

Heart failure decreases quality of life and increases mortality. The objective of drug treatment is to reverse both these trends by:

a. restoring day-to-day function by increasing the capacity for cardiac output

b. interfering with the mechanism contributing to long-term deterioration identified above.

It is noteworthy that some treatments improve cardiac function, but do not increase longevity. This can in part be understood by relating the mode of action of these therapeutic agents to the mechanisms that establish heart failure outlined above, and in this way the response of a patient such as Den in Workbook 4 can be interpreted at the level of his cellular and physiological responses to the drugs administered.

7.5.1 RAAS modifying drugs

ACE inhibitors are first-line drugs in the management of heart failure. These drugs inhibit the final step in the synthesis of angiotensin II, as explained in Chapter 5,

where they are introduced as antihypertensive agents. Their beneficial action in heart failure can be explained by reference to Figure 7.6; start by reversing the arrow in front of angiotensin II so that a fall is indicated, and then follow the consequences through by reversing the subsequent arrows. The result can be usefully summarized as a fall in both preload and afterload, bringing short-term benefit in terms of an adequate cardiac output decreasing symptoms, and long-term benefits from interrupting the progression of left ventricular disease.

All heart failure patients should be considered for ACE inhibitor therapy. Examples are the same as those encountered for hypertension in Chapter 5, e.g. **lisinopril** and **enalapril**.

ACE inhibitors are generally well tolerated. However, we have previously seen (Chapter 5) that a minority of patients develop an intolerable cough and that for such patients the angiotensin receptor **AT-1 antagonists** (**ARBs**, **A2RAs**) are an alternative way of downregulating the influence of the

RAAS without the problems of cough. In the treatment of heart failure these drugs (e.g. **candesartan**) are becoming accepted therapy for such patients.

The aldosterone antagonist **spironolactone**, a diuretic (Chapter 5), also has a role to play in reducing the influence of the RAAS in heart failure. It is mainly held in reserve for those patients remaining symptomatic despite first-line therapy.

Eplerenone is a newer aldosterone antagonist which may be used for patients diagnosed with left ventricular failure after an MI.

7.5.2 Diuretics

Diuretics should be routinely used for patients with heart failure where congestive and fluid retention symptoms are seen. Thiazide diuretics may be beneficial, but loop diuretics, such as **frusemide**, are likely to be the drug of choice. As well as relieving symptoms it is likely that a reduction in central venous pressure will help to slow the progression of the disease.

7.5.3 Positive inotropic drugs

A positive inotropic drug is one that increases the force of contraction of the ventricle. The main positively inotropic drug used for long-term treatment of heart failure is digoxin.

Digoxin

Digoxin has already been mentioned in the control of arrhythmias, where it was indicated that it has two modes of action: slowing atrioventricular conductance and inhibition of the Na^+/K^+ pump. Only the latter mechanism will be further discussed here.

Figure 7.8, panel A, illustrates the normal role of the Na^+/K^+ ATPase (the Na^+/K^+ pump) in maintaining a low intracellular Na^+ with high extracellular Na^+, and how this Na^+ gradient then drives the Na^+/Ca^{2+} exchanger. When the Na^+/K^+ pump is blocked by digoxin, this mechanism for removal of Ca^{2+} from the cytosol is downregulated and Ca^{2+} rises.

This reduced removal of Ca^{2+} when Ca^{2+} channels are opened during the plateau of the ventricular myocyte action potential (Figure 5.3) will result in an increased force of contraction, raising stroke volume and cardiac output. The effect this has on the ventricular function curve of a failing heart can be seen in Figure 7.4—digoxin is able to increase cardiac output for a given end-diastolic volume. As a result digoxin is able to make partial restoration of function, resulting in an increase in quality of life for many patients.

Other positive inotropic drugs

As discussed in Chapter 5, in a healthy heart an increased force of contraction follows from an increased level of cyclic AMP in contracting ventricular myocytes. This is how adrenaline, stimulating ventricular β-adrenoceptors, increases force of contraction. Cyclic AMP is broken down inside the cells by phosphodiesterases.

These comments lead to two ways in which drugs might increase cardiac output in the failing heart (Figure 7.9):

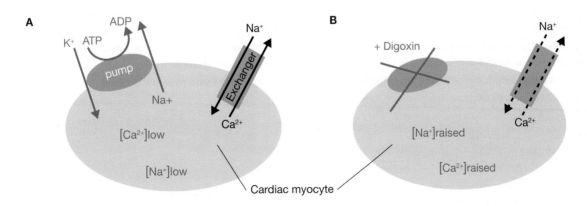

Figure 7.8 Digoxin raises cytosolic Ca^{2+}.

In a normally functioning cardiac myocyte (A) the Na^+/K^+ pump maintains a low intracellular Na^+ level, creating a gradient across the cell membrane. This gradient drives the Na^+/Ca^{2+} exchanger: Na^+ travelling down its gradient results in the removal of Ca^{2+} in the opposite direction, out of the cell. Digoxin inhibits the Na^{2+}/K^+ pump, allowing intracellular Na^+ to rise, reducing the gradient across the membrane and thereby reducing the removal of Ca^{2+} from the cytosol. As a result cytosolic Ca^{2+} rises.

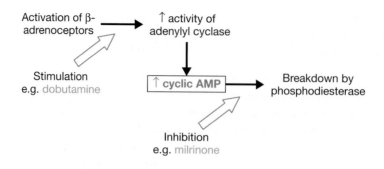

Figure 7.9 Elevation of cyclic AMP levels by stimulating synthesis or inhibiting breakdown.

In a healthy heart: raised cyclic AMP, a raised Ca^{2+} entry plateau in the ventricular action potential (see Figure 5.3) and an increased cardiac output.

a. stimulate cardiac β-adrenoceptors, for example **dobutamine**

b. inhibit phosphodiesterase, for example **milrinone**.

Elevation of cyclic AMP in a failing heart may bring about temporary improvement, but consideration (Figure 7.5) that part of the long-term problem of heart failure is chronic overstimulation of a heart unable to respond effectively will lead to doubts about the benefits of such an approach. Consequently, these drugs do not have a role to play in the long-term management of heart failure.

7.5.4 β-adrenoceptor antagonists

It may seem odd to use a type of drug that we have previously learnt (Chapter 5) will reduce cardiac output to treat a condition characterized by inadequate cardiac output. Indeed the administration of β-adrenoceptor antagonists to heart failure patients has the potential for short-term exacerbation of symptoms. However, by reducing the chronic over-stimulation of the heart by the sympathetic nervous system (Figure 7.5), blocking β_1-adrenoceptors in the heart reduces long-term progression of the disease.

Because of the possibility of short-term worsening, the introduction of β-adrenoceptor antagonists for heart failure patients should be started on a low dose, and only slowly increased with careful monitoring. **Bisoprolol** (β_1-adrenoceptor selective), metoprolol, and **carvedilol** (combined α_1- and β-adrenoceptor blockers) are used in the management of heart failure. Most other β-blockers are contraindicated and should not be used in heart failure.

7.5.5 Strategy in the management of heart failure

An introduction to drug strategy in heart failure is provided in Box 7.3, which indicates that therapy with more than one drug may be anticipated. The management of coexisting arrhythmia and heart failure is illustrated in Den's case in Workbook 4.

Box 7.3

Treatment of heart failure—an introduction

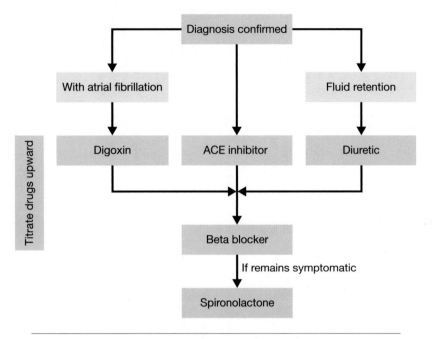

Figure c A possible strategy for the treatment of heart failure.

SUMMARY OF DRUGS USED FOR ARRHYTHMIAS

Therapeutic class	Drugs	Mechanism of action	Common clinical uses	Comments	Examples of adverse drug reactions
Class 1A	Disopyramide Quinidine Procainamide	Blocks Na⁺ channels with intermediate association and dissociation from the channel decreasing rate of depolarization and prolonging repolarization	Arrhythmia	Disopyramide metabolized by hepatic CYP3A4	Nausea Diarrhoea Hypotension Lupus erythematous Arrhythmia
Class 1B	Lignocaine	Blocks Na⁺ channels with fast association and dissociation from the channel allowing normal firing rate but not faster firing rates	Ventricular arrhythmias	Has a short half-life	Dizziness Paraesthesia Confusion Drowsiness
Class 1C	Flecainide	Blocks Na⁺ channels with slow association and dissociation from the channel reducing all excitation decreasing rate of depolarization and prolonging repolarization	Arrhythmia 'pill in the pocket'	Metabolized by hepatic enzyme CYP 3A4, leading to interactions	Nausea Vomiting Arrhythmia
Class II β-blockers	Propranol Sotalol Esmolol	Antagonist at β-adrenergic receptors, leading to reduction in chronotropic, inotropic, and vasodilator responses to β-adrenergic stimulation	Arrhythmia Angina Myocardial infarction Thyrotoxicosis	Sotalol may induce torsade de point	Bradycadia Heart failure Hypotension Bronchospasmdyspnoea Sleep disturbances Cold extremeties Sexual dysfunction
Class III	Amiodarone	Blocks myocardial potassium channels leading to delayed repolarization	Arrhythmia	Extremely long half-life	Nausea Taste disturbances Raised serum transaminases Hypothyroidism Phototoxicity
Class IV	Verapamil Diltazem	Selectively blocks the transmembrane influx of calcium ions into arterial smooth muscles, including conductile and contractile myocardial cells, by inhibiting L-type calcium channel	See Drug summary table for Chapter 5		
A typical anti-arrhythmic drugs	Digoxin Adenosine	Inhibits sodium–potassium ATPase, which increases intracellular sodium concentration, leading to increased intracellular calcium concentration. Aganist at A1-adenosine receptors, which are coupled to K⁺ channel opening, causing hyperpolarization and reduction in pacemaker slopes	Heart failure Atrial fibrillation Supraventricular archythmia Rapid and short-term control of paroxysmal supraventricular tachycardias	Reduce dose in in renal impairment Intravenous injection, rapid onset of action. Very short half-life (seconds). Not for asthmatics	Nausea Vomiting Diarrhoea Transient Facial Flush Cheat pain Bronchospasm Choking sensation Nausea Light-headedness Severe bradycardia

SUMMARY OF DRUGS USED FOR HEART FAILURE

Therapeutic class	Drugs	Mechanism of action	Common clinical uses	Comments	Examples of adverse drug reactions
Angiotensin converting enzymes (ACE inhibitors)	Lisinopril Enalapril Ramipril Captopril Perindopril	See Drug summary table for Chapter 4			
Angiotensin II antagonists (ARBs, A2RAs)	Candesartan Losartan Irbesartan Valsartan				
Aldosterone antagonists	Spironolactone	Competitively inhibits the effect of aldosterone by competing for the aldosterone-dependent sodium-potassium exchange site in the distal tubule cells	Heart failure Refractory oedema Hirsutism in females		Hyperkalaemia Headache Nausea Vomiting Gynaecomastia
	Eplerenone	Blocks the binding of aldosterone by binding to mineral corticoid receptor, a component of the RAAS	Heart failure		Hyperkalaemia Hypotension Dizziness Altered renal function
Loop diuretics	Loop diuretics Furosemide Bumetanide Torasemide Ethacrynic acid	Blocks the reabsorption of sodium and chloride in kidney tubules (proximal and distal tubules and loop of Henle), causing a profound increase in urine output	Heart failure Hypertension Oedema	See Drug summary table for Chapter 5	
Thiazide diuretics	Bendroflumethiazide Chlortalidone Indapamide Metolazone	Increases excretion of sodium and chloride, resulting in loss of potassium and bicarbonate in renal tubule	Oedema hypertension	See Drug summary table for Chapter 5	
Cardiac glycosides	Digoxin	See above table of summary of drugs for arrhythmia			
β-adrenoceptor antagonists	Bisoprolol, carvedilol, metoprolol, and nebivolol	See Drug summary table for Chapter 5		Used in stabilized patients concomitantly with ACE inhibitors	See Drug summary table for Chapter 4

Therapeutic class	Drugs	Mechanism of action	Common clinical uses	Comments	Examples of adverse drug reactions
Cardio sympathomimetic	Adrenaline Dobutamine Dopamine	Partially or completely mimic agonistic actions of noradrenaline or adrenaline on the α- and/or β-adrenoceptors The effect of a specific agent is determined by receptor specificity, compensatory reflexes evoked and the dose		All have inotropic effect Adrenaline is vasodilator at low dose and vasoconstrictor at high dose	Tachycardia Headache Palpitations Tachycardia
Other drugs for heart failure	Milrinone Amrinone	Inhibit phosphodiesterase 3, preventing intracellular degradation of cAMP and leading to increased myocardial contractility		Not used commonly because they improve haemodynamics but worsen survival	Supraventricular and ventricular arrhythmias angina Hypotension Headache Nausea

RAAS, renin-angiotensin-aldosterone-system; ACE, angiotensin converting enzyme.

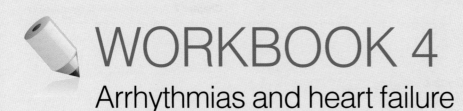

WORKBOOK 4
Arrhythmias and heart failure

Den, a serial heart disease patient: first ischaemic heart disease, then heart failure, and finally atrial fibrillation

The patient: a simplified case history

Sunita and her mum are getting more and more frustrated as their pleas for Eoin to reduce the speed of the car are completely ignored. In fact, urged on by Den, Sunita's dad, who always calls him 'Schumacher', Eoin has steadily been increasing his speed.

All four of them are in Eoin's red Aston Martin, heading for Heathrow airport to board their flight to Trinidad.

They are extremely excited for three reasons:

1) It will be their first transatlantic flight (except for Eoin).

2) Eoin's Formula 1 championship race in Trinidad is in 10 days' time.

3) Eoin and Sunita's wedding is in 2 weeks' time!

Unfortunately they get stopped by the police and Eoin is berated by the female police officer, who is unimpressed when her male partner points out that Eoin is a famous Formula 1 driver.

However, as she starts writing out the ticket, her partner notices that Den appears to be struggling to breathe, as he tries to talk.

Sunita tells the police that her father has a heart condition and insists that an ambulance is called.

At the hospital, Den can just about manage to answer the doctor's questions.

A table of clinical clerking abbreviations is given on page xi.

CLINICAL CLERKING FOR DEN BURTS

Age: 65 years

Weight: 72 kg

PC: Shortness of breath and dizziness

HPC: Shortness of breath while trying to convince police officer not to issue speeding ticket to daughter's fiancée

PMH:

1) Hypertension for 20 years

2) Ischaemic heart disease (IHD) 10 years

3) Chronic heart failure (HF) 5 years

> Note: Heart failure as suffered by Den is also commonly referred to as congestive heart failure, reflecting the congestion in the circulation.
>
> 1. Den suffers from HF, which implies his heart is weakened and failing to supply his body with enough blood and hence oxygen. His HF probably resulted from his IHD.
>
> 2. Den has suffered from IHD for 10 years, which would have placed demands on his heart and then led to HF.
>
> 3. Hypertension is the initial condition Den suffered from. Hypertension is a risk factor for both IHD and HF.

SH: Retired and lives with his wife and two daughters.

DH:

1) Furosemide

2) Bendroflumethiazide

3) Lisinopril

> Furosemide: To reduce the fluid retention also called oedema, caused by HF. Fluid retention in the lungs causes difficulty in breathing and shortness of breath, which Den experienced.
>
> Bendroflumethiazide: To reduce blood pressure.
>
> Lisinopril: To reduce oedema.

O/Q:

Den admits he has been experiencing the following for 2 weeks:

1) dyspnoea – shortness of breath; happens mostly on exertion

2) orthopnea – shortness of breath on lying down; he needs to elevate his head with several pillows before sleeping

> These are both a result of fluid retention in the lungs (oedema) as a result of backflow from the right ventricle, resulting from HF.

O/E:

1) Blood pressure = 140/85 mm Hg (<140/90 mm Hg)

> His blood pressure is not elevated.

2) Pulse = 130/minute and irregular (<60/minute)

> His pulse is extremely elevated and the time between each beat varies irregularly (conventionally described as irregularly irregular).

Biochemistry:

1) Sodium 140 mmol/L (135–145)

2) Potassium 3.5 mmol/L (3.5–5.5)

These are both within the recommended range.

Investigations:

1) Electrocardiogram

- Irregularly irregular QRS complexes

- Absent P waves

An electrocardiogram (ECG) measures the electrical activity within the heart. The ECG changes in the presence of abnormalities in the heart. These include severe IHD and arrhythmia. P waves normally represent depolarization of the atria. When P waves are absent on the ECG, this is an indication of a dysrhythmia of the atrio-ventricular node.

2) Chest X-ray

- Enlarged heart

A chest X-ray was ordered. This will show the size of Den's heart and be used to determine if his HF has worsened. It will also exclude other causes of shortness of breath, e.g. chest infection.

Den's enlarged heart confirms his history of HF and indicates that his condition is worsening.

3) Echocardiogram

- Left ventricular ejection fraction (LVEF) = moderately depressed (30–40%)

A two-dimensional echocardiography test was carried out. It uses sound waves to visualize and measure ventricular wall thickness, chamber size, valve function, and pericardial thickness. The LVEF is estimated based on changes in the ventricle size between diastole and systole.

The LVEF is used to determine the severity of HF.

Den's LVEF of 30–40% indicates deteriorating systolic function.

Diagnosis: Atrial fibrillation (with continuing HF)

Plan:

Admit and commence:

- digoxin 500 mcg IV and then 6 hourly for two further doses

- furosemide infusion (also called frusemide).

Obtain chest X-ray and echocardiogram results from previous admission and compare with current results to determine rate of deterioration of congestive heart failure (CHF).

The doctor explains to Den that he is suffering from what is called atrial fibrillation, which is a type of arrhythmia.

PART 1: EXPLORING DEN'S ARRHYTHMIA

1a) What is the meaning of arrhythmia?

1b) What is the meaning of dysrhythmia?

Den listens as the doctor and nurse discuss his ECG reading. He was told that the ECG was the recording from the pads attached to his chest and his legs.

2) Carefully draw a typical normal ECG recording, illustrating the P, QRS, and T waves (Box 7.1).

Den overhears as the doctor and nurse discuss the 'absence of P waves'

2b) What do P waves correspond to?

They also talk about QRS complexes being irregularly irregular.

2c) What do QRS complexes correspond to?

They continue talking about different arrhythmias and although Sunita, who is a pharmacist, seems to understand what they are talking about, her parents and Eoin do not understand a word.

3a) Define atrial fibrillation (AF).

3b) List two other types of arrhythmias.

3c) What are the main three subtypes of AF, and what are their characteristic features?

Den has heard about arrhythmias causing sudden death.

4a) What does the doctor say to him?

4b) Is AF normally life threatening in the short term? Explain.

4c) Den's ECG has no P waves. What does this tell us about the malfunctioning of his heart and why is it not fatal?

Den is told by the doctor that he might have to be prescribed a drug called warfarin, which he will have to take for life.

5a) Why might someone with atrial fibrillation have to take warfarin?

_____

_____

_____

5b) What alternative should the doctor have considered?

_____

_____

_____

5c) Do you think that in Den's case warfarin was the right choice? Why?

See Box 7.2.

_____

_____

_____

5d) Why do you think low-dose aspirin is normally not as effective as warfarin in the reduction of risk of embolus and stroke?

Clue: Where else have you encountered the danger of stationary/pooled blood?

_____

_____

_____

Den would like to know how long he will be in hospital for and what will happen to his daughter's wedding and all their plans.

The doctor explains that Den will have to be treated with certain intravenous drugs initially and then later on he will be commenced on some oral medication.

The ECG monitor starts bleeping and the doctor tells Den he will have to call the senior doctor because it appears the current intravenous drug does not seem to be working.

The registrar comes and tells Den that because the digoxin does not seem to be working, he will discuss with the consultant whether to add another drug called amiodarone.

6a) Anti-arrhythmic drugs are classified according to mechanism of action. To which of the classes does amiodarone belong?

6b) What is the mechanism of action of this class?

6c) List two other classes of anti-arrhythmics and their mechanism of action.

7) Drug treatment of AF may be aimed at rhythm control or rate control. Explain what these two terms mean.

Rhythm control is:

Rate control is:

8) Which classes of anti-arrhythmic drugs (give examples) are used in each of these two cases and how do they work?

Drug classes and examples used in rhythm control:

Drug classes and examples used in rate control:

9) Which of these strategies has been used so far in the treatment of Den's arrhythmia?

....

....

10a) Describe two main mechanisms of action of digoxin on the heart.

....

....

10b) Which of these effects explains its benefit in atrial fibrillation?

....

....

Sunita asks about the safety of using both amiodarone and digoxin together. She knows that the effect of digoxin could be increased by amiodarone.

The doctor is surprised that she knows this. He reassures her by arranging that the dose of digoxin be halved.

PART 2: DEN'S HEART FAILURE GETS WORSE. MANAGING HEART FAILURE AND ATRIAL FIBRILLATION

Eoin and Sunita agree that their wedding will need to be postponed, but Eoin still needs to go to Trinidad for his championship.

Although they are disappointed, they are happy that Den is receiving treatment.

The next day, the doctors come to see Den and unfortunately have some bad news for him. They tell him that his chest X-ray and echo results have been compared with the results from his last admission. The comparison showed that his CHF has worsened significantly.

11a) What is the underlying abnormality in CHF?

....

....

11b) What determines preload and afterload? How are these affected in CHF and how does this contribute to the development of CHF?

The doctor tells Den the size of his heart has changed significantly when compared to its size during his previous admission.

12a) Does heart size increase or decrease in CHF?

12b) Explain how this happens.

---

13) List two possible causes of CHF in Den.

The doctors explain to Den that the IHD he has had for years has gradually reduced cardiac output, which ultimately led to fluid retention, a key sign of CHF.

14a) What is cardiac output? What determines cardiac output?

15) List the steps through which reduced renal blood flow caused by reduced cardiac output ultimately leads to fluid retention (oedema).

16) What is the effect of oedema on preload and subsequently cardiac output?

Den complains that he feels even more tired and experiences more shortness of breath.

The doctor explains that the shortness of breath is as a result of the fluid retention (oedema). He also explains the origin of the other symptoms.

17) List two other symptoms of CHF.

The doctor tells Den that the dose of furosemide, the drug that is being used to get rid of the excess fluid, will be increased.

18a) To what class of drugs does furosemide belong?

18b) Explain the mechanism by which this class of drug reduces fluid retention.

_____

_____

_____

Sunita tells Den that digoxin is a good drug to have for CHF as well as for atrial fibrillation.

19) Is Sunita right? Explain with reference to the mechanism(s) of action of digoxin.

_____

_____

_____

Sunita, talking things over with the doctor, says that it's a good job Den hasn't been previously put on β-blockers for his hypertension, since she know that this will reduce cardiac output and so will make HF worse. The doctor says this is not correct: some β-blockers could be prescribed specifically to help in the management of CHF.

20a) Explain what is meant by chronic overstimulation of the heart by the sympathetic system.

i) How does it come about?

_____

_____

_____

ii) What is the effect on cardiac β-adrenoceptors and how does this affect cardiac function?

_____

_____

_____

20b) What would be the effect of giving a β-adrenoceptor agonist on the cardiac output of a CHF patient?

i) Immediately

_____

_____

_____

ii) In the long term

20c) What would be the effect of giving a β-adrenoceptor antagonist (β-blockers) on the cardiac output of an HF patient?

i) Immediately

ii) In the long term

Sunita asks why Den is not going to be put on β-adrenoceptor antagonists. The doctor explains that Den's symptoms are not sufficiently under control, given that there is a risk of short-term worsening with these drugs. They remain an option for longer-term management.

Instead the doctor tells Den that the dose of the drug called lisinopril, which he was taking at home, will also be increased.

Den is not too happy because he says he has got a persistent dry cough, which started soon after he commenced the lisinopril. His GP advised him to persevere until the cough improved. The cough had not improved and he had thought it was pointless to tell the GP this because he had got the impression from the GP that there was no other drug that could replace the lisinopril.

The doctor tells Den that actually there is another drug he can try as a substitute to lisinopril, if the cough is causing Den a lot of distress. He explains that the lisinopril will be changed to another drug belonging to a class called angiotensin antagonists (or angiotensin receptor blockers, ARBs).

21a) Which class of drug does lisinopril belong to and by what mechanism of action does it work in the treatment of CHF?

21b) Explain why the ARBs are less likely to cause a dry cough.

Den improves significantly after 2 days and his infusions are changed to tablets. The doctor approaches Sunita and tells her that he has decided, with respect to their earlier discussion about drugs acting as β-adrenoceptors, that he has now decided that Den is suitably controlled to justify the use of a tablet called bisoprolol. He also decides to stop the amiodarone tablets because of the risk of all three drugs (amiodarone, digoxin, and bisoprolol) causing bradycardia and possible heart block. He explains to Den that bisoprolol also has anti-arrhythmic effects.

22a) What class of drug does bisoprolol belong to?

22b) What is the likely mechanism of action by which β-blockers help in CHF?

After 3 weeks in hospital, Den is discharged home on the following medication:

- warfarin tablets
- candesartan tablets
- furosemide tablets
- digoxin tablets
- bisoprolol tablets.

Den improves significantly over the next 8 weeks. The wedding is rescheduled for April the following year.

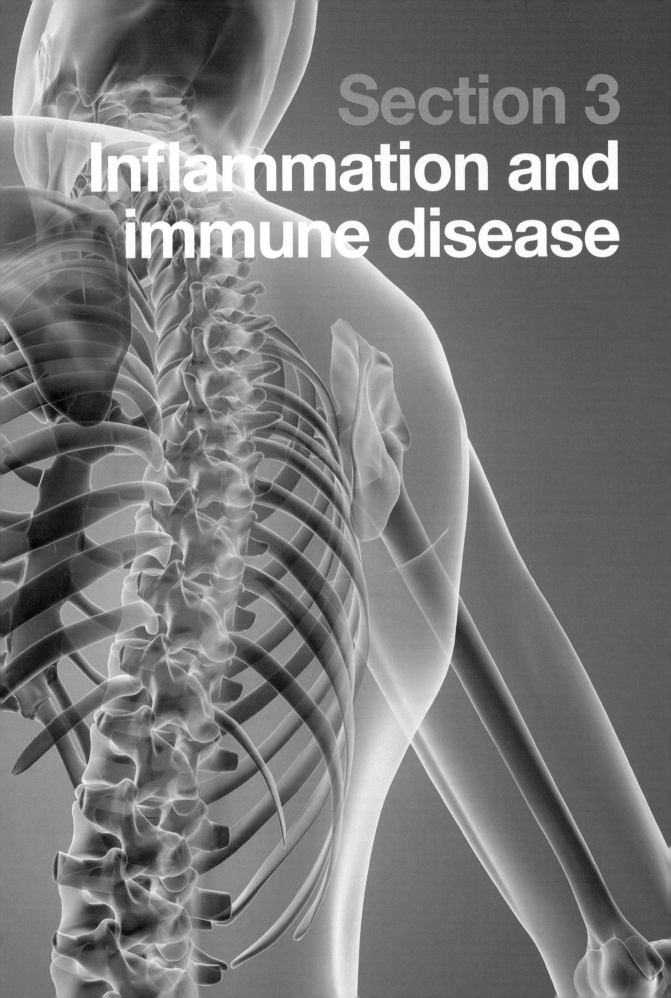

Section 3
Inflammation and immune disease

It may seem surprising that our bodies, being warm, damp, and full of nutrients, don't rapidly rot from the inside out. After all, we provide perfect conditions for the growth of bacteria, fungi, etc. Indeed, as we all know, we do from time to time become cultures of these and other unwanted small life forms, and when this happens we need to consider drugs that will help us overcome infections; this situation is described in Chapter 21. Here we are going to introduce some of the mechanisms in the body which protect us from damage because they can also create a whole range of medical conditions, both common and unusual, and ranging from minor to life-threatening. The protective mechanisms that we all need to survive are inflammation and the immune response, and we need to summarize these processes before we can consider patients and their drug treatment.

The body is protected from invasion by several mechanical and chemical barriers. The most obvious of these is the skin, which stops surface organisms and chemicals that we come in contact with from penetrating the body by providing a waterproof, physical barrier. Some examples of chemical barriers are the acid of the stomach (see Chapter 12) and lysosomes (enzymes that break down the cell walls of bacteria) in our tears. Other protective responses include sneezing, coughing, crying (tearing), and vomiting, all of which try to expel the substance before it can penetrate into the body. If these mechanical and chemical barriers fail it is up to the immune system to protect us.

The immune system, and the inflammatory response, is critical to the body in protecting itself from invasion from foreign bodies (e.g. bacteria) and from damage from within the body (e.g. inflammation after tearing ligaments or tendons). Without it we would succumb to infections, as can people who have inherent (i.e. inborn) or acquired (e.g. HIV or immunosuppressant drug) deficiencies in their immune system. While the immune system is vital to maintain life, sometimes the immune and inflammatory responses react to relatively harmless substances (e.g. pollens) or to proteins normally found within the body, and when the inflammatory response is prolonged it can lead to local pathologies: in the skin it may give rise to the discomfort of eczema; in the joints the result is pain, joint destruction, and permanent loss of movement, such as in rheumatoid arthritis; the nose and eyes may suffer from allergies like hay fever; and in the lungs the result may be asthma. These disease states are commonly modified with drugs; we also try to modify the immune response to maintain life, such as stopping organ rejection after transplantation (e.g. heart transplants). To understand how we can treat or modify inflammation and immune reactions it is important to understand how they interrelate.

Broadly speaking the immune response is divided into innate and adaptive responses. The major differences in these two responses are outlined in Table S3.1.

Table S3.1 The features of innate and adaptive immunity

Innate response (non-specific immunity)	Adaptive response (specific immunity)
Does not rely on an antigen	Requires an exposure from a specific antigen
Quick onset	Slow and delayed onset
Does not result in any immunologic 'memory'	Results in an immunologic 'memory'
Operates from birth	Is acquired after birth
Does not change response with subsequent exposure	Often increases in response to subsequent exposure

S3.1 Innate immune response

The innate response involves humoral (blood borne), chemical, and cellular components. The major constituent of the humoral response is the activation of the complement system, which comprises over 20 different proteins. This contributes to the immune system in a number of ways (hence it is called complement, because it 'complements' the other immune responses), including:

- increasing vascular permeability (resulting in fluid leaking from the bloodstream into the area)
- attracting and activating inflammatory cells such as polymorphonuclear cells and macrophages
- stimulating de-granulation (release of histamine granules) from basophils and mast cells
- opsonizing invading organisms (make changes to the outside of bacteria so that they are targeted and more easily removed by macrophages).

The major chemical constituents of the innate response are eicosanoids, and the principle ones are prostaglandins and thromboxanes (collectively called prostanoids), and leukotrienes. These are synthesised from arachidonic acid via lipoxygenases and cyclooxygenases (Figure S3.1).

The effects of the eicosanoids are outlined in Table S3.2.

The cellular components of the innate response involve neutrophils, macrophages, natural killer (NK) cells, and eosinophils. The neutrophils and macrophages are recruited to phagocytose (engulf the particle and destroy) the invader. In addition,

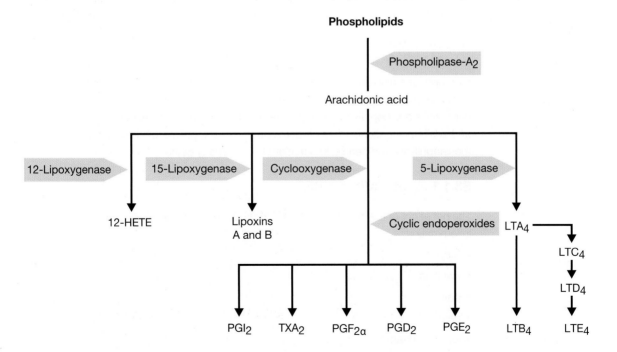

Figure S3.1 Eicosanoid sythesis.

HETE, hydroxyeicosatetraenoic acid; PG, prostaglandin; TX, thromboxane; LT, leukotriene.

Table S3.2 Effects of eicosanoids

Eicoisanoid	Effect					
	Vascular smooth muscle	Vascular permeability	Platelet aggregation	Respiratory smooth muscle	Pain	Other
Prostaglandin I_2	↑		↓		↑	
Thromboxane A_2	↓		↑			
Prostaglandin $F_{2\alpha}$				↓		↑ uterine contraction
Prostaglandin D_2	↑		↓			
Prostaglandin E_2	↑				↑	↓ gastric acid; ↑ gastric mucous
Leukotriene B_4						↑ movement of cells (chemotaxis)
Leukotriene C_4		↑		↓		↑ respiratory mucous
Leukotriene D_4		↑		↓		↑ respiratory mucous
Leukotriene E_4		↑		↓		↑ respiratory mucous
12-HETE						↑ movement of cells (chemotaxis)
Lipoxins						↓ the actions of LTB_4

↑ = increases/dilates; ↓ = decreases/constricts

macrophages also act as antigen-presenting cells and can be involved in the adaptive response (see later). Natural killer cells non-specifically destroy viruses and tumour cells, while eosinophils release granules containing proteins (i.e. major basic protein and eosinophil cationic protein), peroxidases (eosinophil peroxidase), and neurotoxins (eosinophil-derived neurotoxin) that are toxic to many cells.

S3.1.1 Acute inflammation

The net effect of the innate response is to produce the cardinal signs of acute inflammation:

• redness

• swelling

• pain

• heat

• loss of movement.

Redness and heat at the sight of infection/damage occur because of increased blood flow to the region due to vasodilatation. The increased vascular permeability, along with increased blood flow, results in leakage of fluid into the tissues, resulting in swelling, while pain is caused by the sensitization of nociceptors (pain receptors) by prostaglandins. Loss of movement occurs because of the pain and swelling around the joint (if that is the location of the injury/infection).

It is important to remember that these acute effects are protective, aimed at removing invading organisms or preventing further damage by restricting movement, thus allowing the body to start to repair an injured area. For example, when we treat acute inflammation after a sporting injury with injections of corticosteroids, it is important to still allow the body to repair by resting the area (i.e. stopping movement) otherwise further damage may occur (which can be masked by the injection of a powerful antiinflammatory).

S3.2 Adaptive immune response

The adaptive, sometimes called the acquired, immune response occurs because of exposure to specific pathogens. The advantage of adaptive immunity is that it allows a tailored response to an organism or substrate that can increase in intensity with subsequent exposure due to the ability to 'remember' the invader (immunologic 'memory'). The adaptive response underpins the basis of vaccinations.

The three steps or stages in the adaptive response are:

- recognition of a foreign (non-self) antigen
- activation of a specific response to that antigen by recruiting specific cells and/or the production of antibodies, which involves lymphocytes
- development of a 'memory' for future invasions.

S3.2.1 Antigens

Antigens are proteins or polysaccharides that cause the production of antibodies and induce the immune response. Microbial sources include fragments from the outer coats or membranes of bacteria, moulds, or viruses. These are usually produced by cells absorbing the microorganism (phagocytosis) and then breaking down the outer coat or membrane. The cells involved in this process are called antigen-presenting cells and include dendritic cells and macrophages. Dendritic cells are found in tissues that are exposed to the elements, including the skin (called Langerhans cells), and the lining of the nose, lungs, stomach, and intestines, while macrophages develop from monocytes that circulate in the bloodstream. Non-infective sources of antigens include eggs, nuts, and pollens. All of these antigens are called 'non-self' antigens.

Host cells produce antigens that are called 'self' antigens and the immune system distinguishes between 'self' and 'non-self' antigens, thus stopping the body from attacking its own cells. However, this system can sometimes break down, and this produces what are called autoimmune diseases. Examples include coeliac disease (a gastrointestinal disorder attacking the lining of the intestine), systemic lupus erythematosus (causing chronic inflammation in a range of tissues, including the heart, lungs, and kidneys), and multiple sclerosis (a condition where the myelin sheath that surrounds neurones and enables normal electrical transmission is affected, leading to neurological complications).

S3.2.2 Lymphocytes

Lymphocytes are a class of white blood cells that fall into two main types: B- and T-lymphocytes (called B- and T-cells). They are central to mounting an adaptive immune response. The role of B- and T-cells in this process is explored in Figure S3.2.

S3.2.3 Memory cells

An important feature of the adaptive immune response is the ability to 'remember' an antigen and then respond quickly the next time the antigen appears. After B- and

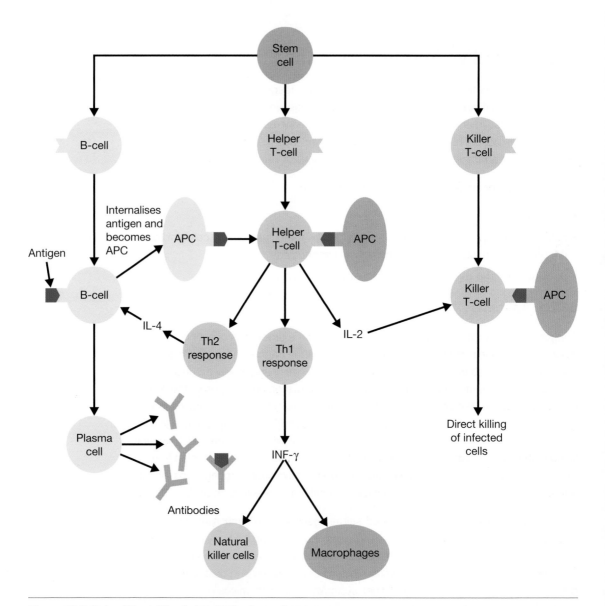

Figure S3.2 Role of B- and T-cells in adaptive immunity.

APC, antigen-presenting cell; IL-4, interleukin-4; IL-2, interleukin-2; INF-γ, interferon gamma; Th1, type 1 helper T-cell; Th2, type 2 helper T-cell.

T-cells are activated by an antigen most will die and be removed from the body. However, a few B- and T-cells will remain within the body and form the basis of the 'memory' databank for the body. The next time the same antigen is encountered these cells will reactivate and the response will be faster and stronger than on the first exposure. This is called 'active memory' and is the basis of vaccination. Newborn babies experience 'passive memory' from their mother through the passage of antibodies across the placenta and in breast milk. However, this memory is short lived, lasting a few days to months, and is aimed at providing early protection from bacteria and other organisms.

S3.3 Mast cells, eosinophils, and mediators of inflammation

You will encounter mast cells and eosinophils at various times when considering inflammation-related disorders and drugs. Mast cells are permanently present within tissues in contact with the outside world, such as the skin and lungs. Eosinophils are another type of white blood cell—they migrate into tissues from the circulation (passing through the blood vessel walls) when attracted by certain mediators that are released from other cells within the tissue. These mediator-releasing cells are themselves resident mast cells or eosinophils already within the tissue.

S3.4 Cytokines and chemokines

Cytokines and chemokines are signalling molecules involved in the inflammatory process. The cytokines are a large group of proteins, peptides, and glycoproteins that attach to specific cell surface receptors. Examples of cytokines are outlined in Table S3.3.

Chemokines are a subset of cytokines. They are involved in the migration of inflammatory cells and help to coordinate the immune response. The chemokines are classified based on the spacing of the first two cystine molecules, and the main groups are CC chemokines (two adjacent cystine molecules), which act on monocytes and lymphocytes and are involved with chronic inflammation, and CXC chemokines

Table S3.3 Examples of cytokines

Family	Examples	Role/function
Colony-stimulating factors	Granulocyte monocyte colony-stimulating factor (GM-CSF)	Differentiation and growth of monocytes and dendridic cells
Interleukins	Interleukin 1a/1b (IL-1) Interleukin 4 (IL-4)	Pro-inflammatory Anti-inflammatory
Interferons	Interferon γ (INF-γ)	Proliferation T-helper cells; viral replication
Grow factors	Tumour growth factor β (TGF-β)	Stimulate cytokine synthesis
Tumour necrosis factors	Tumour necrosis factor α (TNF-α)	Cytokine expression and apoptosis (cell death)

(the two cystine molecules are separated by another molecule), which act on neutrophils and are involved in acute inflammation.

S3.4.1 Immune and inflammatory illnesses

Disorders of the immune system can affect nearly every part of the body. They range from acute, self-limiting conditions such as soft tissue injuries, through to severe, chronic, and disabling illnesses such as rheumatoid arthritis. This section will provide an account of allergic and inflammatory skin conditions (psoriasis and urticaria), allergic and inflammatory respiratory conditions (hayfever and asthma), and inflammatory joint disease (rheumatoid arthritis). We shall consider the major drugs used to manage these conditions, and will introduce some individual patients who struggle with their disease and with the correct treatment.

Chapter 8
Inflammation and the skin: dermatitis, acne, and psoriasis

In Workbook 5 we will meet Elvis, who is 13 years old and scratches away, night and day, at his scaly and cracked skin until it is bruised and bleeding. We should take pity on poor Elvis. As a baby he was tortured by red and swollen rashes at the back of his neck and the inside of his elbows. In addition to his **dermatitis** he developed asthma at an early age, so he was awake at night wheezing and scratching. He was a typically **atopic**[1] child. As he grew up he seemed to leave these childhood complaints behind, until he entered the teenage years, when his dermatitis returned. Now, not only did he have to cope with the discomfort, but also with the embarrassment.

Then think of Elvis's 18-year-old cousin Eimear, who has about 10 lesions on her chin, forehead, and nose, some of which are pus filled. She was diagnosed with acne and has tried several different treatment options. She is extremely shy and only leaves the house to go to school because her acne has led to social rejection.

Or put yourself in the shoes of one of Elvis's teachers, who has psoriasis. His shirt or jacket is always covered with embarrassing white flakes that have fallen off the silvery white scaly plaques on his head, ears, and elbows. They look even worse with the exposed bleeding points that are evident when he scratches them (which he does very often because they itch all the time).

These three individuals are amongst the millions of patients who visit their doctors and pharmacists every year seeking answers and help to alleviate their symptoms. Ten to twenty per cent of consultations in general practice are for skin conditions. Some skin conditions are long term and extremely difficult to cure. For these chronic conditions, treatment is used to reduce their severity and the associated discomfort, improve appearance, and reduce the psychological distress that could be caused by social rejection. Most of the patients dislike the treatment for varying reasons, including the messiness, awkwardness, and side effects. These patients and their carers need encouragement, education, and counselling. Correct management of skin conditions will not only alleviate discomfort and pain but also go a long way to relieve the huge psychological impact of skin conditions.

In order to achieve this, prescribers must have a good understanding of the symptoms and underlying causes of skin conditions, and the way in which these can be treated by the many preparations and drugs available. A firm understanding of the underlying cause of skin conditions will help with accurate diagnosis and provision of individualized treatment.

Some of the major skin diseases are set out in Table 8.1.

In this chapter we shall start by describing the structure and function of the skin, followed by some general comments on the use of medications for direct application to the skin. We shall then concentrate on the first three of the common skin conditions set out in Table 8.1—**dermatitis**, **acne** and **psoriasis**—setting out the underlying mechanisms of these conditions before moving on to their treatment. Finally, in Workbook 5 we end the chapter with examples of the management of individual patients presenting with each of these three conditions.

---

1. Atopy is an inherited tendency to develop an elevated immune responsiveness. It is associated with increased IgE levels. The result is a general hypersensitivity to substances that may be innocuous in most people (e.g. pollen, house mites, cat hairs), leading to allergic reactions such as hay fever, asthma, and atopic dermatitis.

Table 8.1 Most common skin conditions

Clinical diseases	Common locations	Prevalence (%)
Dermatitis and eczema	Seborrhoeic[a] dermatitis: scalp, face, and ears	10
	Dermatitis: neck and elbows	7–30
Acne	Face, chest upper back, and arms	22–33 (almost 90% in teenagers)
Psoriasis	Head, ears, and elbows	1–3
Viral warts	Hands and feet	1–16
Skin cancer	Exposed skin	0.3
Fungal and bacterial infections	All over	10–20

[a] Seborrhoeic means an abnormal discharge from the sebaceous glands, resulting in an oily coating, crusts, or scales on the skin.

8.1 Anatomy and physiology of the skin

The skin is the body's largest organ, constituting about 16% of body weight. The main functions of the skin are:

- protection against heat, light, injury and infection
- regulation of body temperature
- retention by the body of water
- biochemical synthesis (e.g. vitamin D is produced in skin exposed to sunlight)
- sensory detection of painful and pleasant stimulation
- social and sexual communication.

The three main layers of the skin are the epidermis, dermis, and subcutis (subcutaneous layer). The function and characteristics of the various layers of the skin, and sublayers of the epidermis, are illustrated and summarized in Box 8.1.

Thin skin, thick skin

The skin provides a two-way barrier, preventing absorption of substances from the surroundings as well as loss of water and electrolytes from beneath the skin. The skin's thickness, colour, and texture vary throughout the body. For example, the head contains more hair follicles than anywhere else, whilst the palms of the hand contain none; the skin is thicker on the soles of the feet and palms of the hand than elsewhere. Of the layers of the skin, it is the epidermis which is thicker in thick skin—the sublayers of the epidermis responsible for this are set out in Box 8.1. The issue of thick skin and thin skin is important in clinical pharmacology, in part because absorption of topically applied drugs (think of the steroid creams used to treat eczema) into the circulation is significantly greater with thin skin. In dermatology this is usually undesirable.

8.2 Drugs and vehicles: medication for topical use

Treatments of skin conditions aim to alleviate the underlying cause of the damage, and restore and optimize the skin's normal function. Preparations to treat skin conditions are chosen to either treat the specific disease or increase skin protection from the environment.

The preparations used to treat skin disease include those we can obviously label as drugs, such as steroids, but also medications with therapeutic responses that are not due to a drug interacting with specific proteins within cells. An example is the **emollients**, which are absorbed in bulk into

the skin, softening and moisturising it. Their mechanism of action differs fundamentally from that of the majority of drugs discussed in this book. We will see that these preparations are used alongside drugs best understood at the cellular and molecular level, e.g. the steroids discussed later.

8.2.1 Vehicles used in topical preparations

Here, the term 'topical preparation' means one formulated to be applied to the skin. Preparations of drugs for topical use usually consist of the active

Box 8.1

The skin layers and their various functions

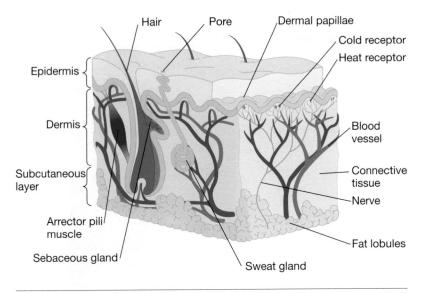

Figure a The structure of the skin.

The three layers of the skin and associated structures such as a hair follicle with sebaceous gland.

The epidermis.

The epidermis is the outer layer of your skin (see Figure a).

1. It is mainly made up of **keratinocytes**, a type of epithelial cell.

2. It acts as the initial protective barrier.

3. It is metabolically active.

4. It has five distinct sublayers (see Table B8.1 and Figure b).

Table B8.1 The main layers and sublayers of the skin

Layer	Function	Sub-layer/contents
Epidermis	Barrier against the penetration of chemicals and other substances Reduces loss of water from skin and underlying tissues	Stratum corneum
		Stratum lucidum
		Stratum granulosum
		Stratum spinosum
		Stratum basale
Dermis	Provides strength Protects from mechanical injury Supports appendages and epidermis Assists temperature regulation Provides nutrition (e.g. vitamin D synthesis) Transmits touch and pain sensations Water storage	Capillary and lymph network
		Nerves
		Sweat and sebaceous glands
		Hair follicles
Subcutaneous (hypodermis)	Fat storage, temperature regulation, nutritional support, cushion for outer skin layers	Adipose tissue and fibrocollagenous septa

Box 8.1 **The skin layers and their various functions**

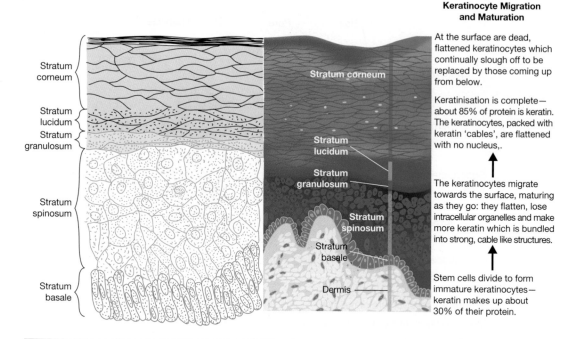

Keratinocyte Migration and Maturation

At the surface are dead, flattened keratinocytes which continually slough off to be replaced by those coming up from below.

Keratinisation is complete—about 85% of protein is keratin. The keratinocytes, packed with keratin 'cables', are flattened with no nucleus,.

The keratinocytes migrate towards the surface, maturing as they go: they flatten, lose intracellular organelles and make more keratin which is bundled into strong, cable like structures.

Stem cells divide to form immature keratinocytes— keratin makes up about 30% of their protein.

Figure b The five layers of the epidermis.

The arrows indicate the migration of immature keratinocytes continuously being formed in the stratum basale to the surface of the skin, where in mature form they make up the majority of the stratum corneum. From Wikipedia http://en.wikipedia.org/wiki/Stratum_granulosum.

The **epidermis** is mainly made up of **keratinocytes**, which are cells that originate from the stem cells in the stratum basale from where they mature and migrate to the surface (Figure b). On the surface, they become flattened and die off, forming the stratum corneum. As this process occurs the cells become more and more packed with the protein **keratin**, which forms itself into thick, tough cable-like structures that have connections between cells, giving enormous strength to the epldidermis. This process is called **keratinization**. The stratum corneum is crucial for barrier function. The whole process normally takes about a month, but may be accelerated in a disease such as psoriasis (see below). The process of keratinocyte maturation and migration begins in the stratum basale and ends in the wearing away of dead cells at the surface of the skin in the stratum corneum, passing through each of the five sublayers of the epidermis in the process:

Stratum basale (stratum germinativium). The origin of keratinocytes, which form from the division of stem cells, which divide, replenishing themselves and forming a daughter immature keratinocyte.

Stratum spinosum. The migrating keratinocytes begin the process of keratinization, forming keratin fibres that give the cytoplasm a 'spiny' appearance. This layer is thicker in thick skin.

Stratum granulosum. By now the keratinocytes have taken on a polygonal shape, with a more granular cytoplasm and more keratin, and begin to flatten. The cells begin to lose intracellular organelles (e.g. nucleus). The layer is three to five cells thick.

Stratum lucideum. Apparent in thick skin only, the cells by now have lost their nucleus and are passing upwards.

Stratum corneum. Typically between three and twenty cell layers in depth, depending on thickness of the skin. The final layer, so cells which have lost their organelles are flattened, fully keratinized and in the outer layer are dead and continuously being sloughed off. These mature keratinocytes are laterally attached to each other, are strong by virtue of their keratinizatin, and give a toughness to the skin.

The dermis

The dermis is the layer located underneath the epidermis. Its main role is to provide strength, protection from mechanical injury, and support for the appendages and epidermis. This layer also plays a part in the provision of nutrition (e.g. vitamin D synthesis). The dermis hosts the capillaries, lymphs, nerves, sweat, and sebaceous glands as well as the hair follicles. These structures provide a varying number of functions for the body, including temperature regulation, transmission of touch, and pain sensations.

The glands of the skin are located in the dermis to secrete sweat or sebum through the epidermis to the surface. The sweat glands can be divided into two groups:

1. Those with ducts passing directly to the surface (these are called eccrine glands). They are the most common sweat glands, producing a thin watery sweat, particularly abundant in thick skin such as the palms, with a major function being cooling. Secretion is stimulated by parasympathetic activity (with released acetycholine acting on M_3 muscarinic acetycholine receptors), and it is this which underlies the unwanted sweating response seen with some medications (e.g. the muscarinic agonist bethanacol, which has limited use for urininary retention) and more commonly the dry skin seen with the muscarinic antagonist atropine.

2. Those that connect to the upper part of hair follicles (apocrine glands). These have a thicker, protein and lipid-rich, secretion that is under the control of the sympathetic system.

The sebaceous glands are intimately connected to the hair follicles. They secrete sebum, which is made up of triglycerides, cholesterol, squalene, wax diesters, proteins, and inorganic salts. They are under hormonal control, with increased secretion at puberty, and it is these glands that are involved in the genesis of acne (see Section 8.6).

The subcutaneous layer

The subcutaneous layer (also called the subcutis or the hypodermis) is made up of adipose tissue and fibrocollagenous septa. These assist the subcutis to fulfil its role of fat storage, temperature regulation, nutritional support, and providing a cushion for the outer skin layers.

---

ingredient mixed in a bulk phase, known as the **vehicle**. The vehicle, and the way it is applied, is almost as important as the active ingredient in the treatment of skin conditions, and must be suitable for the type of lesion for which it is used. For example, ointments are generally better for the treatment of dry skin conditions. The choice of vehicle should also take into account patient preference and acceptability because these factors will influence compliance.

An example of this is when Elvis, the imaginary patient we will encounter in Workbook 5, is prescribed emollients for his dermatitis—he stopped using them because they were too greasy. His pharmacist counselled him to use the greasy ones at bedtime and to use the cream, which is more cosmetically acceptable, in the daytime.

Box 8.2 explores the different types of vehicle, giving some comments on characteristics and common uses.

Box 8.2
Choice of vehicle in the treatment of skin conditions

Different vehicle types may logically be chosen for the same condition, for example creams during the day because they are cosmetically better, and ointments, which are more greasy, at night.

Other determinants of vehicle choice are:

- Does it carry an active drug, and if so how soluble and stable is the active drug in the vehicle?

- How much could the vehicle hydrate the stratum corneum and thereby enhance absorbtion?
- How able is the vehicle to reduce evaporation from the surface?
- Where and when will the preparation be applied?

Table B8.2 Details the various vehicles used in skin conditions

Vehicle	Physical and chemical properties	Characteristics and uses	Examples
Ointment	Water miscible; can be washed off	Lubricates, as in burn dressings. Aids penetration of drugs	Macrogels and PEG mixtures. Emulsifying ointment
	Water insoluble; not easily washed off	Chronic dry skin conditions. Messy	White Soft Paraffin. Paraffin-based ointments
Creams	Oil in water; vanish easily, washable	Cosmetically acceptable. Can act as the vehicle for water-soluble drugs	Aqueous cream. Cetomacrogol cream
	Water in oil; acts similarly to ointments. Increases skin hydration	Less greasy than ointment. Can act as the vehicle for fat-soluble drugs	Oily cream. Zinc cream
Pastes	Thick with insoluble powders. Very adhesive	Can absorb discharges (e.g. pus or oozing fluid) from skin.	Zinc pastes
Powders	Drying and cooling. Absorb moisture and create increased area for evaporation	Intertriginous[a] areas and chronically damp areas (e.g. feet and under diapers	Talc. Antifungal powders
Gels	Semi-solid emulsions, non-greasy, clear, and quick drying, leaving no residue	Useful in hairy areas or where it is unacceptable to have residue of vehicle, e.g. face	Polymers and copolymers
Lotions	Suspensions of powder in water or a dilute emulsion of oil in water	Supercifial oozing dermatoses. Intertriginous areas, inflammation and tenderness, e.g. sunburn, acute contact dermatitis	Calamine lotion

[a] Intertriginous areas: where two surfaces of the skin are normally in contact, such as between fingers and toes, under fold of breasts, armpits.

8.2.2 Absorption of drug from topical preparations

When a drug (e.g. the steroids mentioned below) with its vehicle (see Box 8.2) is applied to the skin there are a number of factors that determine the rate and extent of absorption.

1. The characteristics of the drug, such as water solubility and molecular weight (low molecular weight drugs (e.g. 600 Da) are better absorbed than larger molecules).

2. The vehicle used (see Box 8.2 for some comments).

3. Body site, e.g. more drug is absorbed from thin skin (e.g. scalp and face) than from thick skin (e.g. palms and soles of the feet).

4. Skin hydration, e.g. vehicles that are oil-in-water emulsions will increase hydration. Applying after a bath will increase absorption.

5. Skin condition: more absorption occurs through damaged skin. e.g. in burns or psoriasis.

8.2.3 Is absorption to bloodstream from topical preparations good or bad?

It is worth noting that in some cases drug delivery through the skin into the general circulation may be the objective (e.g. in patches used to deliver fentanyl for pain relief, see Chapter 20), but in the treatment of skin diseases what is needed is for the drug to remain in the skin and not get into the circulation.

An example is the topical use of steroids: we don't want them to get distributed around the body, having unwanted effects.

> This is why, in Workbook 5 at the end of this chapter, our patient Elvis was told by the pharmacist to avoid using the potent steroid on his face because it could lead to more absorption into the bloodstream and more side effects.

Another interesting example is the drug pimecrolimus (see section 8.4.3), used as a cream for atopic eczema. Its molecular weight of 810 means it is above the normal guideline of less than 600 for penetration into the skin. However, in atopic eczema the skin barrier is not fully effective, allowing penetration of the drug into the epidermis but no further, so it cannot get into the bloodstream. This means that complications from systemic effects are unlikely.

8.3 Eczema and dermatitis

Eczema and dermatitis are widely used as synonyms. They refer to a chronic inflammation of the epidermis and dermis that is accompanied by itching (pruritus) and localized oedema of the epidermis, that is the accumulation of fluid between the cells of the epidermis, creating a swollen patch of skin, called spongiosis. Other features include redness of affected areas of skin, dry skin, which is often thickened in the areas that have been scratched, red lumps or blisters in affected areas, and oozing, weeping, or crusty deposits (Figure 8.1). The term 'eczema' may be used for the endogenous inflammatory state and dermatitis when the condition is a response to an outside agent. In fact this distinction is commonly not made and the two terms are used interchangeably.

8.3.1 There are different types of dermatitis

Although the skin's appearance and treatment are predominantly the same for all types of eczema/dermatitis, dermatitis is often subdivided based on the causative factor or irritant. The main groups of dermatitis are set out below.

- **Atopic dermatitis** is the 'allergic' type often seen in people who also have hay fever and asthma (called the 'atopic triad'). About 5–10% of children are affected by atopic dermatitis. Underlying mechanisms of atopic dermatitis, some elements of which are outlined in the introduction to this section (see Box S3.2) and in Box 8.3,

are believed to include an IgE-mediated hypersensitivity reaction, which occurs when mediators of inflammation are released by sensitized mast cells and basophils. This type of account makes it clear that atopic dermatitis has a great deal in common with asthma (Chapter 11). Itching is the most common symptom of atopic dermatitis, often preceding the appearance of rash. Open lesions may follow spontaneously or as a result of scratching (Figure 8.1). Atopic dermatitis does not require local skin contact with the precipitating agent—the patient may, for example, contact the allergen through inhalation or food.

- **Allergic contact dermatitis:** Due to skin contact with a substance to which the individual is sensitive. The same substance does not cause dermatitis in a person who is not sensitive to it.

- **Irritant contact dermatitis**: Due to skin contact with irritating chemicals, powders, cleaning agents, etc. Contact with such a substance is likely to cause dermatitis in any person, although a degree of individual variation still exists.

- **Photoallergic/phototoxic dermatitis:** Due to chemicals being turned into allergens or toxins in the skin when exposed to UV light.

- **Seborrhoeic weeping dermatitis:** Common in infants, where it appears in the nappy area and the scalp. In adults it also appears on the scalp, hands, and in the skin creases between the nose and sides of the mouth. Can be caused by yeast infection.

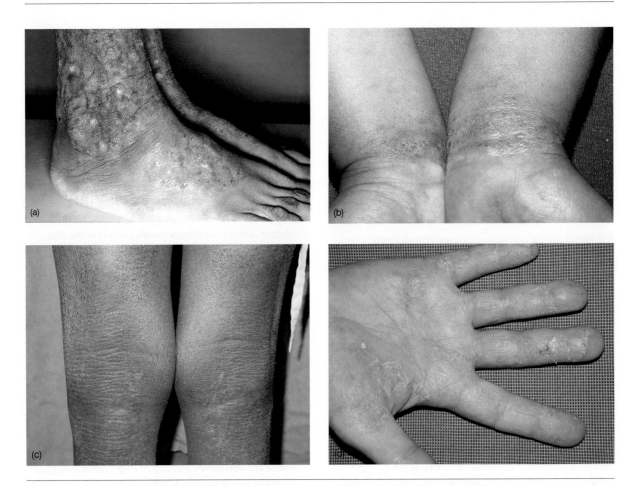

Figure 8.1 Some common appearances of eczema/dermatitis.

A, Typical dry scaly skin with redness in affected area, as also seen more extensively in B, with open lesions. Open weeping lesions are apparent in acute eczema in C, and D gives an example of chronic eczema with extensive well-established weeping lesions resulting in crusty deposits.

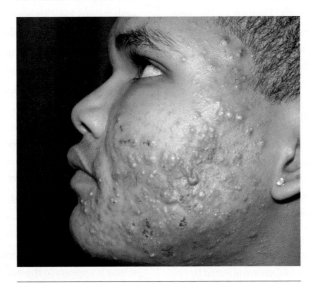

Figure 8.2 A case of acne.

A variety of lesions can be seen.

Box 8.3

Mechanisms of atopic eczema and drug treatment

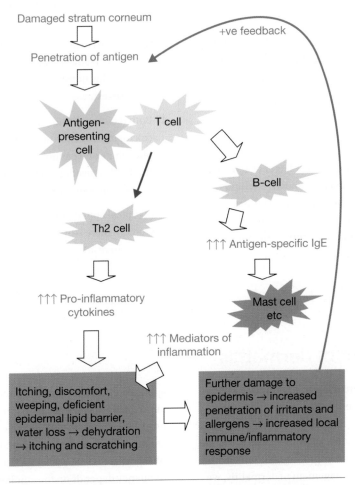

Damaged stratum corneum

Penetration of antigen

+ve feedback

Antigen-presenting cell

T cell

B-cell

Th2 cell

↑↑↑ Antigen-specific IgE

↑↑↑ Pro-inflammatory cytokines

Mast cell etc

↑↑↑ Mediators of inflammation

Itching, discomfort, weeping, deficient epidermal lipid barrier, water loss → dehydration → itching and scratching

Further damage to epidermis → increased penetration of irritants and allergens → increased local immune/inflammatory response

Figure c This is a simplified scheme, and alternative models for the development and maintenance of atopic eczema are possible.

Figure c provides a simplified illustration of how damaged epidermis, immune responses, inflammatory cells, and mediators of inflammation can all contribute to the symptoms of eczema and set up a self-perpetuating feedback.

Medications are used to suppress the mechanisms illustrated.

Emmolients restore the condition of the epidermis, rehydrating and permitting the establishment of an effective lipid barrier against water loss, and further strengthening barrier function, which reduces penetration of allergens and irritants. This reduces itching and scratching, restoring comfort and normalizing the appearance of the skin.

Anti-inflammatory steroids inhibit the processes illustrated at several levels by changing gene expression, giving an increase in anti-inflammatory proteins and a decrease in inflammatory proteins. The result is a dampened down inflammatory response at the level of both recruitment of inflammatory cells and mediators of inflammation.

Calcineurin inhibitors such as **tacrolimus** and **pimecrolimus** also change gene expression, but the mechanism is more restricted than that of the steroids, resulting in the expectation of fewer unwanted effects.

How do calcineurin inhibitors work in the treatment of skin disease?

In summary:

1. When a protein called nuclear factor of activated T-cells (NFAT) is found in the nucleus it binds to DNA and controls gene expression (i.e. it is a transcription factor). It is necessary for the expression of pro-inflammatory cytokines such as IL-2, TNF-α, IL-4, and IL-5 by activated T-cells.

2. When NFAT has a phosphate attached to it (by a protein kinase) then entry into the nucleus is blocked.

3. Calcineurin is a phosphatases. This means it is an enzyme that removes the phosphate, leading to NFAT protein being transported into the nucleus, where it increases expression of immune response genes.

4. Both tacrolimus and pimecrolimus inhibit this calcineurin. The result is that the NFAT keeps its phosphate and cannot enter the nucleus, and so the T-cell activation and inflammatory cytokine expression is suppressed.

With topical application these drugs enter the skin, but remain there—they do not get spread around the body, so there are no systemic effects.

8.4 Treatment of dermatitis

There are two main approaches to treating dermatitis. The first is to remove or minimize contact with the cause/irritant for atopic, allergic/contact, photoallergic/toxic, and irritant dermatitis, and the second is the use of medications. While both approaches should form part of the strategy for management of dermatitis, we shall only consider the medication approach. Here, medication means emollients, two classes of drugs (corticosteroids and calcineurin inhibitors), and topical antibacterials.

8.4.1 Emollients

Emollients are creams and ointments that often hydrate and soothe the skin. Emollients are the first-line treatment for dermatitis. Adequate rehydration of the stratum corneum will help restore the skin's barrier function, protecting against the effects of allergens and irritants, and reducing itching.

The selection of available emollients is quite wide. They range from light emollients (aqueous creams), which are cosmetically acceptable but require more frequent application, to more occlusive[2] but greasy and messy ointments. Some preparations contain urea and propylene glycol to improve penetration by loosening the keratinocyte layer, while others contain humectants (things that draw in water) such as glycerine. Application frequency depends on the emollient, with creams requiring more frequent applications than ointments.

Emollients should be applied liberally—patients may be told to 'slap it on'—and this means that such issues as appearance on the skin, smell, effect on clothing, and ease of removal play a major role in choosing which preparation to use to ensure patients will use as directed.

8.4.2 Corticosteroids

Where dermatitis is failing to respond to emollients, topical preparations of corticosteroids (often referred to simply as steroids) are the mainstay of treatment.

---

2. Occlusive here means a preparation which, when applied to the skin, acts as a physical barrier between the skin and the outside world. This is achieved by thick and greasy preparations.

Mode of action of corticosteroids in reduction of dermatitis

Corticosteroids are anti-inflammatory steroids, with a mode of action essentially as described in Chapter 9 (e.g. Box 9.2). This mechanism involves the steroid drug entering cells, binding to intracellular receptors which act within the nucleus to change gene expression, suppressing inflammatory genes, and increasing expression of anti-inflammatory genes (see Box 9.2). Elements of this alteration of gene expression by steroids also inhibit the immune response, modifying the allergy responses of atopic patients. The overall outcome is a dampening-down of the processes generating dermatitis (see Box 8.3).

We can identify two consequences of this mode of action of steroids for treating dermatitis.

1. The drugs modify the underlying mechanisms generating the disease, providing long-term relief, but they do not cure the patient. For example, an atopic patient remains atopic—the tendency to develop dermatitis will not be modified by the topical use of steroids, and it may be expected that over time symptoms will recur when treatment is stopped.

2. The onset of the drug effects is slow (modification of gene expression and its consequences all have to be given time to have an effect) and so the therapeutic response will be seen over days—the drug should normally be applied twice a day for a sustained period.

Not all topical steroid preparations are the same

The action of all corticosteroid preparations has a lot in common. One way in which they differ is in terms of the vehicle in which the steroid is dispersed. For example, the same steroid may be available as a cream or as an ointment (see Box 8.2 for the significance of different vehicles). Of great important is the potency of the preparation, often referred to as low, medium, or high strength. Potency of preparation depends both on the concentration of the steroid and on which steroid is present. Some preparations are set out in Table 8.2.

What are the key principles of corticosteroid use?

The following comments provide a guide to the use of topical steroid preparations.

- They should only be used when sustained and appropriate use of emollients has proved ineffective.

Table 8.2 Different steroids in topical preparations for dermatitis

Potency	Drug
Mild (low strength)	Hydrocortisone 0.1–2.5% Hydrocortisone acetate 1% Fluocinolone acetonide 0.0025%
Moderate (medium strength)	Betamethasone valerate 0.025% Clobetasone butyrate 0.05% Fluocinolone acetonide 0.00625% Desonide 0.05% Triamcinolone 0.02%
Potent (high strength)	Betamethasone valerate 0.1% Hydrocortisone butyrate 0.1% Methylprednisolone 0.1%
Very potent (high strength)	Clobetasone propionate 0.05% Diflucortolone valerate 0.3% Halcinonide 0.1%

It should be noted that altering the salt could change the potency of a steroid preparation, e.g. clobetasone *propionate* is more potent than clobetasone *butyrate*.

- They should be applied on hydrated skin (after bathing or after use of an emollient) for maximum penetration and maximum effect.

- Usual frequency is twice daily; more frequent application is usually unnecessary and may increase the risk of unwanted effects.

- Use low or medium strength preparations for long-term treatment.

- Use low strength steroids on areas where the skin is thin (e.g. face) to avoid excessive absorption that could lead to side effects.

Anti-inflammatory steroids may be combined with the use of emollients

It would be normal and good practice to continue use of emollients alongside steroids when the emollient alone has proved inadequate.

In Workbook 5 we will see that Elvis was prescribed a mild steroid to use alongside his emollients because the emollients alone had not been effective. During his flare up a potent steroid was prescribed for short-term use.

Side effects of topical steroids

There are two types of unwanted effects from the use of steroids. The first, caused by absorption and distribution around the body (systemic effects), is mostly restricted to the use of high strength preparations, and with careful use is likely to be uncommon (see Chapter 9). More commonly encountered are unwanted effects at the site of application. The local suppression of the immune response may lead to problems with infections, and some patients may suffer from local thinning of the skin, striae (stretch mark-like damage), and telangiectasias (visible dilated blood vessels). Corticosteroids have also been known to precipitate acne. Rebound effects, with enhanced symptoms when treatment is stopped, are also of concern with topical steroids.

8.4.3 Topical immunomodulators (calcineurin inhibitors)

Calcineurin inhibitors are a relatively new class of topical drugs used in dermatitis, usually when other treatments have failed. Two calcineurin inhibitors available are **tacrolimus** and **pimecrolimus**.

Mode of action of calcineurin inhibitors

Calcineurin inhibitors are a class of drug called immunomodulators, that is drugs that directly target the immune response (see also Box 8.3). Calcineurin is an enzyme that removes specific phosphate groups from proteins. It activates a protein called NFAT by dephosphorylating it. The activated NFAT is a transcription factor that then enters the nucleus, where it upregulates the expression of inflammatory cytokines such as interleukin 2 (IL-2), which, in turn, stimulates T-cell responses. Calcineurin inhibitors interfere with this activation of T-cells. This can be useful in other clinical situations (e.g. tacrolimus is used to suppress the

rejection of transplanted organs). In dermatitis the topical use of calcineurin inhibitors suppresses the contribution of allergic responses to the development of the condition (Box 8.3), therefore, like steroids, they target the underlying mechanisms that give rise to the disease. Since both classes of drug suppress the immune response it is not surprising that calcineurin inhibitors, like steroids, may exacerbate local infections, although this may be minimal since calcineurin inhibitors do not inhibit antigen-presenting cell (APC; see the introduction to this section (Box S3.2) and Box 8.3) function and so largely leave the local immune response intact.

Use of calcineurin inhibitors

Calcineurin inhibitors should be used for short-term treatment of patients over 2 years old who do not respond to emollients and topical steroids. They do not share with steroids the unwanted effects on the skin seen with some patients (mentioned above). With topical application they do not distribute themselves around the body and so should be free of systemic effects.

8.4.4 Topical antibacterials

In addition to medication directly targeting the dermatitis process, medication may include topical antibiotics, since open lesions, particularly with the use of anti-inflammatory steroids, may lead to vulnerability to local infections. Compound preparations combining a steroid with an antibacterial are popular. Such preparations are probably best used for short-term (7–10 days) treatment.

8.5 Acne

Acne affects 90% of all adolescents and accounts for more physician visits than any other skin disease. Acne is a disease of the sebaceous glands associated with the hair follicles (see Figure 8.3 and Box 8.1). The burden of acne is illustrated by remembering that its presence on the face is characterized by blackheads, pimples, spots, and pustules (see Figure 8.2), and recalling that it is particularly common in adolescence.

Blackheads (also called open comedones) are caused by an accumulation of oils and keratin that have plugged the sebaceous gland—the oils darken as they oxidize

with time. Whiteheads (closed comedones) occur when this darkening does not happen. These diseased states of hair follicles are illustrated in Figure 8.3. Eimear, our imaginary patient in Workbook 5, suffers from acne with a combination of black and white heads.

The engorged blocked follicles may become infected with bacteria. Chronic long-term acne can be viewed as an inflammatory condition. Scaring is a long-term complication of acne and could lead to psychological problems. It should therefore be avoided by early initiation of treatment.

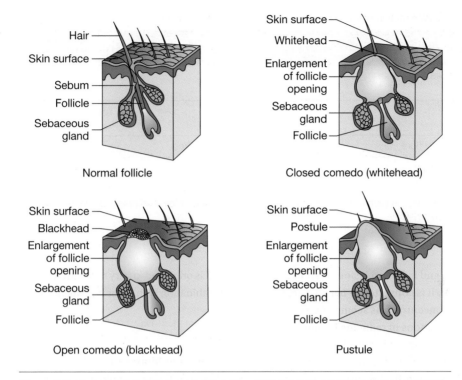

Figure 8.3 Diseased hair follicles are the origin of blackheads, whiteheads, and pustules.

Development of acne

The development of acne occurs in the following stages.

1. Accelerated proliferation of keratinocytes and accumulation of sticky, horny cells in the sebaceous of canal hair follicle.

2. Accumulation of keratinocytes plugs sebaceous follicle.

3. Sebum accumulates in follicle, enlargement occurs, and a closed comedone is formed (Figure 8.3).

4. Keratinization and expansion of closed comedone changes it to open comedone.

5. Pressure caused by accumulating sebum leads to rupture of wall and subsequent inflammatory reaction.

6. Lymphocytes, monocytes, macrophages are recruited and release cytokines and mediators of inflammation, setting off a local, chronic (long-term) inflammatory response.

8.6 Drug treatment of acne

Although there is no cure for acne, treatment can reduce its severity and should be commenced early to prevent scarring. Patients need to be counselled that an improvement may not be seen for a couple of months. The choice of treatment is based on whether or not the acne is predominantly inflammatory as well as on the severity of the acne. Topical drugs are prevalent in treatment, although some may be used orally. Table 8.3 details the site of action of drugs used in acne. An introduction to some of the drugs available follows.

8.6.1 Benzoyl peroxide

Used topically benzoyl peroxide is effective in mild to moderate acne. It has an antibacterial action, reducing the fatty acid levels in sebaceous gland secretions.

Table 8.3 Mechanism of action of some drugs used in the treatment of acne

Mechanism of action	Benzoyl peroxide	Azelaic acid	Retinoids	Antibiotics	Hormone manipulation	Salicylic acid
Normalising follicular keratinization	Yes	Yes	Yes			Yes
Decreasing sebum production			Yes		Yes	
Suppressing bacterial flora	Yes	Yes	Yes	Yes		
Preventing inflammatory response			Yes			

Some drugs combine more than one mechanism of action (e.g. the retinoids are the most potent but are not used commonly because of their adverse drug reactions).

Both comedones and inflamed lesions respond well to benzoyl peroxide. It is converted to benzoic acid in the skin. The lower concentrations seem to be as effective as higher concentrations in reducing inflammation. Treatment should be started with a lower strength and the concentration increased gradually. If the acne does not respond after 2 months then use of a topical antibacterial should be considered. It is even more effective in combination with miconazole.

> In Workbook 5 Eimear used benzoyl peroxide incorrectly initially, suffered side effects (dry skin) and it proved ineffective. Her doctor recommended her to give it a second try. The pharmacist advised her on how to use it correctly.

8.6.2 Azelaic acid

This is a dicarboxylic acid which is an alternative for acne management. It has significant antimicrobial activity, as well as an effect on keratinization and the stratum corneum. It may be an alternative to benzoyl peroxide or to a topical retinoid for treating mild to moderate acne, particularly of the face, and has been shown to be as effective as oral antibiotics.

It should be applied twice daily and continued for several months because its benefit is not seen for up to 4 weeks. Some patients prefer it because it is less likely to cause local irritation than benzoyl peroxide, and will not bleach hair and clothing like benzoyl peroxide.

8.6.3 Salicylic acid

An established keratinolytic, salicylic acid is used in concentrations of 3–6% for acne to help open up pores. It is less effective than benzoyl peroxide and azelaic acid,

and is only used in very mild cases, usually in combination with other ingredients, such as sulfur.

8.6.4 Antibiotics

Topical antibiotics are as effective as benzoyl peroxide and/or tretinoin for mild to moderate acne. However, using them long term should be avoided to reduce resistance. The most commonly used topical antibiotics are **clindamycin** and **erythromycin**. **Systemic antibiotics** are reserved for moderate to severe acne and are more effective than topical formulations. The usual oral antibiotics are tetracyclines such as doxycycline. Patients taking tetracyclines must be careful when out in the sun as they can cause phototoxic dermatitis.

8.6.5 Retinoids

Retinoids are a class of chemical compounds chemically related to vitamin A. Their use in dermatology is primarily due to the way they regulate epithelial cell division, growth, and proliferation. Their role also includes moderation of immune function, inhibition of neutrophil migration, and activation of tumour suppressor genes. Intracellularly they stabilize lysosomes and increase prostaglandin, cyclic AMP, and cyclic GMP concentrations. Their action is mediated by retinoic acid receptors.

Topical retinoids include tretinoin (and its isomer isotretinoin) and adapalene. They should be applied regularly for a minimum of 4 months. Redness and peeling that occur initially will normally settle. Treatment should continue until no new lesions appear.

Isotretinoin is also used orally in the treatment of acne. It is reserved for severe and late onset acne. It is a toxic drug and reserved for use only by specialists. It is teratogenic, and female patients need to be warned to use adequate contraception while on treatment, and for acitretin for at least 2 years after ceasing therapy because of the incredibly long half-life of one of the drug's metabolites (etretinate—half-life of 120 days!)

8.6.6 Hormone treatment

Estrogen (specifically **ethinyl estradiol**), through its antiandrogen effect, has been shown to improve acne in female patients. This effect is exerted through protein synthesis stimulation, increasing the amount of sex-hormone binding globulin, which decreases amount of testosterone. The resultant effect is decreased sebum secretion. This is especially beneficial in women with hirsutism. It should be avoided in pregnancy, male patients, and where there is a predisposition to thrombosis. You will see that in Workbook 5 Eimear was finally put on hormone treatment after all other options failed. This worked for her, and was ideal because it had the extra contraceptive effect!

8.6.7 Corticosteroids

Although steroids can worsen acne, they are occasionally used in extremely severe resistant cases.

Injections of triamcinolone (a synthetic steroid) into the lesions, or a short oral course of steroid, have been shown to be effective in quickly improving acne. Topical steroids are not very effective, although they could be used in combination with isotretinoin in severe inflammatory acne.

8.7 Psoriasis

Psoriasis is a chronic disease affecting both the skin and joints which commonly causes red scaly patches to appear on the skin. These subsequently become silvery-white. Called psoriatic **plaques**, they are characterized by inflammation and increased skin growth. They are common on the skin of the head, elbows, and knees, although they could affect any area. Psoriasis is thought to be immune-mediated and is not contagious. It is a recurring condition and can vary in severity from minor localized patches to complete body coverage. Psoriasis can also cause inflammation of the joints; this is known as psoriatic arthritis and it occurs in 10–15% of people with psoriasis. By far the most common form is plaque psoriasis—this is the only type considered here.

Factors that are thought to aggravate psoriasis are stress, excessive alcohol consumption, and smoking. Psoriasis could lead to depression and loss of self-esteem. Although there are many treatments available, because of its chronic recurrent nature psoriasis remains a challenge to treat.

8.7.1 Pathogenesis of psoriasis

Psoriasis is thought to be an autoimmune process mediated by T-lymphocytes, leading to vascular and inflammatory changes followed by changes in the epidermis. A central feature is rapid skin growth. This means that the stem cells in the stratum basale (Box 8.1) divide more rapidly, increasing the production of cells destined to be keratinocytes. These then travel through the epidermal layers to the stratum corneum within about 3–4 days, rather then the normal 28 days or more. This is insufficient time for cells to mature and for keratinization to occur.

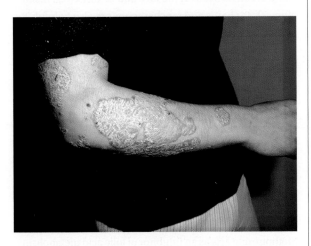

Figure 8.4 An example of plaque psoriasis.

Thickened and raised red plaques can be seen, with the appearance of white surfaces.

8.8 Treatment of psoriasis

The treatment should be individualized for each patient. When it is localized, topical treatment is sufficient. There are a number of common treatment options. Here we give some examples: emollients, vitamin D derivatives, steroids, anthralin, tar preparations, acitretin, and ciclosporine. It may also be noted that non-pharmacological treatment includes phototherapy, and this is incorporated in the brief comments on strategy in psoriasis treatments at the end of this section.

8.8.1 Emollients

These have a crucial role to play in easing discomfort by rehydration and restoration of barrier function (see dermatitis above). They should be considered for use alongside more specific interventions for psoriasis indicated below.

8.8.2 The vitamin D derivatives

Dihydroxy-vitamin D3 (calcitriol), calcipotriol, and tacalcitol are used in the treatment of psoriasis. Vitamin D and its analogues are used topically as for plaque psoriasis, and have the advantage that they do not smell or stain, and therefore may be more acceptable than tar or dithranol products (see below). However, they can be slow to take full effect (taking up to 6 weeks to work). Of the vitamin D analogues, tacalcitol and calcitriol are less likely to irritate. They act by suppressing keratinocyte proliferation, and also have anti-inflammatory properties.

8.8.3 Topical corticosteroids

Corticosteroids in the form of creams, ointments, and gels are widely used treatments for psoriasis. They have anti-inflammatory, immunosuppressive, and antiproliferative properties. They may be most effective when combined with other treatments. The more powerful steroid preparations can have dramatic effects in clearing psoriasis but have some serious side effects and should not be used on certain areas of the body or for long-term treatment. Concerns about the unwanted effects of stronger topical steroids have been mentioned above in the context of dermatitis, and not surprisingly

these same concerns also exist for the treatment of psoriasis.

8.8.4 Dithranol (anthralin)

Dithranol is effective in widespread discrete plaques. It should be applied to chronic plaques only; normal skin should be avoided. It is not generally suitable for widespread small lesions and should not be used on the face. It inhibits DNA synthesis in the stem cells of the stratum basale and other processes related to mitotic activity. The therapeutic response develops slowly, but is longer lasting than seen with steroids—there are none of the rebound exacerbations possible when treatment with steroids is stopped. Dithranol stains skin and clothing yellow, however, and so may be unpopular.

8.8.5 Tars

Tar preparations are very complex, and could contain up to 10,000 constituents. Crude coal tar is the most effective form, but few outpatients tolerate the smell and mess. The cleaner extracts of coal tar included in proprietary preparations are more practicable for home use but they are less effective and improvement takes longer. Contact of coal tar products with normal skin is not normally harmful and they can be used for widespread small lesions; however, irritation, contact allergy, and sterile folliculitis can occur. The milder tar extracts can be used on the face and flexures (e.g. inside elbows). Tar baths and tar shampoos are also helpful. Tar has an antipruritic (anti-itch) effect and can also be used in dermatitis.

8.8.6 Retinoids

Tazarotine should be specifically applied to the plaques. **Acitretin** is taken orally. Although some cases of psoriasis respond well to acitretin alone, it is only moderately effective in most cases and is therefore normally combined with other treatments.

8.8.7 Methotrexate

Methotrexate acts as an inhibitor of folic acid metabolism in the synthesis of DNA, giving it a powerful antiproliferative effect long utilized in cancer chemotherapy. To reduce proliferation in severe psoriasis that cannot be effectively treated with other approaches it is administered systemically (mouth, intramuscular, or intravenous) once weekly. There is danger of severe systemic side effects, which restricts its use (for details see Chapter 9).

8.8.8 Immunomodulators

Cyclosporine, administered by mouth, has positive effects but its toxicity restricts its use in psoriasis to severe unresponsive conditions. It is of interest because its mechanism of action includes inhibition of calcineurin (see comments on calcineurin inhibitors see above) and the growth of keratinocytes.

Infliximab, a monoclonal antibody against tumor necrosis factor-alpha (TNF-α), is also used for the treatment of severe, unresponsive psoriasis. TNF-α is a potent inflammatory cytokine involved in a number of immune reactions. For details of its action and use see Chapter 9.

8.8.9 Phototherapy and photochemotherapy

Phototherapy is exposure to UVB light, resulting in a reduction in psoriatic plaque formation. It extends from natural sunlight to repeated whole body exposure to light in a cabinet. It has disadvantages, including extreme inconvenience, skin burning, and increased danger of melanoma. Phototherapy can be used in conjunction with the medications described above. An alternative is photochemotherapy, when a compound called psoralen is taken 2 hours before exposure to UVA light, resulting in photomodification of psoralen in the skin (psoralen + UVA is often abbreviated to PUVA treatment). Patients may require multiple treatments for very long periods of time, so again development of skin cancers is a significant problem.

8.8.10 Strategy in the treatment of psoriasis

An escalating strategy is justified, taking into consideration the increasing toxicity of treatments, with choice depending on the severity of the condition and whether is it localized or affects a large area.

Level 1   Topical drugs, tar, dithranol (anthralin), vitamin D derivatives, steroids

Level 2   Phototherapy, PUVA

Level 3   Systemic drugs, retinoids, methotrexate, immunomodulators

It is noteworthy that treatments from different levels may be combined.

8.9 Other dermatologic conditions

Other common dermatological conditions include fungal infections, parasitic infections, viral infections, bacterial infections (cellulitis), and alopecia

The drugs and adverse reactions are summarized in Table 8.4. (See Chapter 21 for more details of the antifungal and anti-infective agents.)

Table 8.4 Other skin conditions and drugs commonly used to treat them

Dermatological condition	Drug class (topical)	Action	Adverse effects
Fungal infections Dermatophyses	Imidazoles, griseolfulvin, terbinafine, amorolfine,undecenoates, compound benzoic acid, tolnaftate	Kill or inhibit growth of fungi	Contact dermatitis Rash Skin burning, itching, and redness Skin dryness Stinging
Pityriasis versicolor	Ketoconazole, selenium shampoos, topical imidazoles, terbinafine		
Candiadiasis	Topical imidazoles, nystatin		
Angular cheilitis	Miconazole and nystatin ointments		
Bacterial infection Cellulitis	Systemic antibacterial treatment	Kill or inhibit the growth of bacteria	As above
Erysipelas	Systemic antibacterial treatment		
Infected burn wounds	Silver sulfadiazine		
Impetigo (longstanding/extensive)	Systemic flucloxacillin or erythromycin		
Rosacea	Metronidazole	Soften crust	
Impetigo (simple)	Fusidic acid, or mupirocin if MRSA Polymyxins, neomycin, povidone-iodine		
Viral infections Herpes simplex	Acyclovir cream, idoxuridine	Inhibit growth of virus	As above
Herpes labialis	Acyclovir,penciclovir, idoxuridine		
Parasite infections Scabies	Permethrin, malathion, benzyl benzoate	Act on parasite nerve membranes	Contact dermatitis
Headlice	Carbaryl, malathion, permethrin, phenothrin	and disrupt sodium channel, causing	Hypersensitivity reaction
Crablice	Carbaryl, malathion, phenothrin	paralysis.	Respiratory allergy reaction

SUMMARY OF DRUGS USED FOR ECZEMA (DERMATITIS) ACNE AND PSORIASIS

Therapeutic class	Drugs/vehicle	Mechanism of action	Common clinical uses	Comments	Examples of adverse drug reactions
	Ointment	1) Moisturisers moisturise, soothe, smooth, and hydrate the roughened surface of the stratum corneum by filling the spaces between dry skin flakes with oil droplets, thereby restoring skin barrier function and protecting against effects of allergens and irritants and reducing itching 2) Humectants attract transepidermal water to the stratum corneum and retain it	Eczema Psoriasis	Suitable for dry, thickened skin Not suitable for weeping eczema	
	Creams			Daytime use in eczema, easy to spread Commonly contains preservatives that could irritate Requires more frequent applications	Could cause sensitization
Emollients	Lotion			Used for weeping eczema or hairy parts	
	Gel			Has cooling effect	
	Bath/shower oils			Traps water under oil film and prevents skin from drying out	
	Soap substitutes			Are usually creams that cleanse as good as soap but have less drying effect on skin	
	Humectants: glycerin polyethylene glycols urea and propylene glycol				
Topical corticosteroids	Hydrocortisone Fluocinolone Betamethasone Clobetasone Desonide Triamcinolone Methylprednisolone Diflucortolone Halcinonide	Enters the cell, binds to intracellular receptors within nucleus to change gene expression, suppressing inflammatory genes and increasing expression of anti-inflammatory genes Also inhibits the immune response, modifying the allergy responses of atopic patients, leading to overall dampening-down of dermatitis generating processes	Eczema Psoriasis Extremely resistant acne	Reserved for when sustained and appropriate use of emollients has proved ineffective Should be used twice daily	Local skin thinning, infection Systemic steroid effects for potent steroids.
Topical calcineurin inhibitors	Tacrolimus Pimecrolimus	Interfere with activation of T-cells through inhibiting the enzyme calcineurin, which removes specific phosphate groups from proteins Calcineurin activates a protein called NFAT by dephosphorylating it The activated NFAT is a transcription factor that then enters the nucleus, where it up regulates the expression of inflammatory cytokines such as interleukin 2 (IL-2), which, in turn, stimulates T-cell responses, thereby suppressing the contribution of allergic responses to the development of dermatitis	Atopic eczema	Used for short-term treatment of patients over 2 years old who do not respond to emollients and topical steroids Long-term risk of causing lymphoma or skin cancer not established	Local irritation Burning sensation Itch Erythema Skin infections

Therapeutic class	Drugs/vehicle	Mechanism of action	Common clinical uses	Comments	Examples of adverse drug reactions
Topical benzoyl peroxide	Benzoyl peroxide	Metabolized to free radicals on skin, which oxidizes bacterial wall proteins, thereby suppressing bacterial flora. Causes keratinolysis and increases cell turnover. Also reduces sebum production and lowers free acid concentrations	Acne	Mild to moderate acne. Start with lower concentration and increase concentration	Skin dryness or peeling. Feeling of warmth, mild stinging or erythema
Topical azelaic acid	Azelaic acid	Normalizes follicular keratinization and suppresses bacterial flora	Mild to moderate acne	Improvement seen after 4 weeks. Should be used for 6 months to see effect	Scaling. Itch. Mild burning. Mild transient erythema
Topical salicylic acids	Salicylic acids	1) Normalizes follicular keratinization by dissolving the intercellular cement binding the epithelial cells together, which leads to the reduction in the cell adhesion. 2) Comedolytic effect by facilitating peeling of epidermis, leading to opening of plugged follicles and ultimately skin renewal.	Mild acne. Psoriasis	Topical use of salicylic acid has resulted in salicylate intoxication (symptoms include confusion, dizziness, headaches, rapid breathing, tinnitus). His could be fatal especially in children	Local irritation. Ulceration. Intoxication
Retinoids	Topical: tretinoin isotretinoin adapalene. Oral: tretinoin	1) Normalizes follicular keratinization by promoting detachment of cornified cells and enhancing shedding of corneocytes and increasing the mitotic activity of follicular epithelia. 2) Suppresses bacterial flora. 3) Decreases sebum production. 4) Prevents inflammatory response	Severe acne. Psoriasis	Avoid in pregnancy	Teratogenicity. Severe dryness of skin. Erythema. Peeling. Irritation. Burning
Hormone treatment	Co-cyprindol	Decreases sebum production	Severe acne. Hirsutism. contraception	Useful in women who also require contraceptives	VTE. Oedema. Weight gain
Antibiotics	Topical: erythromycin clindamycin	Suppressing bacterial flora by killing or inhibiting growth of bacteria	Moderate to severe acne	Long-term use required	Dry or scaly skin. Itch. Stinging or burning feeling
	Oral: tetracyclines and macrolides		Severe acne		See Chapter 21

Therapeutic class	Drugs/vehicle	Mechanism of action	Common clinical uses	Comments	Examples of adverse drug reactions
Vitamin D derivatives	Dihydroxy-vitamin D3 (calcitriol), calcipotriol and tacalcitol	Suppresses keratinocyte proliferation and prevents inflammatory	Mild to moderate psoriasis	Can take up to 6 weeks to take effect	Local skin irritation
Dithranol	Dithranol	Inhibits DNA synthesis in the stem cells of the stratum basale and other processes related to mitotic acitivity.	Mild to moderate psoriasis	Chronic isolated plaque psoriasis Start with low concentration	Acute inflammation Stains skins and clothing yellow
Tars	Tars	Inhibits enzymes involved in mitosis and inflammation	Mild to moderate psoriasis	Could stain	Photosensitivity Dermatitis Stains
Methotrexate	Methotrexate	Inhibits metabolism of folic acid in the synthesis of DNA, leading to antiproliferative effects	Severe psoriasis	Used once weekly	See Chapter 22
Immunomodulators	Cyclosporine	1) Inhibits calcineurin 2) Thought to inhibit production and release of interleukin-2, inhibiting the induction of cytotoxic T lymphocytes	Severe unresponsive psoriasis	Normally used once weekly	See Chapter 9
	Infliximab	Is a monoclonal antibody against TNF-α, resulting in prevention of action of IL-1 and IL-6 as well as migration of leukocytes	Severe recurrent disabling psoriasis	Third line use only	Itch Nausea Erythema Premature skin ageing Cutaneous carcinogenesis
	Etanercept	Is dimeric soluble form of p75 TNF receptor and specifically binds TNF-α and TNF-β rendering TNF inactive			
	Efalizumab	Monoclonal antibody against CD11a alpha subunit of LFA-1 blocking interaction between LFA-1 on lymphocytes and ICAM-1 on APCs, resulting in inhibition of T-cell activation			
Phototherapy and photochemotherapy	UVB light	Prevents DNA synthesis	Third line use in severe psoriasis		
	UVA and psoralen	Psoralen Intercalates between base pairs in adjacent DNA strands after which UVA thought to causes photocycloaddition that cross link DNA strands			Phototoxicity pruritus Skin ageing, increased risk of squamous cancer

ICAM-1 = intracellular adhesion molecule-1

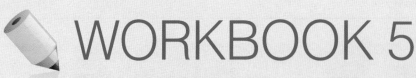

WORKBOOK 5
Dermatology: dermatitis, acne, and psoriasis

Elvis, Eimear and a teacher: three cases of chronic skin diseases and their management

Patient 1, Elvis: a simplified case history

Sunita has taken Elvis, one of their triplets to yet another GP appointment. Sunita has now been married to Eoin for many years and the couple have had several ups and downs as detailed later in chapters 15 and 19 later, when Sunita is the patient.

Elvis has had another sleepless night scratching his neck and trunk and actually has bruises and cuts from scratching. Sunita feels like she lives at the surgery because each week, one of the family needs to be seen by the doctor for one thing or another.

A table of clinical clerking abbreviations is given on page xi.

SUMMARY OF CLINICAL CLERKING FOR ELVIS KAISER AT GP SURGERY

Age: 13 years

PC: Itchy red and swollen areas at the back of neck, inside of elbows, and trunk. Inside of the elbow is painful and weeping.

HPC: The itching started 6 months ago and has become progressively worse. Mum says all different types of emollients have been used as prescribed. They all provide some relief, but overall there has been no improvement. It seems to be worse in spring and summer.

1 Symptoms of acute dermatitis:

- *skin itchy, red, hot, dry and scaly*
- *skin could be wet and weeping and swollen*
- *there may be infection with bacteria*

2 Symptoms of chronic dermatitis:

- *skin dry and thickened*
- *skin could be scaly or cracked, as a result of continual scratching.*

The most common areas affected are the skin creases such as the front of the elbows and wrists, backs of knees, and around the neck. However, any areas of skin may be affected.

PMH: Eczema from 1 month till 3 years. Asthma from 12 months till 4 years.

He had dermatitis and asthma as a child. These were diagnosed as atopic. Atopic dermatitis is the most common type of dermatitis and is linked to hay fever and asthma (called the 'atopic triad'). Being atopic means being extra sensitivity to substances (allergens).

Atopic dermatitis is thought to be IgE (immunoglobulin E)-mediated and patients usually have high levels of Ig E antibodies as a result of interaction with the antigen (allergen). The most common allergens are house dust mites, feathers, pollen, cat or dog fur, and sometimes foodstuffs, e.g. cows milk, eggs, or nuts.

Both conditions improved in childhood. However, the dermatitis seems to have re-occurred.

Atopic dermatitis affects approximately 15–20% of young children in the UK. It clears up in approximately 70% of children by the time they reach their teens and in many it largely clears up by 4–5 years of age. If it persists into adult life, it usually affects the body creases, the face, and the hands.

DH:

1) Oilatum bath additive

2) Aqueous cream as a soap substitute

3) Diprobase cream

4) Hydrocortisone 0.1%

1 Oilatum is an emollient bath oil.

2 Aqueous cream and diprobase are both emollients.

3 Hydrocortisone cream 0.1% is a steroid cream of mild potency.

The cornerstone in the treatment of dermatitis is the use of emollients (moisturisers), including soap substitutes, bath oils, and general moisturisers, and topical corticosteroids (steroids) for flare-ups. Emollients are often underused and the most suitable emollients should be chosen in consultation with the patient to improve compliance.

FH: His grandfather and brother both have asthma. His brother suffers from hay fever.

Inherited factors are important in dermatitis. These inherited factors make patients more sensitive to allergens in the environment and increase the risk of developing dermatitis, asthma, or hay fever.

Other factors that may trigger a dermatitis flare-up are:

- *specific allergies to foods*
- *overheating*
- *secondary infection (usually Staphylococcus aureus)*
- *wool next to the skin*
- *cat and dog fur*
- *soaps and detergents*
- *house dust mites and pollen*
- *extreme hot and cold*
- *humidity (moisture in the area)*
- *hormonal changes in women (caused by the menstrual cycle and pregnancy).*

O/E: Oozing and crusted lesions inside of elbow. Dry thickened and scaly skin all over back, neck, and back of knees.

The elbow lesion could be infected; the others observations are all symptoms of chronic dermatitis. However, scabies needs to be excluded. Patient should be asked if other members of the household have the same symptoms. If they do, it could be scabies, which is infectious, unlike dermatitis.

O/Q: A general approach to a patient with dermatologic symptoms should begin with evaluation of the answers to the following questions.

1) When did the itching start and how long has he had this?

   Answer: See HPC above.

2) What factors make it worse?

   Answer: Spring and summer (?pollen and heat?).

3) Have the lesions recently changed in size, appearance, and severity?

   Answer: See HPC above.

4) What types of lesions are present and how are they distributed?

   Answer: See HPC above.

   Many lesions will present in a characteristic distribution or pattern. The lesions' consistency, borders, and colour are all very important.

5) Where are they located?

   Answer: See HPC above.

   Certain lesions or conditions will almost always appear in certain locations. Atopic dermatitis appears most commonly in flexor areas, e.g. inside of elbow or neck. Lesions involving the eye, mouth, genitalia, and rectal areas should be referred immediately.

6) What is the patient's medical or dermatological history?

   Answer: See HPC above.

   Pre-existing condition may aid assessment. Elvis' history of asthma and dermatitis indicates atopy and likelihood of recurrence. Certain diseases, e.g. diabetes, cancer, and alcoholism, could predispose to dermatologic conditions. Self-neglect could also pre-dispose to certain conditions.

7) What medications have been used in the past?

   Answer: See HPC above.

   A previously ineffective medication should not be used again. However, it must be assessed if the regime was properly followed; a more potent product could be required.

Diagnosis: Infected chronic atopic dermatitis

Plan:

Add to emmolients:

- betamethasone valerate for 7 days and for flare-ups

- bactroban ointment three times a day for 7 days

- paraffin ointment.

  All the emollients should still be used.

  Betamethasone valerate 0.1%, a stronger steroid, should be used for 7 days initially and then during flare-ups.

  Bactroban contains mupirocin, an antibiotic, which should be used on the infected area for 7 days. The most likely bacteria is staphylococcus aureus.

PART 1: ELVIS' DERMATITIS AND ITS TREATMENT

1a) What is dermatitis?

1b) What is the difference between eczema and dermatitis?

2) Explain the pathogenesis of dermatitis. Explain what you expect to be happening within the skin layers in the areas of Elvis' skin that suffer from dermatitis.

3) Does inflammation cause dermatitis or does dermatitis cause inflammation? Explain.

4) What are the symptoms of dermatitis that Elvis experienced?

5) What are the main approaches in the treatment of dermatitis?

6) Which approach was used for Elvis? Was this the right approach?

7) Which classe(s) of drugs besides those used for Elvis are available to treat dermatitis?

Elvis was prescribed a stronger steroid (glucocorticoid) cream than he was previously on.

8) What effects of glucocorticoids make them the mainstay of treatment of dermatitis?

9) How are corticosteroids classified (see Table 8.3)?

Sunita takes the prescription to the pharmacy. The pharmacist confirms that her son has been prescribed a stronger steroid—betamethasone valerate 0.1% in place of hydrocortisone 0.1%—and advises Elvis to apply the steroid thinly and not more often than prescribed because it is a potent steroid which if absorbed could cause side effects. She also advised him not to apply it to his face.

10a) Do you think it is important to prescribe the lowest strength steroid that will do the job? Explain why.

10b) Why was advice given not to apply the stronger steroid to the face?

10c) What are the side effects of topical steroids?

The antibiotic and steroid cream help so much Elvis decides he is cured and he refuses to use his emollients.

His dermatitis flares up 2 weeks later.

The itching is also very bad and his mum goes to the chemist to enquire about what to give him for the itching.

11) What is the role of emollients in the management of dermatitis?

12) Are emollients pharmacologically active? Explain your answer, using Box 8.2 to help.

The pharmacist counsels Elvis to continue using his emollients even when he is without symptoms.

His mum tells her that he hates the greasiness of the ointment.

13a) Which form of emollient could Elvis be advised to use on his face?

13b) When would be the best time for Elvis to use his ointment?

13c) Which is more effective, cream or ointment? Explain why.

> Elvis asks the pharmacist what 'vehicle' means, explaining that this is mentioned on the website he has been looking at.

14) What does 'vehicle' mean? Is it important which vehicle is used? Explain.

> The dermatitis gets a lot worse over the months and Elvis is sent to see a consultant dermatologist. The dermatologist tells Sunita about some more potent drugs used in dermatitis, but advises her that these are only used when all the other treatments fail.

15a) Give two examples of drugs that affect the immune system and are licensed to be prescribed by specialists for dermatitis.

15b) Are these drugs used topically or systemically?

15c) When stronger steroids are given topically there is concern over their systemic effects. Should we have the same concerns with topical use of a drug such as pimecrolimus? Explain your answer.

16) What is the mechanism of action of these immunomodulatory drugs?.

_____

_____

_____

After Elvis admits that he was not compliant with his previous treatment, the dermatologist and specialist nurse both counsel him about the importance of regular and correct use of his medications. They decide that the best option would be to use the same medication that was used in the previous flare-up: betamethasone valerate 0.1% for 7 days was prescribed.

After 1 week, Elvis should stop using the betamethasone valerate and continue using the following emollients:

- oilatum bath additive
- aqueous cream as a soap substitute
- diprobase cream
- paraffin ointment at bedtime.

Sunita is dismayed at the lack of long-term progress with her son, despite the best efforts of the medical profession.

17a) Can atopic dermatitis be cured?

_____

_____

_____

17b) What do you think is the likely long-term prospect for Elvis and his skin condition?

_____

_____

_____

One year later Elvis' dermatitis is well controlled and he is happy he does not have to use his emollients as often because they used to soil his clothes. He always felt self-conscious about the greasiness of the emollients.

PART 2

> During a follow-up appointment, Elvis' GP is surprised when Elvis asks him the difference between dermatitis and psoriasis. He says one of his teachers has psoriasis and one of his classmates has been teasing him and saying that his dermatitis would turn to psoriasis in middle age. Elvis is now worried this will happen to him.

18a) What is psoriasis?

_____

_____

_____

18b) Describe the pathogenesis in terms of keratinocyte proliferation.

_____

_____

_____

19) What are the characteristics of psoriatic skin?

_____

_____

_____

_____

> The GP explains to Elvis that these two skin conditions are not related and dermatitis will not lead to psoriasis. Some of the classes of drugs used in dermatitis are also used in psoriasis. However, the majority of treatment options for the two conditions are different. We see this when the teacher, whose name is Tom, visits his GP for ongoing advice concerning his psoriasis.

20a) Consider the three treatment options for localized psoriasis listed below. Give a single sentence to comment on their usefulness.

Calcitriol_____

Acitretin_____

Dithranol_____

20b) Explain the role of emollients (citing examples) in the treatment of psoriasis.

_____

_____

_____

21a) What are the effects of the vitamin D analogues used in psoriasis?

21b) Explain their mechanism of action.

22a) What are therapeutic tars?

22b) List two characteristics of therapeutic tars that make them effective in psoriasis treatment.

22c) What are the disadvantages of tars?

23) Indicate some treatment options for patients with psoriasis that is unresponsive to the first-line drugs. Suggest why they are not more commonly used.

Elvis is relieved that his dermatitis will not lead to psoriasis. His dermatitis continues to improve steadily. He is extremely happy and grateful that his skin is almost completely normal, which is why he can empathize with his 18-year-old cousin Eimear, who now seems to be suffering from a skin condition. She has been diagnosed with acne. She has what she calls blackheads all over her face and some on her back.

24a) Describe the characteristics of acne.

24b) What is its pathogenesis?

Eimear has been using an over-the-counter benzoyl peroxide for her acne. She does not use it regularly because it dries out her skin. The acne seems to be getting worse. After refusing several times to go out with her friends because of the condition of her face, Monique, her mum, takes her to see the GP. At the surgery the GP examines her and notes that she has a few lesions on her face and her back. They are blackheads with a few whiteheads; this is called comedonal acne. She has mild acne.

After discussing her condition, her GP recommends that the right treatment for Eimear would be regular use of benzoyl peroxide. Although she used this already, she uses in incorrectly. Because her acne is mild, regular use of this drug should be sufficient. He recommends a cream containing benzoyl peroxide 2.5%. The pharmacist counsels Eimear on how to use the benzoyl peroxide. The advice she gives is to use it once a day at night-time for 2 months over the entire affected area. Before starting, she gets Eimear to test her sensitivity by applying a small amount behind her ear and looking for a reaction.

25) What are the actions of benzoyl peroxide that make it effective in acne?

After 2 months, Eimear's acne has got progressively worse. Some spots are filled with pus. The redness and dryness is also very upsetting to her. Monique, who has been reading about options, asks the GP if he could prescribe azelaic acid. The GP recommends that the benzoyl peroxide be discontinued and azelaic acid with an antibiotic cream be used instead. He says that it should cause less drying and irritation.

26) What are the effects and properties of azelaic acid that make it effective in acne?

Eimear returns to the GP after 3 months because there has been no improvement with using the azelaic acid and topical antibiotic.

The GP replaces the azelaic acid with a retinoid cream to be used once daily.

27a) What is the mechanism by which retinoids work to improve acne?

27b) How are they used? How effective are they?

When she goes to collect the retinoid cream, the pharmacist advises Eimear to avoid exposure to light, or at least use a good broad spectrum suntan lotion, while using the cream to reduce the risk of skin irritation. She also advises that it should be used at bedtime.

A while later Eimear leaves her medicine at home when she goes to visit her cousin Elvis for the weekend. She asks a local pharmacist if she could borrow her cousin's steroid cream and use it short-term to tide her over. One of her friends has told her that steroids will treat everything.

28a) Can steroids be used for acne? For which skin conditions should steroids not be used?

28b) What advice do you think the local pharmacist should have given to Eimear when she asked about using her cousin's steroid cream to treat her acne?

However, in the end, the acne remains a problem. The doctor knows that in female patients an anti-androgen hormone will often reduce acne, therefore when Eimear approaches him to discuss contraception, he is able to freely suggest a form of oral contraceptive that will also offer her the prospect of more effective control of her acne. This takes advantage of the anti-androgen effect of oestrogen or oestrogen-mimicking contraceptives. This works, the acne is largely resolved, and Eimear is happy.

Chapter 9
Rheumatoid arthritis

Imagine if your mum's hands are so deformed she struggles to hold her keys and has had to give up driving. Although she takes regular medication for her arthritis, she still suffers from pain in her joints and muscles. What is more, the medication she has to take causes nasty side effects such as cataracts and osteoporosis. If this were the case, your mum would be like Gwen and Pamela, who we will meet in Workbook 6, one of the 1% of the population who suffer from rheumatoid arthritis (RA).

As we will see, RA is a debilitating condition characterized by intermittent worsening of the symptoms (called 'flares'). Effective treatment requires a multidisciplinary team of doctors, physiotherapist, nurse specialists, pharmacist, occupational therapist, and social workers. It is crucial that each member of this team has an understanding of the disease process and treatment options to ensure the patient gets the best possible care.

In this chapter we will cover the pathogenesis of RA, the cellular and molecular basis of action of the commonly used drugs, and available strategies for treatment. We will also discuss the main adverse drug reactions and contraindications, since these play a major role in determining which drug treatments are used. At the end of the chapter we will discuss the management of our two fictional patients, Gwen and Pamela, who have RA.

9.1 What is rheumatoid arthritis?

Rheumatoid arthritis is a chronic disease that predominantly affects synovial joints (joints with spaces between the bones). The most common joints affected are those of the hands and wrists. However, the elbows, neck, shoulders, hips, knees, as well as the feet could also be affected.

The fundamental signs of RA are swelling, stiffness, and pain in the joints, the same as the signs of acute inflammation due to any injury (see section Introduction). Over time, this acute inflammation becomes a chronic condition and leads to loss of function in the affected joints. Sufferers also experience other symptoms, including fatigue, fever, and a general sense of feeling unwell.

Rheumatoid arthritis is three times more common in females than males. The onset of RA is usually around 30–50 years, and the diagnosis is generally based on clinical criteria because the biochemical markers in the blood, in particular rheumatoid factor (RF), do not appear until late in the disease progression. The key diagnostic criteria are as follows:

- symptom duration of >6 weeks
- early morning stiffness of >1 hour
- three or more regions affected
- bilateral compression tenderness of the metatarsophalangeal joints
- symmetry of the areas affected
- RF present (late disease)
- anticyclic citrullinated peptide (antiCCP) antibody present
- bony erosions evident on radiographs of the hands or feet (late disease).

The cause of RA is unclear, although there is evidence that it is immune-mediated. The initial stimulants for the immune reaction are uncertain, but may include auto-antigens, infections, and environmental factors.

9.1.1 What abnormal changes occur in the affected joints in RA?

As discussed above, the parts of the body affected by RA are the synovial joints. A key feature of these joints is the synovial membrane, or synovium (see Figure 9.1). The synovium is a thin membrane that has a number of roles in protecting and maintaining these joints. First, it provides a physical barrier to stop things entering the joint space. Second, cells within the synovial membrane produce fluid, which fills the joint space and keeps the ends of the bones apart, allowing the joint to move freely. It also helps in providing nutrients to the cartilage, a thick, dense, translucent material that covers the end of the joints (you probably have come across it as 'gristle' in meat) to protect them. In RA a number of immune reactions occur that affect this joint, leading to inflammation, joint destruction, and ultimately a loss of motion in the joint.

As outlined in the introduction to this section, the body has a range of defences against invasion from foreign particles and organisms, including the immune system. Normally the immune system can detect the difference between foreign ('non-self') cells and substances, and those of the host ('self'), using a variety of proteins. However, occasionally the body fails to detect the difference and starts to produce antibodies against the host cells (called autoantibodies)—this is the basis of autoimmune diseases. The reason the immune system does this is not well understood, but genetic factors, and possibly environmental factors such as viral infections, may play a role. In RA, the autoantibodies are formed by activated B-cells that convert to plasma cells, and are called RF. The RF binds to immunoglobulin G to form an immune complex, which deposits in the joints. While RF can be tested for, and about 80% of people with RA will have evidence of RF, in early disease the levels may not be elevated. Also, RF can be elevated for a number of reasons other than RA, such as hepatitis, viral infections, and in patients with systemic lupus erythematosis (another autoimmune disease similar to RA but affecting a range of tissues other than joints). Levels of RF are therefore not terribly useful by themselves in diagnosing RA, but can be helpful in conjunction with other symptoms suggestive of RA.

> In the workbook at the end of this chapter our fictional patient Pamela tested positive for RF, and in combination with her signs and symptoms, plus elevation in other inflammatory markers (e.g. C-reactive protein), it helped confirm the diagnosis of RA.

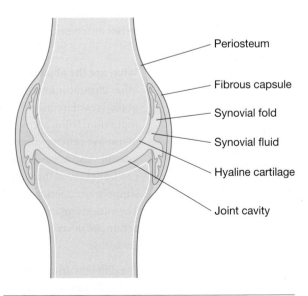

Periosteum

Fibrous capsule

Synovial fold

Synovial fluid

Hyaline cartilage

Joint cavity

Figure 9.1 Synovial joint.

The production of RF occurs in response to the activation of T-cells. In addition to stimulating the plasma cells to produce antibodies, the T-cells produce cytokines that activate the macrophages and fibroblasts in the synovium. This leads to proliferation of these cells as well as chondrocytes (the cells in the cartilage), leading to thickening of synovium and cartilage fibrosis. The cells of the synovium then stimulate the release of various enzymes that break down collagen and stimulate destruction of the bone at the end of the joint. The T-cells also increase the activity of osteoclasts (the cells in bone responsible for reabsorbing the bone matrix) by the expression of receptor activator of nuclear factor κβ ligand (abbreviated to RANKL). A summary of the immune process can be seen in Box 9.1.

Over time the net effect of these immune reactions is the formation of granulation tissue at the edges of the synovium (called pannus formation), destruction of the joint, and fibrosis of the cartilage. If this continues it can lead to ankylosis (loss of movement of the joint). The thickening of the synovium and the infiltration of inflammatory cells cause increased demand for oxygen, which the body responds to by increasing the number of blood vessels (called angiogenesis). Unfortunately, this only serves to deliver more inflammatory cells to the region, exacerbating the problem. As we will see in the chapter on chemotherapy (Chapter 22), many of the features of chronic inflammation mimic those seen in cancers (e.g. rapidly dividing cells and angiogenesis), therefore, not surprisingly, we will see later that several chemotherapy drugs are now used to treat RA.

9.2 Rheumatoid arthritis and its drug treatment

At the start of this section we discussed inflammatory and immune responses and the various inflammatory markers that play a role during the inflammatory response. The pharmacological treatment of RA targets various aspects of these inflammatory processes.

The agents used to treat RA can be broadly classified into anti-inflammatory drugs and disease-modifying antirheumatic drugs (**DMARDs**). The anti-inflammatory drugs are divided into non-steroidal anti-inflammatory drugs (**NSAIDs**), and corticosteroids (**glucocorticosteroids**). The DMARDs can be further subdivided into immunosuppressants/modulators, cytokine blockers (biologics), and antirheumatic drugs (a collection of drugs with various and often uncertain modes of action in RA!).

First-line therapy – DMARDs or anti-inflammatories? Anti-inflammatory drugs, particularly the NSAIDs, were considered the first-line, early treatment for RA for many years. However, we can now see this as an example of concentrating on treating the symptoms while leaving the disease process more or less intact. Early treatment with the DMARDs leads to much better response, so NSAIDs and corticosteroids are largely reserved for pain management (NSAIDs) and acute flares (corticosteroids). For an established diagnosis of RA the first-line recommendations are early initiation of

DMARDs. However, while awaiting a diagnosis (which can take several weeks while tests are conducted) symptoms are treated with NSAIDs (and/or steroids). NSAIDs are still used with the DMARDs because the DMARDs do not offer pain relief. The therapeutic response to DMARDs can be slow (months), which may make it necessary to offer symptomatic relief with NSAIDs during this time. Using NSAIDs alone in a patient with a diagnosis of RA and then adding DMARDs later if things worsen (the old-fashioned 'step up' sort of approach) is no longer advised, as there is good evidence that early DMARD therapy produces better outcomes.

What are the objectives of treating RA? Similar to other chronic inflammatory diseases, the two main objectives of treatment of RA are pain relief followed by remission. Other secondary objectives include control of disease activity, making daily living as normal as possible and maximizing the quality of life. These goals can be achieved through rest, exercise, emotional support, occupational therapy, and drug treatment. The various treatments used in RA and their sites of action are described in Box 9.1 and summarized in Table 9.1.

The different drugs used in RA, in their anti-inflammatory and DMARD categories, are summarized in Table 9.2.

Box 9.1

Processes involved in rheumatoid arthritis

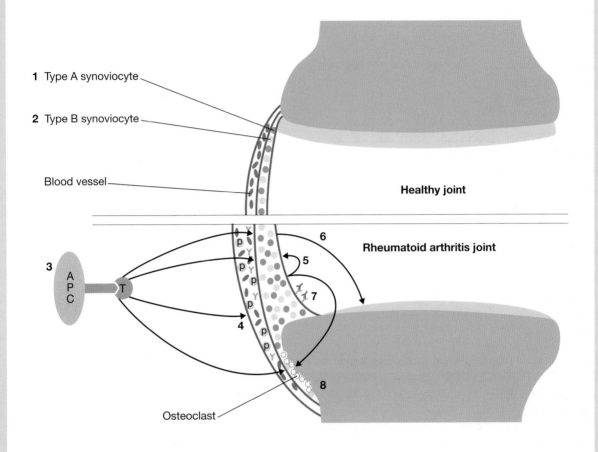

1 Type A synoviocyte

2 Type B synoviocyte

Blood vessel

Healthy joint

Rheumatoid arthritis joint

3 APC

T

Osteoclast

Figure a

1. Type A synoviocytes are macrophage-like cells that phagocytose potential invaders.

2. Type B synoviocytes are fibroblast-like cells and produce the synovial fluid.

3. T-cells are activated after presentation of an antigen. They produce interleukins and interferon gamma, stimulate B-cells to differentiate into plasma cells, stimulate macrophages (Type A) and fibroblasts (Type B), and directly stimulate osteoclasts through receptor activator of nuclear factor β (RANKL). **This is a site of action** for the immunosuppressive drugs and methotrexate.

4. The plasma cells produce the autoantibodies called rheumatoid factor (RF).

5. Macrophages that are activated by the T-cells produce interleukin-I (IL-1) and tumour necrosis factor α (TNF-α). These stimulate osteoclasts and fibroblasts, as well as promoting the release of other cytokines and chemokines. This is a site of action for the corticosteroids, anti-IL-1 drugs (e.g. anakinra), and the antiTNF drugs (e.g. etanercept).

6. The fibroblasts produce enzymes such as collagenase and elastase, which cause destruction of the collagen.

7. Rheumatoid factor binds with immunoglobulin G to form an immune complex that deposits in the joint.

8. Osteoclasts are activated by RANKL and cause removal of the mineralized matrix of the bone, leading to bone destruction.

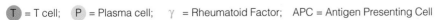

T = T cell;   P = Plasma cell;   γ = Rheumatoid Factor;   APC = Antigen Presenting Cell

Table 9.1 Mediators of inflammation and pharmacological agents

Inflammatory/ immune mediator	Effect	Sources	Pharmacological agent(s)
Prostaglandins	Inflammation	Endothelial cells	NSAIDs Glucocorticoids
Interleukins	Activation of lymphocytes, fibroblasts, and osteoclasts; activation of T-cells and B-cells	Macrophages, T-cells	Glucocorticoids Methotrexate Azathioprine Ciclosporin Cyclophosphamide Leflunamide Anakinra Abatcept
TNF-α	Prostaglandin production; activation of fibroblasts and osteoclasts	Macrophages	Infliximab Etanercept Adalimumab Glucocorticoids
Interferons	Multiple	Macrophages, endothelial cells, T-cells	Glucocorticoids

Mediators of inflammation and inflammatory cells, and cells involved in the immune response are discussed in the introduction to Section 3.
TNF-α, tumour necrosis factor-alpha.

Table 9.2 Major pharmacological agents used to treat rheumatoid arthritis

Anti-inflammatories		Disease-modifying antirheumatic drugs		
NSAIDs	Corticosteroids	Immunosuppressant/ immune-modulators	Antirheumatics	Cytokine blockers
Aspirin	Prednisolone	Methotrexate	Gold salts	Adalimumab
Celecoxib*	Prednisone	Azathioprine	Penicillamine	Etanercept
Diclofenac	Triamcinolone	Ciclosporin	Antimalarials	Infliximab
Etoricoxib*	Methylprednisolone	Cyclophosphamide	Sulfasalazine	Anakinra
Ibuprofen	Hydrocortisone	Leflunamide		
Indomethacin	Dexamethasone	Rituximab		
Ketoprofen		Abatacept		
Ketorolac				
Mefenamic acid				
Meloxicam*				
Naproxen				
Parecoxib*				
Piroxicam				
Sulindac				
Tiaprofenic acid				
Valdecoxib*				

NSAIDs, non-steroidal anti-inflammatory drugs. NSAIDs marked * are COX-2 selective.

9.3 Anti-inflammatories

As mentioned above, the role of anti-inflammatories as first-line drugs has diminished, but they retain a major role in the management of this condition.

9.3.1 Non-steroidal anti-inflammatory drugs

The NSAIDs include a wide range of drugs with different chemical structures but similar pharmacologic effects, including:

- antipyretic: they reduce a high temperature
- analgesic: they reduce the sensation of pain
- anti-inflammatory: they reduce inflammation

These three effects result from the inhibition of cyclooxygenase (COX) and subsequent inhibition of the production of prostaglandins and thromboxanes (collectively called prostanoids). Details of the synthesis and action of prostanoids are covered in the introduction to this section (see Figure S3.1 and Table S3.2) and are summarized in Figure 9.2.

COX-1 or COX-2 inhibitor?

Cyclooxygenase is central to the inflammatory response leading to the synthesis of the prostanoids as described in Figure S3.1 in the introduction to this section.

Cyclooxygenase appears in one of three isoforms, with COX-1 and COX-2 being the most common. COX-1 is called a 'constitutive' enzyme (meaning that it is expressed all of the time) and produces prostanoids that maintain the stomach lining, promote renal blood flow, and alter platelet aggregation. It is a ubiquitous enzyme found in many cells and is important in maintaining normal function. COX-2 is an 'inducible' enzyme involved in inflammatory reactions. While present in small amounts all of the time, the presence of the enzyme increases in response to inflammatory mediators (hence 'inducible'). The prostanoids produced by COX-2 include prostaglandin I_2 (PG-I_2) and prostaglandin E_2 (PG-E_2). The inflammatory effects of these include:

- direct vasodilatation and potentiation of other vasodilators such as bradykinin and histamine, leading to increased blood flow and redness
- potentiation of the effects of bradykinin and histamine on vascular permeability, leading to oedema and swelling
- sensitization of the pain fibres (afferent C fibres), leading to increased pain sensation
- ability to 'reset' the body's thermostat in the hypothalamus, leading to fever (referred to as being pyrogenic).

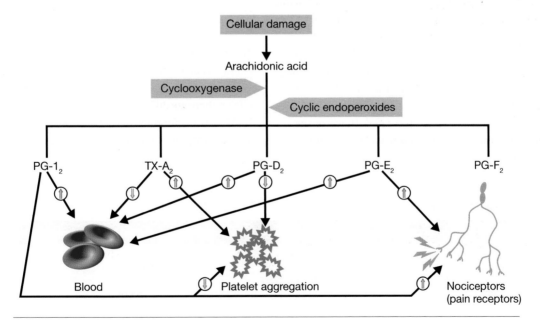

Figure 9.2 Role of cycloxygenase in the inflammatory response.

⇓, decreases/constricts; ⇑, increases/dilates. PG-I_2, prostaglandin I_2; TX-A_2, thromboxane A_2; PG-D2, prostaglandin D_2; PG-E2, prostaglandin E_2; PG-$F_{2\alpha}$, prostaglandin $F_{2\alpha}$.

Theoretically the inhibition of COX-2, while sparing COX-1, will maximise the anti-inflammatory effects while maintaining the protective effects of prostanoids. The older NSAIDs are non-selective and block both COX enzymes, thereby exerting anti-inflammatory properties in RA, but also increasing the patient's risk of gastrointestinal (GI) and renal side effects. There are a large number of older NSAIDs, including **ibuprofen**, **diclofenac**, and **naproxen.** The newer NSAIDs are more COX-2 selective, and include **celecoxib**, **parecoxib**, **valdecoxib**, and **meloxicam** (in low doses—at high doses meloxicam acts like a non-selective NSAID). A list of non-selective and selective NSAIDs can be found in Table 9.2. The COX-2 selectivity comes about from their structure. The COX-1 enzyme will only accommodate relatively small, narrow chemical structures, while the COX-2 can accommodate bulkier molecules, as demonstrated in Figure 9.3. It should be noted that paracetamol is reported to act on COX-3, located in the brain. Because of its lack of effects on COX-2 or COX-1, it doesn't have the anti inflammatory effects of the NSAIDs, but does have antipyretic and analgesic effects.

There is nothing to distinguish the various NSAIDs based on efficacy, with the main differences being the frequency of dosing, routes of administration, and side effects. Table 9.3 summarizes the dosing of the various NSAIDs.

All NSAIDs, with the exception of **parecoxib**, are available in oral formulations. A few, such as **indomethacin**, **ketoprofen** and **diclofenac**, are available in rectal formulations, and ketorolac and parecoxib can be given by injection. These are useful in patients who are unable to swallow. Many of the NSAIDs are also available in topical formulations. These have the advantage of reduced systemic side effects (see later). However, the evidence for the efficacy in RA is so far limited, although

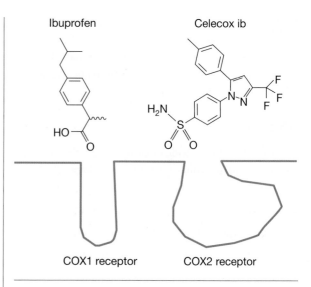

Figure 9.3 Cyclooxygenase enzymes.

The chemical structures above illustrate the narrow form of ibuprofen, which fits into the narrow pocket of COX-1 or the open pocket of COX-2, hence this drug inhibits both types of enzyme (a non-selective COX inhibitor). Contrasting with this, the celecoxib structure cannot enter the narrow pocket of COX-1 because it is too wide, but will fit into its site in COX-2. Hence celecoxib is a COX-2 selective NSAID.

they can be useful in other musculoskeletal inflammatory conditions (e.g. sprains, strains, and soft tissue injuries).

Unwanted effects of NSAIDs and some drug combinations to avoid

The most prominent side effect of the non-selective NSAIDs is their effect on the GI tract (see Chapter 12). While all non-selective NSAIDs have the potential for GI effects, there are differences among the non-selective NSAIDs, with ibuprofen having the lowest risk, and agents such as ketoprofen and piroxicam having the greatest risk.

Table 9.3 Dosing of common NSAIDs

Dosed three or four times a day	Dosed three times or twice daily	Dosed once or twice daily
Aspirin	Diclofenac[b]	Celecoxib
Ibuprofen	Mefenamic acid	Etoricoxib
Indometacin[a,b]	Tiaprofenic acid	Meloxicam
Ketoprofen[a,b]		Parecoxib
Ketorolac		Piroxicam
Naproxen[a]		Sulindac
		Valdecoxib

[a] Can also be dosed twice a day in some instances.
[b] Rectal preparations given once or twice a day.

Other side effects include inhibition of platelet aggregation, leading to increased bleeding, and precipitation of heart failure and/or renal failure due to their effects on the kidneys. The latter effect is particularly important when combining NSAIDs with other drugs that reduce kidney function. These include angiotensin-converting enzyme inhibitors (ACEI) and angiotensin II receptor antagonists (A2RAs), and diuretics. The combination of ACEI/A2RA + diuretic + NSAID is sometimes called the 'triple whammy' and is an important interaction as increasingly combination products of ACEI/A2RAs + diuretics are being used. People prescribed these products can inadvertently add in the NSAID by purchasing it at a pharmacy or supermarket. It is therefore important that patients on ACEI/A2RA + diuretic products be warned about using over-the-counter headache and cold and flu preparations that might contain an NSAID (usually ibuprofen). Another rare side effect of NSAIDs is to precipitate asthma in susceptible individuals (see Chapter 11).

COX-2 selective NSAIDs reduce GI side effects

The main advantage of the newer COX-2 selective NSAIDs is reduced GI effects (see Chapter 12 for more details). However, if your risk is already low (e.g. you are a young, fit, healthy footballer!) it is not cost-effective to use the COX-2 specific agents, and older NSAIDs are the appropriate choice (not many people with RA are footballers, but these drugs are used for other inflammatory conditions such as soft tissue injuries). So far, no other advantage has been found for the COX-2 selective NSAIDs. One serious side effect with the newer COX-2 selective agents is an increase in cardiovascular (CV) events. The exact mechanism of this effect is still uncertain. One theory is that the COX-2 selective agents, by inhibiting the production of PG-I$_2$ (which inhibits platelet aggregation and causes vasodilatation), tilt the balance towards increased production of thromboxane (which causes platelet aggregation and vasoconstriction). There also appears to be a dose response, with higher doses increasing the risk. This finding of increased CV events led to the removal of one agent (rofecoxib) from the market, and means these agents should be used with caution in patients who have an increased risk of CV events. Interestingly, a study has found that diclofenac may also increase your risk of CV events, and it is probably best avoided if you are at increased risk.

In Workbook 5 Pamela is prescribed a COX-2 inhibitor after she develops GI side effects with diclofenac.

Selecting an NSAID

When selecting an NSAID the main considerations are the person's risk of GI complications and their CV risk. Conditions that put you at increased GI risk include existing GI conditions (e.g. peptic ulcers or gastrooesophageal reflux), GI events in the past while on NSAIDs, therapy with other drugs that effect the GI tract (e.g. corticosteroids, see below), and old age. Your CV risk is increased if you have existing CV disease (e.g. have angina, have had a myocardial infarction, etc) and adverse lifestyle factors (e.g. obesity, smoking, type II diabetes), and increases with increasing age.

The recommended treatment choices, considering these factors, are outlined in Table 9.4.

All NSAIDs should be used cautiously in patients with heart failure and hypertension, and in some patients with asthma (see Chapter 11).

9.3.2 Corticosteroids

The corticosteroids mimic the actions of the steroids that are produced by the adrenal gland in the body. The adrenal gland, located on top of the kidneys, secretes catecholamines (from the medulla) and steroids (from the cortex, hence **cortico**steroids) that are essential for life. The corticosteroids have mineralocorticoid (affecting water and electrolyte balance) and glucocorticoid (those that affect metabolism) effects. The main mineralocorticoid is aldosterone, which affects sodium and water reabsorption in the kidney. A number of glucocorticoids are produced, with the most common being **cortisol** (also called **hydrocortisone**). We use glucocorticoids for their anti-inflammatory effects in RA and other inflammatory conditions, and so they will be the focus of this section.

Steroids, the brain, the pituitary, and the adrenals

Release of adrenal hormones is controlled by adrenocorticotrophic hormone (ACTH) secreted by the pituitary. The release of ACTH is increased in response to corticotrophin-releasing factor (CRF) secreted by the hypothalamus. CRF release is inhibited in the presence of increased levels of corticosteroids and ACTH (called a negative feedback loop), as outlined in Figure 9.4. This interrelationship is referred to as the hypothalamic–pituitary–adrenal axis (HPA axis).

An important clinical consequence of the negative feedback loop is that if you give a patient glucocorticoids

Table 9.4 Selection of NSAIDs based on gastrointestinal and cardiovascular risks

Cardiovascular risk ⟍ Gastrointestinal risk	Low	High
Low	Non-selective NSAID, probably ibuprofen as it has lowest GI risk	Non-selective NSAID, probably avoid diclofenac as it may also increase CV risk and ibuprofen as it blocks the effects of low-dose aspirin
High	COX-2 selective NSAID	Non-selective NSAID plus a proton pump inhibitor (see Chapter 12), probably avoid diclofenac as it may also increase CV risk and ibuprofen as it blocks the effects of low-dose aspirin

NSAID, non-steroidal anti-inflammatory drug; GI, gastrointestinal; CV, cardiovascular.

in a manner that allows them to enter the circulation (intentional, as in oral therapy, or undesirable, as in treatment of skin conditions, see Chapter 8) then activity in the HPA axis will be suppressed. This has widespread consequences for the clinical use of glucocorticoids, and warrants particular care on withdrawal from the drug.

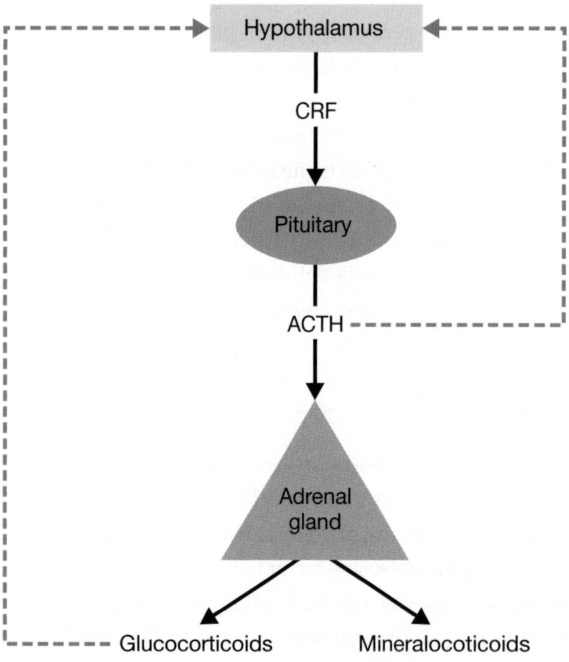

Some aspects of the effects of glucocorticoid steroids on the body are developed in Box 9.2. Notably this includes an introduction to the effects of glucocorticoids on the immune response. This is important because it accounts for both the desirable (therapeutic) and unwanted effects of these steroids when they are used as drugs.

Steroids as drugs in the treatment of RA

In RA, oral and intra-articular (injected directly into the joint) corticosteroids are most commonly used. Topical, intranasal, and inhaled corticosteroids are used for inflammatory skin conditions (see Chapter 8), allergic rhinitis (see Chapter 10), and asthma (see Chapter 11), respectively. The main differences in the glucocorticoids are their potency on a per milligram basis. A summary of the comparative potency and usual routes of administration of the corticosteroids used in RA is given in Table 9.5.

Figure 9.4 Control of corticosteroid production.
Dotted line shows the negative feedback loop. CRF, corticotrophin-releasing factor; ACTH, adrenocorticotrophic hormone.

Table 9.5 Comparison of corticosteroids commonly used in RA

Corticosteroid	Glucocorticoid potency	Oral	Intra-articular
Hydrocortisone	1	✓	
Prednisolone	4	✓	
Prednisone	3.5	✓	
Triamcinolone	5		✓
Betamethasone	25		✓
Methylprednisolone	5		✓

Box 9.2

Effects of corticosteroids on the body: focus on the immune response

The effects of steroids differ from many drugs in that they attach to receptors inside cells, rather than to receptors on the membranes of cells. The receptors for corticosteroids are called nuclear receptors and they are found in the cytoplasm of cells bound to proteins and the cytoskeleton of the cell. Once glucocorticoids enter the cell they bind to these receptors and then are translocated to the nucleus, where they can either induce or repress the transcription of certain genes.

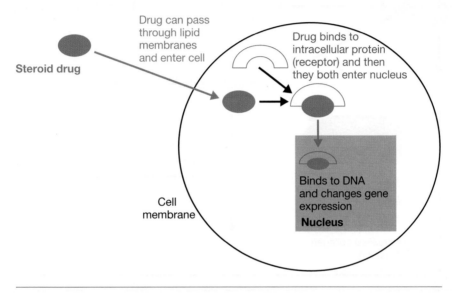

Figure b Effects of corticosteroids on the immune response.

Table B9.1 The effects of corticosteroids in the body

Glucocorticoids	
Carbohydrate	Reduce uptake of glucose and increase gluconeogenesis → hyperglycaemia
Proteins	Increase breakdown and decreased synthesis of proteins → muscle wasting and thinning of skin
Fat	Lipase activation → redistribution of fat ('buffalo hump' and 'moon face')
Calcium	Decreased oral absorption and increased renal excretion of calcium → osteoporosis
Mineralocorticoids	
Kidneys	Increased sodium reabsorption and potassium loss → sodium and water retention

The common metabolic and renal effects of corticosteroids are outlined in Table B9.1.

The glucocorticoids have particularly powerful effects on the immune and inflammatory responses of the body. When used as drugs this is sometime desirable, bringing about the therapeutic response, and sometime undesirable, producing unwanted effects that limit the clinical use of these powerful drugs. The steroids work by affecting both cellular events and the production of inflammatory/immune mediators. The effects are summarized in Figure c. The net effect is that they can suppress the early and late phases of the inflammatory response, including wound healing (which is an example of a side effect of therapy).

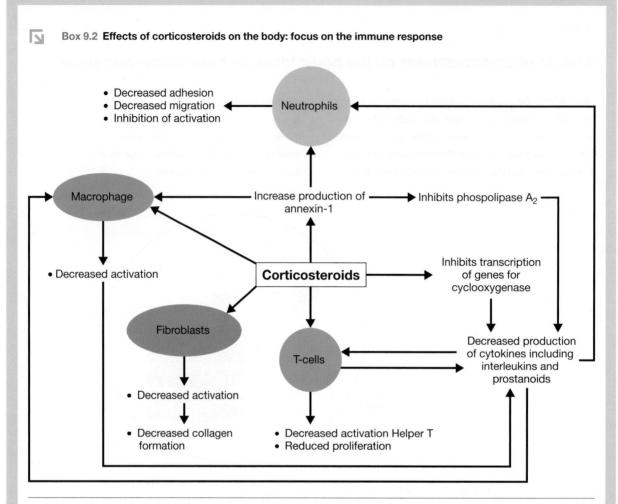

Box 9.2 Effects of corticosteroids on the body: focus on the immune response

Figure c Effects of corticosteroids on the immune response.

The most common corticosteroids used are either oral **prednisolone** or **prednisone**, as they are easy to administer. These two drugs are interrelated and appear to undergo complex reversible metabolism to each other (i.e. prednisolone is converted to prednisone and vice versa in the liver). The equivalent oral dose is therefore the same (i.e. 5 mg predisone = 5 mg prednisolone). Oral corticosteroids are usually given in the morning to mimic the normal circadian production of corticosteroids by the adrenal gland.

Intra-articular steroids have the advantage of reduced systemic side effects and less HPA suppression (see below), but are usually used when only a few joints are affected, and for a limited time.

Pamela was prescribed intra-articular triamcinolone after she had increasing pain in both wrists.

The main side effects of long-term oral corticosteroid use are outlined in Table B9.1 in Box 9.2. The immune-suppressing effects mean patients can be at increased risk of infection, and their wounds may heal more slowly. The corticosteroids also affect your mood and can produce depression or psychotic symptoms. A serious adverse outcome of oral steroid therapy is suppression of the HPA axis (see Figure 9.4), therefore if you stop oral corticosteroids abruptly you can get adrenal insufficiency, sometimes called an '**Addisonian crisis**' because it resembles the symptoms of Addison's disease. It is recommended that anyone on prolonged and high doses corticosteroids (>20 mg prednisolone equivalent for >3 weeks) should have their doses slowly reduced. The rate of tapering depends on the duration of treatment and dose of the corticosteroid.

As the corticosteroids also inhibit the production of cyclooxygenase, with some similarity in outcome to the inhibitory effects of non-selective NSAIDs, they can also cause GI effects, including peptic ulcers. It is recommended that if patients use corticosteroids at doses above 15 mg prednisolone/predisone for more than 1

month they should also be prescribed a proton pump inhibitor to reduce acid in the stomach (see Chapter 12). Given their metabolic effects, patients may also need to have their blood glucose levels and bone mineral density monitored with long-term therapy.

Because of their potent immunosuppressive effects, the wide range of potentially serious side effects, and the possible suppression of the HPA axis, oral corticosteroids are generally reserved for severe flare-ups of RA.

9.4 Disease-modifying antirheumatic drugs

While disease-modifying antirheumatic drugs (DMARDs) used to be reserved as second or third line after NSAIDs, they have now become the cornerstone of the treatment of RA and should be commenced within 3 months of diagnosis.

DMARDs are broadly divided into immunosuppressants/immune-modulators, anti-rheumatics (a catch-all group of agents with varied but largely unknown mechanism of action in RA), and cytokine blockers (also called 'biologics' because they are derived from biological sources, including DNA and antibodies).

Although the exact mode of action of many DMARDs is unclear, most of them exert their effect through the inhibition of cytokine production/release, blocking cytokine action on cells, and/or the proliferation of inflammatory cells (in particular T-cells). The sites of action of various DMARDs are outlined in Figure 9.5.

It is important to note that while DMARDs do modify the disease progression, they may have limited effect on the pain associated with RA. The patient will therefore often require an NSAID for pain relief while taking DMARDs.

9.4.1 Immunosuppressants and immune modulators

These agents have become the first-line treatments in moderate to severe RA and include **methotrexate**, **azathioprine**, **ciclosporin**, **cyclophosphamide**, **abatacept**, and **rituximab**. As their name implies they modify the body's immune response through a variety of mechanisms. Not surprisingly, given this effect, as a group they can produce serious side effects because they prevent the body from mounting its usual defence against invaders.

Methotrexate

Methotrexate is considered to be one of the most effective DMARDs available. It is an analogue of folic acid and inhibits dihydrofolate reductase (DHFR) in cells. The DHFR is involved in DNA synthesis by converting dihydrofolic acid to tetrahydrofolic acid, which is required to produce thymine (one of the essential four bases of DNA). It has been used for many years in high doses in cancer chemotherapy for this action (Chapter 22), which inhibits rapidly dividing cells (like the ones you get with cancer). However, inhibition of DHFR is not thought to be the mechanism of action in RA, as evidenced by the fact that folic acid supplementation (which antagonises the cytotoxic effect of methotrexate) will reduce the side effects of methotrexate without altering its effectiveness in RA. Current theories are that it may increase the production of adenosine, an anti-inflammatory autocoid (locally acting hormone). It may also decrease other cytokines, such as IL-1 and tumour necrosis factor-alpha (TNF-α), and increase levels of the inhibitory cytokine IL-10. However, convincing evidence for this is still lacking.

Methotrexate is given only once a week, orally or by subcutaneous injection. It is very important that patients realize that they only take it once a week as severe toxicity can occur if it is taken daily. The sustained effect from weekly dosing, despite being cleared from the blood reasonably quickly, occurs because the methotrexate is stored intracellularly.

Side effects of methotrexate. Nausea and stomatitis (inflammation of the lining of the mouth) are the most common side effects of methotrexate, but these can usually be managed by giving low-dose folic acid or by dividing the dose across the day (e.g. if the dose is 15 mg

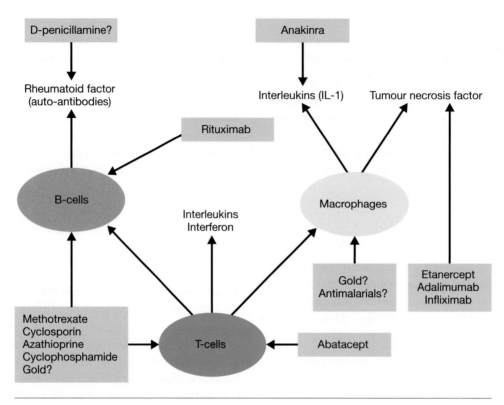

Figure 9.5 Sites of action of DMARDs.

then the patient takes 5 mg three times a day on one day a week). The most serious side effects are those affecting the liver, bone marrow, and lungs. Patients require regular liver function tests and full blood counts. As methotrexate can cause pneumonitis (inflammation of the lung tissue), patients should report any significant coughing or shortness of breath. The administration of NSAIDs with methotrexate can lead to reduced renal clearance of methotrexate and potential toxicity. However, with low-dose methotrexate it is usually safe to continue to use NSAIDs provided careful monitoring for toxicity is done when methotrexate is started, or when doses are increased (or if NSAIDs are introduced later).

Methotrexate has the advantage of having a relatively fast onset of action (about 1 month) compared to many other DMARDs (up to 6 months). If no effect has been seen with oral therapy after 2 months, consider stopping or changing to the subcutaneous route (some patients have poor oral bioavailability of methotrexate).

Pamela was initially prescribed sulphasalazine and because it was ineffective it was replaced with methotrexate.

Azathioprine

Azathioprine is a prodrug, which when converted in the body to 6-mercaptapurine stops the production of purines that are required for RNA and DNA synthesis (Figure 9.6).

Azathioprine inhibits the proliferation of lymphocytes, including T-cells and B-cells, and has been used for decades to stop organ rejection after transplantation. In the treatment of RA it may take 2 to 3 months before an effect is seen, and if no effect is seen at the maximum tolerated dose after 6 months it should be stopped.

The side effect profile of azathioprine is worse than methotrexate, with nausea, vomiting, and diarrhoea being reasonably common. It can also cause bone marrow suppression and liver toxicity. Patients need to report signs of bone marrow suppression, including bleeding and bruising (due to decreased platelets), and fever or other signs of infections (due to over suppression of the lymphocytes). Given that side effects are more serious and more common with azathioprine, it will tend to be used only in patients who have failed on other DMARDs.

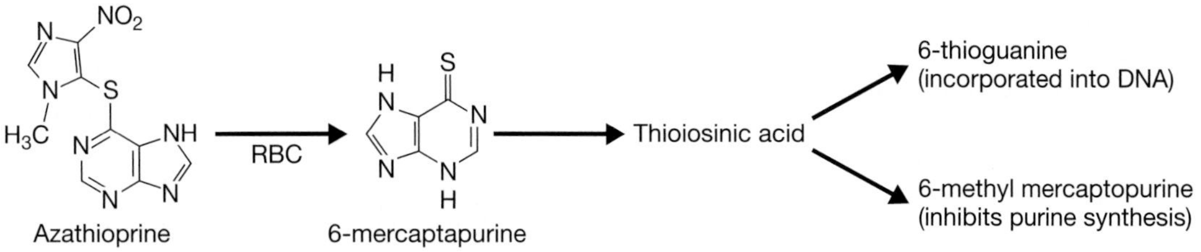

Figure 9.6 Metabolism of azathioprine.

RBC, red blood cells.

Ciclosporin

Ciclosporin is a complex molecule produced by the fungus *Tolypocladium inflatum Gams.* Like azathioprine, it has been largely used to stop organ rejection after transplantation. Ciclosporin works by diffusing into cells and binding to proteins called cyclophillins. This complex then inhibits calcineurin, an enzyme responsible for transcription of interleukins IL-2 and IL-4, and interferon-γ in T-cells. As discussed in the introduction to this section, these cytokines are responsible for T-cell proliferation and differentiation, and the proliferation and differentiation of B-cells (see Figure S3.2). Thus, ciclosporine has a potent effect on the immune system.

Just like azathioprine, ciclosporin may take several months to have an effect, and if insufficient response is seen after 6 months it should be stopped. It also has a range of serious adverse effects, including nephrotoxicity (ironic given that it was used as first line for many years in patients who had kidney transplants), hypertension, liver toxicity, and bone marrow suppression. Most effects are dose related and can be reversed on dose reduction. Patients need to undergo regular screening of their creatinine level, blood count, and liver function tests. Ciclosporin is metabolized in the liver by the cytochrome P-450 system (CYP3A4), therefore there are a number of significant drug interactions, including the azole antifungal agents (e.g. ketoconazole: increases ciclosporin levels) and carbamazepine (inducer: decreases ciclosporine levels). Again, like azathioprine, ciclosporin will tend to be reserved for severe RA where patients have not achieved sufficient response to DMARDs such as methotrexate.

Cyclophosphamide

Cyclophosphamide, like methotrexate, was used mainly in cancer chemotherapy. It is metabolized in the liver into two active metabolites (4-hydroxycyclophosphamide and aldophosphamide), which undergo further metabolism to produce a number of agents, including phosphoramide mustard. The phosphoramide mustard crosslinks DNA and produces cell death, and in RA it reduces T-cell and B-cell proliferation (see Chapter 22 for more details).

Cyclophosphamide is more toxic than methotrexate and can cause bone marrow suppression, increasing the risk of infections. One of the metabolites, acrolein, is toxic to the cells of the bladder and it can cause haemorrhagic cystitis (a severe inflammation of the bladder wall). Patients should be encouraged to drink plenty of water and empty their bladder frequently to reduce their risk of this. Because of its toxicity it is also only used when other treatments have failed.

Leflunomide

Leflunomide is a new agent that inhibits dihydroorotate dehydrogenase, an enzyme that is involved in pyrimidine production. It alters DNA and RNA synthesis, causing inhibition of T-cell and B-cell proliferation and suppression of immunoglobulin production. It is given orally and is converted in the liver into its active form. The active metabolite has a long half-life of 2 to 4 weeks so a loading dose is given for 3 days, followed by a lower maintenance dose. Liver damage is possible and regular liver function tests are recommended. It has also been associated with rare but severe skin conditions, such as Stevens–Johnson syndrome, and patients should report any changes in their skin. Because of the effect on the immune system patients should not receive any live vaccines while on therapy and for 6 months after stopping. Leflunomide is also reserved for patients who have failed on other DMARDs.

Abatacept

Abatacept is a new biological agent that consists of a fusion protein linked to a portion of human immunoglobulin A1. It works by modifying the co-stimulatory signals that are required to fully activate the T-cell. To activate a T-cell two things must occur. First, the antigen-major histocompatibility complex (MHC) on the antigen-presenting cell (APC) must attach to the T-cell receptor. Second, a co-stimulatory signal must occur because of binding between the CD28 protein on the T-cell and the CD80/86 proteins on the APC (Figure 9.7). Abatacept blocks the binding of CD80 and CD86 proteins and thus T-cells cannot become fully activated.

Abatacept is given by intravenous infusion every 2 weeks for three doses, then once a month after that. Side effects include infusion-related reactions such as dizziness and headache, and an increased risk of infection. As this is a very new agent, long-term safety is not established. While it appears to be safe to use with the non-biologic DMARDs (e.g. methotrexate), it should not be used in combination with the new biologic cytokine blockers (e.g. etanercept) because of the increased risk of serious infections.

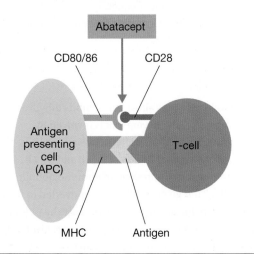

Figure 9.7 Site of action of abatacept.

MHC, major histocompatibility complex.

Rituximab

Rituximab is a monoclonal antibody against the CD20 surface phospoprotein found on mature B-cells. Once attached to the CD20 it prevents the B-cell from proliferating and differentiating, resulting in removal of the B-cell. It is administered as two intravenous infusions given 2 weeks apart. If there is a response, a repeat dose can be given after 6 to 12 months. The main side effects are infusion-related, and it is recommended that paracetamol, an antihistamine, and methylpredinisolone be given before administering the rituximab to reduce the risk. Patients should still be observed for signs of anaphylaxis after the infusion. Rutiximab has similar efficacy to some of the biologic cytokine blockers (e.g. etanercept, see later), but, like the cytokine blockers, it is very expensive. It is therefore reserved for people who have failed other DMARDs, and must be used in combination with methotrexate (as efficacy has only been shown in trials in combination with methotrexate).

9.4.2 Anti-rheumatic drugs

As discussed previously, this is a heterogeneous group of drugs that have uncertain modes of action in RA. It includes gold salts, antimalarials, penicillamine, and sulfasalazine.

Gold salts

Gold compounds have been used for over 70 years in the treatment of RA and for centuries in the treatment of infections. The currently used gold salts are **aurothiomalate** (given by intramuscular injection) and **auranofin** (given orally). A large number of effects have been attributed to gold salts, although the evidence is sometimes contradictory. The proposed mechanism of action includes:

- inhibition of prostaglandin synthesis
- modulation of phagocytic cells (including uptake into macrophages)
- inactivation of complement
- disruption of the MHC
- inhibition of IL-2 and IL-1 biosynthesis
- reduction of T-cell activity
- inhibition of neutrophil migration.

Authothiomalate is given by intramuscular injection weekly until signs of remission, and maintenance treatment usually involves injections every 4 to 6 weeks. The injection can be associated with a severe vasomotor reaction (fainting, sweating, nausea, and heart palpitations) and patients need to be kept lying down for at least 10 minutes after the injection is given. The main side effect with auranofin is severe diarrhoea, which can sometimes be reduced with the use of bulk-forming laxatives (e.g. psyllium husks) or a reduction in dose. Both agents can produce significant immunosupression, and patients need to report signs and symptoms such as mouth ulcers, sore throats, bruising, fever, and malaise. They must also have regular blood cell counts, and must be monitored for signs of renal dysfunction. Although they are very effective in inducing remission in RA, gold compounds are rarely used because of their serious side effects. Like many other DMARDs they may take up to 6 months to have a full effect.

Antimalarials

Chloroquine and **hydroxychloroquine** are both used in RA. Both drugs have very long half-lives because they are taken up and stored in tissues. This means it takes several months for the drugs to reach steady state and even longer to have a clinical effect. As for gold salts, there are a number of proposed mechanisms of action, some with contradictory evidence, including:

- uptake into lysosomes resulting in inhibition of proteases
- inhibition of neutrophil function
- reduction in phospholipase-A$_2$ activity
- inhibition of IL-1 and TNF-α.

Both chloroquine and hydroxychloroquine are better tolerated than many of the other DMARDs. They are taken orally daily, and the most common side effects are GI upset. Both can cause retinopathy, and patients must undergo regular eye examinations while on therapy. Patients should also report any vision changes and should use sunglasses when out in sunlight to reduce potential damage.

While the antimalarials are well tolerated, they are not as effective as the other DMARDs, and are generally only used in mild disease, although arguably sulfasalazine would be a better choice because it is more effective and acts more quickly.

Penicillamine

Also known as D-penicillamine, this is a product of penicillin hydrolysis. Penicillamine contains three functional groups (α-amine, carboxyl, and sulfhydryl) and is a metal chelator (it is used to treat heavy metal poisoning such with mercury and lead). It does not appear to affect cytokine production or macrophage activation, and its effect in RA appears to be unrelated to its chelating properties. It is thought to possibly reduce T-cell activity, and may inhibit immunoglobulin from binding to form immune complexes (i.e. inhibit rheumatoid factor interacting with immunoglobulin in RA).

Although as effective as sulfasalazine, penicillamine it is not as well tolerated, and GI upset, rash, stomatitis, and taste disturbance are common. Significant immunosupression with penicillamine is rare, but regular blood tests to check are still recommended. Penicillamine therefore has a limited role in mild RA.

Sulfasalazine

Sulfasalazine is frequently chosen as the first choice in mild RA because it is relatively effective, cheap, convenient (administered orally), and has fewer side effects compared to the other DMARDs. It is a combination of 5-aminosalicylic acid (5ASA, an anti-inflammatory) and sulfapyridine (a sulfonamide antibiotic) joined by a diazo bond. This bond is cleaved in the colon by bacteria releasing the 5ASA and sulfapyridine. Although the 5ASA is thought to have local anti-inflammatory effects in ulcerative colitis (another use of sulfasalazine), it is the sulfapyridine molecule that is responsible for the DMARD effect in RA, with the 5ASA playing a limited role. It has also been suggested that intact sulfasalazine may also be involved. The exact mechanism of action of sulfasalazine in RA is still unclear, but theories include modification of lymphocyte proliferation (possibly because of sulfapyridine, which like methotrexate acts on folate metabolism) and reduction in cytokine production (possibly by sulfasalazine and/or 5ASA).

Sulfazalazine is taken orally and the main side effect is GI upset. This can be reduced by taking it with food and by using preparations that are enteric coated. Many of the side effects are related to the sulfapyridine molecule and include allergic reactions (you have probably heard of people having a 'sulfur allergy', usually from sulfonamide antibiotics) and blood dyscrasias.

9.4.3 Cytokine blockers: biological DMARDs

The cytokine blockers represent the greatest advance in the treatment of RA in the last decade or so. These agents directly target specific cytokines (**etanercept**, **infliximab**, and **adalimumab** all target TNF-α; **anakinra** targets IL-1) and are called biological because they are derived from DNA or human antibodies. Their manufacture is complex and therefore they are extremely expensive, costing hundreds of times more than some of the older DMARDs. Some of the cytokine blockers, in particular etanercept, have been shown to have similar efficacy to methotrexate in clinical trials. However, most of the agents have been trialled in combination with methotrexate, where they have been shown to improve outcomes by 20–50% over methotrexate alone. A common side effect of all cytokine blockers is, not surprisingly, immune suppression leading to increased risk of infection. Patients on these drugs must therefore report any signs of infection and stop therapy immediately if a serious infection develops. Patients should also not receive live vaccines while using these therapies. The agents targeted against TNF-α can worsen or precipitate heart failure and must be used with caution, or not at all, in patients with existing heart failure. Given their cost, inconvenience of administration (all have to be given by injection, although, as with people with diabetes who have to have insulin, some of them can be self-administered by subcutaneous injection), and side effect profiles, they are reserved for very severe RA or third-line treatment when other DMARDs have been ineffective.

Etanercept

Etanercept is a fusion of two proteins: a soluble TNF receptor bound to a fragment of human immunoglobulin G1 (IgG1). Two types of TNF receptor exist: one form is bound to cells and when activated by TNF-α it causes release of cytokines; the second can become soluble and 'mop up' excess TNF-α to help dampen down the immune response. Etanercept mimics the latter of these two forms, but has a longer life in plasma because of being bound to IgG1.

Etanercept is given by subcutaneous injection once or twice a week. As well as increased infections and

worsening heart failure, a local injection site reaction is among the most common side effects.

> Our patient Gwen (Workbook 6) was initially prescribed etanercept, which she tolerated really well and learned to self-administer at home. Her specialist nurse advised her to rotate sites of injection. She only had to go to hospital once monthly for blood tests and could easily arrange this around work and family. However, after she developed heart failure she was told she would have to come off the drug.

Infliximab

Infliximab is a chimeric (containing both mouse (murine) and human components) monoclonal antibody against TNF-α. Monoclonal antibodies attach to circulating TNF-α and stop it interacting with its receptor. It is given initially as three intravenous infusions given at zero, 2, and 6 weeks, and then repeated every 8 weeks. It has efficacy and side effects similar to the other TNF-α agents, but patients can also have infusion-related reactions (reduced by the pre-administration of paracetamol, an antihistamine, and a corticosteroid), and occasionally have a delayed hypersensitivity reaction. Patients should also have their liver function and blood counts monitored.

Adalimumab

Adalimumab differs from infliximab in that it is a fully human monoclonal antibody, not chimeric, against TNF-α. It is given by subcutaneous injection weekly or every second week. It has a similar efficacy and side effect profile to etanercept and infliximab.

Anakinra

Anakinra is recombinant form of human interlukin-1 (IL-1) receptor antagonist, and competitively binds to the IL-1 receptor blocking the effect of IL-1. It is also given by subcutaneous injection, but given daily. It has similar efficacy and side effects to the TNF-α blockers, but the data on efficacy is not as convincing. You should not combine TNF-α inhibitors with anakinra as you may get serious immune suppression.

Table 9.6 summarizes the DMARDs in the treatment of rheumatoid arthritis.

Table 9.6 Efficacy, safety, and cost of DMARDs

Drug	Route	Efficacy	Toxicity	Monitoring	Cost
Hydroxychloroquine	Oral	+	+	Retinal examination	+
Chloroquine	Oral	+	++	Retinal examination	+
Sulfasalazine	Oral	++	+	FBC; LFT	+
Penicillamine	Oral	++	+++	FBC; E&C; LFT	+
Gold salts	Oral; IM	++	++	FBC; Urinalysis	+
Methotrexate	Oral; SC	++	+	FBC; LFT	+
Azathioprine	Oral	+	+	FBC; LFT	+
Ciclosporin	Oral	++	++	FBC; LFT; E&C; BP	++
Cyclophosphamide	Oral	++	+++	FBC; LFT; E&C; Urinalysis	+
Leflunomide	Oral	++ (+++)a	+	FLC; LFT	++
Abatacept	IV	++ (+++)	++	Infusion reaction; infections	+++
Rituximab	IV	++ (+++)	+/++	Infusion reaction; infections	++++
Etanercept	SC	++ (+++)	+	FBC; LFT; E&C; infections	++++
Infliximab	IV	++ (+++)	+/++	FBC; LFT; E&C; infections	++++
Adalimumab	SC	++ (+++)	+	FBC; LFT; E&C; infections	++++
Anakinra	SC	+ (++)	+	FBC; LFT; E&C; infections	++++

IM, intramuscular; SC, subcutaneous; IV, intravenous.
FBC, full blood count; LFT, liver function tests; E&C, electrolytes and creatinine; BP, blood pressure.
a Results in brackets are the efficacy in combination with methotrexate.

9.5 What is considered when choosing the right drug for RA?

When choosing therapy for RA a number of factors are taken into consideration, including:

- joint function
- patient age and gender
- occupation
- patient preference
- family responsibility
- severity of disease
- previous treatment
- costs
- side effects of therapy.

A general approach to managing RA is outlined in Figure 9.8.

9.5.1 Starting therapy

It is important to commence DMARDs within 3 months of making the initial diagnosis of RA. If the disease is only mild then sulfasalazine is a reasonable first choice. However, if the disease is moderate or severe then methotrexate is the DMARD of choice in most patients.

As noted previously, the DMARDs do not provide immediate pain relief, and may take months to have a full effect. NSAIDs are therefore often prescribed to provide immediate pain management. The choice of NSAID is dependent on the patient's CV risk and risk of GI events (see Table 9.4).

9.5.2 Monitoring therapy for response

Baseline measurements of the disease severity should be taken to allow assessment of progression. These include:

- degree of joint pain (using a visual analogue scale)
- degree of morning stiffness
- number of swollen joints
- limitation of function
- erythrocyte sedimentation rate or C-reactive protein levels
- radiographic findings
- patient's and physician's global assessment of disease activity
- quality of life (using standard questionnaires).

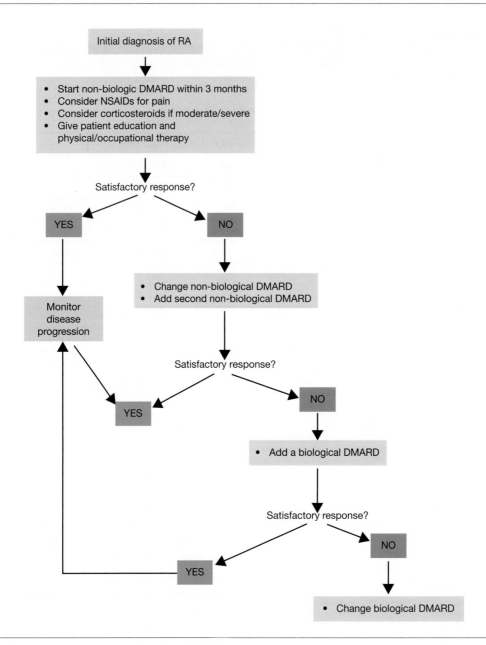

Figure 9.8 Algorithm for treating rheumatoid arthritis.

RA, rheumatoid arthritis; DMARD, disease-modifying antirheumatic drugs; NSAIDs, non-steroidal anti-inflammatory drugs.

Monitoring needs to take account of the delay before many of the DMARDs take effect (from 2 to 6 months). However, for most DMARDs progression of the disease despite 6 months of therapy at the maximal tolerated dose necessitates a change in therapy.

9.5.3 Useful combinations of DMARDs

If patients do fail on a DMARD, a number of combinations have been found to be useful, including:

- sulfasalazine + methotrexate
- methotrexate + leflunomide
- methotrexate + TNF-α antagonist biologicals
- methotrexate + anakinra.

Any combination increases the risk of serious immune suppression, and combinations of anakinra + TNF-α antagonists must be avoided. However, trials with the above combinations have been shown to improve response by 20–40% over methotrexate alone, with acceptable side effect profiles.

9.5 What is considered when choosing the right drug for RA?

227

SUMMARY OF DRUGS USED FOR RHEUMATOID ARTHRITIS

Therapeutic Class	Drugs	Mechanism of action	Common clinical uses	Comments	Examples of adverse drug reactions
NSAIDS	COX 1 and COX 2 inhibitors Aspirin diclofenac Ibuprofen Indomethacin Ketoprofen Ketorolac Naproxen Diclofenac Mefenamic acid Tiaprofenic acid Piroxicam Sulindac COX 2 Selective inhibitors Celecoxib Etoricoxib Meloxicam Parecoxib Valdecoxib	Inhibits cyclooxygenase (COX) and subsequently production of prostaglandins and thromboxanes	Rheumatoid arthritis Osteoarthritis Other inflammatory arthropathies Acute gout inflammatory pain and tissue injury Fever	Hugely variable pharmacokinetics COX-2 selective inhibitors and diclofenac associated with increased risk of thrombotic events Avoid in patients at increased risk of CV events Lowest effective dose should be prescribed for shortest period	Nausea Diarrhoea Bleeding Ulceration Hypersensitivity reactions (rash, angiodema, bronchospasm)
Corticosteroids	Prednisolone Dexamethasone Triamcinolone Methylprednisolone hydrocortisone	They enter the cell, and bind to Glucocorticosteroids receptors, then are translocated to the nucleus, induce or repress the transcription of certain genes, ultimately leading to anti-immune and anti-inflammatory effects	Anti-inflammation in Rheumatoid arthritis Allergies Respiratory disorders Autoimmune disease Neoplastic diseases	Usually reserved for 2nd line use in RA Local injections could be injected into joints Side effects dependent on dose, duration and route	Increased susceptibility to infection oedema hypertension, hyperglycaemia, dyslipidaemia, osteoporosis dyspepsia delayed wound healing skin atrophy hirsutism growth retardation in children fat redistribution (producing cushinoid appearance) weight gain, amenorrhoea psychiatric disturbances

Therapeutic Class	Drugs	Mechanism of action	Common clinical uses	Comments	Examples of adverse drug reactions
Immunosuppresssant/ Immuno-modulators (DMARDs)	Azathioprine	1) Converted in the body to 6-mercaptapurine and stops the production of purines that are required for RNA and DNA synthesis. 2) Inhibits lymphocyte proliferation	Autoimmune diseases Transplant rejection	Monitoring for myelosupresion essential in long term treatment	Nausea Vomiting Diarrhoea Bone marrow suppression Liver toxicity
	Cyclosporine	Diffuses into cells and binds to proteins called cyclophillins forming complex that inhibits calcineurin, an enzyme responsible for transcription of IL–2, IL–4, and INF–γ in T-cells, resulting in decreased proliferation and differentiation of T and B cells	Severe RA Autoimmune diseases Transplant rejection	Partly metabolised by hepatic Cytochrome P450 (Cyp 3A4), leading to interactions. Long elimination half-life of 10–27hrs.	Nephrotoxicity Hypertension Liver toxicity Bone marrow suppression
	Cyclophosphamide	Metabolised to phosphoramide mustard which cross-links DNA and produces B and T lymphocyte cell death	Rheumatoid arthritis cancer	A metabolite of cyclophosphamide called acrolein can cause haemorrhagic cystisis. This is prevented by administering Mesna and hydration. Cyclophosphamide metabolised by hepatic enzymes CYP2B6 and CYP3A4 leading in interactions	Haemorrhagic cystisis Infertility Bone marrow suppresion pulmonary fibrosis Stephen Johnson's syndrome
	Methotrexate	1) Thought to increase the production of adenosine, an anti-inflammatory autocoid (locally acting hormone). 2) May also decrease other cytokines such as IL-1 and TNFα, and increase levels of the inhibitory cytokine IL-10	Rheumatoid arthritis Cancer Psoriasis	Taken once weekly Folic acid supplementation required to reduce side effects Different mechanism of action in cancer	Pneumonitis Stomatitis Nausea Diarrhoea Bone marrow suppression
	Leflunomide	1) Inhibits dihydroorotate dehydrogenase, an enzyme involved in pyrimidine production. 2) Alters DNA and RNA synthesis causing inhibition of T-cell and B-cell proliferation, and suppression of immunoglobulin production	Rheumatoid arthritis	Metabolite inhibits hepatic CYP2C9 leading to interactions Long half life making loading Necessary at initiation of treatment Avoid life vaccines whilst taking and for six months after	abdominal pain diarrhoea nausea vomiting liver toxicity Steven-Johnson's syndrome

Therapeutic Class	Drugs	Mechanism of action	Common clinical uses	Comments	Examples of adverse drug reactions
	Abatercept	modifies the co-stimulatory signals required to fully activate the T-cell by binding to CD80 and CD86 on antigen-presenting cells which prevents full activation of CD28 T lymphocytes thus reducing cytokine production and inflammation	Moderate-to-severe rheumatoid arthritis	Used 2nd line Consists of fusion protein linked to immunoglobulin	Headache dizziness raised liver enzymes, dyspepsia weakness
	rituximab	As a monoclonal antibody it attaches to the CD20 surface phosoprotein on the B-cell and prevents it from proliferating and differentiating.	Severe rheumatoid arthritis	Reserved for patients with inadequate response, or intolerance, to a TNF-alpha antagonist	Infections Musculoskeletal pain weakness Anaphylaxis
	Anakinra	Binds to the IL-1 receptor blocking the effect of IL-1 which is involved in acute inflammatory response	Severe rheumatoid arthritis	Is recombinant form of human interleukin	Headache Serious infection neutropenia
Cytokine blockers (DMARDs)	Etanercept	Mops up excess TNF-α to help dampen down the immune response	Severe Rheumatoid arthritis Psoriatic arthritis Ankylosing spondylitis Active polyarticular juvenile chronic arthritis Plaque psoriasis	Blood count needs to be monitored	Injection site reaction allergic reactions Abdominal pain Dyspepsia
	Infliximab	Chimeric monoclonal antibody against TNF-α	Rheumatoid arthritis Psoriatic arthritis Ankylosing spondylitis Crohn's disease, Ulcerative colitis, Plaque psoriasis, s	2nd line use	Nausea abdominal pain fever vertigo flushing
	Adalimumab	Human monoclonal antibody against TNF-α	Moderate-to-severe active rheumatoid arthritis psoriatic arthritis Ankylosing spondylitis Crohn's disease, Plaque psoriasis, s	2nd line use	Nausea Weakness flu-like syndrome, injection site hyperlipidaemia

Therapeutic Class	Drugs	Mechanism of action	Common clinical uses	Comments	Examples of adverse drug reactions
Antirheumatics (DMARDs)	Aurothiomalate auranofin	Thought to 1) Inhibit prostaglandin synthesis 2) Modulate phagocytic cells 3) Inactivate complement 4) Disrupt MHC 5) Inhibit IL-2 and IL-1 biosynthesis 6) Reduce T-cell activity 7) Inhibit neutrophil migration	Rheumatoid arthritis	Elimination half-life is 42–128 days Aurothiomalate is injection Auranofin is table	diarrhoea (mainly with auranofin), dyspepsia stomatitis nausea taste disturbance, rash alopecia conjunctivitis blood dyscrasias, nephrotoxicity, elevated liver enzymes
	Chloroquine Hydroxychloroquine	1) Inhibits proteases in lysosymes 2) Inhibits neutrophil function 3) Reduces phospholipase-A_2 activity 4) Inhibits IL-1 and TNF-α	Rheumatoid arthritis Lupus erythematous Malaria	Long Elimination half-life of 40 days	Gastrointestinal disorders Headaches Skin reactions ECG changes Visual changes
	Penicillinamine	1) Reduces T-cell activity 2) May inhibit immunoglobulin from binding to form immune complexes	Rheumatoid arthritis Wilson's disease Lead poisonning	Usually used when patients have extra-articular features eg vasculitis Blood count need monitoring	Nausea Anorexia Taste loss Mouth ulcers Male and female breast enlargement
	Sulfasalazine	1) Modifies lymphocyte proliferation 2) Reduces cytokine production	Rheumatoid arthritis Ulcerative colitis	Blood count monitoring required	Rash Gastrointestinal disturbances Loss of appetite Fever Blood disorders

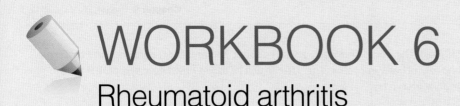

WORKBOOK 6
Rheumatoid arthritis

Pamela and Gwen: battling with joint disease. Rheumatoid arthritis and its management

Patient 1, Pamela: a simplified case history

Whilst struggling out of bed at 7.30am, Pamela makes a mental note to finally take her husband's advice and consult her GP about the pain and general tiredness she has been experiencing. After 4 months of trying to cope it's become worse, and she is ready to admit to herself that her symptoms cannot be entirely attributed to the demands of being a wife and a mum to three children. She wonders is this has anything to do with her recent road traffic accident, which resulted in three broken ribs and sepsis. She gets an appointment and heads to the surgery after dropping the children off at school.

Her GP refers her to a rheumatologist after asking some questions regarding her symptoms and examining her. All these questions and investigations were repeated in clinic followed by more investigations.

A table of clinical clerking abbreviations is given on page xi.

SUMMARY OF CLINICAL CLERKING IN PAMELA'S CLINICAL NOTES

Age: 41 years

PC: Morning stiffness lasting for hours accompanied by fatigue, anorexia, muscle, and joint pain

  The symptoms of rheumatoid arthritis (RA) are as follows:

  - *Joints are red, swollen, tender, warm, and stiff, leading to decreased use.*
  - *Symptoms usually symmetrical.*
  - *Joints commonly affected are hands, feet, and cervical spine.*
  - *Less common are larger joints, e.g. shoulder and knee.*
  - *Patient experiences localized warmth and restricted movement.*
  - *Range of movement decreased and deformity with finger bent towards little finger.*
  - *Stiffness worse on waking is a key distinguishing feature of RA from ostheoarthritis.*

HPC: Progressing symptoms of stiffness, pain and general malaise. Inflammation and swelling around both knee joints and finger joints.

During a medical history, the doctor normally enquires about the presence, duration, and pattern of joint symptoms and any other symptoms. The patient will be asked how these symptoms have impacted on their daily activities.

Presentation of RA

There are three main presentations:

- *First group of patients experience mild intermittent symptoms that resolve and reappear over weeks.*

- *Second group of patients have a sudden onset of symptoms followed by a prolonged remission.*

- *Third group of patients have progressive uninterrupted symptoms that result in disabling joint deformities.*

The early symptoms are usually non-specific, including fatigue, malaise, diffuse musculoskeletal pain, and stiffness. The most obvious symptoms are joint pain and loss of function.

The list below summarizes the criteria used to diagnose RA developed by the American Rheumatism Association (ARA) and referenced by the British Society of Rheumatology. Rheumatoid arthritis diagnosis if four of the criteria are present.

Criteria for diagnosing RA

- *Morning stiffness in and around joints lasting >1 hour for >6 weeks.*

- *Arthritis (soft tissue swelling) of more than three joint areas +/- exudate for >6 weeks.*

- *Arthritis of hands and joints (metacarpophalangeal or interphalangeal) >6 weeks.*

- *Symmetrical arthritis in minimum one area lasting >6 weeks.*

- *Subcutaneous nodules seen by doctor.*

- *Serum test for rheumatoid factor = positive.*

- *Radiographic findings: positive in films of wrist and hands.*

PMH: Sepsis (blood infection) following road traffic accident 5 months ago

Stress

Although patients often report episodes of stress or trauma preceding the onset of their rheumatoid arthritis, stress is extremely difficult to measure. However, some studies do suggest that stressful life events, e.g. divorce, accidents, bereavement, etc., within 6 months are more common in people with RA.

Infection

Although there is no direct evidence linking the two, there is a suspicion that infection with bacteria or viruses may be one of the factors that initiates rheumatoid arthritis.

The doctor must use the criteria listed above to rule out the aftereffects of an accident as diagnosis.

Pam has had both an infection and stress. Pam's history of a gastric ulcer after using ibuprofen should influence the choice of treatment.

DH: Nil significant

Pamela does not take any regular medication.

FH: Pamela's mother and grandmother both suffered from RA

It is important to enquire about family members who have suffered from arthritis or any other inflammatory joint disease because epidemiological data suggest that genetic factors could cause RA.

Both her mother and grandmother had arthritis, increasing the probability that this could be RA. Although there is evidence that RA is immune-mediated, other possible stimulants include:

- *infection and stress*
- *environmental*
- *genetic.*

O/E: Bilateral symmetrical swelling, warmth, tenderness and redness of metacarpophalangeal joints of hands. Subcutaneous nodule is seen when forearm is extended.

During a physical examination, the joints are examined to observe:

- *their range of motion*
- *redness*
- *warmth*
- *swelling (swelling can be a sign of an effusion, a collection of excess fluid inside the joint, or synovitis, an inflammation of the joint lining)*
- *nodules*
- *if the affected joints are symmetric.*

Muscles are also examined for signs of muscle loss.

This presentation shows progression from mild to severe RA.

Biochemistry:

Erythrocyte sedimentary rate (ESR)	elevated
Haemoglobin (Hb)	decreased
C-reactive protein (CRP)	89 (0–10 mg/L)
Rheumatoid factor (RF)	positive
Antinuclear antibodies (ANR)	positive
Platelet count	raised
Serum albumin	decreased
Serum iron concentration	decreased
Total iron binding	normal

Biochemistry

Laboratory tests help to confirm the presence of RA, differentiate it from other conditions, and predict the likely course of the condition and its response to treatment.

Inflammatory markers

The ESR and levels of CRP are non-specific markers of inflammation. A high ESR and CRP suggest the presence of inflammation, but they do not indicate the cause of this inflammation. These markers are useful for distinguishing inflammatory arthritis, such as RA, from non-inflammatory arthritis, such as osteoarthritis.

A normal marker does not exempt RA. Pamela's markers are all raised.

Anaemia

Anaemia resulting from a failure of iron release from the reticuloendothelial tissues is usually present in RA (normochromic, normocytic anaemia).

Testing both serum iron and iron binding capacity would help narrow down the exact form of anaemia.

Although Pamela's serum iron level is decreased, her iron-binding capacity is normal, indicating that her anaemia is not iron-defiency but normocytic. Her anaemia will therefore not respond to treatment with iron.

Alkaline and albumin (liver function tests)

Liver function tests could be deranged in RA.

Pamela 's albumin and alkaline phosphate are deranged.

Rheumatoid factor

An antibody (usually IgM or IgG) called rheumatoid factor (RF) is present in the blood of 70–80% of people with RA.

It forms a complex with the Fc portion of the antigen.

RF is also found in people with other types of rheumatic disease and in a small number of healthy individuals.

Antinuclear antibody test

Between 30 and 40% of people with RA have autoantibodies (antibodies against the body's own tissue) called antinuclear antibodies (ANAs). However, many healthy people also have a positive ANA test.

Pamela's RF and ANA were both positive.

Other investigations:

1) Synovial fluid analysis: positive

Synovial fluid analysis

Small samples of synovial fluid (the fluid around the joint) can be withdrawn and analysed. The joint fluid of people with RA usually contains inflammatory cells and substances.

2) X-rays: No visible changes

X-rays

In people with RA, X-rays can show evidence of changes in the structure of cartilage and bone. These changes show the destruction and loss of bone or cartilage that occurs as RA progresses. Although X-rays are useful for monitoring the status of RA over time, they are usually not helpful for diagnosing RA in its early stages.

Pamela had no changes visible on X-ray, as is usually the case in mild early disease.

About 15–30% of people with RA will have changes on X-rays in the first year of this condition. However, after the first 2 years of RA, more than 90% of people have changes on X-rays. X-rays can also help to measure bone mineral density, which is often decreased in the later stages of RA.

3) Magnetic resonance imaging: not performed on Pamela

Magnetic resonance imaging (MRI) scans are more sensitive than X-rays for detecting the bone damage caused by RA, therefore MRI scans may be more effective than X-rays for detecting the early changes of RA. MRI scans are also useful for assessing changes in the synovium (the joint lining) and for assessing compression of the cervical spinal cord. However, the cost of MRI scanning is much greater than that of plain X-rays, so MRI is not widely used to diagnose or follow the course of RA.

Because Pamela's other investigations and symptoms were quite conclusive, an MRI scan was thought to be unnecessary in her case.

Diagnosis: Early mildly active RA

No single clinical, radiologic, or serologic test exists to help diagnose RA. Similar to other autoimmune rheumatic diseases, the diagnosis is made following review of the symptoms, signs, laboratory data, and radiological findings. The criteria detailed above are commonly used.

Pamela's symptoms, history, family history and results of tests make the diagnosis straightforward.

Plan:

Diclofenac

Sulphasalazine

Diclofenac

This is an non-selective NSAID used in RA. NSAIDs have both a lasting analgesic and an anti-inflammatory effect, which makes them particularly useful for the treatment of continuous or regular pain associated with inflammation.

Sulfasalazine

This is a disease-modifying anti-rheumatic drug (DMARD) and has a beneficial effect in suppressing the inflammatory activity of RA. The initial dose is 500 mg and could be increased at weekly intervals to maximum 2–3 g daily in divided doses.

PART 1

1a) What is rheumatoid arthritis?

1b) Describe the pathogenesis of RA.

2) What are the initial approaches to treatment of RA?

After 2 months Pamela goes to her chemist and requests Gaviscon® for indigestion. The pharmacist, who happens to know she is a regular customer, checks her history on the computer for interactions and realizes that Pamela had lansoprazole listed in her drug history 3 years ago.

On enquiry she ascertains that Pamela suffered from gastritis as a side effect after using ibuprofen 3 years earlier. Pam says she had not mentioned this fact to the rheumatologist when he had enquired about drug reactions because she had bought the ibuprofen over the counter and not realized it was a 'real' drug.

The pharmacist asks Pamela to describe her exact symptoms, after which she recommends that Pamela must be seen by her doctor as an emergency because she suspects Pamela might have a recurrence of her gastritis or worse.

3) Explain how NSAIDs produce their gastrointestinal (GI) effects.

Pamela 's GP enquires about her GI symptoms and orders blood tests to investigate their severity.

Signs and symptoms: Upper abdominal pain occurring 1–3 hours after meals.

This is relieved by food/antacids.

No melena (tarry stools) or haematemesis (blood in vomit).

Based on these symptoms and her history the GP is certain Pamela is suffering from gastritis. Luckily, it has not progressed to an ulcer as yet.

Plan: Stop diclofenac.

Commence lansoprazole 8 weeks.

Refer back to rheumatologist.

After 2 weeks Pamela's RA symptoms are so severe in her wrist joints that she is admitted to hospital via A&E. Her rheumatologist is informed she has been admitted to hospital and he comes round to review her and prescribes injections of triamcinolone (a corticosteroid) to be injected into the two wrist joints.

4a) What is the role of corticosteroids in RA?

4b) Describe their exact mechanism of action.

_____

_____

_____

The rheumatologist also prescribes celecoxib.

5) Explain, with reference to their actions at cellular level, the difference between diclofenac and celecoxib.

_____

_____

_____

6a) List two patient groups who should not be prescribed celecoxib.

_____

_____

_____

6b) Explain why.

_____

_____

_____

Pamela is discharged home on celecoxib and sulfasalazine.

7a) What are the advantages of sulfasalazine over the other DMARDs?

_____

_____

_____

7b) What is the mechanism of action of sulfasalazine?

_____

_____

_____

7c) What monitoring is required for patients treated with sulfasalazine?

At her next clinic appointment, Pamela's symptoms and investigations indicate that she is not responding well to the sulfasalazine. The parameters used to asses this are:

- duration and intensity of morning sickness
- number of painful or tender joints
- number of swollen joints and severity of joint swelling
- range of joint motion
- time to onset of fatigue
- ESR or CRP
- radiographic changes
- subcutaneous nodules.

Her rheumatologists stops the sulfasalazine and prescribes methotrexate.

8) Explain why methotrexate is a good DMARD.

At the pharmacy, when she goes to collect her tablets, she is asked by the pharmacist if she has been told how often to take her tablets. The pharmacist explains that the prescription reads: Methotrexate 10 mg daily.

Pam is unsure and the pharmacist explains that she will need to ring the doctor to confirm because the prescribed frequency is unusual.

9) Why did the pharmacist query the dosing? What is the usual frequency of administering methotrexate in RA?

The doctor is apologetic and asks the pharmacist to alter the prescription.

10a) What is the mechanism of action of methotrexate?

10b) What are the side effects of methotrexate?

10c) What monitoring is required with methotrexate?

After 1 week blood tests show that Pamela's liver function tests are elevated. She is also suffering from mouth ulcers. The rheumatologist prescribes folic acid.

11a) Why has Pamela been prescribed folic acid?

11b) Explain the mechanism of action of folic acid when used with methotrexate.

Pamela's symptoms improve gradually. However, she is upset about the impact of the disease on her life. She has to regularly request time off work to go to clinic for the blood tests required with methotrexate treatment. She reads up on RA on the Rheumatoid Arthritis Society website and decides to contact the volunteer

PART 2

Through her work at the Rheumatoid Arthritis Society she gets to meet others with similar experiences. She chats to Gwen, who also suffers from RA, although Gwen's disease is more advanced. Gwen is on a drug called leflunomide as well as methotrexate.

12a) Explain the mechanism by which leflunomide modifies the disease process of RA.

12b) What are the side effects of leflunomide?

Pam reads up on this and wonders why the first three doses are 100 mg followed by a maintenance dose of 10–20 mg.

13) Explain why this loading dose is required.

Gwen tells Pam about other drugs she tried before she was prescribed leflunomide. One was called penicillinamine

14) Discuss the advantages and disadvantages of penicillinamine and hydroxychloroquine.

One year later Gwen's arthritis gets a lot worse. She has had two trials of DMARDS and asks the doctor if she could be prescribed etanercept or infliximab, which she has read are very effective. The doctor has to check to ensure she fits the criteria according to the guidelines. He wonders if azathioprine, cyclosporine, or gold should be used first.

15a) What is the mechanism of action of azathioprine and cyclosporine?

15b) Describe the place of gold in the treatment of RA.

The doctor decides etanercept would be appropriate but before commencing the drug Gwen is checked to ensure she does not suffer from tuberculosis. Her leflunomide is stopped. She is also seen in clinic by the specialist RA nurse, who tells her about treatment with etanercept and teaches her how to self-administer. Initially she has to have her blood tested every 2 weeks, but after 8 weeks she only needs monthly checks.

16a) What is the mechanism of action of etanercept?

16b) How is etanercept administered?

16c) What are the side effects of etanercept?

After 2 years taking etanercept and methotrexate, Gwen is diagnosed with heart failure and told she must stop taking etanercept. The doctor has to commence her on another biological DMARD. He considers infliximab, anakinra, adalimumab, and abatacept.

17) Explain how the mechanisms of action of these four drugs differ.

_____

_____

_____

The rheumatologist discusses these options with Gwen, who is concerned about regular injections and wants to know how these drugs are all administered.

18a) How does the administration of these four differ?

_____

_____

18b) How should treatment with these drugs be monitored?

_____

_____

Chapter 10
Allergies and antihistamines: allergic rhinitis and urticaria

Most of us look forward to spring after the dullness and cold of winter. There are quite a lot of people, however, who dread the arrival of spring. Why would anyone dread this colourful season? Dorothy, who we encounter in the workbook later, is one of these seemingly unusual people. By the end of this chapter, we realize she is not unusual at all, she has just found she could only survive spring and summer locked up indoors trying to avoid exposure to pollen. Unlike most kids, her two toddlers have to spend most summer days indoors with her because she cannot be outside to supervise them playing. Dorothy is one of the millions of people who suffer from allergic rhinitis. Dorothy turns down all invitations to summer barbecues because she knows that as soon as she steps out her nose will start running (**rhinorrhea**), her nostrils and eyes will start itching, and she will be unable to do anything but sneeze.

Allergic rhinitis is the term used to describe symptoms like nasal congestion, sneezing, and rhinorrhea resulting from exposure allergens in individuals who are susceptible to them. Examples of common allergens are pollen, dust mites, animal dander, and mould. Hay fever is the common name for allergic rhinitis resulting from pollen. Allergic rhinitis is the most common form of chronic rhinitis. Acute rhinitis, on the other hand, is often non-allergic, and is usually caused by viral infections such as the common cold or by exposure to changes in temperature (called vasomotor rhinitis, this is when your nose runs when you go out into the cold air).

In this chapter we will focus on allergic rhinitis, examining the underlying pathophysiology of the disease and its pharmacological management. If allergic rhinitis is managed correctly, patients like Dorothy could live a normal life.

Then there is Bradley, who like Dorothy dreads going out with his friends, but for a different reason. He finds it embarrassing because, he always has to patiently explain to the waiters why no eggs or peanuts can come in contact with his meal. This is because if Bradley eats anything containing eggs or peanuts, he develops skin wheals all over his arms and chests a few minutes later, which can last up to several weeks. These skin wheals are called urticaria, or anaphylaxis of the skin, and could be caused by lots of different things or conditions in hypersensitive individuals such as food, stress, heat, drugs or cold weather. In this chapter we will also look at how urticaria develops and how it should be managed.

10.1 How does self-protection turn to self-destruction?

In the introduction to this section, the inflammatory and immune responses are described in detail. A quick revisit of this will help you understand where allergic rhinitis and urticaria fit in. The human body is like a little country complete with an 'army' equipped to defend it self against any invasion or fight any attacker. This 'army' is known as the immune system, and it produces the inflammatory response. The immune system and inflammatory response have the key role of protecting the body by recognizing and defending it against invading organisms or substances called pathogens. The immune system is made up of 'soldiers', cells that deploy weapons to fight invasion. To assist them in their role, after activation, some of these cells (the B-cells) produce

Table 10.1 Mediators of inflammation

Mediator	Actions
Histamine	Gastric secretion, itching
Prostanoids	Vasodilatation, vasoconstriction, platelet aggregation, bronchoconstriction
Leukotrienes	Spasmogenic
Platelet activating factors	Vasodilatation, platelet aggregation
Bradykinin	Vasodilatation
Nitric oxide	Vasodilatation, pro-inflammatory
Neuropeptides, e.g. substance P and neurokinin A	Pro-inflammatory
Cytokines, e.g. interleukins, interferons, CSF, TNF	Pro-inflammatory

CSF, colony-stimulating factor; TNF, tumour necrosis factor.

immunoglobulins, which are proteins commonly called antibodies. The antibodies will identify and inactivate parts of foreign objects (for example bacteria or a virus) called antigens, which find their way into the body. This involves a series of complicated processes during which the antibodies antigen interactions lead to production or release of wide variety of mediators of inflammation (see Figure S3.2). Examples of mediators of inflammation are histamines, leukotrienes, and prostaglandins (Table 10.1). These mediators are often the targets of drugs used to control symptoms of allergic diseases.

Sometimes the immune system, like any army, misinterprets data, prepares itself for attack (becomes activated), and deploys soldiers inappropriately. This can result in self-destruction.

Inappropriate activation could be directed against body substances (endogenous) and this is referred to as an autoimmune response. Inappropriate activation could also be against harmless substances from outside the body (exogenous) like pollen or dust, and this is what happens in allergies such as allergic rhinitis and allergic urticaria.

In order to treat, educate, and counsel patients correctly, you must have a good understanding of the symptoms and underlying causes of allergic rhinitis and urticaria, and the ways in which these could be prevented or treated by the available drugs.

10.2 Allergic rhinitis

Allergic rhinitis is very common globally and is estimated to affect 10–25% of the population. Because the symptoms are predominantly self-managed, it is thought that statistics probably underestimate the exact prevalence. The number of people affected appears to have increased dramatically over the last two decades. AR has been identified as one of the top 10 reasons for visits to GPs, and is classified as intermittent or persistent. This classification is based on the frequency of symptoms and the responsible allergen. Intermittent (previously called 'seasonal') allergic rhinitis often occurs at certain times of the year, as is the case with patients where pollen is the allergen (commonly called 'hay fever'). Persistent (previously called 'perennial') allergic rhinitis occurs all year round, and examples of common allergens are dust mites, animal dander (e.g. cat hair), and mould. The severity of both intermittent and persistent allergic rhinitis ranges from mild to severe. In order to choose the right treatment, it is crucial that the severity and type are correctly determined. Table 10.2 details the classification of allergic rhinitis.

Although allergic rhinitis is not life threatening, the condition can affect social and family life, school performance, and work productivity.

Dorothy, our patient, and her poor toddlers were virtually prisoners in their home during spring and summer, when the pollen count was high.

Like patients with asthma, sufferers of allergic rhinitis sometimes have an inherited predisposition to be hypersensitive (called atopy). They easily react and

Table 10.2 Classification of allergic rhinitis

Type/severity	Duration of symptoms	Features
Mild intermittent	<4 days per week or <4 weeks	Normal sleep and daily activities No troublesome symptoms
Moderate–severe intermittent	<4 days per week or <4 weeks	Presence of at least one of the following: • disrupted sleep • disturbed daily activities • troublesome symptoms
Mild persistent	>4 days/week or for >4 weeks	Normal sleep and daily activities No troublesome symptoms
Moderate–severe persistent	>4 days/week or for >4 weeks	Presence of at least one of the following: • disrupted sleep • disturbed daily activities • troublesome symptoms

develop symptoms when exposed to certain allergens, such as pollen or house dust mites.

There is also evidence to suggest that **allergic rhinitis**, **atopic dermatitis** and **asthma** are interlinked, and it is not uncommon for an infant to develop atopic dermatitis, then asthma as a small child, and allergic rhinitis as an adolescent/adult (this is called the 'atopic triad'). The pathophysiology and management strategies for asthma and allergic rhinitis share some similarities, and this has lead to the concept of 'one airway, one disease', i.e. clinicians who subscribe to this concept believe that allergic rhinitis and asthma are different manifestations the same disease.

10.2.1 The anatomy and physiology of the nose

The main functions of the nose are smell, speech, and the conduction and conditioning of air. During the process of nasal conditioning of air, the nose filters, humidifies, and warms the air as it makes its way to the lungs. The nose contains certain structures to enable it fulfil these functions. These structures are illustrated in Figure 10.1.

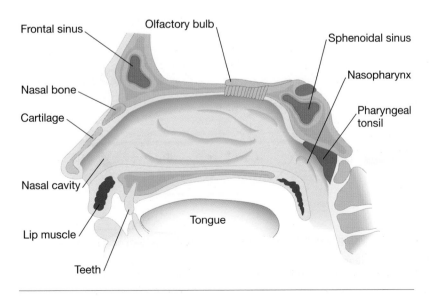

Figure 10.1 Anatomy of the nose.

The nose is shaped like a pyramid and has two openings, called nostrils, which lead into its two halves. The wall separating the two halves of the nasal cavity is called a septum and is made of bone and cartilage, with projections into the nasal cavity called conchae or turbinates. These projections increase the surface area of the septum, providing more space for conditioning of air as it is breathed in. The septum and turbinates are covered by the mucosal membrane, which is covered with mucous. This membrane has two key functions:

1) It provides a physical barrier against microbes and other particles in the air that is breathed in

2) It provides immunologic defence against 'invaders' with the aid of immunoglobulin A.

The mucous is produced by goblet cells, which are interspaced with the epithelial cells that make up the mucous membrane. The epithelial cells contain little finger-like projections called cilia, whose main function is to transport mucous into the pharynx. During normal breathing, inspired air moves through the pharynx and larynx into the lower airway, facilitated by the turbinates. The inflammatory process occurring in the nostrils of an allergic rhinitis patient leads to disruption of this coordinated air movement. The result is that the patient starts experiencing symptoms of congestion.

10.2.2 Role of the autonomic nervous system

The nose relies on the autonomic nervous system to assist it in the conduction and conditioning of air. The autonomic nervous system utilizes neurotransmitters, mainly acetylcholine (Ach) and noradrenaline (NA).

When the sympathetic system is stimulated it leads to release of Ach from the brain stem. The ACh is transmitted to the nicotinic receptor at the ganglion, which is followed by the release of NA by the postganglionic neuron. The NA binds the α receptors on the vascular muscle wall and results in transduction of a signal through inositol triphosphate and camodulin (Figure 10.2). This signal results in muscle contraction, which causes vasoconstriction of the nasal blood vessels. The effect is similar to that seen with Ach on smooth muscle in the bronchi (see Chapter 11).

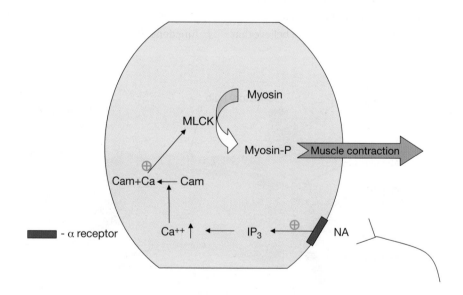

Figure 10.2 Actions of the sympathetic nervous system on vascular smooth muscle.

NA, noradrenaline; InsP$_3$, inositol triphosphate; Cam, camodulin; MLCK, myosin light chain kinase; Myosin-P, phosphorylated myosin; ⊕, stimulates.

A prominent feature of rhinitis is inflammation and hyper secretion in the nasal cavity. This causes vasodilation in the nasal mucosa, leading to symptoms of congestion. **Sympathomimetic** drugs (drugs that mimic the effects of adrenaline and noradrenaline) are commonly used to relieve this congestion through vasoconstriction.

Stimulation of the parasympathetic system leads to release of ACh from the brain stem. The ACh is transmitted to the nicotinic receptor by the preganglionic neurone. This activates release of more ACh, which is transmitted along the postganglionic neuron to the M3 receptors on the goblet cells. Stimulation of these receptors results in the increased release of mucous. Thus, anticholinergic agents are also used to treat simple rhinorrhea associated with rhinitis.

10.2.3 What processes are involved in the development of allergic rhinitis?

A series of events, which can be subdivided into three phases, occur in the development of allergic rhinitis.

Sensitization phase

This is the initial phase during which the antigen-presenting cell (APC) has an initial contact with the allergen such as pollen or mould. The APC ingests the pollen and produces an antigen complex, which activates T-cells (see Figure S3.2 in the introduction to this section for details).

Early response

When someone who is predisposed to allergies is exposed to an allergen that they have encountered in the past, it invokes what is called an 'early response'. During this phase, the allergen comes in contact with

immunoglobulin E (IgE), which is present on the surface of mast cells. This leads to mast cell degranulation involving release of mediators of inflammation, predominantly histamine (see Chapter 11, Box 11.1 for further details). Histamine is a basic amine that acts as an agonist on histamine type 1 (H_1), 2 (H_2), and 3 (H_3) receptors. The H_1 receptors are primarily involved in allergic reactions, and H_2 in gastric secretions; the H_3 receptors are found pre-synaptically in the central nervous system (CNS). The effects of histamine are shown in Table 10.3.

Late response

This usually develops in about one-third of patients approximately 8 hours after the allergen exposure and can last for up to 4 hours. The inflammatory process for the late phase is very complex and congestion is a key symptom. The cells involved are T-cells, eosinophils, neutrophils, macrophages, and mast cells. The mediators involved are cytokines, prostacyclin, and leukotrienes, which all have different roles. The longer the exposure to the antigen the longer the duration of the late response.

All of these events are similar to those seen in asthma, and the cellular events are described in more detail in Box 11.1 in Chapter 11.

10.2.4 Who is likely to develop allergic rhinitis?

Both the patient's genetic makeup and their environment are implicated in the development of allergic rhinitis. Having one or more parents with atopic symptoms (e.g. asthma, rhinitis, and/or atopic dermatitis) increases the risk of developing rhinitis (and other diseases associated with atopy). Excessive hygiene and sterilization of a

Table 10.3 Effects of histamine

	H_1	H_2	H_3
Stimulation of gastric secretion		✓	
Contraction of smooth muscle (except vascular)	✓		
Vasodilatation	✓		
Increased vascular permeability	✓		
Cardiac stimulation		✓	
Central nervous system arousal and wakefulness	✓		
Inhibition of neurotransmitter release in the central nervous system			✓

child's environment is also thought to increase the chances of becoming hypersensitive and to develop allergic conditions like asthma or allergic rhinitis. This is called the hygiene hypothesis. The hygiene hypothesis is centred on the differentiation of Th0 lymphocytes to Th2 lymphocytes in early life, which usually happens after exposure to allergens. Bacteria and viruses in a child's environment will stimulate response of Th1 lymphocytes. This leads to down regulation of responses by Th2 lymphocytes. A child with little exposure to bacteria and viruses will have little stimulation of Th1 lymphocyte responses and reduced down regulation of Th2 lymphocyte response. This will result in hyperactive Th2 lymphocyte response, leading to allergic disease.

> Both of Dorothy's parents had asthma and were considered atopic. With two parents with atopy, Dorothy's chance of having allergic illnesses is increased to 66%.

> The common allergens in her environment to which Dorothy was exposed to during her early life probably influenced the course of her allergic rhinitis.

10.2.5 Common triggers of allergic rhinitis

Pollen from grasses, trees, and weeds is the most common trigger of intermittent allergic rhinitis. The amount of these triggers at different times varies among geographical locations. This is measured and reported as the pollen count. Sufferers often plan their day based on the predicted pollen count.

On the other hand, patients with persistent allergic rhinitis develop symptoms after exposure to allergens like house dust mites, indoor moulds, and animal dander. Less common triggers are allergens in the workplace, including flour, wood and detergents.

10.3 Treatment of allergic rhinitis

Antihistamines, anti-inflammatory drugs, anticholinergics, and decongestants are the main classes of drugs used to manage the symptoms of allergic rhinitis. Other agents used include immunomodulators such as leukotriene antagonists and monoclonal antibodies. The antihistamines, anticholinergics, and decongestants are effective in modifying the early response, whilst the nasal anti-inflammatory drugs and leukotriene antagonists modify the late-response reactions.

10.3.1 Routes of treatment

The most common routes of administering drugs for allergic rhinitis are topically (nasal spray) and orally (tablets). The subcutaneous route as an injection is used for the monoclonal antibody. However, as we will see later, this is used only in rare, unresponsive cases.

Antihistamines and decongestants are used both orally and as a nasal spray. The anti-inflammatory drugs used are predominantly given as nasal sprays (corticosteroids and mast cell stabilizers). Leukotriene antagonists are the only oral anti-inflammatory drugs used, and they are reserved for resistant patients because of their cost.

The choices of any particular drug or route should be based on the patient's symptoms (e.g. severity and duration) and preference. Drugs could be used either regularly (for persistent allergic rhinitis) or just when required (for intermittent allergic rhinitis).

10.3.2 Antihistamines

As noted previously, histamine is the major mediator released in rhinitis. It is an agonist on the H_1 receptor on the nasal mucosa as well as on the H_2 and H_3 receptors found predominantly in other parts of the body. The effect of histamine on the H_1 nasal receptors results in the symptoms of itching, rhinorrhea (runny nose), and sneezing experienced by the patient in the early phases of rhinitis.

Antihistamines make up a huge class of drugs and are used for a variety of clinical conditions, including allergic rhinitis. This class is further divided into H_1-type and H_2-type antihistamines. H_1-type antihistamines are used in allergic rhinitis, while the H_2-type antihistamines are used for gastrointestinal hyperacid conditions (see Chapter 12 for details). In practice, the term 'antihistamine' is generally associated with agents that modify the effect of histamine on H_1 only.

Antihistamines are commonly used drugs in the management of allergic rhinitis and have been the first-line agents for decades. However, evidence now indicates that for people who get persistent (i.e. >4 weeks) moderate/severe

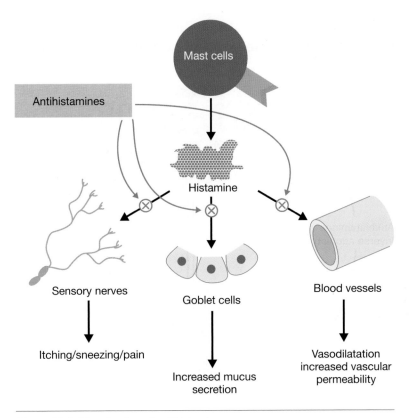

Figure 10.3 Site of action of antihistamines.

symptoms of allergic rhinitis, the intranasal corticosteroids are superior (see later). The sites of action for antihistamines are described in Figure 10.3.

Although antihistamines were thought in the past to work by blocking the histamine receptors (antagonist), H_1-type antihistamines are currently thought to have another mechanism of action. The theory is that they act by stabilizing the inactive histamine receptors, thereby preventing their activation by histamines. This action is what is referred to as an inverse agonist effect (Box 10.1).

H_1-type antihistamines are also subdivided into sedating and less-sedating antihistamines. There is a lot of evidence showing that less-sedating antihistamines lead to a bigger improvement in the quality of life of patients and should therefore be used first line in mild allergic rhinitis.

Sedating antihistamines

As already noted, these are the oldest members of the antihistamines and are referred to as first-generation

antihistamines. This group can be further subdivided into five classes based on structure (Table 10.4).

Apart from interacting with histamine receptors, many drugs also inhibit acetylcholine, 5-hydroxytryptamine (serotonin), and α-adrenoceptors. This leads to a range of positive and negative effects. The effects on both histamine and acetylcholine make some of these preparations (e.g. dimenhydrinate and cyclizine) useful in the prevention and treatment of nausea and vomiting, in particular motion sickness (see Chapter 12).

The effects of first-generation antihistamines on acetylcholine receptors is also used to advantage in cough and cold preparations. Apart from helping you sleep (a first-generation antihistamine is often put into 'night time' tablets, see later), the anticholinergic and antihistamine effects help 'dry up' a runny nose by reducing rhinorrhea.

One of the most prominent effects of the first-generation antihistamines is CNS depression, cognitive impairment, and sedation (which is why they are called 'sedating antihistamines'). First-generation antihistamines readily

Box 10.1

Action of agonists and reverse agonists on histamine receptors

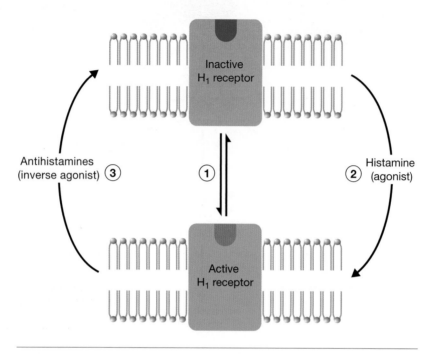

Figure a

1. The H_1 receptor is a g-protein coupled receptor that exists in dynamic equilibrium between active and inactive forms.

2. Agonists (histamine) occupy the receptor and drive the equilibrium towards the active form.

3. Antihistamines do not block the receptor; rather they cause a change in the receptor that drives the equilibrium towards the inactive state.

cross the blood–brain barrier and can easily cause these effects by attaching to receptors in the brain. While this is a problem when they are used for treating allergies such as allergic rhinitis (no point stopping the sneezing if you are going to sleep all day!), it has been used as an advantage in the short-term treatment of insomnia, with several over-the-counter hypnotics based on antihistamines available. First-generation antihistamines will also interact with other drugs and substances that depress the CNS, such as hypnotics and alcohol, producing an additive effect.

Dorothy would not give up her red wine and therefore stopped taking her chlorpheniramine!

Less-sedating antihistamines

This relatively newer class of H_1-type antihistamines (often called the 'second generation' or 'third generation') have a better H_1 receptor selectivity and fewer effects on the 5-hydroxytryptamine, α-adrenoceptors, and acetylcholine receptors associated with sedation and other CNS side effects. They also do not cross the blood–brain barrier as readily as the first generation. Originally these were called the 'non-sedating' antihistamines, however the term 'less-sedating' is more accurate, as some still cause significant sedation, with cetirizine being the most sedating and fexofenadine the least sedating. A list of second- and third-generation antihistamines is given in Table 10.5.

Table 10.4 First-generation antihistamines

Class	Examples	Other uses		
		Sedation	Cough, cold, and flu	Nausea/vomiting
Ethylenediamines	Mepyramine	++		
	Antazoline			
Ethanolamines	Diphenhydramine	++	++	
	Clemastine			
	Dimenhydrinate			++
	Doxylamine	++		
Alkylamines	Pheniramine			+
	Chlorphenamine		++	
	Dexchlorpheniramine		++	
	Brompheniramine		++	
	Triprolidine		++	
Piperazines	Cyclizine			++
	Hydroxyzine			
	Meclizine			++
Tricyclics and	Promethazine	+		+
tetracyclics	Trimeprazine	+		+
	Cyproheptadine			
	Azatadine			
	Ketotoifen			

+, Indication; ++, major indication, with preparations specifically for this indication.

Some of the second-generation antihistamines, specifically terfenadine and astemizole, were shown to cause serious cardiac arrhythmias and have been withdrawn from the market. This led, in part, to the development of the third-generation agents, which are closely related to many of the second-generation antihistamines. For example, fexofenadine is the active metabolite of terfenadine, but does not have the cardiac effect of the parent compound. Similarly, desloratadine is the active metabolite of loratadine, while levoceterazine is the active isomer of cetirizine (cetirizine is a racemic mixture of D- and L- isomers; the L- is active).

Table 10.5 Less-sedating antihistamines

Generation	Example
Second generation	Loratadine
	Cetirizine
	Terfenadine[a]
	Astemazole[a]
Third generation	Fexofenadine
	Desloratadine
	Levocetirizine

[a] Now discontinued.

Another advantage of the newer antihistamines is their prolonged duration of action, with most being given once or twice a day. In contrast, several of the older antihistamines must be dosed up to four times a day, unless given as a sustained-release preparation.

Most guidelines recommend that oral less-sedating antihistamines should be used in preference to the sedating antihistamines for allergic rhinitis, despite their higher cost. It is argued that improved patient quality of life and productivity adequately offset the cost.

Intranasal antihistamines, such as levocabastine and azelastine, are also available. They have the advantage of an even lower risk of sedation. However, they may be needed more frequently (up to four times a day) and they have little effect on other symptoms of allergic rhinitis that people often suffer from, such as itchy eyes.

10.3.3 Intranasal corticosteroids

For many years corticosteroids were reserved as second- or third-line agents behind antihistamines for most types of allergic rhinitis. However, current evidence has shown them to be the drug of choice for patients with moderate to severe rhinitis that lasts more than a few weeks.

The corticosteroids used in allergic rhinitis are glucocorticoids (for details of the different types of corticosteroids and their mode of action see Chapter 9). Briefly, they bind to receptors on the surface of cells where they are then translocated to the nucleus. The effects in the cell are to up or down regulate the transcription of various genes. The net effect in inflammation is reduced production of cytokines and inflammatory mediators, and suppression of the recruitment or proliferation of inflammatory cells such as T-cells and macrophages. This makes them among the most powerful anti-inflammatory agents. Unfortunately, they also have the potential for serious adverse events, including thinning of the skin, fat redistribution, osteoporosis, and increased risk of infections (see Chapter 9 for details of their systemic side effects).

The corticosteroids used intranasally are the more potent corticosteroids, and include **fluticasone**, **triamcinolone**, **budesonide**, **beclomethasone** and **mometasone**. The main difference is in their frequency of administration, with fluticasone, mometasone, and triamcinolone used once daily, while beclomethasone and budesonide are used twice daily (although a single daily dose may be possible with budesonide).

Because they are administered directly to the surface of the nose, the dose is much smaller (similar to inhaled corticosteroids in asthma) and the absorption into the bloodstream is limited. This means that they are unlikely to cause the significant systemic side effects seen with oral corticosteroids; the common adverse effects are stinging and nasal irritation.

The main drawback with intranasal corticosteroids is that they are slow to start working and may need to be used for several days before an effect is seen. It may therefore be useful to use a topical or oral decongestant for the first few days while the corticosteroid starts to take effect (more on decongestants later).

10.3.4 Other medications used to treat rhinitis

Although antihistamines and nasal corticosteroids are the mainstay of drugs used to manage allergic rhinitis, there are other classes of medication available. These are reserved as an 'add on' or as second- or third-line options in cases where antihistamines or corticosteroids have not

been fully effective, are not tolerated, or are contraindicated.

Cromolyns

The two drugs belonging to this class are **sodium cromoglycate** (also called cromolyn or cromolyn sodium) and **nedocromil**. Sodium cromoglycate is the cromolyn used as a nasal spray in allergic rhinitis whilst nedocromil is used in eye drops for allergic conjunctivitis.

Cromoglycate is used for persistent allergic rhinitis as a prophylaxis where symptoms can be anticipated. It is also used first line in children with moderate to severe symptoms because, unlike steroids, growth inhibition is not one of its side effects.

Although their mechanism of action is not quite fully understood, they are generally called 'mast cell stabilizers'. This is because in the past they were thought to work by preventing the release of histamine from mast cells. However, a number of alternative theories, including blocking chloride channels and reducing sensory nerve activity, have also been proposed.

Because cromolyns have no inhibitory effect on histamine once it is released, they must be used prophylactically, and must be started several weeks before the anticipated allergy season. This makes them virtually useless for people who get intermittent allergic rhinitis, for example on exposure to cats or other animals. Cromolyns have few side effects and are well tolerated. However, they have a short duration of action and therefore need to be used four to six times a day. This could lead to reduced compliance and effectiveness.

> Sam, Dorothy's son, was taken off his cromoglycate spray because he could only remember to take it twice a day, whilst at home.

Decongestants

These are used both orally and intranasally in allergic rhinitis where congestion is a major symptom. **Ephedrine**, **phenylephrine**, **oxymetazoline**, and **xylometazoline** are examples of intranasal decongestants. Congestion is more common in persistent allergic rhinitis, where oral decongestants could be used in combination with antihistamines or with intranasal corticosteroids at the beginning before the corticosteroid starts to take effect.

Their mechanism of action is through direct stimulation of α-adrenoceptors, where they act as sympathomimetics. This leads to vasoconstriction, which results in reduced tissue swelling and ultimately decreased congestion (Figure 10.2). The overall effect on the nasal mucosa is reduced resistance and increased patency of the airway.

Intranasal decongestants are immediately effective in reducing the symptoms of congestion. However, they can cause rebound congestion when they are withdrawn after prolonged or too much use (as little as 5 or 6 days). This condition is called **rhinitis medicamentosa**. In rhinitis medicamentosa, the α-adrenoceptors are over-stimulated, which causes 'fatigue' of the constrictor muscles of the nasal mucosa, as well as hypoxemia of the mucosa cells resulting from excessive and sustained vasoconstriction. The result is that the mucosa becomes engorged and oedematous (fluid filled). Unfortunately, patients are often tempted to use more decongestants to relieve the congestion of rhinitis medicamentosa, and this leads to a vicious cycle. While ephedrine is less likely to cause this rebound congestion, its availability as a commercial preparation is limited. To prevent rhinitis medicamentosa, intranasal decongestants should not be used for more than 5 days at a time.

Oral (systemic) nasal decongestants are less effective but do not cause rhinitis medicamentosa. The two commonly used oral agents are pseudoephedrine and phenylephrine. They are structurally similar to each other, and are related to ephedrine (Figure 10.4).

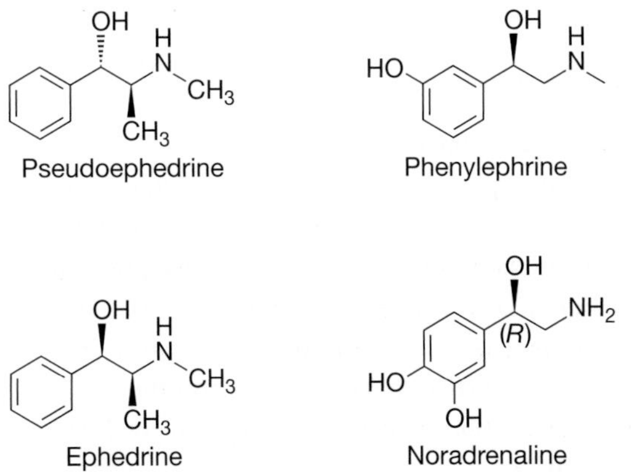

Pseudoephedrine has largely been replaced with phenylephrine in most preparations because psuedoephedrine can be easily extracted from tablets (even those compounded with other drugs such as paracetamol) and converted to methamphetamine (a popular illicit party drug called 'ice', which has stimulatory properties similar to other amphetamines). While generally well tolerated, they can cause irritability and CNS stimulation, leading to difficulty sleeping. They should be used with caution in patients suffering from certain conditions, including hypertension, hyperthyroidism, diabetes, and angle-closure glaucoma. However, the elevation in blood pressure in people who are well controlled may be negligible.

All decongestants interact with **moclobemide**, a mono-amine oxidase inhibitor (MAOI; see Chapter 19). Moclobemide could potentiate the effect of the decongestant by decreasing its metabolism, and could lead to hypertensive crises, therefore they should not be used within 14 days of MAOI therapy.

Anticholinergic drugs

Ipratropium bromide is a short-acting anticholinergic that is used rarely as a nasal spray to reduce excessive rhinorrhea (watery secretions) in allergic rhinitis. The mechanism of action of ipratropium bromide is by blocking the action of acetylcholine at the M3 receptor in the nasal mucosa. Intranasal anticholinergics are well tolerated and their main side effects are local irritation and dry mouth. However, they have to be used three or four times a day.

Leukotriene antagonists

This class of drug is relatively new and their use in allergic rhinitis is based on the theory that the inflammatory processes involved are linked with those in asthma (see Chapter 11 for details). **Montelukast** and **zafirlukast** are examples of leukotriene antagonists. They are recommended third line in allergic rhinitis, and while they reduce congestion, they have minimal effect on itching, sneezing, and rhinorrhea, which are present in allergic rhinitis.

They work by antagonizing the effect of leukotrienes produced by mast cells and eosinophils. Leukotrienes are mediators produced following oxygenation of arachidonic acid by the enzyme lipooxygenase (see Figure S3.1 in the introduction to this section).

Figure 10.4 Structures of common oral decongestants and their relationship to noradrenaline.

Activation of leukotriene receptors leads to an increase in inositol triphosphate and intracellular calcium, which ultimately results in potentiation of the inflammatory reaction.

Their main side effects are gastrointestinal upset and headaches, although these are rare.

Monoclonal antibodies

Omalizumab is the monoclonal antibody, also used in unresponsive moderate to severe allergic rhinitis. Its role in allergic rhinitis is based on the idea of 'one airway, one disease'.

Omalizumab, like all monoclonal antibodies, is a genetically engineered protein. This class of drugs is thought to represent the future of drug therapy. Its mechanism of action is unusual because it prevents the full allergic reaction from happening by blocking the production of mediators during the early and late response phases. It binds to circulating immunoglobulin E (IgE) and prevents it from attaching to mast cells and thereby indirectly prevents mast cell degranulation (see Chapter 11 for more details).

It is administered by subcutaneous injection once or twice a month. The dose is based on IgE levels. It is the most expensive drug option available and it should only be used in resistant cases. Anaphylactic reactions and reactions at the injection site are the main adverse drug reactions.

Immunotherapy or desensitizations

Immunotherapy refers to the immunomodulator techniques used to alter the immune system with the aim of curing or managing some diseases, such as allergic rhinitis. Desensitization is one such technique. This form of treatment is only considered in severe and complicated cases.

The mechanism by which desensitization is achieved is complex. Extremely small doses of the identified allergen are given to the patient and the dose is gradually increased. This gradual increase prompts the patient's immune system to retrain and readapt itself. Following this 'memory', the patient could be exposed in the future to that specific allergen without their immune system producing an allergic response.

Evidence has shown that this technique is most effective when used in younger children. The most common reactions are injection site reactions and anaphylactic shock. Patients can be given antihistamines before the injections to prevent this.

Allergen avoidance

Prevention, though not easy or often possible, is actually the best management option for allergic rhinitis. Patients should try to avoid exposure to the allergens they react to, such as pollen, dust mites, and animal dander. Broadcasts of pollen counts in the media can help limit exposure by informing sufferers when to keep windows shut (on high-pollen count days), as can regular cleaning and the use of a vacuum cleaners with a high efficiency particulate air (HEPA) filter (these filters remove any particles of 0.3 μm or greater, thus extracting 99.97% of airborne particles).

A summary of the treatments of allergic rhinitis is given in Table 10.6.

10.4 Urticaria

Urticaria, commonly called hives, is often referred to as anaphylaxis of the skin. The eruptions seen in urticaria arise as a result of the inflammatory processes in the skin causing small amounts of fluids to leak out from the capillaries to the dermis (skin structure is shown in Box 8.1). This leakage results in oedema (swelling of soft tissue as a result of accumulation of interstitial fluid) of the dermis, which leads to lesions that appear raised and red (Figure 10.5).

In most cases, the lesions appear almost instantly following exposure to the causative substance or condition in a susceptible individual. The lesions cause intense itching and commonly disappear after a few hours. Urticaria can be divided into two main groups based on the cause: allergic urticaria and non-allergic urticaria. There are many other subclassifications of urticaria and these are detailed in Table 10.7.

Table 10.6 Overview of treatments for allergic rhinitis

Class of drugs	Route	Examples	Symptoms controlled
Corticosteroids	Local (intranasal)	Beclomethasone Fluticasone Mometasone Triamcinolone	All symptoms
	Systemic (oral)	Prednisolone/prednisone	
Antihistamines	Local (intranasal)	Azelastine Levocabastine	All symptoms
	Systemic (oral)	Sedating: • chlorpheniramine • diphenhydramine • promethazine Less-sedating: • cetirizine • loratadine • fexofenadine • levocetirizine	
Decongestants	Systemic (oral)	Pseudoephedrine Phenylephrine	Congestion
	Local (intranasal)	Xylometazoline Oxymetazoline Ephedrine	
Mast cell stabilizers	Local (intranasal)	Sodium cromoglicate	All symptoms
Anticholinergics	Local (intranasal)	Ipratropium	Rhinorhea
Leukotriene antagonists	Systemic (oral)	Montelukast	Congestion
Monoclonal antibody	Systemic (subcutaneous injection)	Omalizumab	All symptoms

Table 10.7 Subtypes of urticaria

Urticaria type	Onset	Duration	Cause
Acute	Few minutes following contact	Hours to weeks	Food antigen (e.g. shellfish, nuts, eggs, fish) Virus or bacteria Nickel
Chronic	Few minutes following contact	>6 weeks	Food antigen (e.g. shellfish, nuts, eggs, fish) Virus or bacteria Nickel
Drug-induced	1–4 weeks after ingestion	Weeks	Sulfonamides, sulphonylureas, aspirin, penicillin
Physical	Few minutes to weeks following exposure	Hours to weeks	Water: aquagenic urticaria Heat: cholinergic urticaria Cold: chronic cold urticaria Scratching: dermatographic urticaria Sun: solar urticaria Pressure

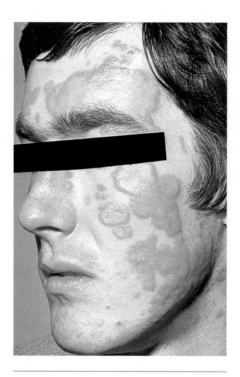

Figure 10.5 Urticaria skin reaction.

10.4.1 Allergic urticaria

Allergic urticaria results following exposure to certain allergens in susceptible individuals. These include food, drugs, dyes, latex, and, less commonly, virus or bacteria. Shellfish, nuts, eggs, and fish are examples of food allergens, whilst sulphonamides, sulphonylureas, aspirin, and penicillin are examples of drug allergens. The most common allergen is nickel, which can be found in cheap jewellery. Allergic urticaria can be either acute or chronic.

> Bradley, a friend of Dorothy, is allergic to latex. He is a dentist, and unfortunately there has been a steady rise in latex allergies among professions that require the wearing of gloves.

The pathophysiology of allergic urticaria is very similar to that of allergic rhinitis. Histamine and other mediators of inflammation are released from mast cells after binding of the allergen to IgE, which is present on the mast cells following sensitization. This results in mast cell degranulation (Figure 10.3).

10.4.2 Non-allergic urticaria

This form of urticaria results from other causes besides allergens. These include drugs, neuropeptides released by stress, porphyria (a disorder of the biosynthesis of heme leading to deposits in the skin), heat, and cold (see Table 10.7). The mechanism differs from allergic urticaria in that histamine release from mast cells is provoked directly without any interaction between allergens and IgE on mast cells.

10.5 Treatment and management of urticaria

The ideal management of urticaria is avoidance of the triggers. This is, however, extremely difficult because there are too many types of urticaria and sufferers often suffer from more than one type. Furthermore, the actual cause is often never determined.

Drug treatment is also difficult because drugs usually require time to get to effective levels in the body. This could happen after the eruption has cleared because of the often quick and intermittent nature of urticaria.

In many cases, the rash will clear up with no treatment. When drugs are used, these are usually antihistamines or corticosteroids.

10.5.1 Antihistamines

As discussed previously, there are two types of antihistamines: H_1-type and H_2-type. The H_1-type antihistamines can be taken alone or in combination with H_2-type. Combining the two has been shown to be more effective than single treatment in urticaria management, although this is currently unlicensed.

The less-sedating antihistamines are usually preferred. However, if night-time itching is a particular problem then the first-generation antihistamines may be better. Antihistamines should be taken regularly as prophylaxis or as required during attacks to reduce symptoms.

10.5.2 Corticosteroids

The oral corticosteroid prednisolone is often used for severe acute urticaria at doses of 0.5 mg/kg for a few days. Using corticosteroids in chronic urticaria is, however, not recommended because of the many side effects of oral corticosteroids.

10.5.3 Tricyclic antidepressants

Certain tricyclic antidepressants, for example **doxepin**, exhibit potent H_1 and H_2 antihistamine effects, and are sometimes used in the management of unresponsive urticaria. The sedative effects can be helpful for nocturnal symptoms.

10.5.4 Other treatments

Clinical trials are currently being undertaken with an analogue of α-melanocyte-stimulating hormone called afamelanotide (for the treatment of solar urticaria, which results following exposure to certain wavelengths of sunlight in susceptible individuals). The leukotriene antagonists (e.g. montelukast) may also have a role, but trial evidence so far is limited.

SUMMARY OF DRUGS USED FOR ALLERGIC RHINITIS AND URTICARIA

Therapeutic class	Drugs	Mechanism of action	Common clinical uses	Comments	Examples of adverse drug reactions
Local antihistamines	Azelastine Levocabastine	Modifies the effect of histamine on H_1, leading to reduced inflammatory mediator effects of histamines	Allergic rhinitis Allergies		Local irritation
Systemic antihistamines	Chlorpheniramine Diphenhydramine Promethazine Cetirizine Loratadine Fexofenadine Levocetirizine		Allergic rhinitis Urticaria Allergies Allergic reactions Nausea and vomiting	Divided into sedating and non-sedating antihistamines Sedating tend to have shorter duration of action	Sedation Dizziness Tinnitus Urinary retention Dry mouth Blurred vision Palpitations Arrhythmias
Intranasal glucocorticosteroids	Beclomethasone Fluticasone Mometasone Triamcinolone	Binds to receptors on cell surface translocated to the nucleus where they up- or down-regulate the transcription of various genes, leading to reduced production of cytokines and inflammatory mediators, and suppression of the recruitment or proliferation of inflammatory cells such as T-cells and macrophages	Allergic rhinitis	Several weeks to take effect Used once or twice daily	Local dryness Irritation Ulceration
Systemic corticosteroids	Prednisolone	See Drug summary table in Chapter 9			
Mast cell stabilizers	Sodium cromoglycate Nedocromil	Theories: 1) prevents the release of histamine from mast cells. 2) blocks chloride channels 3) reduces sensory nerve activity	Allergic rhinitis	Nasal and eye drops Eye drops	Local irritation
Systemic decongestants	Pseudoephedrine Phenylephrine	Stimulates α-adrenergic receptors, leading to vasoconstriction resulting in reduced tissue swelling and ultimately decreased congestion	Nasal congestion	Not as effective as topical decongestants	Irritability Tachycardia CNS stimulation (anxiety, restlessness)
Topical decongestants	Ephedrine Phenylephrine Oxymetazoline Xylometazoline			Instant effect	Rhinitis medicamentosa Local irritation
Anticholinergics	Ipratropium bromide	Blocks the action of acetylcholine at the M3 receptor in the nasal mucosa	Rhinorhea Asthma COPD	See Chapter 11	
Tricyclic antidepressants	See Chapter 19		Urticaria	See Chapter 19	

CNS, central nervous system; COPD, chronic obstructive pulmonary disease

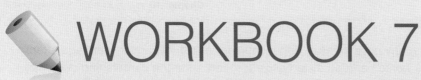

WORKBOOK 7
Allergic rhinitis and urticaria case studies

Dorothy: a simplified case history

Dorothy jumps up with a start when she hears her name called asking her to go to Room 2. She had been deeply engrossed in thoughts whilst waiting in the reception area of her GP surgery. Dorothy was amazed that she had been able to think at all, considering that she could not stop sneezing or blowing her runny nose. She also had a severe headache and felt generally tired and miserable.

She had been sat there thinking how isolated she had become from all her friends and how lonely and depressed she felt.

She and her kids had enjoyed spending time with their friends until 2 years ago, when her symptoms had become much worse soon after they moved house. What had been mild sneezing in the spring months had suddenly become sneezing, runny nose, itchy watery eyes, and headaches. The winter symptoms disappeared after they replaced all the carpets and curtains. However, all the symptoms returned with a vengeance at the end of winter. Now she rarely ventures from the house, and keeps the children inside as she does not want to spend time out in the garden.

She has resisted going to the doctors for 18 months now because she was worried he would put her on those horrible tablets that a chemist had sold to her whilst on holiday in Cyprus, insisting they were the best tablets for her symptoms. Although they had worked wonders and all her symptoms had magically disappeared, she had found all she could do was sleep all day. Then, after having a couple of glasses of wine, as you do on holiday, she had been convinced she was about to die.

Last night she and her husband had argued once again about her refusal to see the doctor. After he had pointed out to her how unhealthy and unfair it was to keep the children indoors all through the summer holidays, she realized she had to do something.

A table of clinical clerking abbreviations is given on page xi.

SUMMARY OF CLINICAL CLERKING FOR DOROTHY AT THE GP SURGERY

Age: 28 years

PC: Itchy and runny nose, sneezing, congestion of nose, itchy watery eyes, headaches and tiredness

HPC: Has had mild itchy runny nose in the spring months for about 4 years. 2 years ago after moving house, symptoms worsen and persisted all year round. After the carpets and curtains were replaced, winter/autumn symptoms vanished. However, as soon as spring started they resurfaced.

Symptoms of allergic rhinitis are:

- *itchy and runny nose, sneezing, congestion of nose, itchy and watery eyes, altered sense of smell*

- *headaches, malaise, and tiredness sometimes present*

- *nasal discharge, which is clear.*

These are the common symptoms of allergic rhinitis. However, because these symptoms are similar to those of acute rhinitis of a cold, the history should be longer, with details about the onset, character, frequency, severity, and duration of the above symptoms. This information is obtained during a detailed patient interview (below).

PMH: Dermatitis as a child

FH: Mum and dad both had asthma. Her 5-year–old, Sam, has asthma.

Dorothy had dermatitis as a child. It was diagnosed as atopic. Atopic dermatitis is the most common type of dermatitis and is linked to hay fever and asthma (called the atopic triad).

Atopic means an extra sensitivity to substances (allergens). Atopic conditions are thought to be immunoglobulin E (IgE) mediated, and patients usually have high levels of IgE antibodies.

The most common allergens for intermittent (seasonal) allergic rhinitis are pollen and mould on trees and herbs. For persistent (perennial) allergic rhinitis they are house dust mites, feathers, animal dander (cat or dog fur), and sometimes foodstuffs, e.g. cows' milk, eggs, or nuts.

Dorothy's family also have atopic conditions. These inherited factors make patients more sensitive to allergens in the environment and increase the risk of developing dermatitis or hay fever.

Allergic rhinitis is very common globally and is estimated to affect 10–25% of the population. Because the symptoms are predominantly self-managed, it is thought that statistics probably underestimate the exact prevalence.

DH: Currently nil. Previously: methyldopa for hypertension in pregnancy, chlorpheniramine for hay fever

DS: Chlorpheniramine – severe sedation and drowsiness

Her history of gestational hypertension is relevant in case she later develops chronic hypertension and is put on medication. She would be best to avoid oral decongestants for congestion symptoms.

Her adverse drug reaction to chlorpheniramine, and the interaction with alcohol, has scared Dorothy so much she has ignorantly refused to consult the doctor. Instead she changed her lifestyle and put her family through a lot of unnecessary isolation.

Antihistamines are important treatments for allergic rhinitis, but chlorpheniramine was definitely not the ideal one!

O/E: Breathing through the mouth. Has oral and dental changes consistent with longstanding breathing through the mouth.

Breathing through the mouth is very common when there is nasal congestion. Breathing through the mouth for long periods can transform the mouth and face, and lead to significant jaw pain.

O/Q:

> *A firm diagnosis of rhinitis is not based on a laboratory test. It can only be reached through reviewing detailed patient interview with information on medication history, family history, and the onset, duration and severity of symptoms, together with some tests and physical examination.*
>
> *A general approach to a patient with suspected allergic rhinitis symptoms should begin with evaluation of the answers to the following questions.*

1) Which symptoms is she experiencing?

> *Answer: See above.*

2) What colour are her nasal secretions?

> *Answer: Clear.*
>
> *Coloured would be another form of rhinitis. Allergic rhinitis shows clear secretion.*

3) When did these symptoms first appear?

> *Answer: See HPC above.*
>
> *This could be correlated to exposure to allergens.*

4) Are the symptoms associated with change in environment?

> *Answer: Some symptoms were worse after moving house. The previous owner had three cats. Once the carpets were replaced the symptoms improved. They also improve outwith the summer months.*

5) How often do the symptoms appear?

> *Answer: See HPC above.*
>
> *This will distinguish between hay fever (intermittent allergic rhinitis) or persistent allergic rhinitis due to dust mites, etc.*

6) For how long do the symptoms persist?

> *Answer: See HPC above.*
>
> *This will help determine if it is hay fever or persistent allergic rhinitis due to dust mites, etc.:*
>
> • *hay fever usually persist through season*
>
> • *perennial allergic rhinitis could persist as long as the allergen is present, which could be all year round.*

7) What precipitates symptoms?

> *Answer: See HPC above.*
>
> *The most common allergens for intermittent (seasonal) allergic rhinitis are pollen and mould on trees and herbs.*
>
> *The most common allergens for persistent (perennial) allergic rhinitis are house dust mites, feathers, animal dander (cat or dog fur), and sometimes foodstuffs, e.g. cows' milk, eggs, or nuts.*

8) Which activities precipitate symptoms?

> *Answer: Gardening and other outdoor activities.*

9) Do symptoms disturb the patient's normal functioning?

> *Answer: Dorothy has been avoiding social activities and keeps the children inside to avoid going into the garden.*

Diagnosis: Moderate allergic rhinitis

Table 10.2 details how this is decided.

Plan:

loratadine

PART 1

1) What is allergic rhinitis?

2) What is the difference between allergic rhinitis and acute rhinitis?

3) Describe the structure of the nose and the function of its various components.

4) Explain the pathogenesis of allergic rhinitis.

5) What is the role of the autonomic nervous system in the functioning of the nose?

6) Explain how older antihistamines cause sedation.

The doctor explains to a worried Dorothy that the new antihistamine is very unlikely to cause sedation like chlorpheniramine does. He tells her that as long as she takes it regularly her symptoms should soon improve.

She is worried about forgetting if she has to take it many times a day, like the chlorpheniramine. The doctor assures her she only needs to take it once a day.

7) What is mechanism of action of antihistamines?

Dorothy goes home. After 2 weeks she goes to the pharmacy and asks if there is anything that would stop the stuffiness in her nose. All her other symptoms have improved, except for the congestion. The pharmacist sells her what she says are decongestant drops, which she should use for a maximum of 5 days.

8) Explain how decongestants work to relieve rhinorrhea.

9) Why must Dorothy not use too much of the decongestant and not for longer than 5 days?

Dorothy is ecstatic when her symptoms improve drastically. For the first time in months her dribbling nose is cleared. She uses the decongestant drops for a month and when she runs out she decides to stop. The congestion returns and is worse than before so she goes to the doctor. He tells her the congestion after she stopped the decongestant was called rebound congestion or rhinitis medicamentosa.

He prescribes the oral decongestant phenylephrine for 1 week only, to help her gradually get over the congestion. He also prescribes fluticasone nasal spray to continue long term. He explains that it will reduce the inflammation that happens in rhinitis medicamentosa.

10) Explain how steroids improve symptoms of allergic rhinitis.

When Dorothy goes to her pharmacy she suddenly remembers she forgot to tell doctor she was pregnant. The pharmacist advises that her medication will have to be altered and she should go back to doctor. The doctor tells her she will have to be taken off loratadine. He advises her to try another old-generation antihistamine because they are considered safer in pregnancy. He tells her that although she suffered from drowsiness on chlorpheniramine it does not mean she will be drowsy with all the older antihistamines, but he promises to stop it if she gets drowsy. She finally agrees. He also stops the phenylephrine.

She improves on pheniramine and fluticasone nasal spray.

PART 2

The following year, at about the same time, Dorothy is back at surgery with her 5-year-old, Sam, who now has similar symptoms to those Dorothy used to have. He also has asthma.

Following an examination as detailed as Dorothy's, Sam is put on cromoglycate nasal spray.

11) What is the mechanism of action of cromoglycate nasal spray?

12) Explain how it should be used and why.

One month later, Sam is not better at all and Dorothy is back at surgery with him. The doctor prescribes montelukast, a leukotriene antagonist.

13) Explain where and how leukotriene antagonists act to reduce the symptoms of allergic rhinitis. Why is montelukast ideal for Sam?

Sam improves significantly. One year later Dorothy is back at the surgery as nothing seems to control her symptoms and she is fed up. She would like a cure.

The doctor talks to her about immunotherapy. She agrees and is referred to the outpatient clinic where it is given and monitored.

14) Explain the theory behind immunotherapy.

15) List the other drugs that could have been tried.

16) Explain the mechanism of action of monoclonal antibodies.

17) How do anticholinergic agents work in rhinitis?

18) What symptom would anticholinergic agents control?

Dorothy improves very much.

Bradley is a friend of Dorothy who also has many allergies. He knows what to avoid on most days. He doesn't suffer from rhinitis; rather he gets urticaria when he is exposed to latex. This is a real problem because he is a dentist and has to wear gloves. Fortunately, he usually has polyurethane gloves to use. However, now and then they run out in the surgery and he has to use latex gloves.

19) What is urticaria? Which layer of the skin is affected?

20) Discuss the initial treatment of urticaria.

21) if Bradley's urticaria is particularly bad at night, what would be the best choice of treatment and why?

Chapter 11
Respiratory disease: asthma and COPD

Three things are needed to sustain life: food (nutrients), water, and air (oxygen). Although we can survive for a few weeks without food, and for a few days without water, we can only last for a matter of minutes without oxygen. The importance of this can be found in the simple first-aid mantra ABC, used when a person collapses: the first and most important thing to do is to establish or maintain an airway (A), the second is to ensure the person is breathing (B), and the third is to check circulation (C).

We all generally take our lungs for granted, but imagine what it must be like to not be able to get air in or out of your lungs? What it must be like to have to stop every few steps to catch your breath, unable to carry on a conversation without pausing for breath between each word? Imagine having to carry an oxygen canister with you for the rest of your life? This is what can happen to people who have lung diseases. In most developed counties lung diseases like asthma and chronic obstructive pulmonary disease (COPD) contribute to a significant burden of illness. What is most frustrating is that COPD, one of the leading causes of morbidity and mortality, could be significantly reduced if people did not smoke!

In this chapter we will review the physiology of the lungs and respiration, and how this relates to two common respiratory diseases: asthma and COPD. We will examine the molecular and cellular events that relate to lung (pulmonary) function and dysfunction, and how drugs used for pulmonary diseases modify these events. The chapter will focus on the primary respiratory drugs, namely bronchodilators and anti-inflammatories, as well as some of the newer agents, such as the interleukin antagonists.

11.1 The respiratory system

The respiratory system is composed of a complex series of structures starting at the mouth and nose, where air enters, and terminating in the alveoli, where oxygen and carbon dioxide are exchanged. Also important to respiration is the diaphragm, a sheet of muscle that divides the chest (thoracic) cavity from the abdomen. Contraction of the diaphragm produces a negative pressure in the thoracic cavity that causes the lungs to expand and air to be drawn in (Figure 11.1).

Basic respiration is initiated and controlled by the respiratory centre located at the base of the brain. Mostly breathing is under autonomic control and we are not conscious of the process. However, it is possible to influence breathing voluntarily because of connections between the medulla and the cerebral cortex, as we do when we hold our breath under water. The rate of ventilation is influenced by the blood levels of carbon dioxide (CO_2) and oxygen (O_2). Increasing concentrations of CO_2 (hypercapnia), as occurs when we exercise, produces increases in the depth and rate of respiration by direct stimulation of the respiratory centre. Changes in O_2 levels are usually less important, unless levels drop very low (hypoxemia). If the oxygen level drops below 60% of normal this triggers chemoreceptors in the carotid and aortic bodies that then stimulate the respiratory centre.

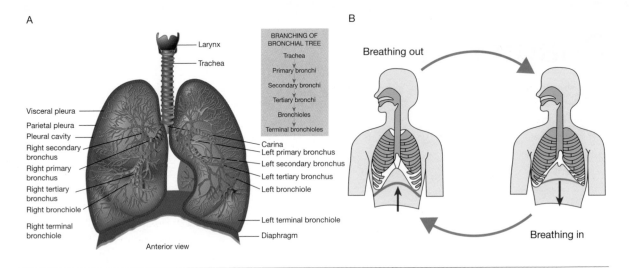

Figure 11.1 The respiratory system.

11.1.1 Protective mechanisms in the respiratory tract

Like the skin, most parts of the respiratory tract are exposed to the elements. This means that in addition to life-giving oxygen, the lungs are potentially exposed to a range of chemicals, microorganisms, and dusts. As a result the respiratory tract has a number of important defence mechanisms. The first of these occurs in the nasal passages, where much of our air is breathed in. Within the nose there are many tiny hairs that help to trap large particles, preventing their entry into the lungs. To assist in this the nose is lined with mucous-producing cells, as is much of the respiratory tract. This sticky mucus further traps small particles for removal.

The second defence mechanism is found in the tracheobronchial tree, the repeatedly branching pipes that start from the single trachea in the throat and end at the alveoli. This tree is lined with cilia, small finger-like projections from cells that continually sweep the secretions produced by goblet cells and bronchial glands up towards the throat to be swallowed. Excessive production of overly sticky mucus, as in patients with cystic fibrosis and asthma, or damage to these cilia, as in patients who smoke, is a significant contributor to respiratory disease.

A third protective response comes from a number of cough receptors located in the tracheobronchial tree that when stimulated produce a reflex cough. These receptors detect noxious stimuli (chemoreceptors) or respond to local inflammation (mechanoreceptors).

11.1.2 Smooth muscle and the respiratory tract

Starting at the trachea the bronchial tree is surrounded by bands of muscles wrapped in a double helix. Lower down the tree (i.e. closer to the alveoli) the amount of muscle increases while the amount of cartilage (the substance that provides rigidity to the upper parts of the respiratory tract) decreases. Both sympathetic and parasympathetic nerves innervate this smooth muscle, providing a balance between contraction (bronchoconstriction) and relaxation (bronchodilation).

Stimulation of the sympathetic system, and the subsequent release of catecholamines such as noradrenaline, is associated with what is sometimes referred to as the 'fight or flight' response. This occurs when we are under stress and is supposed to help us 'fight' or take 'flight' from whatever is causing the stress. In organs such as the heart and peripheral blood vessels the release of catecholamines results in stimulation of mostly β_1-adrenoceptors, resulting in increased heart rate, increased force of contraction of the heart muscles, and increased peripheral resistance to return blood to the muscles and brain (see Chapter 5 for more details). However, in the respiratory tract the catecholamines bind to β_2-adrenoceptors, which are receptors that stimulate adenylcyclase, resulting in increased production of cyclic adenosine monophosphate (cAMP) (Figure 11.2). The cAMP produces relaxation of smooth muscle by inhibiting myosin light chain kinase (MLCK), which is responsible for phosphorylating myosin. The cAMP also enhances intracellular binding of calcium and extrusion of calcium. The net effect is bronchodilatation, which contributes to the 'fight or flight' response by making it easier to get air into the lungs.

Stimulation of the parasympathetic system, through the vagus, causes release of acetylcholine (ACh), which attaches to muscarinic ACh receptors (mAChR) of the M_3 subtype on the smooth muscle of the respiratory tract. Stimulation of M_3 receptors increases the production of inositol triphosphate ($InsP_3$) by increasing the activity of phospholipase C. The $InsP_3$ then attaches to ligand-gated channels on the endoplasmic reticulum and causes the release of calcium. The calcium binds with calmodulin, which then activates MLCK, which produces contraction of the smooth muscle (bronchoconstriction).

The effect of these two systems on the smooth muscle is one of the major targets for treatments for asthma and COPD, as we see in Chris and Ian's cases in Workbook 8.

11.1.3 Other effects of the sympathetic and parasympathetic systems

In addition to bronchodilatation and bronchoconstriction, the sympathetic and parasympathetic systems have other positive and negative effects on respiratory function. Stimulation of β_2-adrenoceptors results in inhibition of histamine release from mast cells. Histamine is formed from histidine and is a potent inflammatory mediator. As we will see later, these actions are important parts of the disease process in asthma.

Acetylcholine, in addition to producing bronchoconstriction, also stimulates the exocrine glands of the lining of respiratory tract, resulting in an increase in the volume of secretions. These two effects, bronchoconstriction and hypersecretion, are protective in that they occur often as a reflex in response to some sort of noxious substance, and are supposed to reduce the entry of the substance into the lungs. However, as we will

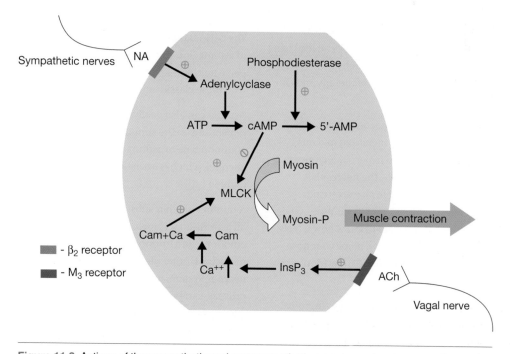

Figure 11.2 Actions of the sympathetic and parasympathetic nervous systems on smooth muscle.

NA, noradrenaline; Ach, acetylcholine; ATP, adenosine triphosphate; cAMP, cyclic adenosine monophosphate; AMP, adenosine monophosphate; $InsP_3$, inositol triphosphate; Cam, camodulin; MLCK, myosin light chain kinase; Myosin-P, phosphorylated myosin; ⊘, inhibits; ⊕, stimulates.

see later, in patients with asthma their airways can respond in this way to substances that would otherwise not affect most people; this is called airways hyperresponsiveness or hyperreactivity.

11.1.4 Common airways diseases: asthma and COPD

Asthma and COPD are collectively the most prevalent respiratory diseases, with each affecting approximately 1 in 10 adults. While they share some common symptoms and some common treatments, there are distinguishing features that set them apart from one another (Table 11.1).

11.2 Asthma

Asthma is the most common lung condition, affecting 10–15% of children and 8–10% of adults. The Global Initiative for Asthma (GINA), an international collaboration involving the World Health Organization, estimates that over 300 million people are affected worldwide. Asthma is associated with significant morbidity, and a considerable number of patients suffer frequent, including daily, attacks. These attacks can disrupt sleep, work, or schooling, and make activities such as sport difficult. If severe enough they can lead to a condition called status asthmaticus, which is unresponsive to normal bronchodilator therapy and can be fatal.

Asthma is characterized by bronchoconstriction, inflammation of the airways, and increased mucous secretions. All of these result from hyperreactive airways that respond to a variety of stimuli. The net result is narrowing of the airways, leading to characteristic wheezing, cough, chest tightness, and dyspnoea (difficulty in breathing). If you want to know how it feels to have asthma, grab a drinking straw, block your nose, and try to breath in and out through the straw (don't try this if you actually have asthma!).

The diagnosis of asthma is a combination of symptoms and standard measures of lung function. The three most common measures are the forced expiratory volume (FEV_1), the forced vital capacity (FVC), and the peak expiratory flow (PEF). The FEV_1 is the forced amount of air expelled in 1 s, while the FVC is the maximum total volume of air that can be exhaled under force. These two

Table 11.1 Comparison of asthma and COPD

	Asthma	COPD
Usual age of onset	Childhood	Middle age
Triggers/causes of the disease	Allergens Exercise	Smoking
Degree of airway reversibility	Reversible[a]	Partially reversible
Time course of symptoms	Episodic	Gradually progressive

[a] Except status asthmaticus, a very severe and potentially fatal form of asthma that may not be reversible.

Because of these differences, we will consider each separately.

measurements are made using a spirometer. The PEF (usually referred to as peak flow) is the greatest airflow that can be sustained for 10 milliseconds on forced expiration. This can be measured with a less complex, hand-held device that can be easily used at home. The PEF is not as accurate as the spirometry measures, but it gives a reasonable estimate of lung function and is often used for self-monitoring of asthma.

The GINA has proposed four classifications for the severity of asthma: intermittent, mild persistent, moderate persistent, and severe persistent. The diagnosis associated with these classifications is shown in Table 11.2.

Asthma can also be divided into different types depending on the stimuli that trigger an attack. The most common type of asthma is extrinsic (also called atopic or allergic), which is associated with a range of allergens (Table 11.3).

A number of other substances and conditions can trigger an asthma attack, including the weather (hot or cold), emotions, and hormones. Apart from allergies to medicines, other medications that affect the sympathetic nervous system, or are involved in the inflammatory process, can precipitate an asthma attack.

β-blocker antihypertensive agents can cause bronchoconstriction due to the blocking of the β_2-adrenoceptors on the smooth muscle of the lungs. As discussed in Chapter 5, β-blockers act by primarily blocking β_1-adrenoceptors in the heart and kidney. Non-selective β-blockers (i.e. those that block both β_1 and

Table 11.2 Classification of asthma severity proposed by GINA

Intermittent

Symptoms less than once a week
Brief exacerbations
Nocturnal symptoms not more than twice a month

FEV1 or PEF ≥80% predicted
PEF or FEV1 variability <20%

Mild persistent

Symptoms more than once a week but less than once a day
Exacerbations may affect activity and sleep
Nocturnal symptoms more than twice a month

FEV1 or PEF ≥80% predicted
PEF or FEV1 variability <20–30%

Moderate persistent

Symptoms daily
Exacerbations may affect activity and sleep
Nocturnal symptoms more than once a week
Daily use of inhaled short-acting β_2-agonist

FEV1 or PEF 60–80% predicted
PEF or FEV1 variability >30%

Severe persistent

Symptoms daily
Frequent exacerbations
Frequent nocturnal asthma symptoms
Limitation of physical activities

FEV1 or PEF ≤60% predicted
PEF or FEV1 variability >30%

Table 11.3 Common allergic asthma triggers

Area	Examples
Outdoor	Pollens: • grasses • flowers Pollution
Lifestyle	Food: • eggs • shellfish • yeasts Occupational: • nickel • latex
Indoor	Moulds and fungi Dust mites Animal dander Cockroach excrement
Other	Drugs: • penicillins and sulphonamides

Adapted from http://www.asthma.org.uk/applications/triggers/.

β_2 receptors), such as propranolol, may precipitate an asthma attack, whereas those selective for β_1-adrenoceptors (sometimes called cardioselective), such as atenolol, have a much lower risk. However, even these have the potential to cause bronchoconstriction in some people and therefore are generally to be avoided in asthmatic patients.

The other class of drugs associated with precipitating asthma is the non-steroidal anti-inflammatory drugs (NSAIDs), in particular aspirin (sometimes called 'aspirin sensitive' asthma). The NSAIDs block the conversion of arachidonic acid into a number of thromboxanes and prostaglandins (see Section 3 for more details). If this pathway is blocked the arachidonic acid is converted preferentially into leukotriene B_4, which is a precursor to a number of leukotrienes that are potent bronchoconstrictors. We will revisit this later. However, not all people with asthma are sensitive to aspirin, and

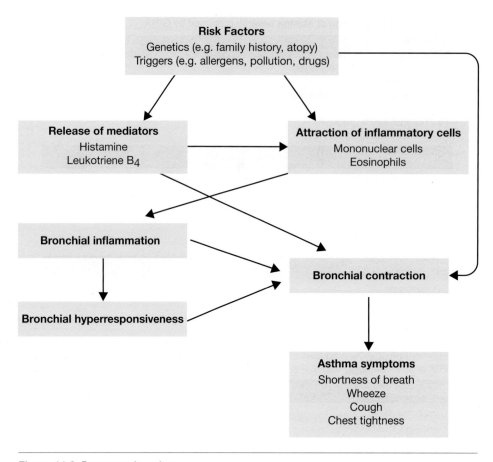

Figure 11.3 Processes in asthma.

estimates put the proportion that are sensitive at between 5 and 20%. Patients who have shown asthma sensitivity to aspirin—usually accompanied with rhinitis and facial flushing a few hours after exposure—should avoid NSAIDs.

11.2.1 Phases in an asthma attack

An asthma attack is broadly divided into an early/acute phase and a late/chronic phase. In the early phase bronchoconstriction and increased secretions dominate. These processes are outlined in Box 11.1. The key mediators involved in the early phase are histamine and leukotriene B$_4$.

Histamine is a basic amine that attaches to one of three types of histamine receptors. Histamine-1 (H$_1$) receptors are responsible for the inflammatory responses seen with

histamine and are found on smooth muscle and blood vessels. Cysteinyl leukotrienes are potent bronchoconstrictors and contribute to the hyperreactivity of the airways in people with asthma (Figure 11.3). Airway hyperreactivity results in airway narrowing in response to a stimulus that would be innocuous in a normal person. It is caused by excessive bronchoconstriction, thickening of the airway walls due to oedema, and sensitization of sensory nerves, resulting in excessive bronchoconstriction in response to stimuli.

The late phase of asthma results in structural changes to the airways. These include:

• hypertrophy (increased size) and hyperplasia (increased number) of the smooth muscles surrounding the bronchial tree

- increased number of blood vessels, resulting in thickening of the airway wall

- increased number of goblet cells, resulting increased mucous secretion and mucous plugging.

Inflammatory cells, such as eosinophils, which are recruited as part of the early phase, play an important role in the late phase of asthma. Eosinophils are polymorphonuclear (multilobed nuclei) cells containing granules that are released as part of the inflammatory response. These granules contain proteins and toxins, including eosinophil major basic protein (EMBP), eosinophil peroxidase (EP), eosinophil cationic protein (ECP), and eosinophil derived neurotoxin (EDN). These substances, particularly EMBP, are thought to produce 'irreversible' damage to airways cells, resulting in increased airways hyper-reactivity.

11.3 Asthma treatments

The two main groups of asthma drugs are bronchodilators and anti-inflammatories. These modify the early phase (bronchodilators and anti-inflammatories) and late phase (predominantly anti-inflammatories) of asthma (see Box 11.1).

11.3.1 Routes of administering treatments

Both bronchodilators and anti-inflammatories can be given orally or by inhalation. Oral bronchodilators are salbutamol and theophylline, while the most common oral anti-inflammatories used are prednisone and prednisolone. Generally inhaled therapy is the preferred route of administration. This is because of the potential for rapid onset of action (e.g. inhaled salbutamol can start working within minutes during an acute attack) and the ability to minimize side effects by being able to use much smaller doses and limiting the systemic absorption. As an example, the usual oral dose of salbutamol is 2–4 mg for an adult, while the inhaled dose is 200 µg (one tenth of the oral dose). The reduction in side effects from using inhaled corticosteroids is particularly important, as we will see later.

Inhaled medications are available in a range of formulations:

- metered dose inhalers

- dry powder

- nebulizer solutions.

The metered dose inhalers (MDIs) are pressurized canisters with the drugs dissolved in a solvent/propellant. Up to a few a years ago the main propellants used were chlorofluorocarbons (CFCs). The use of CFCs has been associated with thinning of the ozone layer and so they have been phased out and replaced with hydrofluoroalkanes (HFAs). The MDIs require skill and coordination to ensure the canister is activated only as the person breathes in. Failure to due this results in reduced efficacy and depositing of the active ingredients on the back of the throat, which can lead to adverse effects. One solution to the coordination problems is to use breath-actuated MDIs. These devices only deliver a dose once the person starts to inhale. Another alternative is dry powder inhalers, but these require a minimum inspiratory flow rate, usually greater than 30–50 L/min, and people with severe airways limitation may not be able to use them.

Nebulizers versus spacers

Corticosteroids and bronchodilators are available as nebulizer solutions. These are given using a nebulizer machine, which vaporizes the liquid into a fine mist that is inhaled through a facemask or mouthpiece. Most nebulizers use compressed air and they are very popular in hospitals, as they require minimal supervision. It is also thought that they deliver the drugs more effectively and do not require the coordination you need to use an MDI. However, MDIs can be given through a spacer. A spacer is a plastic chamber that has a hole for the MDI mouthpiece on one end and a mouthpiece on the other (Figure 11.4). Patients puff the required dose from the MDI into the chamber and then they breathe deeply to get the dose into the lungs. The chamber keeps the mist from the MDI suspended long enough for the dose to be administered without the need to coordinate activating the MDI and breathing. Recent evidence shows that an MDI with a spacer is just as effective as a nebulizer, but at a much lower cost. What is more, it removes the need to be 'tied' to a machine, and this can be important psychologically, particularly for children with asthma.

Box 11.1

Early and late phases of asthma

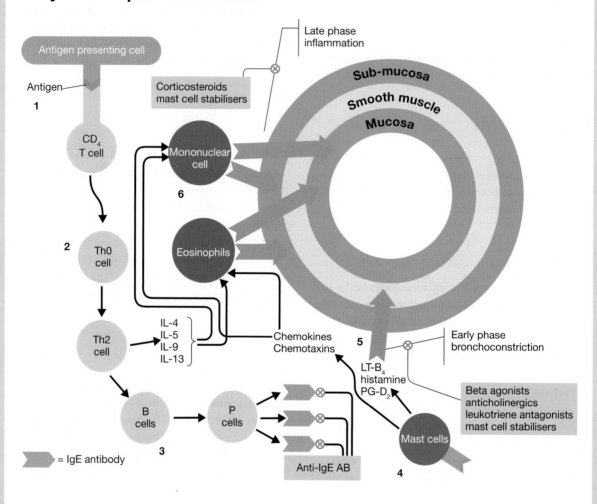

Figure a

1. Antigens that enter the lung are captured and interact with CD_4 T-cells via the antigen-presenting dendritic cells that line the respiratory tract.

2. CD_4 T-cells stimulate the production of T-helper 0 (Th0) and T-helper 2 (Th2) cells from naïve T-cells. These cells release a number of cytokines, including interleukins IL-4, IL-5, IL-9, and IL-13.

3. The cytokines coordinate the release of immunoglobulin E (IgE) by B-cells and plasma cells, as well as attracting other inflammatory cells, particularly eosinophils. The IgE attaches to mast cells.

4. Activated mast cells release mediators, including cysteinyl leukotrienes ($LT-B_4$), prostaglandin D_2 ($PG-D_2$), and histamine. They also release chemokines and chemotaxins that control the migration of eosinophils and mononuclear cells,

5. $LT-B_4$, $PG-D_2$, and histamine attach to receptors on bronchial smooth muscle and cause bronchoconstriction, as well as increasing mucous secretions.

6. Inflammatory cells, including eosinophils and mononuclear cells, migrate into the mucosa and submucosa. Eosinophils release basic proteins that damage the epithelial cells, and may also release growth factors responsible for airway remodelling.

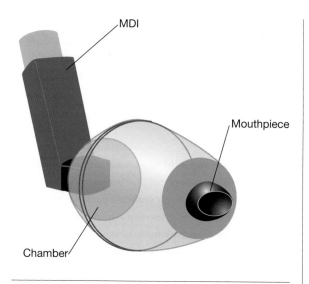

Figure 11.4 Spacer device.

11.3.2 Bronchodilators

Three classes of bronchodilator drugs are used:

- β_2 agonists
- anticholinergics
- methylxanthines.

β agonists

The actions of β-adrenoceptor agonists are described in Figure 11.2. As noted previously, of the two types of β-adrenoceptor found in the body β_2 is largely found on bronchial smooth muscle. Non-selective sympathomimetics (agents that stimulate the sympathetic nervous system), such as noradrenaline (norepinephrine) and adrenaline (epinephrine), stimulate both β_1- and β_2-adrenoceptors, whereas agents selective for β_2, such as salbutamol, are preferred in the treatment of asthma and COPD. However, β_2 agonists are not totally β_2 selective and can stimulate β_1-adrenoceptors, particularly at high doses or if used excessively. Two groups of inhaled β_2 agonists are used: short-acting (**salbutamol** and **terbutaline**) and long-acting (**salmeterol** and **eformoterol**). The short-acting β_2 agonists have a quick onset but short duration of action (3–5 h). They are used on an 'as required' basis and are referred to as 'reliever' medications. The short-acting medications are the drugs of choice for acute exacerbations of asthma and are used prophylactically in patients who get exercise-induced asthma.

The long-acting inhaled β agonists generally have a delayed onset and prolonged action, and therefore are used as 'preventers' rather than 'relievers'. However, eformoterol produces bronchodilatation within a few minutes (similar to salbutamol), compared to 10–20 minutes with salmeterol, and therefore it can be used as a 'reliever' when used in combination with **budesonide** (a corticosteroid). The long duration of action of these agents appears to come from them being more lipophilic (lipid soluble). Salmeterol has a long lipophilic side chain. It has been postulated that this side chain binds to an 'exoreceptor site' located near the β receptor, keeping it in close proximity to the receptor. However, another theory is that salmeterol binds to the β-adrenoceptor by entering the membrane lipid bilayer and attaching to the receptor from within the membrane (Figure 11.5). Although eformoterol also has a long side

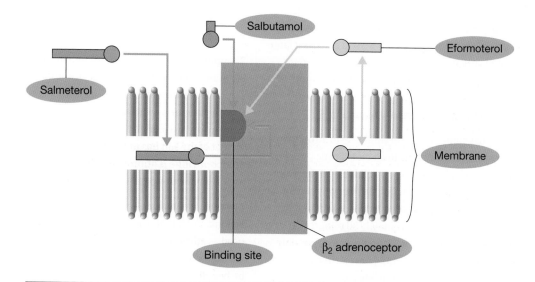

Figure 11.5 Binding of β_2-adenoceptor agonists.

chain it is not thought to have the same binding action as salmeterol, rather it undergoes rapid rebinding to the receptor after displacement because of the eformoterol being 'stored' in the cellular membrane. Because they have a long duration of action (8–12 h) salmeterol and eformoterol are usually given twice a day.

The oral β_2-adrenoceptor agonist used is salbutamol. This has a limited role because of potential adverse effects, which are far greater than for the inhaled β agonists. Because the β agonists are not entirely selective for β_2-adrenoceptors the main side effects are caused by stimulation of β_1-adrenoceptors in the heart and skeletal muscle, and include increased heart rate and tremors. The effects of stimulation of β adrenoreceptors in the liver include glycogenolysis resulting in hyperglycaemia, and hypokalemia as potassium is moved intracellularly with glucose.

Although controversial, there is a possible increased risk of asthma-related death in people using regular rapid acting short- and long-acting β_2 agonists. The mechanism is uncertain, but is thought to be due to a relative refractiveness to β_2 agonists in a small number of people. This may result from deterioration in β-adrenoceptors in people with an unusual genotype of the β-adrenoceptor, therefore short-acting β agonists should only be used on an intermittent 'when required' basis, and long-acting β agonists should only be used in combination with a corticosteroid.

Anticholinergic drugs

Anticholinergic drugs block the action of acetylcholine at the M_3 receptor on bronchial smooth muscle, producing bronchodilatation (see Figure 11.2). Like β_2 agonists they come in short-acting (**ipratropium**) and long-acting (**tiotropium**) forms. However, tiotropium has only been studied in patients with COPD, and we will discuss it later. Only inhaled anticholinergic formulations are used to treat airways diseases, as oral anticholinergics would produce too many systemic side effects, including dry mouth, blurred vision, and urinary retention.

Ipratropium has some structural similarity to atropine, and is non-selective so it binds to all muscarinic receptors. However, it is very water soluble and therefore little enters the bloodstream, reducing the potential for side effects. It has a slower onset of action compared to short-acting β agonists (approximately 30 minutes) and does not produce as greater bronchodilatation, possibly because of inhibition of presynaptic muscarinic receptors (M_2), which increase acetylcholine release thus reducing

the effectiveness. It is therefore only used as a second-line agent, in addition to β agonists, in patients who are not controlled with β agonists alone. Ipratropium is well tolerated, with the main adverse effects being a dry mouth and throat irritation.

Methylxanthine drugs

The best-known, and most consumed, methylxanthine is probably caffeine. Others include theobromine, which is found in chocolate. Although caffeine has been used in medicine for centuries, its use as a respiratory drug today is generally limited to premature infants. The methylxanthine currently used in lung diseases is **theophylline** and its salts **aminophylline** (ethylenediamine salt) and **choline theophyllinate** (choline salt). The methylxanthines are non-selective phosphodiesterase inhibitors. Phosphodiesterase (PDE) is the enzyme responsible for breaking down cAMP (see Figure 11.2) and cGMP. Five main isoforms exist, with PDE_3 and PDE_4 selective for cAMP. The PDE_4 is expressed on inflammatory cells (e.g. eosinophils) and is one of the new targets for asthma treatments. Inhibition of PDE leads to an increase in cAMP in the bronchial smooth muscle, mimicking the effects of β_2 agonists, resulting in bronchodilatation. However, this not thought to be the main mechanism of action of these agents in respiratory disease, as the levels of theophylline present at therapeutic doses produce minimal inhibition of PDE. Methylxanthines also produce direct stimulation of the respiratory centre, resulting in increased respiration. Other effects attributed to methylxanthines include acting as inhibitors of adenosine A_1 and A_2 receptors. The inhibition of phosphodiesterase and adenosine receptors on mast cells may also reduce the amount of histamine and other inflammatory mediators released (see Box 11.1).

Theophylline is available in immediate-release and sustained-release formulations. Aminophylline is available for intravenous administration and choline theophyllinate is available as an oral mixture. When converting between the salts and theophylline, the weight of the salt has to be taken into consideration: 1 mg of theophylline is approximately equivalent to 1.25 mg of aminophylline and 1.54 mg of choline theophyllinate.

Evidence for the long-term efficacy of theophylline is lacking, but it is generally accepted that it should only be used as add-on therapy for patients not managed on corticosteroids. The effects on the respiratory centre may be beneficial in patients with COPD.

The toxicity of theophylline further limits its role in respiratory disease. The unwanted side effects of theophylline result from central stimulation, cardiac, and gastrointestinal effects. Theophylline, like caffeine, increases alertness and can cause tremor and nervousness. In the heart it causes increased rate and force of contraction, and in the gastrointestinal tract it causes nausea and vomiting. Like caffeine it also acts as a weak diuretic. At high doses it can produce serious and potentially fatal cardiac and central effects such as cardiac arrhythmias and seizures. It is therefore a drug of narrow therapeutic index and requires blood levels to be taken to monitor therapy. Ideally trough (pre-dose) levels of the drug should be monitored with the aim of keeping the blood levels between 10 and 20 mg/L (55 and 110 µmol/L); levels on the lower end appear to be effective and may not require monitoring.

To make the use of theophylline even more complicated it is metabolized in the liver by cytochrome P450 (CYP450 1A2), therefore its metabolism is affected by a number of other drugs, including some macrolide antibiotics (e.g. erythromycin) and cimetidine (inhibitors resulting in increased levels of theophylline), and phenytoin and carbamazepine (inducers that lead to decreased levels). Cigarette smoke is a significant inducer of the metabolism of theophylline, with the half-life of theophylline decreased by as much as 60% in smokers. This is a potentially important interaction because if a person stops smoking (as recommended particularly for people with COPD and asthma) while taking theophylline, the blood levels of theophylline can rise and cause toxicity.

11.3.3 Corticosteroids

Corticosteroids are the cornerstone of therapy for all people with asthma, with the exception of those with mild, intermittent symptoms, including exercise-induced asthma. Just as in other inflammatory conditions (see Chapters 8, 9, and 10), it is the glucocorticoids that are used (see Chapter 9 for a discussion of their action). In asthma both oral and inhaled corticosteroids are used.

Potency of corticosteroids used in asthmas

Table 11.4 outlines the comparative doses of the commonly used oral and inhaled corticosteroids.

Oral corticosteroids

The most common oral corticosteroids used in asthma are prednisolone and prednisone, just as they are in rheumatoid arthritis and other severe inflammatory conditions. The common side effects of prolonged and/or high dose use are outlined in Box 9.2. Given these potentially serious side effects, the use of oral corticosteroids is usually reserved for severe acute attacks, where doses of 25–50 mg daily in adults for 7–10 days are often used. The advantage of short courses of high-dose corticosteroids is that there is no need to taper the dose, as the hypothalamic–pituitary–adrenal (HPA) axis is not significantly suppressed (see Chapter 9 for more discussion of HPA suppression).

Inhaled corticosteroids

The inhaled corticosteroids allow the delivery of potent corticosteroids directly to the lung, thus reducing their potential systemic adverse effects (see above). **Beclomethasone** and **budesonide** were the first inhaled corticosteroids, and newer agents include **fluticasone** and **ciclesonide**. Ciclesonide is an unusual corticosteroid in that it is a prodrug, having almost no activity until it is converted in the lungs by esterase hydrolysis to the active form des-ciclesonide. The supposed advantage of this 'on-site' conversion is reduced systemic and local side effects. However, the clinical significance of this is yet to be fully determined.

Although the systemic adverse effects with inhaled corticosteroids are reduced, they are not completely eliminated. There is conflicting evidence that long-term use of corticosteroids may reduce early growth in children, although they tend to still reach their normal adult height. The message of most management guidelines is to use the

Table 11.4 Comparative potency of common oral and inhaled corticosteroids

Corticosteroid	Equivalent oral doses	Equivalent inhaled doses
Hydrocortisone	100 mg	N/A
Prednisolone	25 mg	N/A
Prednisone	25 mg	N/A
Beclomethasone	N/A	100 µg
Budesonide	N/A	200 µg
Fluticasone	N/A	100 µg
Ciclesonide	N/A	80 µg

minimal dose of inhaled corticosteroid that achieves satisfactory relief of symptoms. It is important to note that the inhaled corticosteroids have shown a fairly flat dose–response curve, and pushing the doses above 250 µg fluticasone/beclomethasone daily may achieve little except increased side effects.

The main adverse effects of inhaled corticosteroids are caused by local deposition on the back of the throat and mouth, leading to oral thrush. Using a spacer (see Figure 11.4) and/or washing the mouth (rinsing the mouth with water, gargling, and spitting it out) after use can reduce the risk of oral thrush.

Combination corticosteroids and long-acting β agonists

Puffers are now available that combine a long-acting β agonist with a corticosteroid. The benefit is that the number of puffs a person needs to take each day can be reduced and therefore adherence improved. However, patients should be stabilized on the individual puffers of each type of inhaler first before swapping to the combination puffers; patients should never be initiated on the combination puffers.

11.3.4 Other drugs used for asthma treatment

While bronchodilators and corticosteroids are central to asthma management, a number of other agents have been developed. They are always second- or third-line treatments and are usually used when maximal doses of corticosteroids have been reached. They include:

- cromolyns
- cysteinyl leukotriene antagonists
- IgE antagonists.

Cromolyns

Sodium cromoglycate (also called cromolyn and cromolyn sodium) and **nedocromil** have similar mechanisms of action and are often referred to as 'mast cell stabilizers'. They do not produce bronchodilatation and their exact pharmacology is still uncertain. They were thought to work by inhibiting the release of histamine from mast cells, possibly by blocking calcium channels. Other proposed mechanisms include inhibition of chloride channels, reducing the activation of sensory nerves and neuronal reflexes (i.e. reduced vagal stimulation). This is thought to explain the effect of cromolyns on reducing airway hyper-reactivity. It is

important to remember that they are only useful prophylactically and have no effect in an acute attack.

The cromlyns are generally well tolerated with few side effects except mouth and throat irritation. Because of their short duration of action they have to be given four times a day.

Cysteinyl leukotriene antagonists

These are relatively new agents targeting the leukotrienes released by mast cells and eosinophils. Leukotriene receptors are found on bronchial smooth muscle and when activated have similar effects to the muscarinic receptors by increasing inositol triphosphate and intracellular calcium. The two selective inhibitors used in clinical practice are **montelukast** and **zafirlukast**, which blocks the CysLT1 receptor, inhibiting the effect of leukotriene C_4, leukotriene D_4, and leukotriene E_4 (components of slow reacting substance of anaphylaxis).

Clinical trials have show that these drugs only have a small effect on the airways and are inferior by themselves to inhaled corticosteroids and β agonists. Their role is best in combination with inhaled corticosteroids to reduce the dose of corticosteroid (steroid sparing). Montelukast has a long duration of action and can be given once a day, while zafirlukast is given twice a day.

Both montelukast and zafirlukast are well tolerated, with gastrointestinal upset and headache the main side effects.

IgE antagonists

Omalizumab is a monoclonal antibody that binds with circulating IgE to prevent it attaching to mast cells. It is given by subcutaneous injection and begins to reduce IgE levels within hours, although it takes several days to have a full effect. It has a long duration of action and is usually administered every 2 to 4 weeks, with the dose based on IgE levels. Omalizumab inhibits both early and late phases of asthma, but its role in asthma management is still to be determined. Clinical trials have shown reductions in symptoms, improvements in quality of life, and reductions in doses of corticosteroids in patients with moderate to severe asthma that required corticosteroids. It is extremely expensive compared to other treatments and therefore it is best reserved for patients with moderate to severe asthma, with high levels of circulating IgE levels, who are on corticosteroids.

Omalizumab is generally well tolerated, with injection site reactions being the main adverse effect. However, like any protein, it has the potential to cause anaphylactic reactions.

Table 11.5 Definitions of asthma control from GINA

Symptom or characteristic	Controlled (all of the following)	Partly controlled (any in any week)	Uncontrolled
Daytime symptoms	≤ twice a week	> twice a week	Three or more features of partly controlled asthma in any 1 week
Limitations on activities	None	Any	
Nocturnal symptoms	None	Any	
Use of 'reliever' medication	≤ twice a week	> twice a week	
Lung function (FEV_1 or PEF)	Normal	<80% predicted	

Antihistamines

Although histamine is an important mediator in asthma, antihistamines have not been shown to have any effect in preventing or treating asthma.

11.3.5 Choosing an asthma treatment

Most guidelines, including GINA, recommend a step-wise, additive approach to choosing therapy based on asthma severity and symptom control. The approach of GINA is outlined in Box 11.2.

11.4 Chronic obstructive pulmonary disease

Chronic obstructive pulmonary disease is not a single disease, but comprises a number of chronic lung conditions. The two main components of COPD are chronic bronchitis and emphysema. While these two conditions can exist independently, most people with COPD have both. Bronchitis is literally inflammation of the bronchial tract. Emphysema affects the alveoli, the small air sacs responsible for exchanging oxygen and carbon dioxide. When healthy, the alveoli are like a new balloon—they expand and return to their original size with each breath. When emphysema occurs the alveoli start to break down and merge together, and their walls become hard and resistant—more like blowing up a paper bag!

As discussed previously, COPD and asthma share many common features and treatments (see Table 11.1). Tobacco smoking has a much larger role to play in the aetiology of COPD and, unlike asthma, people with COPD tend to have slowly declining lung function interspersed with 'exacerbations' that are often caused by lung infections (Figure 11.6).

11.4.1 Management of COPD

Smoking cessation

Smoking is the single largest etiological factor in the development of COPD, and the most significant intervention to slow or reverse the decline in lung

function with COPD is to stop smoking. A number of smoking cessation options are available, including nicotine replacement, buproprion, and varenicline.

Short- versus long-acting β_2 agonists

Short acting β_2 agonists have been shown to improve lung function in patients with COPD. Although there has been less experience with long-acting β_2 agonists, there is growing evidence that they too have a role in COPD. The current recommendations are that short-acting β_2

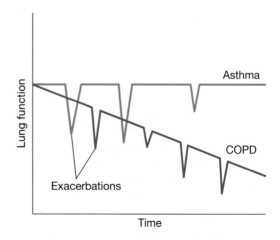

Figure 11.6 Comparison of lung function over time for asthma and COPD.

Box 11.2

Adapted GINA guidelines on asthma management

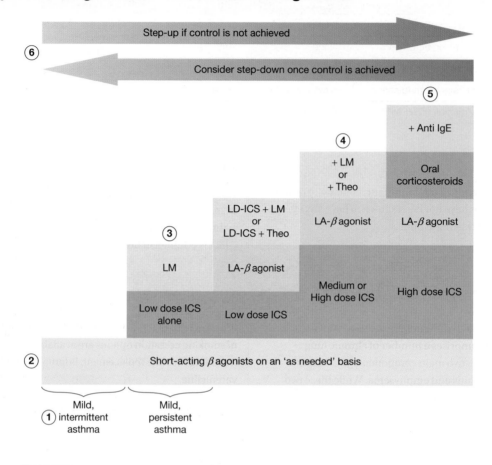

Figure b

1. For definitions of asthma severity see Table 11.2.

2. All patients should receive short-acting β agonists (salbutamol or terbutaline) on an as-needed basis only. Use of these more than twice a week indicates possible loss of asthma control.

3. Low dose ICS is considered to be equivalent to 200–400 μg daily of budesonide (see Table 11.4 for equivalent doses of ICS).

4. Medium dose ICS is considered equivalent to 400–800 μg of budesonide, and high dose 800–1600 μg (see Table 11.4). The addition of leukotriene antagonists or theophylline could be considered to spare the use of corticosteroids.

5. This should be treated as a severe exacerbation of asthma and oral corticosteroids should be used. The lowest dose possible should be chosen (e.g. 25 mg usually for adults). Anti IgE should be instigated only if the patient shows high levels of IgE.

6. Once control is achieved a step down to the next level should be considered. In the case of mild persistent asthma, a reduction in the dose of the inhaled corticosteroid to the lowest dose that maintains control should be tried.

ICS, inhaled corticosteroids; LM, leukotriene modifier (e.g. montelukast); LA-β agonist, long-acting β agonist (e.g. salmeterol); LD-ICS, low dose inhaled corticosteroid; Theo, theophylline; Anti IgE, anti immunoglobulin E agents (e.g. omalizumab). Preferred treatments are in coloured boxes; treatments in white boxes are usually alternatives for patients who cannot tolerate the preferred treatments.

agonists should be started first on an as-needed basis and long-acting agents implemented if this fails to control exacerbations or improve functioning. Unlike asthma, it is recommended that the efficacy of these drugs in COPD should not be assessed using measures of lung function such as FEV_1 alone, but should include measures of functionality such as the ability to undertake daily activities. It should be noted that PEF measurements used in asthma have no role in monitoring COPD.

Inhaled anticholinergic drugs

While the role of these drugs in asthma appears limited, they have been shown to have significant effects in improving COPD. Both the short-acting (ipratropium) and long-acting (tiotropium) agents have demonstrated superiority to placebo, and in some trials superiority to β_2 agonists. Tiotropium is structurally similar to ipratropium but differs in its binding to muscarinic ACh receptors. Whereas ipratropium is a non-selective muscarinic antagonist, binding at M_1, M_2, and M_3 receptors, tiotropium is more selective for M_1 and M_3 receptors because although it binds to M_2, it dissociates from it more quickly than ipratropium. In addition, tiotropium binds more tightly to the M_3 receptor than ipratropium, which gives it a prolonged duration of action (half-life of 35 hours compared to 15 minutes for ipratropium), allowing once-daily dosing.

Corticosteroids

The role of corticosteroids is less clear in COPD than in asthma. The nature of the inflammation in COPD is quite different and less responsive than in asthma. Studies with inhaled corticosteroids have not shown convincing evidence of efficacy, but corticosteroids may be useful in patients who have a documented response to inhaled corticosteroids and are having frequent (more than two) exacerbations a year. Oral corticosteroids produce a very small improvement in lung function. However, the systemic side effects of long-term therapy (see Box 9.2) preclude their use in most patients. There is currently insufficient information to clearly advocate the use of the corticosteroid plus long-acting β agonist combination puffers in COPD. While they may show some benefit, if response is not seen within a month they should be discontinued.

Mucolytics

A predominant feature of COPD is excessive production of sputum. This is often difficult to clear and leads to chronic coughing and breathing difficulties. Bromhexine is an orally administered mucolytic, while N-acetyl cystine (also used as an antidote for paracetamol poisoning) is sometimes given by nebulizer. Mucolytics break down mucoprotein fibres in sputum through hydrolytic depolymerization of the disulphide bonds. This has the effect of reducing the viscosity of the sputum, making it easier to clear. Other effects of bromhexine that have been postulated include increased lysosomal and pulmonary surfactant production, while both are thought to increase bronchial secretions and improve ciliary activity; some of these claims are yet to be proven.

Studies have shown an approximately 20% reduction in exacerbations compared to placebo with the use of mucolytics, and an increase in the chance of being exacerbation free. They are very well tolerated with few side effects, except gastrointestinal upset with bromhexine and, rarely, bronchospasm with N-acetylcystine. Mucolytics may have a role in patients who have significant cough associated with their COPD.

SUMMARY OF DRUGS USED FOR ASTHMA AND COPD

Therapeutic class	Drugs	Mechanism of action	Common clinical uses	Comments	Common adverse drug reactions
Beta agonist	Inhaled: short-acting β agonist salbutamol terbutaline	Selectively stimulates β_2 receptors leading to bronchodilation	Acute exacerbations of asthma and COPD Viral-induced wheeze	Quick onset of action Short duration of action	Tremor Nervous tension Headache
	Inhaled: long-acting β agonist salmeterol eformoterol		Prophylaxis of asthma and COPD	Salmeterol: delayed onset Eformoterol: quick onset used for acute asthma in stable patients in symbicort SMART protocol Both prolonged duration of action	
	Oral: salbutamol		Acute exacerbations (not advisable)	Rarely used	Tachycardia Tremor Arrhythmia Sleep and behaviour disturbances
Inhaled anticholinergics	Ipratropium Tiotropium	Blocks the action of acetylcholine at the M_3 receptor on bronchial smooth muscle, producing bronchodilation	Asthma COPD	Ipratropium: slow onset of action, Shorter duration of action Tiotropium: longer duration of action	Dry mouth Nausea headache Urinary retention Glaucoma
Methylxanthines	Theophylline Aminophylline	1) Non-selectively inhibits phosphodiesterase, the enzyme responsible for breaking down cAMP 2) Directly stimulates the respiratory centre, resulting in increased respiration 3) Inhibits adenosine A_1 and A_2 receptors	Asthma COPD	Theophylline used orally Aminophylline used intravenously Narrow therapeutic window Metabolized by hepatic cytochrome P450, leading to interactions	Tachycardia Palpitations

Therapeutic class	Drugs	Mechanism of action	Common clinical uses	Comments	Common adverse drug reactions
Corticosteroids	Prednisolone Beclomethasone Fluticasone Budesonide Ciclesonide	Binds to receptors on cell surface translocated to the nucleus where they up- or down-regulate the transcription of various genes, leading to reduced production of cytokines and inflammatory mediators, and suppression of the recruitment or proliferation of inflammatory cells such as T-cells and macrophages	See Drug summary table in Chapter 9	Prednisolone used orally Others inhaled Less effective in COPD-higher doses usually used than in asthma Potencies variable, based on dNg preparation	See Drug summary table in Chapter 9
Leukotriene receptor antagonists	Montelukast Zafirlukast	Antagonizes the effect of leukotrienes produced by mast cells and eosinophils	Allergies Asthma	Montelukast metabolized by hepatic CYP3A4 and CYP2CG, and zafirlukast by CYP2C9, leading to interactions Zafirlukast has longer elimination half-life of 10 hours	Gastrointestinal Headache Insomnia Malaise
IgE antagonists	Omalizumab	A monoclonal antibody that binds with circulating IgE to prevent it attaching to mast cells	Severe asthma	Long half-life of 26 days IgE levels measured before treatment commenced	Headache Injection site reactions Nausea Diarrhoea

COPD, chronic obstructive pulmonary disease.

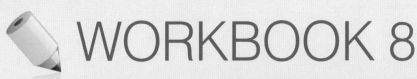

WORKBOOK 8
Chronic obstructive pulmonary disease and asthma case studies

The patient: a simplified case history

Once again Den has been admitted to hospital. His heart failure condition has deteriorated, and he requires review of his heart medication and adjustment of his diuretic therapy. Once in the cardiac ward his condition is stabilized and he is encouraged to take some gentle exercise. While wandering the hospital corridors he runs into Ian, an old friend. Ian and Den used to work together in their youth but they have not seen each other for 10 years.

Den remembers Ian as a person who was very active, very funny but also a very heavy smoker. He is in hospital because he has a condition known as chronic obstructive pulmonary disease (COPD), and he is very short of breath. Ian has been admitted to the respiratory ward, which is one floor above the cardiac ward.

A table of clinical clerking abbreviations is given on page xi.

CLINICAL CLERKING FOR IAN WRIGHT

Age: 68 years, weight 98 kg, height 170 cm

PC: Increasing shortness of breath and productive cough with increased sputum production.

HPC: 6 years history of COPD (dominated by chronic bronchitis symptoms) and hypertension. Exercise tolerance has been good up until recently but he has been in and out of hospital a few times. He also has a wheeze and has been producing phlegm.

Shortness of breath can be a sign of many disease conditions. It could be due to cardiac failure, as in the case of Den. In the case of Ian it is due to a respiratory problem.

Ian suffers from COPD, which is a chronic disease of the lungs characterized by expiratory airflow obstruction. It is a collective term for a number of disease conditions. The two main subtypes are chronic bronchitis and emphysema. These two conditions differ in their underlying pathophysiology and appearance of the patient; patients with emphysema used to be referred to as "pink puffers" because they generally have a reddish complexion and puffing appearance when breathing, due to hyperventilation, whilst chronic bronchitic patients were "blue bloaters" because coexisting signs of heart failure and hypoxenia make then appear big and blue. The conditions coexist in many patients with COPD.

The airflow obstruction is usually progressive, not fully reversible, and does not change markedly over several months. It is most commonly seen in smokers, but it is not exclusive to that group. It causes a progressive decline in lung function leading to breathlessness, particularly on exercise.

DH:

- ipratropium bromide inhaler (four times a day)
- salbutamol inhaler daily and when required
- tiotropium bromide once a day
- oxygen

No known drug allergies.

Ipratropium bromide and salbutamol are both bronchodilators that have different mechanisms of action. They are sometimes used in combination to alleviate breathlessness.

Tiotropium acts in a similar way to ipratropium bromide but is a long-acting bronchodilator.

Oxygen therapy is considered as a drug therapy. In COPD patients, oxygen is recommended to prevent hypoxia (low oxygen saturation in blood), which can improve survival.

SH:

- Ex-smoker, stopped 3 years ago, used to smoke 30/day.
- Married, lives with wife.

O/E:

- Ian was breathless
- "Obese appearance of blue bloater"

Investigations:

1) Relevant blood results:

- white blood cells (WBC): 18.1×10^9/L ($\uparrow$) (normal range 3.5–11 $\times 10^9$/L)
- C-reactive protein (CRP): 56 (normal range <10)
- Hb: 15.6 g/dl (normal 13.5–17 g/dl for males, 11.5–16.5 g/dl for females).

The raised WBC indicates the presence of infection. This is also confirmed by a raised CRP. CRP is secreted by the liver in response to inflammatory mediators. A raised level indicates inflammation, trauma and infection. These two results in combination with Ian's symptoms indicate that he is having an infective exacerbation of COPD.

2) Spirometry

Ian previously had a recorded FEV_1 of 45% of the predicted value, indicating a moderate degree of airflow obstruction.

The measurement of airflow obstruction is necessary for the diagnosis of COPD, and spirometery is used to determine this. However, the results should be interpreted in combination with the patient's ability to function.

Patients are asked to perform a forced expiration (this involved blowing out as hard and as fast as possible into a sealed tube) and the volume of expired air is plotted against time. In COPD patients the volume of air expired in the first second, known as forced expiratory volume (FEV_1), is reduced. Another measured value is the forced vital capacity (FVC), which is used in combination with FEV_1 to determine airflow obstruction and hence diagnosis of COPD.

The values for both FEV_1 and FVC must be compared with normal values, which depend on an individual's age, height, and sex. Tables of normal values are published and for patients in the UK certain European tables are usually used.

Airflow obstruction is confirmed when the FEV_1 < 80% of predicted and the FEV_1/FVC ratio is < 0.7.

Diagnosis: Infective exacerbation of his COPD based on blood results and symptoms.

Plan: Admit.

Commence:

- intravenous amoxicillin
- salbutamol and ipratropium bromide puffer via spacer
- oxygen therapy
- oral steroid-prednisolone.

Nebulisers used to be the preferred method of administering drugs like salbutamol and ipratropium in urgent cases such as this. A nebulised drug is delivered using a nebuliser, which is a device used to reduce or convert a solution of medicine into an aerosol (or fine cloudlike particles) for inhalation. It is extremely useful in delivering medication to deeper parts of the respiratory tract. However, there is increasing evidence that metered dose inhalers (MDIs) used with a spacer are just as effective, but at much reduced cost.

Exploring Ian's condition

The doctor explains that Ian has an infective exacerbation of his COPD, i.e. that the exacerbation is because of Ian having a respiratory tract infection.

The doctor explains to Ian's family that he will need to continue the bronchodilator therapy, but using a spacer to give higher doses of the drugs. He will also have intravenous antibiotics and a course of oral steroids.

1) What is COPD? What are the two subdivisions of COPD?

In your answer identify which parts of the respiratory tract are affected in each subdivision.

----

2) In emphysema, adjacent alveoli are known to become indistinguishable from each other because of the loss of alveolar walls. What physiological airway function is lost due to this (see page 11.2)?

Hint: Consider the functions of alveoli in breathing.

----

3) What is the main cause of COPD and what does it result in?

----

4) Explain what describing COPD as being irreversible and asthma being reversible means.

5) List the main types of bronchodilators used in obstructive airway disease.

6) Salbutamol is one of the most common bronchodilators used. What type of receptor does it act on? Where are these receptors located? Which neurotransmitter/hormone(s) usually acts on these receptors?

7a) What is the final effect of stimulation of β_2-adrenoceptors? What are the events in the smooth muscle cell that produce this effect?

7b) Tremor is one of the main side effects of the β_2-adrenoceptors. Explain pharmacologically why this occurs.

8) What is the difference between adrenaline (epinephrine) and salbutamol that causes the latter to be used in asthma treatment and the former to be used in allergic and anaphylaxis reactions?

The ward pharmacist notes that Ian is prescribed two inhaled anticholinergic bronchodilators; ipratropium bromide and tiotropium. He queries using both simultaneously and explains to the junior doctor that Ipratropium should be discontinued when Tiotropium is commenced. The doctor confirms with the registrar and the Ipratropium is discontinued.

Anticholinergic bronchodilators have more significant effects in COPD than asthma and are commonly used. Ipratropium is short acting and non-selective on muscarinic receptors whilst Tiotropium is more selective and longer acting, offering the advantage of once daily administration. Although inhaled, anticholinergics have a slower onset of bronchodilatation than the β2-agonists, they have a more sustained effect.

9a) What type of receptors does ipratropium act on? Why are these receptors termed as they are?

9b) What are the subtypes of receptor that are blocked by ipratropium bromide, where are they located, and what is the significance of these effects on patients with COPD like Ian?

9c) What are the side effects of anticholinergic agents?

Another group of drugs that can be used in COPD are steroids. **Oral steroids**, like prednisolone, are used for acute exacerbations. **Inhaled steroids** have a role in moderate to severe COPD, where they are recommended to be initiated and followed up but to be discontinued if no response is seen in 4 weeks.

The role of inhaled steroids in COPD is not as clear as in asthma treatment, even though many patients with COPD are on them. Inhaled steroids are not licensed to be used alone in COPD.

10a) If Ian is to be started on an inhaled steroid, what inhaler would be suggested, with consideration to the above information?

10b) Explain why corticosteroids appear to be less effective in COPD compared to asthma.

On day 2 after admission Ian showed improvement and his antibiotics were changed to oral form.

On day 4 after admission it was decided that he should be discharged.

Discharge plan:

Complete course of oral antibiotics.

Complete course of oral steroid prednisolone.

Continue on oxygen therapy.

To continue with inhalers via spacer, these include salbutamol, and tiotropium.

Seretide (compound preparation of fluticasone and salmeterol, see page 9.3) was initiated, benefit will be assessed after 4 weeks by GP and if no improvement will be discontinued. The pharmacist advises that a seretide accuhaler should be used instead of the metered dose inhaler because the metered dose inhaler is a lot more expensive. He counsels Ian on how to use the Accuhaler properly.

CLINICAL CLERKING FOR CHRIS

As Ian was leaving the hospital accompanied by his daughter Rose, they meet one of Rose's colleagues, called Chris, who works with her in the local nursery. Chris has asthma. She was experiencing exacerbation (worsening symptoms) of her asthma and therefore was being admitted to the respiratory ward. Rose could see that Chris was not well; she had a mask around her nose and mouth, which she realized later was high-flow oxygen. She remembered that Chris had complained of a wheeze, which she thought was due to a chest infection.

To wheeze means to breathe hard, with an audible piping or whistling sound.

History of Chris' medical complaint

Chris is a 32-year-old mother of two small children who works as a part-time assistant at the local nursery with Rose.

She lives with her husband and children, who got a new pet cat last week. Chris has been complaining of a wheeze over the last few days.

She has had asthma for few years. She has mostly had no serious problems with asthma as she uses her inhalers regularly. She realizes that asthma can be a very serious condition and if uncontrolled can to lead to life-threatening acute asthma attacks.

She was brought into A&E by her husband as she became very breathless over the last few hours; she was also confused and disorientated.

Diagnosis: Acute exacerbation of asthma due to allergen.

Plan: Admit

High flow oxygen therapy

Nebulised salbutamol

Oral prednisolone

> Once her breathing was stabilized Chris was transferred to the respiratory ward to continue her therapy.

DH:

Salbutamol one to two puffs three to four times a day, when required.

Salmeterol two puffs twice a day

Beclometasone two puffs twice a day, regularly.

Volumatic device (also known as a spacer device, see page 9.8)

> A volumatic is a clear plastic chamber. The patient attaches their puffer to one end and puffs the required doses into the chamber. The patient then breathes in the dose.

> Drug allergy: Aspirin worsens asthma (reminder: not all asthmatic patients are sensitive to aspirin, see page 9.6).

> Asthma is defined as 'A chronic inflammatory disorder of the airways ... in susceptible individuals, inflammatory symptoms are usually associated with widespread but variable airflow obstruction and an increase in airway response to a variety of stimuli. Obstruction is often reversible, either spontaneously or with treatment.'

> In asthma there are two main patterns: atopic and non-atopic. Other patterns of asthma include occupational asthma and drug-induced asthma.

> Useful definitions: Atopy is a form of allergy in which there is a hereditary tendency to develop hypersensitivity reactions. Atopens are allergens.

11) In the table below list the differences between atopic and non-atopic asthma as you would predict the presentation from the above definition and from your reference sources.

	Atopic asthma	Non-atopic asthma
Age of onset		
Family history		
IgE type I hypersensitivity reaction is involved		

12a) Chris had very well controlled asthma. What was likely to be the triggering factor for her asthma attack?

12b) List five other typical triggering stimuli for asthma.

_____

_____

13) The flow chart below represents the process of asthma symptoms. Discuss and complete the flow chart in your groups using the reference sources and your understanding of asthma processes (refer to main text to complete the flow chart).

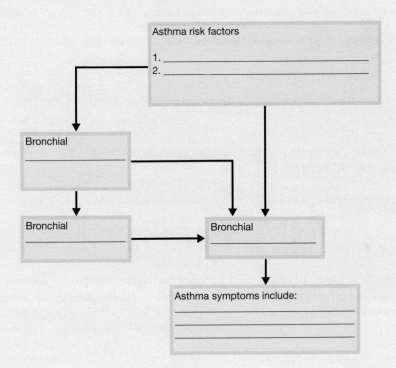

Chris is thought to have an exacerbation of her asthma due to hyper-responsiveness to the fur of their new cat Felix! This is because her asthma was well controlled until the cat was brought to the house, i.e. her asthma was controlled until that point. This type of asthma is commonly known as allergic asthma.

In allergic asthma, those who suffer from it undergo an inflammatory reaction, known as a type I hypersensitivity reaction. The effects of this reaction can be localized. i.e. in the bronchial tree (asthma) or in the nose (hay fever).

Certain inflammatory cells and chemical mediators are responsible for this type of reaction.

14) What are the names of the three immune mediator cells directly involved in this type of immune reaction (see Box 9.2).

_____

_____

_____

In an acute asthma attack, Chris or any sufferer would undergo two phases: an immediate phase and a late phase.

Immediate phase of asthma attack is dominated by bronchospasm.

Late phase is dominated by airway inflammation and airway hyper-reactivity, which further aggravate bronchospasm, wheezing, and cough.

The acute phase occurs as a result of the priming reaction that took place on first exposure to the allergen. It involves the release of chemical mediators by mast cells and eosinophils. Once the individual is re-exposed to the allergen, this substance interacts with mast cell-fixed IgE and causes release of substances known as spasmogens.

A spasmogen is defined as a substance that causes contraction of the smooth muscle.

15a) Name the main spasmogens released by the mast cells and state their effect on a patient like Chris.

....

....

....

15b) Antihistamines (histamine (H_1) receptor antagonists) are not used in the treatment of asthma to reduce bronchospasm. Why is this?

....

....

....

16) Prostaglandins and leukotrienes are mediators of inflammation involved in asthma. Complete the diagram below, which indicates the action of the mediators in inflammation to explain why aspirin can worsen asthma in Chris's case.

....

....

....

As mentioned above, the symptoms of asthma exist in two phases, leading to two main objectives in treating asthma. These include:

- relieving the bronchospasm or problems in breathing
- reducing inflammation, especially in late phase of asthma, to prevent worsening and future attacks.

As a result of this classification anti-asthma drugs are classed as *relievers* and *preventers*.

17) Which of Chris's inhalers is the *preventer* inhaler? Describe the mechanism of action of this inhaler that supports its usage in asthma treatment and give another example of a similar inhaler.

....

....

....

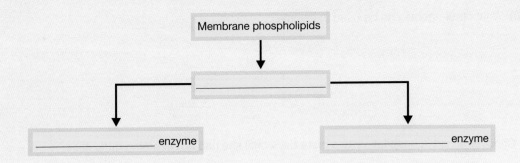

Chris was also initiated on a course of prednisolone. The doctor explained to Chris that prednisolone is similar to the beclometasone used in her inhalers, i.e. it is a corticosteroid. It is given at high doses in acute exacerbations. High doses are needed to suppress the inflammatory reaction seen in the acute exacerbation of asthma.

18) Can a corticosteroid like prednisolone be used on its own to treat asthma exacerbation? Explain your answer.

_____

_____

_____

19a) Why should salbutamol be used when required, whilst beclometasone should be used regularly?

_____

_____

_____

_____

The pharmacist advises that a combination inhaler (e.g. seretide or symbicort) containing both a steroid and a long acting beta agonist could improve adherence by simplifying chris regimen. He informs the junior doctor that symbicort SMART (Symbicort Maintenance and Relieves Therapy) protocol, which contains the steroid called budesonide and beta agonist called Eformoterol can be used as both a reliever and preventer. This would mean using a single inhaler instead of three in select patients with asthma.

19b) Explain why it is possible to use symbicort. When required.

_____

_____

_____

20) What other agents can be used in asthma?

Chris remained in hospital for two more days until she had no breathing difficulties.

On day 3 of admission she was discharged on the following:

- usual inhalers (no changes)
- 30 mg of oral prednisolone for four more days.

21) How do prednisone and predisolone relate to each other?

22) What are the dangers of abruptly stopping an oral corticosteroid? Does this matter in this case and why?

"Chris is seen by her respiratory consultant in the asthma clinic, four weeks after her discharge. During the consultation, the consultant decides to put Chris on the Symbicort SMART regime. He explains to Chris that SMART stands for Symbicort Maintenance and Reliever Therapy meaning Chris would henceforth need just one single inhaler; Symbicort. She should use one puff of the Symbicort when required as a reliever and one puff regularly twice a day as a preventer. He gives her a prescription to collect a Symbicort inhaler from the pharmacy and discard all her old three inhalers. He makes an appointment to review Chris three months later. When Chris collects her inhaler from the hospital pharmacy, the pharmacy technician counsels her on how to use the Symbicort turbohaler properly (Chris has always used a metered dose inhaler in the past).

Chris' children are very happy to have her healthy again, but they are disappointed that they have had to find a new home for Felix! Felix had to leave as he was the cause of the episode of asthma attack that their mum Chris experienced."

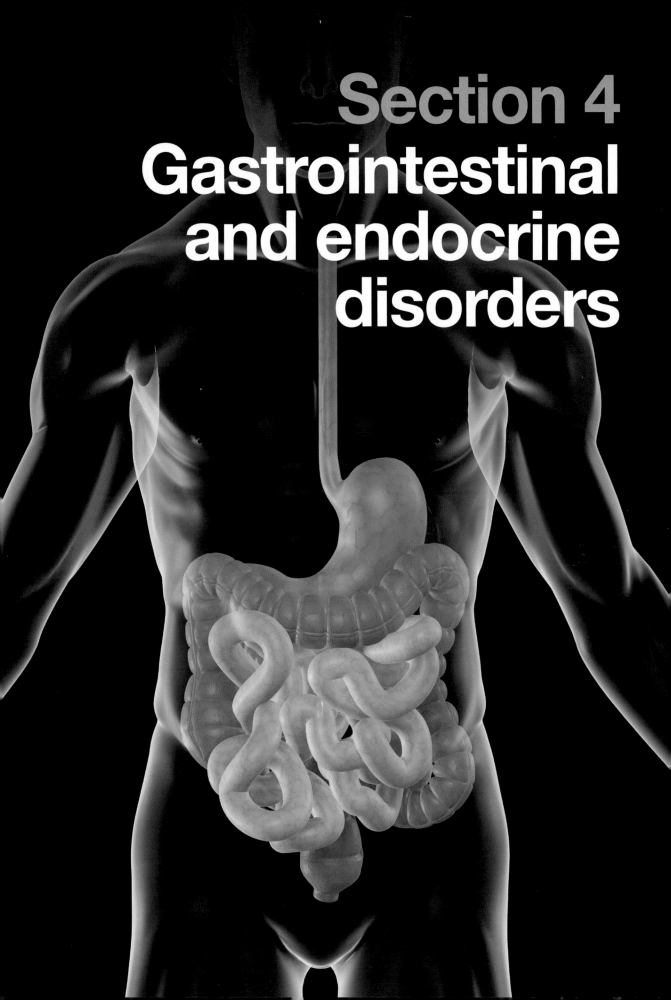

Section 4

Gastrointestinal and endocrine disorders

While the lungs provide us with life-giving oxygen, the other two essentials for life—food and water—come to us via the gastrointestinal (GI) tract. In addition to allowing the body to digest and absorb important nutrients, the GI tract plays a pivotal role in medical treatment as the site where most medicines are administered and absorbed. The other important role of the GI tract is in the elimination of the waste products of digestion and absorption.

As we will see later, an important part of the GI tract is the endocrine system. To function normally the various parts and organs of the body must be able to effectively exchange information with each other. They do this to allow the body to respond and adapt to changes within the body. Two systems are responsible for this: the nervous system, which allows rapid communication and produces a quick response, and the endocrine (or hormonal) system, which produces widespread and more sustained responses.

This section will focus on important GI disorders, including peptic ulcers, gastro-oesophageal reflux disease, nausea and vomiting, diarrhoea, constipation, and irritable bowel syndrome. We will also look at a number of endocrine disorders, including diabetes, obesity, and thyroid disease. Although not a disorder, we will also look at the endocrine system and how we manipulate this system to prevent conception. Before we look at these, we will review the structures and function of the GI tract and the endocrine system.

S4.1 Structure and function of the GI tract

The GI tract is broadly divided into the lower and upper GI tract (Figure S4.1). The upper GI tract starts at the mouth, which connects to the oesophagus. The oesophagus conducts food and other substances from the mouth into the stomach, one of the major parts of the GI tract. The lower GI tract starts with duodenum, which is found at the outlet of the stomach. The duodenum feeds into the small intestine (also called the ileum), which then connects to the large intestine (also called the colon). The lower GI tract terminates at the rectum, where solid wastes are eliminated.

The GI tract uses a combination of motility and secretions to undertake the functions of digestion, absorption, and elimination. These are regulated by both the autonomic nervous system and hormones secreted by cells in and around the GI tract (endocrine system).

S4.1.1 Neural control of the GI tract

The GI tract is regulated by a vast system of nerves called the enteric nervous system, which controls motility, blood flow, and secretions. This nerve system contains over 100 million neurones, which is about the same number as found in the spinal cord, and because of the complex way it controls the GI tract it is referred to as the 'second brain'. The enteric nervous system comprises two major networks called the myenteric plexus and the submucosal plexus. The myenteric plexus is involved primarily with motility, while the submucosal plexus regulates blood flow and secretions. The enteric nervous system comprises both intrinsic and extrinsic components. The intrinsic system controls secretions and motility independent of the central nervous system, and the major neurotransmitters involved include acetycholine, serotonin (5-hydroxy tryptamine), nitric oxide, vasoactive intestinal polypeptide, and substance P. Extrinsic

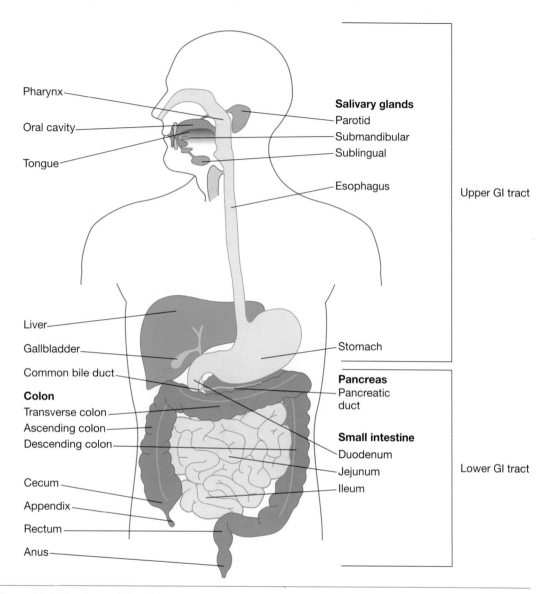

Figure S4.1 Structures of the GI tract.

control comes from the autonomic nervous system and involves both parasympathetic (cholinergic) and sympathetic (adrenergic) neurones. The effects of these are described in Table S4.1.

Table S4.1 Effects of the sympathetic and parasympathetic nervous system on the GI tract

	Parasympathetic	Sympathetic
Salivary glands	Increased secretion (thin/watery)	Increased secretion (thick)
Gut smooth muscle	Increased motility	Decreased motility
Gut sphincters	Dilatation	Contraction
Gut glands	Increased secretion	No effect
Gut blood flow	No effect	Decreased

S4.1.2 Hormonal controls in the GI tract

In addition to the neuronal control, gastric secretions and motility are also influenced by a number of hormones. These hormones can be broadly divided into endocrine and paracrine hormones. Endocrine hormones are secreted into the bloodstream and then have to travel to their site of action (Figure S4.2). Important endocrine hormones are gastrin, cholecystokinin (CCK), secretin, and gastric inhibitory peptide (GIP). Paracrine hormones are secreted by cells close to their site of action (Figure S4.2). Examples of these include somatostatin and histamine.

Gastrin is produced by gastrin cells (G-cells) in the pylorus (see Chapter 12, Figure 12.2) of the stomach. It is released in response to the presence of digested protein in the stomach, distension of the stomach, and by gastrin-releasing-peptide, which is released under the influence of cholinergic vagal nerve fibres. Gastrin release is

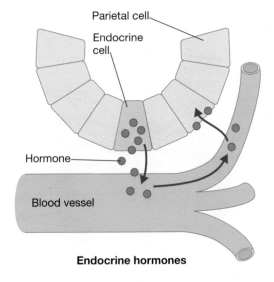

Endocrine hormones

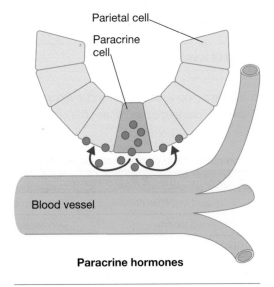

Paracrine hormones

Figure S4.2 Endocrine and paracrine hormonal transmission.

inhibited by somatostatin (see later). The effect of the gastrin is to increase acid secretion and promote the growth of the gastric and intestinal mucosa.

Cholecystokinin and secretin are released in response to chyme in the ileum. Chyme is a mixture of partially digested proteins and fat, and acid, which forms in the stomach and is passed to the intestines for absorption of the nutrients. Cholecystokinin stimulates the production and release of bile from the gallbladder (needed for fat absorption) and the production and release of alkaline fluid from the pancreas. It also reduces gut motility, inhibits gastrin secretion, and inhibits stomach emptying. Secretin has similar effects to CCK on the pancreas and gastrin secretion.

Gastric inhibitory peptide is released by K-cells in the intestine in response to the presence of glucose, fatty acids, and amino acids in the upper small intestine. The effects of GIP are to increase insulin release (hence its other name, glucose-dependent insulinotropic peptide) and inhibit gastric acid secretion.

Somatostatin is released by D-cells in response to raised acid levels in the stomach. It inhibits acid secretion and the release of gastrin. Histamine is released by enterochromaffin-like cells, which are mast-cell-like histamine-releasing cells located near the parietal cells. Both acetylcholine and gastrin promote the release of histamine, which attaches to histamine receptors on parietal cells, producing increased acid secretion. The effects of the various gastric hormones are outlined in Table S4.2.

Thus, the digestion and absorption in the GI tract is coordinated using a balance of the neuronal and hormonal systems. For example, when you smell and see food the parasympathetic nervous system, through the vagal nerves, causes stimulation of the parietal (acid-producing cells, see Chapter 12, Box 12.1) of the stomach and begins to increases the levels of acid in the stomach in anticipation of food. Once

Table S4.2 Effects of gastrointestinal hormones

	Acid and pepsinogen secretion	Pancreas	Gallbladder and bile	Gastric motility and emptying	Other effects
Gastrin	+				Stimulates mucosal growth
Histamine	+				
Somatostatin	−				
Gastrin-releasing peptide	+				
Cholecystokinin	−	+	+	−	Contracts pyloric sphincter
Secretin	−	+		−	
Gastric inhibitory peptide	−				Stimulates insulin release
Motilin				+	
Pancreatic polypeptide		−			

+ = promotes/increases; − = inhibits/reduces.

you swallow the food, the stretching of the stomach wall produces further release of gastrin from G-cells, resulting in more acid being released. Once the partially digested food (chyme) enters the ileum it causes release of CCK, which stops the acid production (it isn't needed anymore because the food has moved on into the intestine) and starts to stimulate the pancreas and gallbladder to begin the process of absorption, as well as 'switching off' the vagal stimulation, which causes the pyloric sphincter (see Chapter 12, Figure 12.1) to close to prevent more chyme entering the intestines.

S4.2 Structure and function of the endocrine system

The key structures involved in the endocrine system are the hypothalamus, pituitary gland, thyroid gland, adrenal gland, pancreas, and gonads (ovaries and testes). At the centre is the hypothalamus, which is located at the base of the brain. Being located within the central nervous system, the hypothalamus provides the essential link between the nervous and the endocrine systems, and it receives input from both the internal and external environments. The hypothalamus produces a range of hormones, most of which promote or inhibit the release of hormones from the anterior pituitary gland (see Box S4.1). The pituitary gland is a marble-sized gland that is connected to the hypothalamus by both a series of blood vessels and by a group of nerves called the hypothalamohypohyseal tract. It is divided into the anterior and posterior region, with the anterior region accounting for most of the gland. The posterior region secretes two hormones: antidiuretic hormone (also called arginine vasopressin) and oxytocin. Antidiuretic hormone is involved in controlling the osmolality (a measure of the concentration of substances such as sodium, chloride, potassium, and other ions) of the blood by changing the permeability of the renal collecting ducts. It increases the permeability of the ducts, leading to increased water reabsorption and urine that is more concentrated. Oxytocin is involved in the contraction of the uterus and in ejecting milk in lactating women.

The hormones of the anterior pituitary are the most significant in controlling bodily functions. A range of hormones that act on other organs and glands, including the adrenal gland, thyroid gland, gonads (testes in men and ovaries in women), liver, bones, and muscles are secreted (see Box S4.1). The most abundant of these hormones is growth hormone (GH), which affects the body's growth and development. GH promotes the lengthening of bones, growth of organs, development of the reproductive organs, and the development of adipose and connective tissues, endocrine glands, and muscles. It therefore plays a pivotal role in childhood and declines after puberty.

Thyroid stimulating hormone is involved in metabolic processes and is discussed in more detail in Chapter 15, along with luteinizing hormone and follicle-stimulating hormone, which are discussed in the context of contraception. Adrenocorticotrophic hormone is responsible for the production of steroids involved with protecting the body from various stresses, including surgery, trauma, and severe infections, and is discussed in more detail in Chapter 9. Prolactin is a hormone associated with lactation. During breastfeeding the action of the baby suckling causes the release of prolactin,

Box S4.1
Major elements of the endocrine system

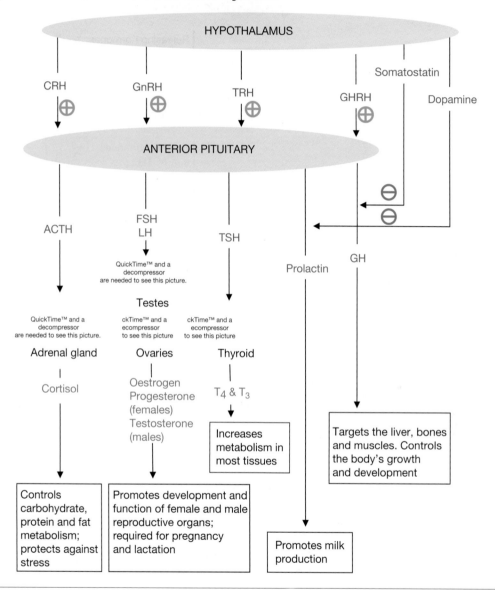

Figure a

CRH, Cortotophin-releasing hormone; GnRH, gonadotropin-releasing hormone; TRH, thyrotropin-releasing hormone; GHRH, growth hormone-releasing hormone; ACTH, adrenocorticotropic hormone; MSH, melanocyte-stimulating hormone; FSH, follicle-stimulating hormone; LH, leutenizing hormone; TSH, thyroid-stimulating hormone; GH, growth hormone; T_4, tetraiodothyronine (thyroxine); T_3, triiodothyronine; $\ominus$, inhibits release; $\oplus$, promotes release.

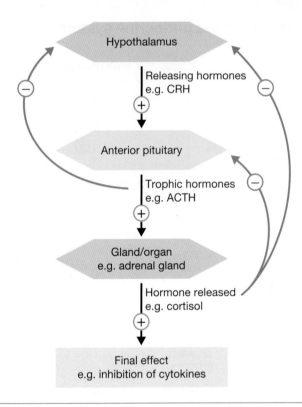

Figure S4.3 Feedback loops in the endocrine system. CRH, corticotropin-releasing hormone; ACTH, adrenocorticotropic hormone; ⊖, inhibits; ⊕, increases/enhances.

which stimulates the mammary glands to produce milk. During pregnancy prolactin levels also rise, resulting in enlargement of the breasts and the production of milk. However, during pregnancy, the high levels of progesterone stop the milk from being ejected; the levels of progesterone drop after birth, thus allowing breastfeeding to start.

The pancreas is an important gland that is not under the influence of hormones from the pituitary. It has both exocrine functions (excreting enzymes into the gut lumen to help digest food, see Chapter 12), and endocrine functions (producing the hormones insulin and glucagon, see Chapter 14).

S4.2.1 Control of hormone secretion

The release of most hormones in the endocrine system is controlled by a series of feedback loops. These feedback circuits generally have a negative effect (i.e. reduce further excretion as levels rise) and can occur at a number of levels (see Figure S4.3). This constant feedback ensures that hormone levels are maintained within normal ranges, and derangement of this system can lead to pathological states such as thyroid disease (see Chapter 15).

S4.2.2 Mechanism of action of hormones

The mechanism of action of various hormones is determined largely by their general molecular structure. Broadly speaking hormones can be divided into lipid-soluble and water-soluble hormones. Examples of lipid-soluble hormones include steroids (e.g. cortisol) and thyroxine. Water-soluble hormones include proteins and polypeptides comprising chains of amino acids, insulin, growth hormone, and prolactin. A list of the different types of hormones and their sources is found in Table S4.3. The fat-soluble hormones are capable of entering the cell and produce their effect, in part, by attaching to receptors within the nucleus of the cell, resulting in changes to gene transcription. Water-soluble hormones must attach to receptors (G-protein coupled receptors) on the surface of cells, and many produce effects through second messengers such as altering cyclic AMP, cyclic GMP, or calcium levels.

Table S4.3 Source and main actions of common water-soluble and lipid-soluble hormones

Hormone	Source	Main action	Secondary messenger
Water-soluble hormones			
Adrenocorticotrophic hormone	Anterior pituitary	Increase steroid production from adrenal gland	cAMP
Follicle stimulating hormone	Anterior pituitary	Stimulate follicle development in women and sperm production in men	cAMP
Growth hormone	Anterior pituitary	Promote body growth and development	JAK-STAT
Luteinizing hormone	Anterior pituitary	Stimulates production of sex hormones in women and production of testosterone in men	cAMP
Prolactin	Anterior pituitary	Controls milk production	JAK-STAT
Thyroid stimulating hormone	Anterior pituitary	Stimulates release of thyroid hormone	cAMP
Somatostatin	Hypothalamus	Inhibits release of GH from the anterior pituitary	cAMP
Thyrotropin releasing hormone	Hypothalamus	Promotes release of TSH from the anterior pituitary	cAMP
Glucagon	Pancreas	Increases blood sugar levels	cAMP
Insulin	Pancreas	Decreases blood sugar levels	Tyrosine kinase
Antidiuretic hormone	Posterior pituitary	Controls water and electrolyte balance	$InsP_3$ and DAG
Oxytocin	Posterior pituitary	Promotes uterine contraction and milk ejection	$InsP_3$ and DAG
Lipid-soluble hormones			
Cortisol	Adrenal gland	Controls protein, carbohydrate and lipid metabolism; protects body from stresses	N/A
Oestrogen	Ovaries	Develops female reproductive organs	N/A
Progesterone	Ovaries	Prepares uterus for pregnancy and mammary glands for lactation	N/A
Testosterone	Testes	Develops the male reproductive organs	N/A
Thyroxine	Thyroid	Controls metabolic function in cells	N/A

GH, growth hormone; TSH, thyroid stimulating hormone; cAMP, cyclic AMP; JAK, Janus family of tyrosine kinases; STAT, signal transducers and activators of transcription; InsP3, inositol triphosphate; DAG, diacylglycerol.

Chapter 12
Upper gastrointestinal tract disorders

Everybody has experiences of upset stomach, indigestion, and nausea. These problems can have obvious physical causes, such as infections, inappropriate diet, or a chronic tendency for excess acid secretions (see below). But what about someone who becomes very stressed studying for exams, aware that time is passing away with little progress despite trying to work long hours, the first exam is getting closer, not everyone passes ... and just when things couldn't seem much worse along comes stomach-derived pain—indigestion, but more and worse. This person is in the common situation of a crossover of a psychological problem, stress, and a physical problem, which in our imaginary case is a real upper gastrointestinal (GI) tract disorder caused by stress. The physical problem in the stomach needs treatment to relieve symptoms now, but also to prevent the physical problem taking on a life of its own, so that it persists even when the stress goes away. Drugs can help enormously for both short- and long-term aspects of GI problems. In the Workbook at the end of this chapter we meet a doctor whose life and stress issues contribute to the persistence of severe GI medical problems. Unlike the anxiety of approaching exams, his stress has no obvious end. In this chapter we will examine the action of different drugs targeting the upper regions of the gut, and with this in mind begin to understand how to optimize the treatment of individual patients, providing a firm foundation for offering advice and counselling as appropriate.

12.1 The stomach

The stomach is a J-shaped, hollow structure surrounded by layers of muscle. It is divided into four regions (Figure 12.1):

- cardia
- fundus
- body (or corpus)
- pylorus (or antrum).

The cardia is where the oesophagus (esophagus in the USA) enters the stomach, and is the site of the lower oesophageal sphincter (LOS), which is a ring of muscle that closes to prevent the stomach contents entering the oesophagus. The LOS is important in the pathogenesis of one of the most common gastric disorders, gastro-oesophageal reflux disease (GORD, or GERD if you are American), as improper closing of this sphincter leads to acid entering the oesophagus, resulting in pain and damage to the mucosa. We will discover more about this later.

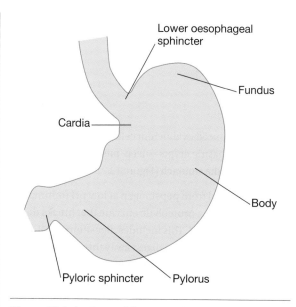

Figure 12.1 Anatomy of the stomach.

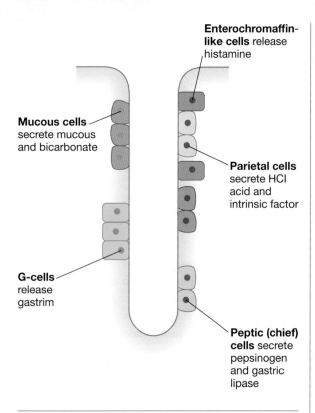

Enterochromaffin-like cells release histamine

Mucous cells secrete mucous and bicarbonate

Parietal cells secrete HCl acid and intrinsic factor

G-cells release gastrim

Peptic (chief) cells secrete pepsinogen and gastric lipase

Figure 12.2 Major cells of the stomach.

The fundus is a pouch-like region at the top of the stomach that allows gases that are formed as by-products of digestion to be stored. Both the fundus and the body of the stomach contain the important secretory cells that produce the substances that make up the gastric juices.

The gastric juices are composed of four main components:

- pepsin
- hydrochloric acid
- mucous
- intrinsic factor.

These are produced by different cells located along what are called the gastric crypts—deep 'pits' that project into the mucosa of the stomach (Figure 12.2).

Pepsin is formed from pepsinogen at low pH (optimally pH < 2). Pepsin is a proteolytic enzyme that breaks down protein for digestion. This includes digestion of cell walls, which means it can digest away the wall of the stomach, contributing to the pathologies described below. To prevent it digesting itself the stomach has protective mechanisms, as discussed below. Mucous and bicarbonate secreted from the mucous cells

produce a gel-like layer on the surface of the stomach. This serves to protect the lining of the stomach from being destroyed by the gastric juices. Importantly for us, the release of mucous and bicarbonate is stimulated by prostaglandins.

One of the most important ingredients of gastric juices, and the one targeted by most pharmacological treatments, is hydrochloric acid. This is produced by the parietal cell from water and carbon dioxide using carbonic anhydrase (Box 12.1). Hydrochloric acid has a number of roles in the stomach. First, it helps to break down proteins by changing their structures (referred to as denaturing). Second, it activates the conversion of pepsinogen to pepsin, which further breaks down protein. Third, it protects the body by destroying many bacteria and other micro-organisms (unfortunately one bacteria, *Helicobacter pylori*, thrives in the acid environment and is associated with peptic ulcers; this will be covered later).

A further point to note about parietal cells is that they produce intrinsic factor, which is essential for the absorption of vitamin B12.

12.1.1 Phases of gastric secretion

There are three main phases of the secretion of gastric juices: cephalic, gastric, and intestinal.

Cephalic phase

This phase occurs in response to senses (e.g. smelling, seeing, and tasting) and thoughts (anticipating eating) about food, and is referred to as a conditioned reflex. These sensations result in stimulation of the medulla oblongata in the brain stem, which in turn stimulates the myenteric plexus via the vagus. This causes release of acetylcholine, which stimulates the parietal cells to start to produce acid and the chief cells to produce pepsinogen. Vagal stimulation also causes the release of gastrin-releasing peptide, which stimulates the release of gastrin from G-cells. The gastrin then further stimulates the production of acid by parietal cells.

Gastric phase

This occurs once food has entered the stomach. The presence of food causes distension of the stomach, which causes further stimulation of the vagal nerves and the release of acetylcholine and gastrin, resulting in increased

Box 12.1

Influences on gastric acid secretion by parietal cells

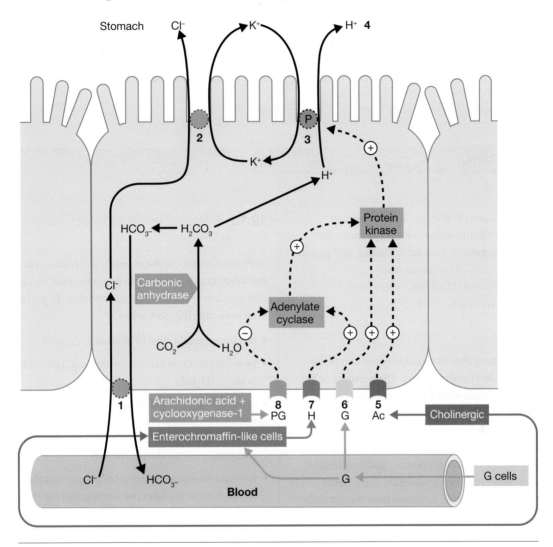

Figure a

1. Chloride and bicarbonate ions are exchanged via an antiport.

2. Chloride and potassium are released into the stomach lumen by a co-transporter.

3. The proton pump is H^+/K^+ ATPase. This 'pumps' H^+ out in exchange for K^+. This is the site of action for the proton pump inhibitors (e.g. omeprazole), which irreversibly block this pump.

4. H^+ in the stomach can be neutralized by combining with hydroxide (OH^-) or bicarbonate (HCO_3^-) ions. This is the site of action for simple antacids (e.g. sodium bicarbonate).

5. Acetycholine from cholinergic nerves stimulates muscarinic (M_2) receptors on the parietal cells, causing an increase in intracellular Ca^{++}, which stimulates the proton pump through protein kinase. Acetylcholine also increases the release of histamine from enterochromaffin-like cells. This is the site of action for anticholinergic agents (e.g. atropine), which reversibly block this receptor.

6. Gastrin released from endocrine cells (G-cells) attaches to gastrin receptors, causing an increase in intracellular Ca^{++}, which stimulates the proton pump through protein kinase. Gastrin also stimulates the release of histamine from enterochromaffin-like cells. There are no gastrin-inhibitors used therapeutically for gastrointestinal (GI) conditions.

acid and pepsinogen production. The presence of digested proteins in the stomach also stimulates the G-cells to release gastrin. Both acetylcholine and gastrin also cause the release of histamine from enterochromaffin-like (ECL) cells, which further stimulates acid secretion.

Intestinal phase

This occurs as partly digested food (chyme) leaves the stomach and enters the duodenum. The presence of fats and acid in the duodenum causes inhibition of the parasympathetic (cholinergic) nervous input to the stomach, causing a decrease in acid production and slowing of gastric motility. The arrival of chyme also causes the release of three hormones: gastric inhibitory peptide, secretin, and cholecystokinin. These cause further inhibition of gastric secretion from the stomach. Distension of the duodenum also causes releases of serotonin from ECL cells, which is involved in intestinal motility.

12.1.2 Protecting the stomach cells from self-digestion

The main function of the stomach is digestion. However, the substances it produces to digest the food we eat will also attack the cells that line the stomach. To prevent this from occurring the stomach:

- produces bicarbonate to neutralize the acid

- produces mucous to form an unstirred layer that protects the cells

- cells of the gastric mucosa produce prostaglandins E and I, through cyclooxygenase 1 (COX-1), which stimulate the production of bicarbonate and mucous, and inhibit the production of acid

- has tight junctions between cells to prevent the stomach contents from penetrating into the stomach wall

- has a high turnover of cells, and therefore continually replaces damaged cells to maintain a barrier.

12.2 Disorders of the upper gastrointestinal tract

Upper GI conditions are among the most prevalent illnesses in western countries. It is estimated that the lifetime prevalence of gastro-oesophageal reflux disease (GORD, or GERD in the USA) is 20%, and for peptic ulcers it is about 10%. However, the exact prevalence is uncertain as many people fail to seek medical help, particularly for GORD, relying on self-treatment with simple antacids they can buy in the supermarket.

Another common disorder is nausea and vomiting. Although not always caused by a disorder in the upper GI tract, it involves the stomach, as we will see later.

12.2.1 Gastro-oesophageal reflux disease

The two main symptoms of GORD are retrosternal pain (pain behind the sternum, about the middle of the chest, referred to as heartburn) and regurgitation (tasting the contents of the stomach at the back of the throat, sometimes called 'sour mouth'). Approximately one-third of patients may also suffer from dysphagia (difficulty in swallowing) because of strictures (narrowing of the oesophageus) or changes in the normal peristalsis in the oesophageus caused by chronic inflammation. Mild intermittent GORD is not a serious or life-threatening condition. However, chronic GORD can lead to a number of complications, including aspiration pneumonia (inhaling some of the stomach contents) and Barrett's oesophagus. Barrett's oesophagus results from continual damage to lower end of the oesophagus because of repeated exposure to the acid of the stomach. Initially inflammation of the oesophagus occurs. However, over time this causes changes in the structure of the cells lining the oesophagus, can result in strictures (permanent narrowing of the end of the oesophagus), and predisposes to oesophageal cancer. It is therefore important that people who get repeated GORD get medical advice and do not self-treat.

Initial treatment of chronic GORD is aimed at lifestyle changes. These include losing weight, eating smaller meals, not eating just before lying down, and reducing foods and medicines that reduce the lower oesophageal sphincter (LOS) tone. Being overweight and being pregnant increases the pressure inside the thoracic cavity, putting pressure on the stomach and making it easier for the stomach contents to be pushed up the oesophageus. As noted previously the LOS helps to keep the stomach contents from coming back up the oesophagus. Drugs that cause smooth muscle to relax, such as calcium channel blockers and nitrates (see Chapter 5), can exacerbate GORD. Foods such as peppermint and caraway (called carminatives, i.e. agents that help gas to escape from the stomach), and garlic and onions, also reduce LOS tone and can make GORD worse. Smoking, alcohol, and spicy or acidic foods (e.g. fruit juices) are also possible risk factors for GORD, and stopping or decreasing their consumption may help. Foods that slow the digestive process, such as fatty foods, may also worsen GORD. Although the evidence for these risk factors is poor, the lifestyle changes, such as reducing weight, stopping smoking, and reducing alcohol intake, have other health benefits.

> Our patient in Workbook 9, Dr Brown, has a number of risk factors for GORD, including being overweight (BMI of approximately 36), smoking, and consuming large amounts of alcohol.

Pharmacological management of GORD is aimed at relieving symptoms, increasing healing, and reducing complications of GORD (e.g. Barrett's oesophageus). The main approaches protect the lining of the oesophageus tract either directly (e.g. with alginates that form a protective coat) or indirectly (by reducing the acid levels in the stomach). Agents that increase the motility of the

GI tract (called prokinetic agents) have also been used. However, they have largely fallen out of favour because of their limited efficacy, and **cisapride**, the only agent with any evidence of efficacy, has been withdrawn from the market.

The main agents used are:

- simple antacids (with or without alginate)
- H_2-receptor antagonists
- proton pump inhibitors.

Antacids

Antacids work by neutralizing the acid in the stomach. One of the simplest antacids is sodium bicarbonate ($NaHCO_3$, baking soda). The chemistry behind the reaction in the stomach is as follows:

$$NaHCO_3 + HCl \rightarrow NaCl + H_2O + CO_2$$

While sodium bicarbonate is quick acting, unfortunately the reaction is short lasting and soon more acid is produced and the pH starts to drop again. The other problems with sodium bicarbonate come from the by-products of the neutralizing reaction. First, if you have ever added baking soda to vinegar (a weak acid) you will know that it fizzes as gas is produced by the reaction, namely carbon dioxide. This can cause bloating and distension of the stomach. Second, the sodium released as part of the reaction is absorbed and can cause problems in large amounts in people with hypertension.

Calcium carbonate is another simple antacid that, like sodium bicarbonate, is quick acting. However, it is less soluble than sodium bicarbonate and therefore longer lasting, giving 2–3 hours of relief compared to only about 30 minutes to 1 hour with sodium bicarbonate. Calcium carbonate has an added bonus in that it is a source of calcium, which is important, particularly as we get older and start to suffer from osteoporosis (thinning of the bones). However, this can also be a problem if you have kidney failure, as you are not able to excrete excess calcium. The main side effect people suffer from with calcium carbonate is constipation.

The most commonly used antacids are combinations of magnesium and aluminium hydroxide, $Mg(OH)_2$ and $Al(OH)_3$. These have the advantage over calcium carbonate and sodium bicarbonate that they do not produce gas as a side product, and are the longest lasting of the simple antacids, giving 4–6 hours of relief. However, to maximize the duration of effect they should be taken 2 hours after eating. They are well tolerated, but like calcium carbonate if you have severe kidney failure you may accumulate aluminium and magnesium. The main side effect of magnesium hydroxide is diarrhoea, while aluminium hydroxide causes constipation. The rationale is therefore that a combination of the two will cancel these side effects out. However, it is possible to get either diarrhoea or constipation with the combination products (more about constipation and diarrhoea in Chapter 13).

Aluminium-, magnesium-, and calcium-based antacids all have the potential to reduce the absorption of some drugs due to chelation (binding or complexation with other molecules). Important examples of drugs that may have reduced absorption with antacids include tetracyclines (e.g. doxycycline) and quinolone (e.g. ciprofloxacin) antibiotics. The antacid needs to be taken at least 2 hours before the interacting drug.

Another interaction occurs with antacids (and all other drugs that reduce acidity, including histamine-2 (H_2) receptor antagonists and proton pump inhibitors, see below) and with drugs that require an acidic environment to be absorbed. Examples include the azole antifungals, such as ketoconazole, and some antiretrovirals, such as azatanavir. Again, administering the antacid 2 hours before the drug will reduce this interaction.

Many simple antacids contain additional ingredients, such as simethicone and alginate. Simethicone alters the surface tension of gas bubbles in the stomach, causing them to join into larger bubbles, which are easier to get rid of (usually by burping). Alginate is extracted from seaweed and forms a thick viscous gum when exposed to gastric juices. It is added to antacids to produce a protective 'raft' that floats on the top of the gastric juices. When the stomach contents enter the oesophagus this 'raft' sticks to the inner surface first, thus protecting the oesophagus. Unfortunately, neither simethicone nor alginate has been proven convincingly to provide any advantage over antacids alone, but they produce no real adverse effects either.

Histamine-2 receptor antagonists

Histamine-2 receptor antagonists (known as H2RAs) were the first major advances on simple antacids. Histamine is a basic amine formed from histidine, and is stored in granules inside mast cells, basophils, and the enterochromaffin-like cells (ELC) of the stomach. There are three main types of histamine receptors in the body. The location and function of these receptors are described in Table 12.1.

Table 12.1 Location and function of histamine receptors

	Location	Function
H_1	Smooth muscle, CNS, and endothelium	Contraction of smooth muscle (e.g. bronchoconstriction), vasodilatation, and increased vascular permeability.
H_2	Parietal cells and heart	Increased acid production and increased heart rate
H_3	Presynaptic on neurones	Inhibits neurotransmitter release (noradrenaline, acetylcholine, and serotonin)

CNS, central nervous system.

The H_1 receptors are primarily involved in allergic and inflammatory reactions (for more details see Chapter 10) and in nausea caused by vestibular (inner ear) problems (see more on this under nausea and vomiting later). The role of the H_3 receptor is less clear. However, it may be an important target for sleep disorders and as an anti-inflammatory in the future.

The H_2 receptor on parietal cells is a G-protein coupled receptor, which when activated by histamine increases adenylyl cyclase, producing an increase in cyclic adenosine monophosphate (cAMP). The cAMP then stimulates the H^+/K^+ ATPase, or proton pump, causing the excretion of hydrogen ions into the stomach (see Box 12.1). Histamine is released by the ELCs under the influence of gastrin and acetylcholine (causing increased release), and somatostatin (inhibiting release).

Four H_2 receptor antagonists are used clinically:

- ranitidine
- famotidine
- cimetidine
- nizatidine.

They are all competitive inhibitors of the H2 receptor and only differ in their pharmacokinetics, with **cimetidine** given three to four times a day (although high single-daily doses can sometimes be used), and **ranitidine**, **famotidine**, and **nizatidine** being given once or twice a day. All inhibit acid secretion by at least 90%. They are generally very well tolerated with very few adverse effects. The most problematic H2RA is cimetidine, which has some affinity for androgen receptors and is occasionally associated with gynaecomastia (development of enlarged breasts) in men. Also, cimetidine is an inhibitor of cytochrome P450, which results in a number of potential interactions with drugs such as phenytoin, theophylline,

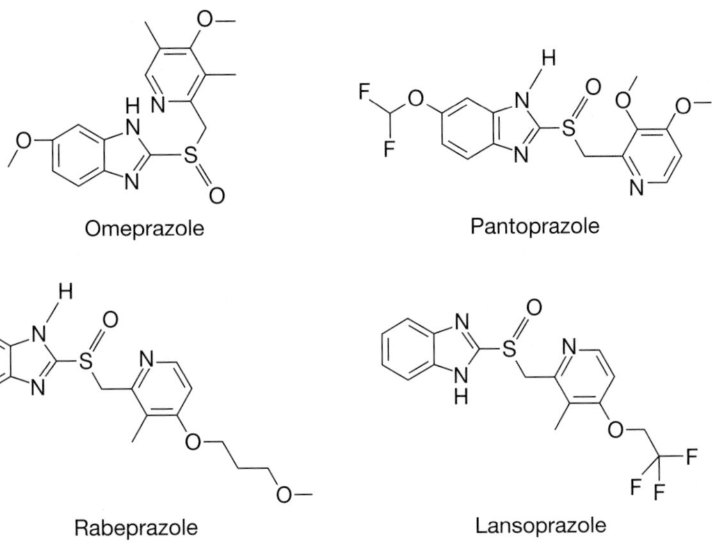

Figure 12.3 Structures of common proton pump inhibitors.

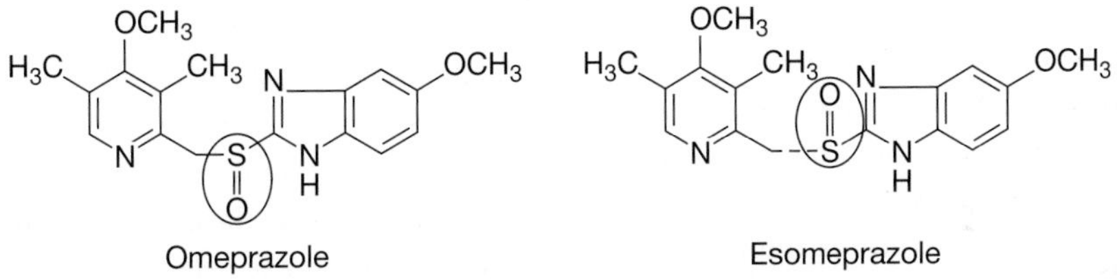

Figure 12.4 Structures of omeprazole and esomeprazole.

and warfarin. For these reasons cimetidine has largely fallen out of favour as a H_2 receptor antagonist.

While the H_2 receptor antagonists lack the chelation interactions of the large-cation antacids, they can reduce the absorption of drugs that require an acidic environment for absorption (e.g. ketoconazole). However, their longer duration of action (up to 12–24 hours) makes managing the interaction more difficult, therefore increased doses of the interacting drug may be required and clinical effect needs to be monitored.

Proton pump inhibitors

The proton pump inhibitors (PPIs) are the latest advance in the treatment of GORD (and peptic ulcers). Five PPIs are used:

- omeprazole
- esomeprazole
- pantoprazole
- rabeprazole
- lansoprazole.

The PPIs irreversibly bind to cysteine residues on the H^+/K^+ ATPase (proton pump) on the luminal side of the parietal cell (see Box 12.1). All, except esomeprazole, have slightly different structures compared to omeprazole (the first PPI) (Figure 12.3).

However, there are no clinical differences between PPIs and all can be given once a day because of the irreversibility of their binding with the proton pump. Esomeprazole is simply the S-isomer of omeprazole (Figure 12.4), therefore 10 mg of esomeprazole is equivalent to giving 20 mg of omeprazole (as each milligram of omeprazole contains 50% R-omeprazole and 50% S-omeprazole in a racemic mixture). The PPIs are more potent than the H_2 receptor antagonists at maintaining the pH above 4, probably because of the irreversible blocking of the proton pump, and that blocking of the histamine receptors still allows the stimulation of acid secretion through other routes (e.g. cholinergic). This gives them a clinical advantage over H2RAs.

All of the PPIs are degraded, ironically, in acidic environments, yet paradoxically require an acidic environment to be active. They are all given in enteric-coated oral formulations. This means that their absorption increases as they start to take effect, with maximal effect seen after 5 days of therapy. It also means that patients should not crush or chew their tablets or capsules, as this will destroy the enteric coat.

The PPIs are generally very well tolerated, with few side effects. They also lack significant interactions due to inhibiting metabolism or chelation. There is an interaction with clopidogrel, with the activity of clopidogrel reduced by PPIs; the combination should be used with caution. However, as noted previously, all drugs that raise pH can reduce the absorption of drugs that require acidic environments to be absorbed and, like the H2RAs, managing this with PPIs is more difficult because of their prolonged (>24 hours) duration of action. It must be remembered that the long-term effects of suppressing acid secretion to the extent that PPIs do is uncertain. Potential problems include increasing the risk of infections due to reducing the protective effect that stomach acid has on eliminating micro-organisms, and possible osteoporosis because of reduced calcium absorption (calcium requires an acidic environment to be absorbed). In addition, because of their powerful effect on acid secretion there is the possibility of masking the signs of gastric carcinoma. When used for GORD it is generally recommended that short courses should be tried (4 to 8 weeks) and if control is achieved then consider swapping to an H2RA or cutting back the PPI to 'when required'.

12.2.2 Peptic ulcer disease

Peptic ulcers are breaks in the protective mucosal lining of the stomach and duodenum. They can range from small erosions of only a few millimetres through to large ulcers of several centimetres, and can range from superficial (producing few symptoms) through to deep enough to erode through the wall of the stomach/ duodenum, leading to perforation and bleeding (this can be life threatening). Men were more likely to get ulcers than women were, but the gap is narrowing. Duodenal ulcers are more prevalent than gastric ulcers, with a lifetime prevalence of approximately 20% compared to 10%.

Helicobacter infections and ulcers

For many years it was thought that ulcers were caused only by increased acid in the stomach and compounded by factors such as stress and smoking. However, in the last couple of decades the role of *Helicobacter pylori* has become the focus of the prevention and treatment of peptic ulcers, particularly duodenal ulcers. *H. pylori* is present in 60–80% of patients who get gastric ulcers, and in most if not all patients who get duodenal ulcers. *H. pylori* is a helix-shaped gram negative, microaerophilic (meaning it requires oxygen, but at lower levels than that found in the atmosphere) bacteria that inhabits the stomach and duodenum. It damages the gastric epithelial cells by converting urea to ammonia using urease, and by excreting other substances such as protease and phospholipase. This damage results in chronic gastritis (inflammation of the stomach lining) and ulcers. The inflammation leads to increased activity of the G-cells that secrete gastrin, leading to an increase in acid production. Furthermore, the elevated gastrin levels cause an increase in the number of parietal cells, leading to more acid being secreted. The organism also appears to decrease D-cells, which secrete somatostatin; Somatostatin inhibits gastrin release and acid production.

Non-steroidal anti-inflammatory drugs and ulcers

Aspirin and other non-steroidal anti-inflammatory drugs (NSAIDs) have been implicated in the production of peptic ulcers for decades. Their contribution to mucosal damage comes from their effect on the production of protective prostaglandins, as well as local toxic effects. The NSAIDs inhibit the cyclooxygenase enzymes that convert arachidonic acid to prostaglandins and thromboxane (see Section 3 and Chapter 9 for more details). The cyclooxygenase enzyme exists in three isoforms, with cyclooxygenase 1 (COX-1) and cyclooxygenase 2 (COX-2) being the most important. COX-1 is referred to as constitutive enzyme. It is found on most cells all of the time, and is responsible for producing protective prostaglandins. In the GI tract prostaglandins have two effects. First, they inhibit acid production by stimulating receptors on parietal cells, which results in inhibition of adenylyl cyclase, a reduction in cAMP, and reduced proton pump activity (see Box 12.1). Secondly, prostaglandins stimulate mucous cells to secrete mucous and bicarbonate, which forms the lining on top of the surface of the mucosal cells in the GI tract to keep acid and other enzymes away from the cells.

Aspirin and most NSAIDs (e.g. ibuprofen, diclofenac, and naproxen) are inhibitors of both COX-1 and COX-2, and therefore have negative effects on the GI tract by inhibiting the protective effects of the prostaglandins produced by COX-1. Newer NSAIDs have been developed that are COX-2 selective, such as celecoxib, parecoxib, and meloxicam (in low doses). The COX-2 selectivity comes from having large side chains that cannot fit into the 'narrow' COX-1 receptor, but fit nicely into the larger COX-2 receptor (See Chapter 9, Figure 9.3 for details).

> Dr Brown in Workbook 9 was taking ibuprofen before presenting with a peptic ulcer.

It is claimed that the COX-2 selective agents produce less GI irritation, including ulceration. However, the absolute benefits are much greater for gastric upset than for ulceration, perforations, or bleeds. There have also been concerns raised about the negative cardiovascular effects of COX-2 selective agents (e.g. causing myocardial infarction) and this has resulted in one of these agents, rofecoxib, being withdrawn from the market around the world (see Chapter 9 for details).

In addition to their systemic effects on COX, the NSAIDs also have local irritant effects on the mucosa. They are weak organic acids and thus are non-ionized at low pH. This allows them to easily cross the lipid membranes of cells, where in the more neutral environment of the cell they become ionized and are trapped; this can lead to cellular damage.

The treatment of peptic ulcers is aimed at removing the cause, preventing further damage, and allowing the GI tract to heal. Acid reduction is important to allow healing and is usually achieved with PPIs (see above). Other treatments specific for peptic ulcers are aimed at eliminating *H. pylori* and agents that target the negative effect of NSAIDs on prostaglandin production.

H. pylori eradication

The significant role of *H. pylori* in duodenal ulcers has resulted in many guidelines recommending eradication therapy in all cases of duodenal ulcer. The role of *H. pylori* in gastric ulcers is less clear and some argue for a 'test and treat' approach, while other advocate for empirical

treatment in anyone who is suspected of a gastric ulcer. The presence of *H. pylori* can be detected by either non-invasive tests or endoscopy with biopsy. The least invasive tests are urea breath tests, which are based on the production of urease (an enzyme that breaks down urea into ammonia and bicarbonate, which is then expelled as carbon dioxide) by *H. pylori*. The patient is given radiolabelled urea (using ^{13}C or ^{14}C)—infected people with *H. pylori* then excrete radiolabelled CO_2 in their breath. The more invasive tests using gastroscopy are indicated where there is suspicion of more sinister pathologies such as gastric cancer.

Eradication therapy for *H. pylori* is a combination of acid suppression and antibiotics, and because the use of two antibiotics is recommended to improve eradication rates and reduce possible resistance, it is referred to as 'triple therapy'. A number of combinations have been recommended, including:

- PPI twice a day + amoxicillin 1 g twice daily + clarithromycin 500 mg twice a day for 7 days or
- PPI twice a day + clarithromycin 500 mg twice daily + metronidazole 400 mg twice daily for 7 days or
- PPI twice a day + amoxicillin 500 mg three times a day + metronidazole 400 mg three times a day for 14 days.

Selection of which 'triple therapy' is based on patient characteristics (e.g. allergies to penicillin), cost, local *H. pylori* resistance patterns, and duration of treatment (shorter treatments will improve compliance).

Efficacy rates are reasonably high (80–85%) for all triple-therapy combinations. If a patient does fail it may indicate bacterial resistance. Ideally, the organism should undergo sensitivity testing and another course of triple therapy, using different antibiotics, should be used. Quadruple therapy, using a combination of bismuth subcitrate (a cytoprotective agent we will discuss later), metronidazole, tetracycline (or doxycycline) plus a PPI has also been recommended. However, this combination is more complicated to give and has more side effects than the commonly used triple therapy regimens. An alternative is using the bismuth salt of ranitidine instead of a PPI and using another combination of antibiotics.

Misoprostol

Misoprostol is an analogue of prostaglandin E_1 (PGE_1), which can be given orally (Figure 12.5).

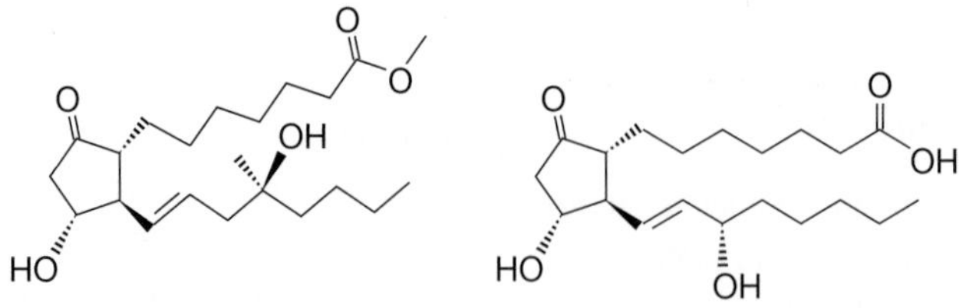

Figure 12.5 Structures of misoprostol and prostaglanin E$_1$.

It is used to reduce the effects of NSAIDs on gastric protection by attaching to the prostaglandin receptor on parietal cells (see Box 12.1), as well as increasing mucosal blood flow and stimulating the production of bicarbonate and mucous by mucous cells. However, the use of misoprostol is often limited by side effects, which include diarrhoea and abdominal pain. Misoprostol should also not be used in pregnancy as the effects of prostaglandins on the uterus can cause premature labour and abortions.

Other cytoprotective agents

A range of somewhat older cytoprotective (protecting the cells) agents are sometimes used. These include bismuth salts and sucralfate. Bismuth salts are given as a suspension of bismuth as the citrate salt (bismuth subcitrate). At neutral and alkaline pH the bismuth subcitrate remains suspended. However, in an acidic environment, like the stomach, the bismuth salt precipitates out, forming a protective coating on the top of the mucosa. Bismuth salts may have a number of other effects, including stimulating the production of prostaglandin E$_2$ (protective prostaglandin), neutralization of pepsin, and antibacterial properties against *H. pylori* by disruption of the bacterial coat and inhibiting adherence by *H. pylori* to the stomach wall.

Bismuth subcitrate can be given alone or in combination with H2RAs (particularly ranitidine). It is used as part of *H. pylori* eradication, but only when standard triple therapy has failed. It has a few unpleasant side effects, including turning the tongue and stools black. The black stools can be disturbing as this is also a possible sign of an upper GI bleed—called melena—and is something that people who have peptic ulcers are told to look for.

Our patient, Dr Brown, suffered from melena prior to presenting with a peptic ulcer—this should have been an early warning sign!

Sucralfate is a complex of aluminium hydroxide with sulphated sucrose (a type of sugar) and works in a similar way to bismuth subcitrate. The complex forms a protective coating in the stomach, which is selective for ulcer craters, because of bonds between the negatively charged molecules in the complex and the positively charged protein molecules of the mucosal lining. The formation of these bonds is pH dependent, and is reduced in pH greater than 4, therefore sucralfate is less effective for duodenal ulcers. Sucralfate is generally better tolerated than bismuth salts, with constipation and nausea the most common side effects. Because of the development of better agents, in particular the H2RAs and PPIs, these agents are considered second-, or more often third-line.

12.2.3 Nausea and vomiting

Nearly everyone suffers at least one bout of nausea, with or without vomiting, in his or her lifetime. The actual prevalence is not known because in most cases people do not seek care. However, certain conditions and medicines are associated with high rates of nausea and vomiting, such as some chemotherapy treatments. Further, nausea and vomiting, like pain, are considered one of the most distressing sensations that a person can suffer. Although nausea and vomiting are not always caused by disorders of the GI tract, the consequences of nausea and vomiting, particularly vomiting, are certainly felt in the upper GI tract.

Nausea and vomiting, like coughing (see Chapter 11) and diarrhoea (see Chapter 13), are often protective mechanisms. They can occur in response to the body sensing that something that has been swallowed is potentially harmful, and therefore the body is prompted to expel the potential toxin by vomiting. However, there are a number of other causes of nausea and vomiting. An outline of the neural and sensory inputs into producing nausea and vomiting is given in Box 12.2.

Box 12.2

Process involved in nausea and vomiting

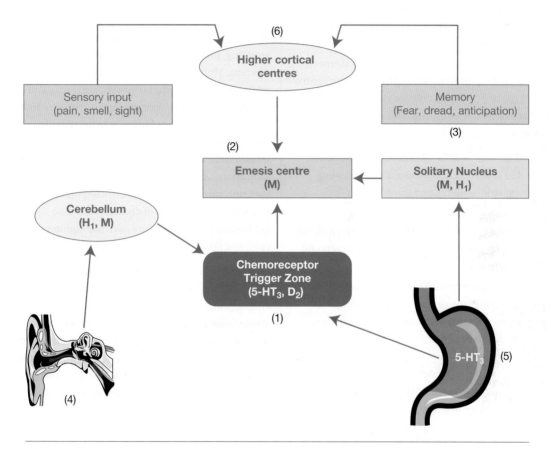

Figure b

1. The chemoreceptor trigger zone lies in the medulla and senses chemicals and toxins in the bloodstream. It also receives input from the stomach through 5-HT$_3$ released by enterochromaffin cells, and from the vestibular nuclei in the cerebellum. This is a site of action for the dopamine entagonists (e.g. metoclopramide) and the 5-HT$_3$ antagonists (e.g. ondansetron).

2. The emesis centre (also called the vomiting centre) coordinates neural output to produce nausea and vomiting. It receives input from the chemoreceptor trigger zone, the solitary nucleus, and from higher cortical centres. This is a site of action for the anticholinergic drugs (e.g. hyoscine).

3. The solitary nucleus is located along the medulla. It receives inputs from a variety of chemoreceptors and mechanoreceptors in the heart, lung, and gastrointestinal tract, and is involved in the gag reflex that results in vomiting. This is a site of action for the anticholinergic drugs (e.g. hyoscine) and the antihistamines (e.g. promethazine).

4. The labyrinth is a series of fluid-filled canals within the vestibular system that contributes to our sense of balance. Stimulus from this system, through the vestibular nuclei, can produce motion sickness. This is a site of action for anticholinergic agents (e.g. hyoscine) and antihistamines (e.g. dimenhydrinate).

5. Enterochromaffin cells in the gastrointestinal tract release serotonin in response to stimuli/damage such as after radiation or chemotherapy. This is a site of action for 5-HT$_3$ antagonists (e.g. ondansetron).

6. A number of emotional and sensory factors can stimulate nausea and vomiting, including seeing certain things (e.g. major trauma or other unpleasant sights), smelling certain smells (e.g. the smell of vomit!), or very strong pain.

M, muscarinic acetylcholine; H$_1$, histamine-1; D$_2$, dopamine-2; 5-HT$_3$, 5-hydroxytrptamine (serotonin).

The chemoreceptor trigger zone (CTZ) and the vomiting centre are crucial to producing nausea and vomiting. The CTZ is located outside the true blood–brain barrier and therefore is exposed to all chemicals, toxins, and drugs that circulate through the body. In addition, it receives input from visceral afferents from the GI tract. Stimulus of the CTZ through this mechanism can arise from distension of the stomach or irritation of the gastric mucosa. The vomiting centre (or emesis centre) is responsible for coordinating the events that can lead to vomiting. The stages are usually as follows:

- Feeling of nausea—a difficult to describe experience, but one that is extremely unpleasant. When feeling nauseous gastric motility often slows.

- Retching—also called dry heaving. When retching there is contraction of the abdominal muscles, often without actual vomiting. During this the antrum contracts and the pyloric sphincter closes.

- Vomiting—this is a series of coordinated events that lead to expulsion of the stomach contents (and sometimes the contents of the small intestine). First, there is a deep intake of breath, followed by closure of the glottis (where the vocal cords are located) to protect the airways, and the soft palate in the mouth rising to block of the nasal passages. Next, the diaphragm contracts to produce negative pressure in the abdomen, thus opening the lower oesophageal sphincter. Finally, there is strong contraction of the abdominal wall, squeezing on the stomach, causing the contents to be expelled through the mouth.

While occasional bouts of vomiting are not necessarily dangerous, it is exceptionally unpleasant. However, prolonged attacks of vomiting can lead to serious consequences such as dehydration, electrolyte disturbances, and occasionally tears to the oesophagus (called Mallory–Weiss tears). Dehydration and electrolyte changes can be particularly important in the very old, infants, and pregnant women.

The main neurotransmitters involved in nausea and vomiting are histamine, acetylcholine, 5-hydroxytryptamine (5-HT; serotonin), substance-P, and dopamine, and these are the targets of anti-emetic therapy. Opiate receptors are also implicated in nausea and vomiting. However, these are not major targets in the therapy of nausea and vomiting, but are probably the cause of nausea and vomiting associated with opiates.

Antihistamines

Antihistamines refer to antagonists at the H_1 histamine receptor (see above and Chapter 10), distinguishing them from the histamine H_2 antagonists described above. Only the older, first-generation, sedating antihistamines are used in the prevention or treatment of nausea and vomiting, primarily for the prophylaxis of motion sickness. Motion sickness is a disorder caused by a mismatch between what your eyes are seeing and what your inner ear thinks your position is. The labyrinth system in the ear sends impulses to the vomiting centre, with histamine and acetylcholine being the primary transmitters, hence the use of antihistamines for these indications. Among the antihistamines that are used are cyclizine, promethazine, and dimenhydrinate (the chlorotheophylline salt of diphenhydramine—an antihistamine used in many over-the-counter cough, cold, and flu medications).

Because the first-generation antihistamines cross the blood–brain barrier they produce central nervous system effects, primarily sedation. However, the older antihistamines such as promethazine and dimenhydrinate, have the advantage that they are safe to use in pregnancy, during which nausea and vomiting can be significant (particularly in the first trimester, when it is known as 'morning sickness'). For more details on antihistamines see Chapter 10.

Anticholinergics

Hyoscine hydrobromide (called scopolamine hydrobromide in the USA) is an alkaloid with anticholinergic effects closely related to atropine. It can be given orally or as a transdermal patch. It appears to be effective against most causes of nausea and vomiting, although like antihistamines it tends to be used mainly for motion sickness, where it may be more effective than antihistamines. Hyoscine also produces sedation, but to a lesser extent than antihistamines. However, it produces other anticholinergic side effects including dry mouth, blurred vision, and constipation.

Dopamine antagonists

Older antipsychotic agents, such as chlorpromazine, droperidol, and haloperidol, are used as anti-emetics for their dopamine antagonist activity (see Chapter 18). In addition, some possess antihistamine and anticholinergic activity, which may add to their effectiveness. The most popular of these is prochlorperazine, which is marketed primarily as an anti-emetic. However, these agents have a range of unpleasant side effects, including sedation and extrapyramidal side effects such as tardive dyskinesias (involuntary movements that can be seen after high and prolonged doses of dopamine antagonists and can be irreversible).

Metoclopramide is a commonly used dopamine antagonist related to the phenothiazine antipsychotics (although it is not used as an antipsychotic). In addition to its effect on the CTZ, metoclopramide has direct effects on the GI tract by releasing acetylcholine, resulting in increased peristalsis (called prokinetic properties), which adds to its role as an anti-emetic. Unfortunately, like the older antipsychotics, it can produce movement disorders, in particular torticollis (the head tilts to one side while the chin is elevated) and oculogyric crises (where the eyeballs roll upwards into the eye socket). These adverse effects seem to be more common in females and young adults.

Domperidone is another dopamine antagonist that is similar to metoclopramide, but does not pass through the blood–brain barrier. Thus, it has few central nervous system effects, including less sedation and less risk of movement disorders.

Selective 5-HT$_3$ receptor antagonists

The discovery of the selective 5-HT$_3$ receptor antagonists was one of the greatest breakthroughs in the management of nausea and vomiting caused by highly emetogenic chemotherapy drugs such as cisplatin, by radiotherapy for cancers, and post-operatively. They target the CTZ and have been shown to be superior to metoclopramide for the immediate emesis (first 24 hours) in patients

Table 12.2 5-HT receptor subtypes

5-HT	Receptor type and messengers	Location	Major effects/role
1 (A, B, D—? e, f)	GPCR—cAMP$\ominus$	CNS Vascular tissue	Anxiety Temperature regulation Vasoconstriction
2 (A, B, C)	GPCR—InsP$_3$/DAG$\oplus$	CNS Stomach Vascular smooth muscle Platelets Fundic smooth muscle Cardiac valves Choroid plexus	Smooth muscle contraction Platelet aggregation Increased vascular permeability Hormone release (e.g. ACTH) Hallucinations Contraction of gastric fundus Vasodilatation
3 (A, B, C)	Ligand-gated cation channel	Sensory neurones Peripheral autonomic neurones CNS	Gastric motility Intestinal secretions Anxiety Nausea/vomiting Memory
4	GPCR—cAMP$\oplus$	CNS Peripheral nerves	Modulates neurotransmitter release Gastric motility Cardiac contraction force Memory
5 (A, B)?	GPCR—cAMP$\oplus$?	CNS?	Acquisition of adaptive behaviour under stress?
6 ?	GPCR—cAMP$\oplus$?	CNS?	Control of central cholinergic function, e.g. Alzheimer's? Feeding-related behaviour?
7	GPCR—cAMP$\oplus$	Non-vascular smooth muscle CNS Vascular system	Vasodilatation Mood/affective disorders

GPCR, G-protein coupled receptor; cAMP, cyclic adenosine monophosphate; InsP3, inositol triphosphate; DAG, diacylglycerol; CNS, central nervous system; ACTH, adrenocorticotropic hormone;$\oplus$, increases;$\ominus$, reduces; those areas marked with ? are still under investigation and are uncertain at this stage.

receiving highly emetogenic chemotherapy; for less emetogenic chemotherapy, or for other causes of nausea and vomiting (except from radiotherapy) they are no better than simpler alternatives such as metoclopramide or prochlorperazine.

Over 90% of the 5-HT in the body is located in the ELCs in the gut. There are seven main groups of 5-HT receptors, although some have only recently been discovered and their roles are still to be established. With the exception of 5-HT_3, they are all G-protein coupled receptors (GPCR), using either cAMP, inositol triphosphate ($InsP_3$), or diacylglycerol (DAG) as second messengers to exert their effect. Some of these are further divided into subunits. For example, the 5-HT_2 receptor has three subunits: 5-HT_{2A}, 5-HT_{2B}, and 5-HT_{2C}. Further information on the 5-HT receptors is found in Table 12.2. The 5-HT_3 receptors are intrinsic ligand-gated channel receptors, and are similar to the nicotinic acetylcholine and gamma amino butyric acid ($GABA_A$) receptors. Activation of the receptors, found on

neurones, causes calcium influx and potassium efflux, and results in rapid depolarization. The major role of the 5-HT_3 receptors is in nausea and vomiting. However, they are also involved in gastric motility and secretions, anxiety, and memory, although use for the latter is in its early stages of investigation.

Four selective 5-HT_3 receptor antagonists are used in clinical practice: ondansetron (the first developed), granisetron, dolesetron, and tropisetron. They are all equally efficacious, with the only difference being that ondansetron has to be given two or three times a day, while the others are only given once a day.

The selective 5-HT_3 receptor antagonists are generally very well tolerated, with the main side effects being constipation, headache, and a rise in liver enzymes (transaminases). They do not produce the extrapyramidal effects seen with the antipsychotics and their derivatives, and they appear to be free of any clinically significant drug interaction.

SUMMARY OF DRUGS USED FOR GASTRIC ULCERS AND GASTRO-OESOPHAGEAL REFLUX DISEASE

Therapeutic class	Drugs	Mechanism of action	Clinical uses	Comments	Examples of adverse drug reactions
Antacids	Sodium bicarbonate Calcium carbonate Magnesium and aluminium hydroxide combinations	Neutralize acid in the stomach through chemical reaction (for sodium bicarbonate) $NaHCO_3 + HCl \rightarrow NaCl + H_2O + CO_2$	Dyspepsia	Relatively short-lasting effect Chelates with some drugs and reduces their absorption Sometimes contains simethicone/dimethicone	Bloating and distension Diarrhoea (magnesium) Constipation (aluminium)
H$_2$-receptor antagonists	Ranitidine Famotidine Cimetidine Nizatidine	Competitively inhibits H$_2$-receptor	Gastric and duodenal ulcer GORD Zollinger–Ellison syndrome *Helicobacter pylori* eradication	Could reduce absorption of drugs requiring acidic environment for absorption Cimetidine inhibits cytochrome P450, leading to interactions	Gastrointestinal Altered liver function test Headache Cimetidine: gynaecomastia
Proton pump inhibitors	Omeprazole Esomeprazole Pantoprazole Rabeprazole Lansoprazole	Irreversibly binds to cysteine residues on the proton pump (H$^+$/K$^+$ ATPase) and inhibits it	Gastric and duodenal ulcer GORD Zollinger–Ellison syndrome *H. pylori* eradication	Could reduce absorption of drugs requiring acidic environment for absorption	Gastrointestinal Headache Dizziness
Prostaglandin analogues	Misoprostol	1) Attaches to the prostaglandin receptor on parietal cells 2) Increases mucosal blood flow 3) Stimulates the production of bicarbonate and mucous by mucous cells	Gastric and duodenal ulcer	Contraindicated in pregnancy	Gastrointestinal Rashes Menorrhagia
Bismuth salts	Bismuth subcitrate	1) Precipitates out, forming a protective raft coating on the top of the mucosa 2) Stimulates the production of prostaglandin E$_2$ (protective prostaglandin) 3) Neutralizes pepsin	Gastric and duodenal ulcer *H. pylori* eradication	Usually reserved for second-line usage	Blackens tongue and stools
Sulphated aluminium hydroxide	Sucralfate	Precipitates out, forming a protective coating on the top of the mucosa	Gastric and duodenal ulcer	Not effective in duodenal ulcer	Constipation and nausea

Therapeutic class	Drugs	Mechanism of action	Clinical uses	Comments	Examples of adverse drug reactions
H. pylori eradication medication	PPI, H$_2$-receptor antagonists, Bismuth salts	See individual classes above	*H. pylori* eradication	1–2-week course of a combination of three of these	Diarrhoea, Nausea, Taste disturbances, Dizziness
	Antibacterial: amoxicillin, clarithromycin, metronidazole	See Chapter 21			

SUMMARY OF DRUGS USED FOR NAUSEA AND VOMITING

Therapeutic class	Drugs	Mechanism of action	Common clinical uses/comments	Comments	Common adverse drug reactions
Older antihistamines	Cyclizine, Promethazine, Dimenhydrinate	Inhibits histamine	See Chapter 10		
Anticholinergics	Hyoscine hydrobromide	Anticholinergics effects centrally and in periphery	Nausea and vomiting, Vertigo, Excessive secretions	Available as patch	Dry mouth, Blurred vision, Sedation
Dopamine antagonist	Older generation: chlorpromazine, droperidol, haloperidol	Inhibit dopamine receptors	Nausea and vomiting, Psychoses, Hiccup, Movement disorders	Some have anticholinergics and antihistamine effects	Sedation, Extrapyramidal side effects (see Chapter 17)
	Metoclopamide		Nausea and vomiting, Motility stimulant	Induces acetylcholine secretion, causing peristalsis and therefore used as pro-kinetic	
	Domperidone			Does not cross blood–brain barrier, so fewer CNS side effects	
Selective 5-HT$_3$ receptor antagonists	Ondansetron, Granisetron, Dolesetron, Tropisetron	Antagonists of 5-HT$_3$ receptor	Nausea, Vomiting, Motility stimulant	Superior to others for highly emetogenic chemotherapy/post surgery	Constipation, Headache, Rise in liver enzymes

GORD, gastro oesophageal reflux disease; PPI, proton pump inhibitor; CNS, central nervous system.

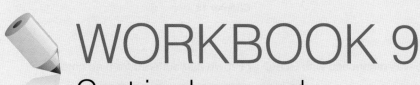

WORKBOOK 9
Gastric ulcers and gastro-oesophageal reflux disease

Dr Brown: a simplified case history

After a short stay in accident and emergency, Dr Carter Brown was being wheeled to the gastrointestinal ward at Glenfield Hospital, where he had been admitted.

He had been too unwell to protest when his mother had bundled him into the car and driven him to the hospital. He was uncomfortable with the idea of being a patient in that hospital because he had worked there in the past.

His mum had realized how pale he was when she had stopped by for a quick visit. He had recently been divorced and she had been concerned about him. He hadn't been looking after himself since his wife left. He was having far too many takeaways in her opinion. When she arrived on this occasion she had found him lying on the sofa and quite obviously in agony. Abdominal pain, he said. She had made him some chicken soup. This reduced the pain initially, but he had then thrown up. The coffee-ground colour of the vomit had alarmed them both. Being a doctor, this had made him realize that he was sicker than he had thought.

Luckily he had been attended to quite promptly because he had been recognized by the staff.

A table of clinical clerking abbreviations is given on page xi.

CLINICAL CLERKING FOR DR CARTER BROWN AT A&E DEPARTMENT

Age: 35 years

PC: Gnawing abdominal pain accompanied by coffee-ground vomit

> *Coffee-ground vomit: This means vomit is the colour of ground coffee and indicates the presence of blood that has coagulated in the gastric juices.*

HPC: Two-day history of intermittent stomach pains that had gradually become more severe. He had actually had similar, although not as severe, pain over the last 6 months. Initially he had used antacids bought from his chemist, then later on his GP had diagnosed gastro oesophageal reflux disease (GORD) and put him on medication, which had helped until this recent episode. Since yesterday, he had passed several loose stools that were dark in colour and smelt foul.

PMH:

• GORD diagnosed by GP

• Recent injury sustained in a domestic incident

This means that until he was diagnosed with GORD Dr Brown had suffered from no chronic medical condition.

DH:

1) Ranitidine for GORD prescribed by his GP

2) Ibuprofen (prescribed by GP for a recent injury sustained when an ex-girlfriend had hit him with a tennis racket)

3) Gaviscon: occasionally

4) No other regular medication

His GORD until recently was controlled by cimetidine and occasional doses of Gaviscon. Since he recently started taking ibuprofen for acute injury these two medications do not seem to control his symptoms anymore.

SH: 35-year-old medical doctor. Recently divorced, he lives alone. Smokes 20 cigarettes a day and drinks about 30 units of alcohol per week.

> *Smoking impairs ulcer healing and promotes ulcer recurrence. Alcohol and stress have been implicated to pre-dispose to peptic ulcer disease.*

O/E:

1) Pale, sweating and shocked

2) Blood pressure =115/60 mm Hg (120/90)

3) Pulse = 98 beats per minute

The diarrhoea and vomiting have led to significant loss of fluids, which has resulted in signs of shock (pale sweaty skin, low blood pressure, and a raised pulse).

4) Abdomen = tender

5) Rectal examination = melaena

> *Melaena: passage of black tarry stool, a result of haemorrhage (bleeding) into the bowel.*

6) Weight = 120 kg

7) Height = 185 cm

> *He is overweight. Excess weight is a risk factor for GORD.*

Biochemistry:

All within range except:

1) haemoglobin = 10 g/dl (reference 14–18)

2) mean cell volume = 72 femtolitre (reference 78–94)

3) haematocrit = 0.31 (reference 0.36–0.46)

> *1) Haemoglobin: His haemoglobin level is low because of the bleeding leading to loss of red blood cells. This is the most common method of detecting anaemia.*

> *2) Mean cell volume: Average volume of red cell. A low level is called microcytic anaemia and is used to identify iron deficiency anaemia as a result of bleeding.*

3) Haematocrit: The ratio of the volume of occupied by red cells to the total volume of blood. It is low in all forms of anaemia.

All three readings indicate that he has iron deficiency anaemia as a result of bleeding secondary to an ulcer.

Provisional diagnosis: Gastric ulcer

Plan:

Half hourly observations

Endoscopy

Urea breath test

Intravenous fluids

Cimetidine

Metoclopamide and as required

Ferrous sulphate

Stop ibuprofen

1) Endoscopy: A procedure using a tube which allows for complete visualization of the oesophagus, stomach, and duodenum.

2) Urea breath test: urea breath tests which are less invasive and quicker, have replaced CLO-tests as the first line test for H. pylori. The urea breath is based on the production of urease (an enzyme that breaks down urea into ammonia and bicarbonate, which is then expelled as carbon dioxide) by H. pylori. The patient is given radio labelled urea (using 13C or 14C)—and if they colonised with H. pylori they will excrete radiolabelled CO2 from their breath. CLO (Camplyobacter-like organism) test is a more invasive test whereby mucosal biopsy sample from the patient is inoculated into a medium containing urea and phenol red, a dye that turns pink in a pH of 6.0 or greater, which happens when urease containing H. pylori metabolizes urea to ammonia.

3) Metoclopramide: Used to control vomiting. It acts as an antagonist at the D2-dopamine receptors (see Chapter 18) at the base of the brain (the chemoreceptor trigger zone), which controls vomiting.

4) Ferrous sulphate: Used to treat the anaemia caused by blood loss.

5) Ibuprofen: Discontinued because it is a non-steroidal anti-inflammatory drug (NSAID). There is a lot of evidence that NSAIDs induce mucosal damage in the gastrointestinal tract and can cause peptic ulcer, bleeding, and haemorrhage.

Although it's late, Carter's mum insists on staying with him while they wait for the doctors. She is quite worried and cannot understand why her son is so sick. Carter tries to calm his mum down, explaining that the stomach wall normally protects itself from being digested by gastric acid by secreting certain substances.

1) List five ways in which the stomach protects itself from being digested and explain how each of them serves a protective role.

2) List two chemicals normally found in the stomach that would destroy the mucosa in the absence of the above-mentioned protective substances.

3a) List the three main stimuli or endogenous secretagogues leading to the secretion of destructive acids by the parietal cell and explain how they stimulate acid secretion,

3b) Where do each of these stimuli come from and what causes them to be released?

The gastro-enterologist finally comes to see Carter. He confirms Carter's history as documented in A&E.

Although he knows Carter is a doctor, he still explains to him what he thinks has gone wrong. Carter's mum listens to him talk about gastric acid, mucous, and bicarbonate and prostaglandins.

She wonders what they mean when they talk about pumps.

4a) What is the name of the pump involved in the exchange of potassium ions for hydrogen ions during acid secretion in the parietal cell?

4b) What is the source of the H^+ ions moved by this pump?

The doctor goes on to explain to Carter that a combination of factors could have contributed to his developing what they think is an ulcer. Tests results are pending to confirm this and the possible cause.

The doctor talks about an imbalance between the mucosal damaging mechanism and mucosal protecting mechanism. This imbalance could be brought about by a variety of things, such as lifestyle, bacteria, medication, or tumour.

5a) What is *Helicobacter pylori?*

5b) Explain the mechanism by which *H. pylori* leads to peptic ulcer formation.

The doctor also explains that Carter has been given metoclopramide to stop him from vomiting.

6a) Explain the mechanism of action of metoclopramide in vomiting.

6b) What are the main side effects of metoclopramide, and in which groups of patients do they most often feature?

The doctor also explains that the painkiller prescribed for Carter's injury would most probably have contributed to the ulcer.

He said an acid-producing tumour was unlikely to be the cause.

7) Explain how NSAIDS contribute to the development of peptic ulcers.

The doctor asks Carter about the symptoms he had when he had GORD.

8) What exactly is GORD and what are the symptoms of this condition?

_____

_____

_____

9) List five risk factors for GORD and explain how they can contribute to this condition.

_____

_____

_____

_____

Carter explains that cimetidine had been prescribed by his GP to treat his GORD symptoms.

10) Elaborate on approaches to the treatment of GORD.

_____

_____

_____

The doctor explains to Carter that the cimetidine would probably be changed to a combination of drugs if the test results came back positive.

He says he hopes the results will be back in under an hour. He encourages Carter to have a rest. He tells Carter he has to go to a clinic but another doctor in his team will come round later to explain the results.

Carter's mum finally agrees to go home after the nurses explain to her she can call at any time to enquire about how her son is doing.

Two hours later Carter almost passes out when he is woken up by his ex-wife, Dr Knight, who introduces herself as the doctor on the gastroenterology team. She is very professional and does not bother with any chatting.

She explains that the endoscopy has confirmed an ulcer. She also says that the urea breath test has confirmed that _Helicobacter pylori_ was a contributing factor.

Carter's ex-wife explains to him that the cimetidine for his GORD will be discontinued and replaced by what she calls a triple therapy.

Dr Knight explains to Carter that the combination of drugs in his triple therapy are: lansoprazole, clarithromycin, and amoxicillin. Although he knows this, she still explains that two are antibiotics and one is what is called a proton pump inhibitor (PPI).

11) Explain the rational for a triple therapy approach for the treatment of gastric ulcers where *H. pylori* is detected.

12) Explain the mechanism of action of PPIs.

> Dr Knight explains that PPIs are more successful at reducing stomach acid than H_2 receptor antagonists.

13) Why are PPIs more successful than histamine H_2 receptor antagonists in affecting stomach acid?

> Carter said he was actually glad he had to discontinue taking the cimetidine because he had experienced certain embarrassing side effects.
>
> Dr Knight tells Carter that he will have to stay in hospital for a week because of the size of his ulcer. She leaves after instructing the nurses about Carter's medication.
>
> Carter is unhappy about having to stay in hospital but decides to be a good sport about it. To make matters worse, the triple therapy fails to eradicate Carter's *H. pylori* after 14 days.
>
> The combination is changed to ranitidine bismuth citrate, amoxicillin, and metronidazole.

14) What could the side effects he experienced be?

15) Explain the rationale of using bismuth in *H. pylori*-induced peptic ulcer.

After 1 week on this combination, Carter finally gets better and is discharged home.

At home, although he is physically well, he is depressed about the state of his personal life. Although he was told to stop smoking and drinking he finds he is drinking and smoking even more than he used to.

Three months later he starts experiencing symptoms of gastritis. He decides to buy antacids over the counter from his pharmacist. The pharmacist recommends an antacid that combines aluminium and magnesium salts. This makes him feel better.

16) Explain why antacids are beneficial in alleviating symptoms of gastritis.

17) Why are antacids that combine magnesium and aluminium salts better than antacids containing either magnesium or aluminium only?

Carter continues to drink and smoke regularly. After 4 weeks his symptoms of dyspepsia return and he goes to consult his GP. Although he specifically requests that the GP should prescribe a prostaglandin analogue or a mucosal protective agent for him, the GP decides to put him on a PPI instead.

18) What are the properties of mucosal protective agents that make them beneficial in the treatment of gastritis and gastric ulcers?

The GP tells Carter that he will probably have to take the PPI all his life if he does not stop drinking and smoking.

When Carter goes to pick up his prescription, his chemist tells him to take the PPI with breakfast and to swallow the tablet whole.

19) Explain why the PPI tablet should be swallowed whole.

20) What are the potential problems with long-term PPI use?

Carter tries to follow the GP's advice and cut down on alcohol and cigarettes, but cannot. His personal life is still a shambles. To make matters worse he is informed by one of his friends that his ex-wife is very happy in a new relationship!

Do you think medical intervention has more to offer Carter? Can medicine be applied to someone whose life has become a mess? Obviously he should continue to optimize his drugs to help with his physical problems, but perhaps he now needs something else to help him with the root of his problems. Further lifestyle advice and psychological therapy should be considered. One important question: is he chronically depressed? This leads us to the issues considered in Chapter 19.

21) What advice would you give Carter at this juncture, if you were counselling him?

Chapter 13
Disorders of the lower gastrointestinal tract

Are your bowels healthy? Is this a question you are accustomed to asking yourself? The answer may be cultural. Attitudes to bowels and their productions vary among communities around the world. Some cultures display extreme disregard: 'I have a bowel movement once a week whether I need one or not.' Contrasting with this, some health advisors suggest that you should have two bowel movements every day and worry if you don't. Some advise close and regular inspection of your stools (more correctly called faeces); some would regard this as perverse.

It may be thought that lower gastrointestinal disorders are easy to understand because diarrhoea and constipation are so commonplace, but this is not so. For example, constipation can be the cause of diarrhoea due to irritants released from stagnant wastes. Irritable bowel syndrome (IBS) can cause both diarrhoea and constipation, and is itself in many cases caused, and best treated, psychologically. Unrecognized bowel dysfunction is likely to contribute widely to feelings of poor health.

As discussed in the introduction to this section, the lower gastrointestinal (GI) tract is responsible for absorption of nutrients (and other substances such as drugs) and elimination of waste. While a number of disorders affect the lower GI tract, by far the most common are diarrhoea and constipation. IBS is another common, but less clearly diagnosed, problem with the lower GI tract, which as mentioned above can also include diarrhoea and constipation.

13.1 Diarrhoea

Almost everyone has suffered from diarrhoea at some time in his or her life. In western countries, nearly all cases are acute and self-limiting. However, in developing countries diarrhoea can be chronic and/or life threatening, and is one of the leading causes of infant death. Studies have found that 5–7% of people in western countries report having diarrhoea in the previous 4 weeks, with the youngest have the greatest prevalence (almost 1 in 10 in children under 5 years). As a measure of the self-limiting nature, the same studies find that only 1 in 5 seek medical care.

13.1.1 Diagnosis of diarrhoea

Just like constipation, which we will discuss later, diarrhoea is diagnosed in reference to a person's normal bowel habits. The clinical diagnosis of diarrhoea is watery or liquid stools, often with a stool weight above 200 g per day, and increased frequency of motions.

13.1.2 Causes of diarrhoea

Diarrhoea can be broadly classified into three types: osmotic, secretory, and motility. The causes of these are given in Table 13.1.

13.1.3 Treatment of diarrhoea

The most obvious first treatment is to address the possible cause of the diarrhoea (e.g. stop eating so much artificially sweetened food). The most common causes of diarrhoea in western countries are simple viral and mild bacterial infections of the gut, usually after having

Table 13.1 Types of diarrhoea and their causes

Type of diarrhoea	Causes
Osmotic	Non-absorbable substances in the gut cause an osmotic gradient, which draws water into the gut. Often produced by lactase deficiency, this results in lactose remaining in the intestine. Other causes include magnesium salts such as magnesium sulphate and hydroxide (see antacids in Chapter 12), and excess use of foods with the artificial sweeteners such as xylitol and mannitol (see later).
Secretory	Excessive secretion of chloride and bicarbonate, and inhibition of sodium absorption because of disruption of the cells lining the intestine. Commonly caused by bacterial endotoxins such as from *E. coli* and cholera, as found in travellers' diarrhoea.
Motility	Excessive stimulation of muscles around the gut, increasing peristalsis. Can be due to impaired autonomic control (e.g. diabetic neuropathy) or agents that stimulate gut motility, such as sennosides (more about these under constipation).

contaminated food (food poisoning). For most people diarrhoea is just an inconvenience, causing you to run to the toilet every few minutes or hours. Mild to moderate gastroenteritis is usually self-limiting, only lasting for 24–48 hours. However, in the very young and very old and frail, even moderate diarrhoea can be life threatening because of dehydration, therefore the mainstay of the treatment of diarrhoea is maintaining hydration.

Oral rehydration solutions

Oral rehydration solutions (ORS) are the best treatment for mild to moderate diarrhoea in most adults and children. There are many old wives' tales about how to treat diarrhoea, one of the favourites being 'flat lemonade'. However, lemonade, flat or fizzy, can actually make diarrhoea worse, and the reason is the special relationship between glucose and sodium concentrations, and water absorption in the intestine (see Box 13.1).

As seen in Box 13.1 you need a certain concentration of sodium and glucose to maximize the water absorption in the gut. Products like Gatorade® (a sports drink promoted to replace lost fluids and electrolytes) and lemonade have too much glucose and too little sodium to maximize water absorption (Table 13.2). The excess glucose can have the opposite effect by drawing water into the gut lumen to dilute out the glucose, making diarrhoea worse. To solve this a product containing the correct balance of glucose, water, and sodium has been developed called ORS.

A number of different formulations and brands of ORS exist. However, they are all similar in terms of their balance of sodium, water, and glucose, and all have an osmolality of approximately 240–250 mOsm/L. The important thing is to drink as much ORS as you can tolerate, aiming for at least 2–3 L per day for adults.

Table 13.2 Nutritional comparison of Gatorade®, lemonade, Gastrolyte® (ORS), and the WHO ORS

	Gatorade® (per litre)	Lemonade (per litre)	ORS (Gastrolyte®) (per litre)	ORS (WHO) (per litre)
Protein (g)	0	0	0	0
Fat (g)	0	0	0	0
Carbohydrate				
Total (g)	63	80	20	13.5
Sucrose (g)	45			
Glucose (g)	18	80	20	13.5
Sodium (mmol)	18	1	60	75
Potassium (mmol)	3	37	20	20

Box 13.1

Water absorption in the intestine

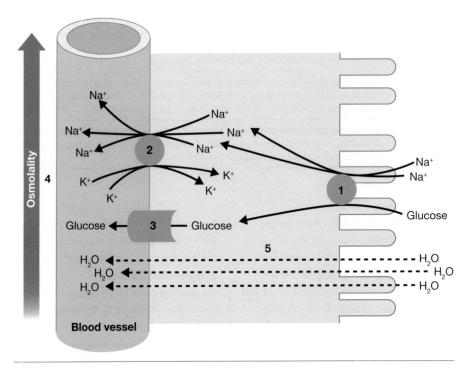

Figure a

1. Sodium and glucose are transported into the cells lining the intestine by SGLUT1, a sodium/glucose co-transporter. Sodium attaches first and causes a conformational change in the transporter so that glucose can bind. The sodium and glucose are then internalized into the cell. The SGLUT1 transports one molecule of glucose and two molecules of sodium.

2. Sodium and potassium are exchanged via a Na^+/K^+ ATPase on the basolateral membrane of the cell, with three molecules of Na+ being pumped out of the cell in exchange for two molecules of K^+.

3. Glucose is moved out of the cell by another glucose transporter, SGLUT2, on the basolateral membrane.

4. The effect of moving glucose and sodium into the blood vessel is to increase the osmotic gradient between the blood vessel and the gut lumen by increasing the osmolality (osmolality is a measure of the amount of dissolved substances in a solution).

5. Water moves passively from the lumen across the cells into the blood vessel to balance the increased osmolality (i.e. to try and dilute out the sodium and glucose).

Helen, our patient in Workbook 10, was initially treated with ORS for a bout of 'food poisoning' that she got on holiday.

Antidiarrhoeal drugs

Although ORS, along with rest, is the best treatment for diarrhoea, sometimes it isn't convenient to just rest at home. If someone needs to travel, or if they need to go to work, short courses of antidiarrhoeal drugs can be used. The reason that antidiarrhoeals are not used routinely is that they work on reducing gut motility, which gives more time for water to be reabsorbed and reduces the frequency of trips to the toilet. However, like coughing, diarrhoea is a protective strategy that

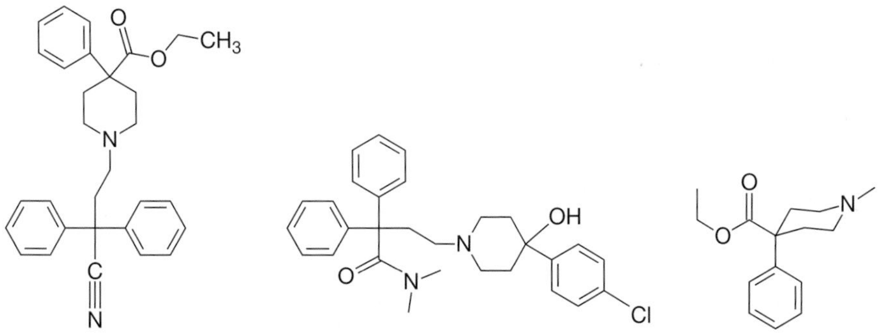

Figure 13.1 Comparison of diphenoxylate, loperamide, and pethidine structures.

aims to 'flush out' whatever toxin is causing the diarrhoea, so using antidiarrhoeals routinely will keep the toxins within the small intestine, possibly doing more harm than good.

Opiate derivatives

Two main opiate antidiarrhoeals are used, **diphenoxylate** and **loperamide**. They are structurally related to pethidine (see Figure 13.1), and their action comes from agonist activity on mu opiate receptors. Other opiates, such as codeine, can also be used. However, because of their lesser potential for abuse, loperamide and diphenoxylate are preferred for the treatment of mild/moderate diarrhoea. The mu receptors are found in the myenteric plexus and activation leads to reduced motility by inhibiting the release if acetylcholine. This slowing of motility allows more time for the gut to absorb water. Codeine and loperamide also have inhibitory effects on secretions in the lower GI tract.

Diphenoxylate crosses the blood–brain barrier and is therefore open to abuse. To combat this it is administered in combination with a small amount of atropine. Although atropine would also have slowing effect on GI motility, the amount given is subtherapeutic and is only used so that if a person takes too many tablets they will get the anticholinergic side effects from the atropine (e.g. dry mouth, blurred vision, etc). The hope is that suffering these effects will deter people from abusing the tablets.

Loperamide acts locally in the gut—it does not cross the blood–brain barrier—therefore loperamide may be preferred because of the lower potential for dependence.

Furthermore, loperamide has a longer half-life than either codeine or diphenoxylate (7–15 hours compared to 2.5 hours). Loperamide also blocks the gastrocolic reflex that increases gastric motility in response to distension of the stomach or chyme entering the small intestine. This reflex is implicated in IBS (see later).

Loperamide is given as an initial dose of two tablets/capsules followed by one capsule/tablet after each loose bowel action; diphenoxylate is usually given as two tablets four times a day. Both loperamide and diphenoxylate are well tolerated, with the main side effects being constipation from overuse, and potential dry mouth and other anticholinergic effects with the diphenoxylate/atropine combination.

Absorbent agents

These products include **kaolin**, **pectin**, and **charcoal**. Kaolin is a natural substance with the formula $Al_2Si_2O_5(OH)_4$. It is a white powder that is mined in tropical parts of the world. Pectin is a polysaccharide found in the cell walls of plants. It is used in the food industry for its ability to cause liquids to become jelly-like (hence it is used in making jam). Charcoal is made by burning organic materials such as wood. The products used clinically are called 'activated charcoal'. They are 'activated' by exposing them to oxidizing substances at high temperature. This produces a large number of pores in the charcoal that increases the surface area available to absorb things (the surface area can be up to 1500 m^2/g, with a 50 g dose of charcoal having the surface area of 10 football fields). The main medical use of activated charcoal is in the treatment of

Table 13.3 Rome III criteria for adult chronic constipation

(1) Two or more of the following for at least 12 weeks in the preceding 6 months:
   - straining in more than 25% of defecations
   - lumpy or hard stools in more than 25% of defecations
   - sensation of incomplete evacuation in more than 25% of defecations
   - sensation of anorectal obstruction or blockade in more than 25% of defecations
   - manual manoeuvres (e.g. digital evacuation) to facilitate more than 25% of defecations
   - fewer than three defecations per week
(2) Loose stools are not present (without the use of laxatives)
(3) There are insufficient criteria for the diagnosis of irritable bowel syndrome

poisonings, where the large surface area is used to absorb drugs and other poisons. The mechanism of action of these agents in diarrhoea is to absorb toxins and bacteria in the gut, and decrease water loss, although the exact role of pectin is uncertain. However, evidence has shown that they are generally not effective and are probably best avoided. Apart from their lack of efficacy, they also have the potential to absorb many drugs, reducing the effectiveness of the drugs.

13.2 Constipation

Like diarrhoea, constipation is a very common condition, and most people do not seek any medical treatment for it. The incidence of constipation has been reported in studies to be between 2 and 28%, but this differs among different ethnic groups as it depends on the definition of constipation used. A diagnosis of constipation needs to be made in reference to a person's normal bowel habits. The normal frequency of defecation in the population ranges from two or three times a day to once or twice a week, therefore constipation is only defined relative to *your* normal frequency and must be accompanied by difficulty in passing a stool. The Rome III criteria, agreed on by an international committee, defines chronic constipation in adults as outlined in Table 13.3.

Although constipation itself is not life threatening, it can lead to significant discomfort. Chronic constipation can lead to faecal impaction (where a large, hard mass of faecal matter cannot be passed and has to be manually removed). It can also cause straining when going to the toilet, which can lead to anal fissures and haemorrhoids (engorged blood vessels around the anus that lead to bleeding and itching, and can become thrombosed, leading to pain and discomfort).

13.2.1 Pathophysiology of constipation

As noted, constipation is related to the frequency of defecation and/or the hardness of the stools, therefore things that slow the gut, or change the content of the stools, can result in constipation. A number of physiological conditions can cause slowing of the gut, including megacolon (an abnormally dilated colon with paralysis of the peristaltic activity of the bowel) and having weak abdominal muscles. Delaying emptying the bowels due to psychological (e.g. fear of using public toilets, which often happens with young children at school) or physiological causes (e.g. painful anal fissures that result in pain passing stools) can lead to constipation.

The most common cause of constipation in western populations is our low-fibre, highly refined diet. The lack of fibre leads to small, hard stools (it is recommended that an adult has 20–35 g of fibre a day, but most of us consume less than half of this in our diet). To make matters worse we often drink insufficient water to maintain soft stools.

A number of other causes, including medicines and psychological conditions such as depression, can result in constipation (Table 13.4).

13.2.2 Treatment of constipation

The mainstay of treating constipation is to correct the underlying cause. As noted, for most people it is due to our highly refined diet, therefore people should try to get more fibre into their diet and increase their water intake. It is important to increase the fibre gradually as a sudden increase can lead to bloating and distension of the gut because of increased gas production from the bacteria in the gut breaking

Table 13.4 Causes of constipation

Causes from within the GI tract	Causes from outside the GI tract
Dysfunction of the colon: • megacolon • colon obstruction (e.g. neoplasm) Anal fissures	Dietary: • low fibre diet • insufficient water intake Medications: • anticholinergics (e.g. hyoscine, TCAs) • opiates • antacids (calcium and aluminium salts) • laxative abuse Diseases: • thyroid dysfunction • diabetes mellitus • depression Sedentary lifestyle

GI, gastrointestinal; TCA, tricyclic antidepressants.

down the fibre. Foods that should be consumed include brown rice, wholemeal breads, and fruit and vegetables that have edible skins (e.g. apples, carrots, pears, etc).

Laxatives

If pharmacological treatment is required then laxatives are the mainstay. They can be grouped into five classes (Table 13.5).

Stool softeners

Stool softeners are the most gentle (or least powerful) laxatives available. Docusate is an anionic surfactant, a

Table 13.5 Classes of laxatives

Class	Examples
Stool softeners	Docusate
Bulk-forming laxatives	Psyllium (ispaghula) husks Sterculia Methylcellulose
Osmotic laxatives	Saline-based: • magnesium sulphate • sodium phosphate Non-saline based: • lactulose • polyethylene glycol • sorbitol • glycerine
Lubricants	Liquid paraffin
Stimulants	Sennosides Cascara Phenolphthalein Bisacodyl Castor oil

type of soap. It works by changing the surface tension around the stool and thus allowing water to penetrate the stool more easily, causing it to become emulsified. Docusate is also a very weak stimulant laxative (see later). It has a very slow onset of action (taking 3 or 4 days to work), and therefore it is generally only used prophylactically when constipation is anticipated due to medications, for example, or in combination with stimulant laxatives such as senna. It has virtually no side effects and can be given safely to children.

Bulk-forming laxatives

The bulk-forming laxatives work by increasing the mass in the stool, which traps water and improves the consistency of the stool. The larger stool then stimulates the peristalsis, causing evacuation. Colonic bacteria also use the fibre as a substrate and they increase in number. This also adds to the softening effect. Bulk-forming laxatives largely come from natural sources and include the husks of seeds, including bran and psyllium. They are actually hydrophobic and can be used, ironically, to reduce diarrhoea in some circumstances.

> Our patient Helen was prescribed bulk-forming laxatives because of the constipation she suffered as a result of her IBS...and the medication she was prescribed!

Bulk-forming laxatives work faster than stool softeners, starting to have an effect in 24–48 hours, but they are not as strong as the stimulant, or some of the osmotic, laxatives. They are very well tolerated, with the main side effects coming from the breakdown of the increased fibre by intestinal bacterial leading to gas being produced, resulting in bloating and flatulence (similar to increasing your intake of high-fibre foods). The retention of water in the bowel can also lead to bloating and pain due to distension (stretching) of the bowel.

Osmotic laxatives

Osmotic laxatives are large molecular weight and/or poorly soluble substances that work by increasing the osmotic pressure within the gut lumen. The presence of these insoluble solutes causes water to be drawn from the blood across the endothelium into the gut lumen, leading to softer stools. There are two main groups: saline osmotic laxatives, based largely on magnesium and sodium salts, and non-saline osmotic laxatives, based largely on poorly soluble sugars.

The saline osmotic agents have been used for years in the form of magnesium sulphate, also known as Epsom salts. Newer agents include sodium phosphate, sodium picosulphate, and magnesium carbonate. They can be given orally as a mixture or as an enema (directly inserted into the rectum).

The three main non-saline agents are sorbitol, lactulose, and polyethylene glycol. Sorbitol is a sugar alcohol that is formed by reduction of glucose, altering the aldehyde group to a hydroxyl group. It is used as a sugar substitute

in 'sugar-free' foods such as confectionary. Lactulose is a synthetic disaccharide made up of fructose and galactose moieties. Some of its activity comes from its metabolism by colonic bacteria (Figure 13.2). Bacteria convert the lactulose to a range of organic acids. These lower the pH of the gut lumen and soften the stool. The acids also trap ammonia from the blood in the gut lumen by converting it from unionized ammonia (NH_3) to cationic ammonium (NH_4^+), which cannot pass back into the blood. This property of lactulose is used in the treatment of hepatic encephalopathy, where increased ammonia can be present because the damaged liver is unable to covert it to urea. However, there is only limited evidence of its efficacy in hepatic encephalopathy.

Polyethylene glycols (PEGs), also known as macragols, are polymers of ethylene oxide having the general formula $HO\text{-}(CH_2\text{-}CH_2\text{-}O\text{-})_n\text{-}H$, where n is the number of repetitions of the ethylene oxide moiety in the chain. They can have large molecular weights, ranging from several hundred to tens of thousands of kilodaltons (kD), and their names usually reflect their average molecular weight (e.g. PEG 4000 has a molecular weight of approximately 4000 kD). Their molecular weights make them virtually impossible to absorb from the gut and they are usually

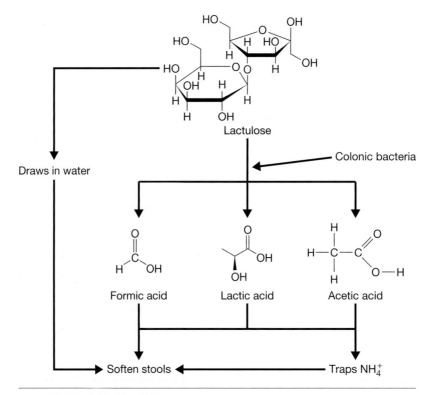

Figure 13.2 Action of lactulose.

given in combination with electrolytes, such as sodium and potassium chloride, and some contain additional saline osmotic agents such as sodium sulphate.

Osmotic agents act more rapidly than the bulk-forming and stool-softening agents. When given orally they usually act within 24 hours; when given rectally they can act in a matter of minutes. The non-saline osmotic laxatives are used for moderate to severe constipation. The PEG laxatives combined with saline osmotic agents and many of the saline osmotic laxatives are usually reserved for bowel preparation prior to endoscopy or bowel surgery. They have a powerful effect on the gut and lead to complete evacuation along the length of the lower intestine.

While these agents are generally well tolerated, the main side effects come from their ability to shift large amounts of water from the blood into the gut. This can lead to fluid and electrolyte disturbances, which can be particularly problematic in the elderly. The risk of this is greatest with the saline osmotic agents, and when patients fail to take sufficient additional water with the products.

Lubricants

Mineral oils, such as paraffin, have been used for decades as a laxative. Their action, as their name suggests, is to lubricate the stool to make it easier to pass. Because they are generally unpalatable by themselves, they are usually made into emulsions (substances similar to milk, which is an emulsion of fat and water) with the addition of flavouring agents. Evidence of their effectiveness is almost non-existent and they do pose potential risks, such as aspiration pneumonia (this occurs if you accidentally inhale the fatty liquid into the lungs because of poor closure of the epiglottis—this is a problem in the elderly, who may take the laxative at night, lie down, and then aspirate), therefore they are generally not used any more.

Stimulants

These agents come from both natural (e.g. sennosides) and synthetic (e.g. **bisacodyl**) origins. Sennosides, or senna glycosides, are anthraquinone derivatives found in a range of plants from the genus *Senna*. Other plants, including *aloe*, *cascara*, and *frangula* species, also contain anthraquinones. These act on the myenteric plexus and have a direct action on the intestinal mucosa, resulting in increased peristalsis. The active constituent of senna

appears to be rheinanthrone, which is formed by bacteria metabolizing sennosides in the gut.

Bisacodyl is a stimulant laxative that has been in use since the 1950s. It has reported effects on the parasympathetic nerves, resulting in peristalsis. It also appears to affect local axon and segmental reflexes in the colon, leading to widespread peristalsis. Another mode of action appears to come from its effect on water and electrolytes, leading to excretion of sodium and water into the gut lumen. Importantly, because its effects occur locally (therefore it is known as a contact laxative) it will work in patients who have spinal cord injuries and therefore do not have normal central nervous system (CNS) input into their bowels. **Phenolphthalein** is also used for similar effects, although its main use is as an acid–base indicator. However, a ruling by the Food and Drug Administration that phenolphthalein is not a safe over-the-counter laxative has lead to it being replaced with senna and other stimulant laxatives in most preparations.

The stimulant laxatives have a rapid onset of action, working in 6–12 hours when given orally and within minutes when given rectally. The side effects include cramping and abdominal pain. A more serious concern is the over-use of stimulant laxatives and their effect on the bowel, leading to what is called a 'lazy bowel' (a bowel that no longer has peristaltic movement and hence does not move faeces through the bowel) because of 'over stimulation'. The evidence for this, however, is poor. That being said, over-use of any laxative should be discouraged, particularly in people who wrongly take them to lose weight (often young girls/women) or those who take them in the mistaken belief that they must have a bowel action every day to be 'normal' (not an uncommon cultural phenomenon).

Prokinetic drugs

Drugs such as **domperidone** and **metoclopramide** increase gastric motility and promote stomach emptying. Their effect is generally confined to the upper parts of the GI tract (stomach and duodenum) and they are used primarily as antiemetics (see Chapter 12); they have no real role in constipation.

Treatment of opiate-induced constipation

Patients with chronic moderate/severe pain may require long-term treatment with opiate analgesics. As discussed above in the treatment of diarrhoea, opiate derivatives such as loperamide and diphenoxylate reduce diarrhoea by slowing gut motility by stimulating mu opioid receptors on smooth muscle in the gut. Not surprisingly, all opiates have the potential to do this and therefore often cause constipation. Traditional treatment was with stimulant laxatives or osmotic laxatives, and, when these failed, the addition of enemas. However, because of the risks of electrolyte disturbances and the possible development of 'lazy bowel', alternative treatments for these patients have been developed. **Methylnaltrexone**, a derivative of naltrexone (the drug used to block the effects of opiates, and used to reverse opiate toxicity and in the treatment of opioid dependence), has been shown to promote bowel actions without reducing the central effectiveness of opiates on pain relief. Its local effect on the bowel comes from the fact that methylnaltrexone, unlike natrexone, is charged and is therefore unable to cross the blood–brain barrier (Figure 13.3).

Alvimopan is another structurally unrelated peripheral mu receptor antagonist that has been studied for the treatment of opioid-induced gastroparesis. It has a greater affinity for the mu receptor than methylnaltrexone, although the significance of this is uncertain. Like methylnatrexone it is poorly lipid soluble and does not

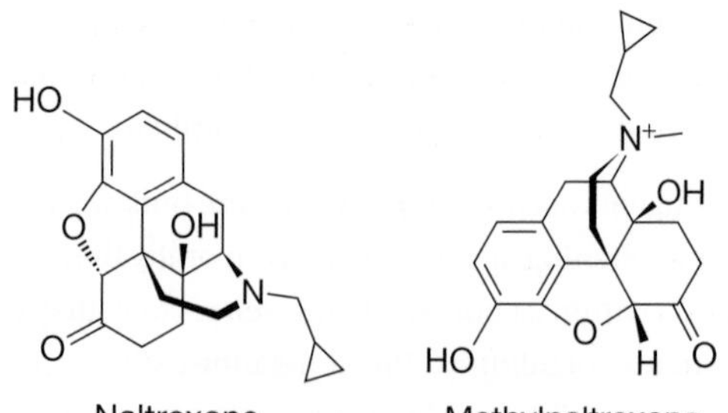

Figure 13.3 Comparison of naltrexone and methylnaltrexone.

cross the blood–brain barrier, thus leaving the analgesic effects of opiates intact.

Methylnaltrexone is given as a subcutaneous injection every second day, whereas alvimopan is given orally once a day. The agents are usually given in addition to laxatives, and are used to delay the use of more severe laxatives such as enemas. Both agents are well tolerated, with the main side effects being abdominal pain, nausea, and flatulence. They are significantly more expensive than the older osmotic and stimulant laxatives, and their exact role in therapy is yet to be determined.

13.3 Irritable bowel syndrome

Irritable bowel syndrome is a common, functional abnormality in GI function that affects up to 20% of the population. It is distinct from inflammatory bowel disease (IBD), where there is a clear association with inflammation around the GI tract. Irritable bowel syndrome is often a diagnosis of exclusion.

13.3.1 Diagnostic criteria for IBS

A number of criteria have been proposed for the diagnosis of IBS. The Rome III criteria, produced by an international body interested in functional GI disorders, are as follows:

Recurrent abdominal pain or discomfort at least 3 days/ month in the last 3 months (occurring at least 6 months prior to diagnosis) associated with two or more of the following:

- improvement with defecation
- onset associated with a change in frequency of stool
- onset associated with a change in form (appearance) of stool.

There are four main types of IBS described: diarrhoea dominant (IBS-D), constipation dominant (IBS-C), mixed diarrhoea and constipation (IBS-M), and alternating diarrhoea and constipation (IBS-A). The usefulness of these classifications is uncertain, and patients often switch between subtypes. The main advantage of classification is that the dominant symptom is the one that is targeted for treatment.

Helen, in Workbook 10, suffers from symptoms consistent with constipation-dominant IBS.

13.3.2 Pathophysiology of IBS

There are three components to IBS: changes in gut motility, visceral hyperalgesia, and a psychiatric component. Gut dysmotility is a prominent feature and can affect the small bowel and colon. Patients with IBS-D show accelerated meal transit time, while those with IBS-C have prolonged meal transit time. In patients with IBS-D the accelerated meal transit time is thought to be due to shorter intervals between migratory motor complexes (MMC, these are the waves of peristaltic action that occur when fasting to push digested food through the intestines).

Visceral hyperalgesia means patients have an enhanced perception of normal gut motility and visceral pain, therefore patients will sense normal gut movements, or the presence of gasses in the gut, as being painful.

Most patients who have IBS also have panic or anxiety disorders, or major depression. However, whether the IBS or the psychiatric disorder comes first remains unclear.

Other pathologies suggested include microscopic inflammation of the gut mucosa, overgrowth of bacteria in the small intestine, and changes in the type of faecal bacteria; these are still being investigated.

Role of serotonin in IBS

As discussed in the introduction to this section, the GI tract is controlled by a complicated interaction between the CNS, the autonomic nervous system (ANS), and the enteric nervous system (ENS). The extrinsic control of the GI tract comes from the CNS and the ANS, while the intrinsic control involves the ENS. The ENS contains intrinsic primary afferent neurones, which respond to stimuli from within the gut, and coordinate motor and secretory responses (e.g. stimulating gut motility in response to distension in the stomach to promote passage of chyme out of the stomach). The ENS also carries nociceptive (painful) stimuli to the ANS, which communicates this to the CNS. Disruptions in this interrelationship are thought to contribute to the symptoms of IBS, and serotonin appears to play a pivotal role. The main source of serotonin (5-hydroxytryptamine, 5-HT) in the gut comes from the enterochromaffin-like (ELCs) cells located in the gastric mucosa.

Seven subtypes of serotonin receptors have been identified. Of these, three subtypes (5-HT_{1p}, 5-HT_3, and 5-HT_4) play a major role in the gastric tract. The 5-HT_3 receptors are primarily involved in transmission of painful stimuli from the bowel to the ANS. Stimulation of receptors on the vagal afferents results in sensations of nausea, bloating, and fullness, and therefore antagonism of 5-HT_3 may be helpful in reducing some of the visceral hyperalgesia in IBS. Serotonin is involved in the initiation of the MMC in the gut, and its release from ELCs is partly controlled as part of a

positive feedback loop by 5-HT_3 receptors. The 5-HT_{1p} and 5-HT_4 receptors augment peristalsis and secretory reflexes by promoting the release of neurotransmitters such as acetylcholine, which have a direct effect on gut motility and secretions. Peripheral 5-HT_4 receptors may also be involved with normalizing pain sensitivity in the colon.

In addition to the release of serotonin, the reuptake of serotonin (the mechanism by which serotonin is deactivated) may also play an important role in the pathophysiology of IBS. In the gut reuptake occurs because of the presence of the serotonin reuptake transporter (SERT) in the plasma membrane. The absence of SERT leads first to prolonged effects of serotonin (causing diarrhoea), followed by inhibition of the effects of serotonin due to receptor desensitization (causing constipation). There is some evidence that some patients with IBS may have decreased SERT expression compared to people without IBS.

13.3.3 Management of IBS

Dietary modification has been suggested in patients with IBS, although the evidence for its efficacy is still being sought.

Other recommendations have included reducing fat, caffeine, alcohol, and spicy foods.

Cognitive behavioural therapy and hypnotherapy have also been through clinical trials. They can help people both with and without obvious psychological pathologies.

However, pharmacological therapies remain an important intervention. There is nothing currently to directly address the causes of IBS, therefore treatment is aimed at what symptoms dominate.

Treatment of constipation-dominant IBS

This is treated in the same way as constipation in patients without IBS, as discussed above. Patients should start by trying to increase the fibre in their diet and their water intake. If laxatives are needed then bulk-forming and non-saline osmotic agents can be used. Caution may be needed in patients who have IBS-C and symptoms of bloating and GI pain, as increasing fibre intake too quickly may exacerbate the bloating.

Tegaserod is a 5-HT_4 partial agonist that was developed for the treatment of IBS-C. By stimulating the 5-HT$_4$ receptors it increases peristaltic and secretory activity in the gut. However, it is associated with serious side effects, including profuse diarrhoea. More seriously, its use was found to be associated with an increased risk of cardiovascular events. This resulted in its withdrawal from markets across the world in 2007.

Lubiprostone is a derivative of prostaglandin E1. It activates the CIC-2 chloride channels found on the basolateral membrane of colon enterocytes, resulting in secretion of chloride ions into the gut lumen. These secretions soften the stool and promote peristalsis. Lubiprostone is given orally twice a day. The main side effect to look for is severe diarrhoea.

Treatment of diarrhoea-dominant IBS

Opiate derivatives, as described above for the management of diarrhoea, are used intermittently for exacerbations of diarrhoea in IBS. Loperamide is the agent of choice as it has fewer side effects compared to diphenoxylate, and reduced dependence potential compared to codeine. Unlike in the treatment of self-limiting gastroenteritis, when used for IBS loperamide is dosed regularly (i.e. one capsule once to three times a day).

Alosetron is a 5-HT$_3$ antagonist used to treat IBS-D in women. Inhibition of 5-HT$_3$ results in slowing of colonic transit time and enhanced fluid and sodium absorption. It also reduces abdominal pain by relaxing the left colon and inhibiting spinal cord reactivity, resulting in reduced perception of distension in the bowel. The 5-HT$_3$ receptors on ELCs are also involved in the positive feedback and their blockage results in reduced serotonin release. The important side effects with alosetron have been constipation-related complications, including ischaemic colitis. As some of these resulted in death, it was temporarily withdrawn from the market in the USA in 2000, and reintroduced in 2002 with new restrictions on its use (the first drug ever to be reintroduced after being withdrawn).

Treatment of abdominal pain associated with IBS

Antispasmodics can be used to treat abdominal pain and may reduce diarrhoea in IBS-D. The main pharmacological agents used, **mebeverine**, **hysoscine butylbromide**, and **dicycloverine** (also called dicyclomine), all have some anticholinergic properties. Mebeverine is a direct-acting smooth muscle relaxant and reduces GI motility and spasm. Mebeverine is thought to block voltage operated sodium channels so less influx of sodium occurs, leading to less calcium influx via voltage-gated calcium channels and consequently less contraction of the smooth muscle cells. Hyoscine butylbromide is a salt of hyoscine, an anticholinergic agent. However, it has reduced central effects compared to hyoscine hydrobromide because it does not readily cross the blood–brain barrier. Dicycloverine is a weak anticholinergic agent, and like mebeverine it is thought to have direct action on smooth muscle cells.

Tricyclic antidepressants (TCAs), such as **amitriptyline** and **imipramine** (see also Chapter 19), are used for their analgesic properties. The exact mechanism of action is unclear. However, theories include reduced peripheral pain sensations, as well as modification of pain perceptions in the anterior cingulate cortex, an area of the brain responsible for processing pain and emotions. Importantly, the effects are thought to be independent of their antidepressant effects, as they occur at doses lower than those used in treating depression, and they also act quicker than when used as antidepressants. An additional use of TCAs is as a result of their anticholinergic effects, which results in slowing of gut motility and therefore can be helpful in IBS-D.

Given the important role of serotonin, the selective serotonin reuptake inhibitors (SSRIs, see Chapter 19) have also been investigated in the treatment of the symptoms of IBS. Like TCAs, their exact mechanism of action is uncertain, but not related to their antidepressant effects. They have been shown in a limited number of trials to reduce the GI pain associated with IBS. Because they do not have anticholinergic effects, they do not cause gut slowing and resultant constipation. Both the TCAs and the SSRIs can be useful because they can treat the psychological symptoms of depression, which are often present in patients with IBS.

Peppermint oil is also used in the treatment of IBS. It contains a significant amount of menthol, which is thought to be the main active constituent. Menthol is a calcium channel antagonist and acts on smooth muscle to produce relaxation. In IBS it acts as an antispasmodic by inhibiting the contraction of smooth muscle in the small intestine. Its main side effect is that it also causes relaxation of the lower oesophageal sphincter, resulting in gastro-oesophageal reflux disease (see Chapter 12). To help reduce this it is given as an enteric-coated capsule, so that the peppermint oil passes through the stomach and is delivered to the lower intestine.

SUMMARY OF DRUGS USED FOR DIARRHOEA

Therapeutic class	Drugs	Mechanism of action	Common clinical uses	Comments	Examples of adverse drug reactions
Oral rehydration solution	Powders containing: 	Constituent	Concentration per litre
---	---
Glucose (g)	13.5–20
Sodium (mmol)	60–75
Potassium (mmol)	20		1) Glucose maximizes water absorption in the gut 2) Sodium and potassium replenish lost electrolytes	Diarrhoea	First-line treatment for diarrhoea Rehydration should be rapid	Wrong glucose concentration could aggravate diarrhoea
Opiate derivatives	Diphenoxylate Loperamide Codeine phosphate	Agonistic effect on mu opiate receptors inhibits acetylcholine release, leading to reduced motility, allowing more time for water absorption	Diarrhoea	Prevents flushing out of toxin so could cause more harm than good Loperamide does not cross blood–brain barrier so fewer side effects Loperamide has longer half-life Diphenoxylate is sometimes combined with atropin	Constipation Dry mouth Anticholinergic effects (diphenoxylate/atropine combination) Nausea Vomiting Drowsiness Respiratory depression
Absorbent agents	Kaolin Pectin Charcoal	Absorbs toxins and bacteria in the gut and decrease water loss	Diarrhoea	Best avoided because little evidence for efficacy Could absorb other drugs, reducing absorption	Black stools

SUMMARY OF DRUGS USED FOR CONSTIPATION

Therapeutic class	Drugs	Mechanism of action	Common clinical uses	Comments	Examples of adverse drug reactions
Stool softeners	Docusate	1) Changes surface tension around the stool, allowing water to penetrate it more easily emulsifying it better	Constipation	3–4 days for effect so best as prophylaxis	Virtually none!
Bulk-forming	Psyllium (ispaghula) husks Sterculia Methylcellulose	1) Increases stool mass, which traps water and improves stool consistency. Larger stool then stimulates the peristalsis, causing evacuation 2) Used as substrate by colonic bacteria, which increase in number, increasing softening effect	Constipation	Requires 24-48 hours to take effect Best taken with plenty of water	Bloating Flatulence

Therapeutic class	Drugs	Mechanism of action	Common clinical uses	Comments	Examples of adverse drug reactions
Osmotic	Saline-based magnesium sulphate Sodium phosphate Non-saline Lactulose Polyethylene glycol Sorbitol Glycerine	Large molecular weight or insolubility Increases osmotic pressure within the gut lumen, causing water to be drawn from the blood into the gut lumen, leading to softer stools	Constipation	<24 hours to take effect following oral administration 4–6 hours to take effect following rectal application Safer if taken with plenty of water	Fluid and electrolyte disturbances
Lubricants	Liquid paraffin	Lubricates the stool to make it easier to pass	Constipation	Hardly used anymore due to adverse drug reactions	Aspiration pneumonia
Stimulants	Sennosides Cascara Phenolphthalein Bisacodyl Castor oil	1) Acts on myenteric plexus and exerts direct effect on the intestinal mucosa, resulting in increased peristalsis 2) Affects parasympathetic nerves, resulting in peristalsis. 3) Appears to affect local axon and segmental reflexes in the colon, leading to widespread peristalsis 4) Increases excretion of sodium and water into the gut lumen	Constipation	Effect within 4–6 hours following oral administration Effect within minutes following rectal administration	Cramps Abdominal pain 'Lazy bowel' (a bowel that no longer has peristaltic movement because of over-stimulation)
Naltrexone derivative	Methylnaltrexone alvimopan	Antagonist at mu receptor	Opiate-induced constipation	Not centrally absorbed	Abdominal pain Nausea Flatulence

SUMMARY OF DRUGS USED FOR IRRITABLE BOWEL SYNDROME

Therapeutic class	Drugs	Mechanism of action	Common clinical uses	Comment	Common adverse drug reactions
Prostaglandin derivative	Lubiprostone	Activates ClC-2 chloride channels on the basolateral membrane of colon enterocytes, resulting in secretion of chloride ions into the gut lumen These secretions soften the stool and promote peristalsis	Constipation dominant IBS	Third-line use	Diarrhoea.

Therapeutic class	Drugs	Mechanism of action	Common clinical uses	Comment	Common adverse drug reactions
5-HT$_3$ antagonist	Alosetron	1) Inhibits 5-HT$_3$, resulting in slowing of colonic transit time and enhanced fluid and sodium absorption 2) Also reduces abdominal pain by relaxing the left colon and inhibiting spinal cord reactivity, resulting in reduced perception of bowel distension 3) blockage of 5-HT$_3$ receptors on ELCs results in reduced serotonin release because positive feedback blocked	Diarrhoea-dominant IBS in women	License was withdrawn in USA but later relicensed	Constipation-related complications, including ischaemic colitis
Antispasmodics	Mebeverine	Blocks voltage-operated sodium channels so less influx of sodium occurs, leading to less calcium influx via voltage-gated calcium channels and consequently less contraction of the smooth muscle cells	Abdominal pain associated with IBS	Commonly used. May reduce diarrhoea	Rarely allergic reactions
	Hyoscine butylbromide / Dicycloverine (also called dicyclomine)	Works as anticholinergic agent, having direct effect on smooth muscles			Anticholinergics side effects
	Peppermint oil	A direct-acting smooth muscle relaxant that reduces gastrointestinal motility and spasm	Abdominal pain associated with IBS	Given as enteric-coated preparation so that the peppermint oil passes through the stomach and is delivered to the lower intestine	Heartburn. Perianal itching or burning
Tricyclic antidepressants	Amitriptyline / Imipramine	Theories include: 1) reduced peripheral pain sensations 2) modification of pain perception in the anterior cingulate cortex, an area of the brain responsible for processing pain and emotions	Abdominal pain associated with IBS	Helpful in diarrhoea-dominant IBS. Effect independent of antidepressant effects. Can treat the psychological symptoms of depression, which are often present in patients with IBS	See Chapter 19
Selective serotonin reuptake inhibitors	See Chapter 19	See Chapter 19	Abdominal pain associated with IBS	Can treat the psychological symptoms of depression often present in patients with IBS. Effect independent of antidepressant effects	See Chapter 19

IBS, irritable bowel syndrome; CIC-2, ; 5-HT3, 5-hydroxytryptamine.

WORKBOOK 10
Irritable bowel syndrome, constipation, and diarrhoea

Helen: a simplified case history

Helen finally decides to see her GP about the symptoms she has been experiencing for some time, which have got worse in the last few weeks. Although the symptoms have been a nuisance she has suffered in silence for so long because they change constantly and are not particularly specific.

The main symptoms alternate between constipation and diarrhoea. She also experiences other non-specific symptoms that are just as irritating.

A table of clinical clerking abbreviations is given on page xi.

CLINICAL CLERKING FOR HELEN JONES AT THE GP SURGERY

Age: 39 years

PC: Abdominal pain, constipation, recurrent heartburn, nausea

HPC: She suffers from painful abdominal cramps, accompanied by bloating and abdominal rumblings, which have been recurrent for 9 months. The abdominal pain is more severe after eating or at night. The constipation is intermittent and sometimes she has diarrhoea instead. She also feels an urgent need to defecate several times in the morning, including during and after breakfast. She has also felt lethargic and quite anxious.

PM: Recurrent heartburn, nausea, and constipation

> *Helen has not suffered from any significant illness in her life.*

DH: Gaviscon, senna, and loperamide occasionally as per pharmacist's recommendations

> *Her pharmacist has recommended the above drugs at different periods when she has requested medication for heartburn, constipation, and diarrhoea, respectively.*

SH: Lives with husband; has two daughters. She is under a lot of stress at work currently. She has been working long hours as she is leading a project that has a deadline to meet

Weight: 60 kg

O/Q: Helen reveals that she finds her urinary frequency has increased. She also thinks that she is depressed. Following further questioning, she gives the following positive answers to the GP's questions:

1) The pain of heartburn is relieved by defecation.

2) The pain is associated with a change of frequency and consistency of stool.

3) Her stool frequency keeps changing from more than three motions per day to fewer than three motions per week.

4) The stool form keeps altering from lumpy/hard to loose/watery.

5) The passage of stool alters from having to strain to urgency with feeling of incomplete evacuation.

6) There is a lot of mucous with her stool.

7) She feels bloated and her abdomen feels distended.

She also gives the following negative answers:

1) She has not experienced weight loss.

2) She has not experienced gastrointestinal (GI) bleeding.

3) She is not anaemic.

4) She does not have an abdominal mass.

5) She does not have a family history of GI malignancy or inflammatory bowel disease (IBD).

> Unlike other illnesses, irritable bowel syndrome (IBS) is a functional disorder and the symptoms are not explained by biochemical or structural abnormalities, therefore diagnosis is often difficult.
>
> GPs tend to use the Rome criteria, which involves asking the patient the above questions.
>
> Alarm symptoms that would prompt further investigations to exclude other diseases (e.g. cancer and IBD) include:
>
> - acute or late onset age > 50 years
> - weight loss
> - GI bleeding
> - abdominal mass or fever, or signs of infection.

Helen has no alarm symptoms; if she had she would have to be referred for further investigations.

In the presence of positive symptoms and the absence of alarm symptoms a diagnosis can be made by the GP.

Diagnosis: Irritable bowel syndrome

The GP explains to Helen that her symptoms are consistent with IBS. He says he will prescribe some medication and she should come back in 2 months' time for a follow up.

He also explains to her that some patients get extracolonic features, e.g. low backache, constant lethargy, nausea, urinary symptoms, and gynaecological symptoms. This could explain the increase in the urinary frequency that she has had and her lethargic feeling.

Helen had compared her symptoms with a colleague at work who had ulcerative colitis. She asks the GP if that is similar to what she has. The GP reassures her that the ulcerative colitis is an IBD while she has IBS, and they are different conditions.

Note: The treatment of IBS has been unsatisfactory and few new drugs have been available in the past 20 years, therefore management of IBS usually involves managing triggering factors, and certain pharmacological and dietary approaches. IBS is one of the ailments seen in community pharmacies for which some over-the-counter products can be recommended. It is therefore important to be familiar with the features of this condition and able to recognize 'red flag' or 'danger' features.

Plan:

Commence peppermint oil capsules

Commence mebeverine tablets

The GP explains that peppermint and mebeverine should help alleviate the symptoms of IBS, but she will have to be patient.

1a) Define the term 'functional disorder' and state why IBS is considered a functional disorder and a syndrome.

_____

_____

_____

1b) Explain the difference between IBS and IBD.

_____

_____

_____

2) List the GI and non-GI symptoms of IBS and their probable causes.

_____

_____

_____

3a) What class of drugs are peppermint oil and mebeverine, and how do they act to relieve the symptoms of IBS?

_____

_____

_____

3b) Explain how mebeve rine achieves smooth muscle relaxation.

_____

_____

_____

4a) What is the second subclass of drugs that can be used to relax smooth muscle? Give two examples of this subclass of drugs.

_____

_____

_____

4b) Explain how the drugs listed in question 4a act to relieve the symptoms of IBS.

_____

_____

_____

5) What is thought to be the physiological basis of IBS?

_____

_____

_____

6a) Name four types of foods that are thought to worsen IBS, and what is the constituent that is thought to cause the problem.

_____

_____

_____

6b) Can IBS be cured?

_____

_____

_____

One week later, Helen returns to the GP. She is feeling really down due to the stress of her job and her IBS symptoms, which have not really improved yet. After assessment, the GP decides that she is suffering from clinical depression and prescribes imipramine.

Three weeks later Helen is back at her GP. Her mixed symptoms of constipation and diarrhoea have changed. She is now suffering very badly from constipation. She tells the GP she has less pain.

7a) What is constipation?

_____

_____

_____

7b) What is the likely reason for Helen's symptoms shifting to predominantly constipation? Explain your reasoning.

_____

_____

_____

8) Does imipramine have a role in IBS therapy?

_____

_____

_____

The GP prescribes Helen a drug called sodium docusate and tells her to take one dose twice a day for 5 days only. He explains that this drug acts in two ways to relieve constipation. He explains that the drug is fast acting and should relieve her symptoms quickly.

9a) Describe the mechanism of action of docusate sodium.

_____

_____

_____

The GP also asks Helen to keep a symptom diary listing which food she eats. This will help to rule out any food triggers for the IBS. He instructs Helen that she needs to drink a lot of water and increase her dietary fibre. Finally he prescribed another drug called ispaghula husk (Fybogel®), asking her to drink one sachet twice a day for a week and as required after the constipation improves.

10a) Ispaghula husk is an example of which type of laxative?

10b) Why would increasing fibre content of the diet be expected to relieve constipation?

10c) What are the risks associated with increasing fibre intake for an IBS sufferer?

The GP reassures Helen that the docusate and isphagula should treat her constipation. He says that in the unlikely event that they don't, she should report back as there are other options available.

10d) What are the other options that could be used to treat constipation? Give an example of each type, explain its mode of action and indicate whether it would be useful in the treatment of constipation predominant IBS.

Helen hopes the drugs she has been given work because she wants to go to her friend Sunita's wedding in Hawaii.

Helen's symptoms improve, she feels better in herself and she makes it to the wedding.

As Helen helps Sunita prepare for her wedding she asks her about other treatments for IBS. Sunita tells her that in the USA alosetron and tegaserod are prescribed to treat diarrhoea-predominant and constipation-predominant IBS, respectively, in cases where other treatments have failed. Both these drugs act at 5-HT receptors.

11) Describe the roles of 5-HT in the gut which would make it a target for IBS therapy.

12a) Which 5-HT receptors are targeted by alosetron and tegaserod? Are they agonists or antagonists at these receptors?

12b) Why would targeting these receptors have differing effects on GI tract motility?

13) What group of medicines that act on the 5-HT uptake mechanism could be useful for treating Helen's condition, considering her past medical history? Give three reasons why they would be suitable.

After the wedding, Helen decides to stay on the island for a holiday to get some quiet away from all the stress.

Although the first couple of days are brilliant, this morning she has hardly left the bathroom. She thinks it might be something she ate as she hasn't had any other IBS symptoms since arriving on the island.

Regardless of the cause of her symptoms, it is still very inconvenient.

14a) The definition of diarrhoea is subjective. What questions would you ask to determine if someone did have diarrhoea and what would you expect them to answer if they did?

14b) What is the clinical definition of diarrhoea?

14c) Describe the three main causes/types of diarrhoea.

15) List some of the causes of acute and chronic diarrhoea and indicate what is the most likely cause in Helen's case.

Helen finds a pharmacy in the town centre. She explains her symptoms to the pharmacist. The pharmacist also asks whether she has any other condition or any other medication started recently that could have caused diarrhoea.

He sells her what he says is called oral rehydration sachets (ORS). He asks her to come back if the diarrhoea does not improve in 3 days' time.

16) What are the three main approaches in the treatment of acute diarrhoea?

17a) The pharmacist recommended an ORS. Is that the right decision? Explain your reasoning.

17b) What is the composition of World Health Organization ORS?

17c) What is the rationale for this composition? How does ingestion of an ORS lead to rehydration?

One day later, although Helen has been taking the ORS and drinking as recommended, she still has diarrhoea and the abdominal cramps she experiences are very painful. She decides to go back to the pharmacy.

The pharmacist recommends a drug called loperamide and also sells her charcoal sachets.

18a) What type of drug is loperamide and why would it improve the symptoms of diarrhoea?

18b) Codeine is another opioid agent used to slow the gut. Which is a better choice for the treatment of diarrhoea: loperamide or codeine? Give three reasons to support your choice.

19) Explain the rationale for using adsorbents such as charcoal in the treatment of diarrhoea. What is the current role of adsorbents?

Helen's symptoms improve 2 days later, which is timely because she will not have to worry about diarrhoea on the long flight back home.

Chapter 14
Diabetes mellitus and obesity

Eating, for most people, apart from being life-sustaining is also at the centre of most important events. Then there is comfort eating, a universal activity that arguably has its advantages when done in moderation. Comfort eating can make us feel temporarily happier, safer, and better. So imagine what it must be like not to be allowed to eat a chocolate bar or a slice of cake, or to have to mentally calculate the amount of carbohydrate in most things you eat. Or imagine having to prick your finger to check your blood sugar levels at least once a day because under certain circumstances, if you fail to do so, you might fall into a coma. Andreas is among the more than 200 million diabetic patients worldwide who do not have to imagine this because it is, or will become, their life. Andreas suffers from type 2 diabetes mellitus and now has to inject himself twice a day with insulin as part of the management of his diabetes.

Diabetes mellitus is a chronic progressive disease caused by either a deficiency of or resistance to a hormone called insulin. This differs from the less common diabetes insipidus, which is caused by a deficiency of another hormone called vasopressin. There are two forms of

diabetes mellitus: type 1 and type 2. Type 2 is more common and so fast growing that it has been designated an epidemic by the Centres for Disease Control and Prevention (CDC) in the USA, a highly unusual designation for a non-infective disease. It is also a risk factor for coronary artery disease, which is the most common cause of death in the developed world, therefore the need to correctly diagnose and manage this disease is extremely important.

To complicate his life even further, Andreas, who is already overweight, becomes obese. At his heaviest, he had the most embarrassing experience of his life: he was so fat that he had to pay for two seats to get on a flight because he could not fit into one seat. The incidence of obesity is also growing quickly and, like diabetes, it is a risk factor for coronary artery disease.

This chapter covers the pathophysiology and management of both diabetes and obesity. In this chapter we will look into the molecular and cellular processes influenced by insulin and other hormones involved in diabetes and obesity, and how these processes are modified by pharmacological agents.

14.1 Blood glucose control

After eating, most of the carbohydrate in food is broken down by the body into glucose. Glucose is the main source of 'fuel' for the body and it provides most of the energy the body needs to function. However, in order for the cells to open up and let glucose in, they need insulin which acts as a 'key' to open the doors of the cell.

14.1.1 Where does insulin come from?

Insulin is normally produced by the pancreas, which is located across the upper abdominal wall of the body. About 1–2% of the pancreas is endocrine and produces hormones whilst the rest of it is exocrine and produces enzymes that aid digestion (see Chapter 13). The hormones are produced in the epithelial cells of a collection of tissues called the **islet of Langerhans**. The islets of Langerhans have a variety of different cells with certain key functions:

- β cells of the islet of Langerhans produce and secrete insulin, which plays a central role in glucose metabolism
- β cells also secrete **amylin**, a polypeptide that works synergistically with insulin
- α cells secrete **glucagon**, a hormone which opposes the action of insulin
- δ cells secrete **somatostatin** (see Chapter 13)
- PP cells (also called F cells) secrete pancreatic polypeptide, which regulates the action of the pancreas.

In order for insulin to be released by the pancreas, glucose must be present. Glucose is produced from carbohydrate-containing food after it has been broken down in the gastrointestinal (GI) tract. The glucose is absorbed from the GI tract into the blood. The blood transports the glucose to the β-cells of the pancreas, where a series of processes ultimately lead to insulin release. Box 14.1 illustrates these processes

14.1.2 Production of insulin

Insulin is a protein consisting of two amino acid chains called the A chain and the B chain. The A chain contains 21 amino acids, whilst the B chain contains 30. Each chain is linked by disulphide bridges. Insulin is synthesized in the endoplasmic reticulum of the β-cells as preproinsulin. This is carried to the Golgi apparatus, where it is broken down to proinsulin and then to insulin. In addition to insulin, a molecule called C-peptide is also produced by hydrolysis, which is stored with insulin, in equimolar concentrations, in granules ready for release. The role of C-peptide is unclear, but it may be responsible for preventing some of the complications of diabetes such as diabetic neuropathy and nephropathy. The mechanism leading to the release is illustrated in Box 14.1.

14.1.3 The actions of insulin

As well as regulating the metabolism of carbohydrate, insulin also plays a very important role in the metabolism of protein and fats. The mechanism of action of insulin in the metabolism of these substances varies from organ to organ. The ultimate effect of all these functions of insulin

is the storage of glucose, amino acid, and fat in the form of glycogen, protein, and fat, which all serve as fuel for the body.

14.1.4 Insulin and carbohydrate metabolism

Insulin increases the uptake of glucose into the muscle and adipose tissue. The initial step of the mechanism leading to this increased uptake is the stimulation of the insulin receptor. This receptor is a tyrosine kinase receptor with four subunits (two α and two β). Stimulation of the receptor leads to phosphorylation of intracellular molecules, which are involved in signalling. These molecules activate kinases and phosphatases, which in turn recruit glucose transporters like Glut4 and transport them to the surface of the cell. The transporters open up and allow glucose to enter the muscle or adipose tissue from the blood, resulting in a drop in the blood glucose concentration. The occupied insulin receptors internalize and are stored in vesicles. This results in down-regulation of the activity of insulin (i.e. it stops the effect on the cell). These vesicles are then broken down by liposomes and the receptors are returned to the plasma membrane.

The absorbed glucose is stored in a polysaccharide (polymer) called **glycogen**. In the liver, insulin increases the quantity of glycogen through various mechanisms. These include prevention of the breakdown of glycogen in a process called **glycogenolysis**, and the prevention of **gluconeogenesis** (the synthesis of glucose from sources that are not carbohydrate). Insulin also increases the use of glucose (**glycolysis**) in the liver.

Insulin and fat metabolism

Insulin increases fatty acid and triglyceride stores in the liver and adipose tissue by preventing the breakdown of fats (lipolysis). The mechanism of lipolysis involves dephosphorylation of enzymes that break down fat called lipases. Insulin also prevents the breakdown of fat by adrenaline, glycogen, and growth hormones.

Insulin and protein metabolism

Protein concentration in muscle is increased by insulin through the stimulation of amino acid uptake. This amino acid uptake leads to increased production of protein. Insulin also stops the breakdown of protein in the liver.

Box 14.1

Insulin release in β-cells

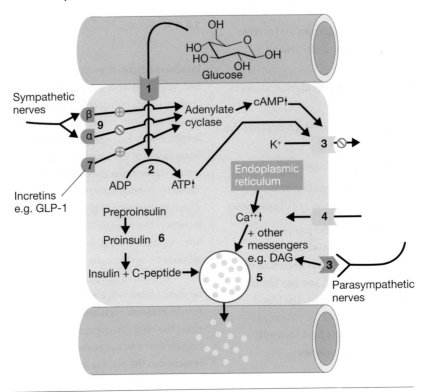

Figure a

1. Glucose enters the b-cells from the bloodstream through GLUT-2, a specific membrane transporter.

2. Glucose is metabolized to pyruvate, which through the tricarbocylic acid cycle in the mitochondria increases production of ATP in the cell.

3. The increase in ATP closes the K_{ATP} channels, which transports K+. **This is the site of action of sulphonylureas and repeglanide**.

4. The shutting of the K_{ATP} channels causes depolarization and opening of voltage-dependent calcium channels. This leads to an influx of calcium as well as the release of calcium from the endoplasmic reticulum.

5. Increase in intracellular calcium causes release of insulin. However, other molecules must be present, including diacylglycerol (DAG) and non-esterified arachidonic acid.

6. Insulin starts as preproinsulin produced in the endoplasmic reticulum. This is cleaved to proinsulin, and then to insulin plus the fragment C-peptide in the golgi body. Both the insulin and C-peptide are collected in granules in the cell prior to release.

7. Incretins are gastrointestinal (GI) tract hormones that promote insulin release. The main incretins are glucagon-like peptide 1 (GLP-1) and glucose-dependent insulinotropic peptide (GIP, also known as gastric inhibitory polypeptide). They attach to receptors on the β-cells and promote insulin release through adenylate cyclase, which increases cAMP and closes the K_{ATP} channels. **This is the site of action for exenatide and sitagliptin**.

8. Innervation from the parasympathetic nervous system through muscarinic receptors leads to an increase in DAG, resulting in insulin release.

Other actions of insulin

Insulin causes cells to take up potassium, and this is used in the treatment of hyperkalemia. It also causes increased secretion of acid in parietal cells and relaxation of arterial smooth muscle tone.

The main actions of insulin are summarized in Table 14.1.

Table 14.1 The action of insulin in carbohydrate, fat, and protein metabolism

Type/organ	Carbohydrate metabolism	Fat metabolism	Protein metabolism
Liver cells	↑ gluconeogenesis (synthesis of glucose from non-glucose) ↓ glycogenolysis (breakdown of glycogen) ↑ glycolysis (degradation of glucose to pyruvate) ↑ glycogenesis (glycogen synthesis)	↑ lipogenesis (simple sugars converted to fatty acids) ↓ lipolysis (breakdown of fat cells)	↓ protein catabolism
Adipose tissue	↑ glucose uptake ↑ glycerol synthesis	↑ triglyceride synthesis ↑ fatty acid synthesis ↓ lipolysis	
Muscle	↑ glucose uptake ↑ glycolysis ↑ glycogenesis		↑ amino acid uptake ↑ protein synthesis

14.2 Diabetes mellitus

Diabetes mellitus is the most common and arguably the most important metabolic disorder with a significantly increased mortality rate for sufferers compared to non-sufferers. It is more common than diabetes insipidus, which is a different disease and not covered in this textbook. Diabetes mellitus is caused by either absolute or relative insulin deficiency (reduced production or resistance of receptors), and is divided into types I and type II. Absolute insulin deficiency, which is present in type I diabetes, is when the β-cells of the pancreas have been destroyed and produce no insulin at all. Type I diabetes was formally known as insulin-dependent diabetes.

In type II diabetes a relative insulin deficiency is present whereby either the pancreas produces too little insulin to meet the body's demands, or the insulin receptors on the target organs are too few or absent. Type II diabetes mellitus was formally known as non-insulin-dependent diabetes. However, given that a significant number of patients with type II diabetes require insulin, this terminology is no longer valid.

Table 14.2 Features of diabetes mellitus

Characteristic	Type I diabetes	Type II diabetes
Common/older names	Juvenile onset diabetes/insulin-dependent diabetes	Adult onset diabetes/non-insulin-dependent diabetes
Initial treatment	Insulin	Diet, followed by oral medication
Insulin treatment	Compulsory	Only needed if oral medication fails
Age of diagnosis	Childhood or adolescent; usually under 30	Commonly mid 30s and over
Body mass index at diagnosis	Below ideal level	Above ideal level
Cause: • genetic predisposition	Moderate/ present	Strong
• autoimmune destruction/presence of islet antibodies	Present	Absent
• environmental causes (e.g. viruses, bacteria, toxin)	Present	Absent
Insulin production	Absent	Variable
Prevalence	5–20% of all diabetes	80–95% of all diabetes
Pathogenesis	Islet cell antibodies causing destruction	Combination of • reduced insulin secretion • increased resistance to insulin due to absent or insufficient insulin receptors • increased production of glucose

Table 14.2 summarizes other key differences between the two types of diabetes.

It is estimated that approximately 5% (1 in 20) of the population in most western countries suffers from diabetes, and more than 80% of patients with diabetes suffer from type II diabetes. With the growing obesity rates, these numbers are likely to rise significantly.

> Andreas, our patient, is suffering from type II diabetes. Andreas is very overweight, which is a significant contributor to the development of diabetes.

14.2.1 Type I diabetes mellitus

In type I diabetes, the pancreas produces no insulin at all and sufferers need insulin to survive. The cause of this is complete destruction of the β-cells of the pancreas. This destruction could either be caused by viral invasion, bacteria, or toxin exposure, or by antibodies produced by the body itself (autoimmune antibodies). These autoimmune antibodies trigger the autoimmune destruction of the Langerhans cells in genetically predisposed individuals. Without externally administered insulin, patients will die either from complications of

hyperglycaemia or from diabetic ketoacidosis. The destruction period ranges from weeks to years, with absolute destruction and insulin deficiency resulting within 8 to 10 years.

Patients are usually young at diagnosis and tend to be undernourished. They exhibit classic symptoms, such as increased thirst (polydipsia), increased hunger (polyphagia), and increased urinary frequency (polyuria). The genetic predisposition of type I diabetes is moderate, which means most patients do not inherit it from their parents.

14.2.2 Type II diabetes

Unlike type I diabetes, type II has a strong genetic predisposition. Age and ethnicity are two other factors that influence the prevalence of type II diabetes, with a higher incidence of diabetes being reported in older and non-Caucasians patients. People with type II diabetes are quite often obese, and have a combination of impaired functioning of their Langerhans cells, insulin resistance, and increased production of glucose by the liver.

> Andreas has many of these features.

Impaired insulin secretion following glucose ingestion develops progressively over time as the Langerhans cells slowly lose their responsiveness to glucose. Insulin resistance occurs most commonly in the skeletal muscle.

The theory is that a combination of decreased number of insulin receptors, decreased affinity of the receptors to insulin, and defects in the signalling pathways results in inadequate response to insulin.

14.3 Complications of diabetes

Untreated diabetes results in several complications that are the main cause of mortality and morbidity in sufferers. Management of these diabetic complications also accounts for most of the high cost of diabetes. The most common complications can be grouped into acute complications and long-term complications.

Acute complications are more common in type I diabetes and are often metabolic emergencies that could be life threatening.

14.3.1 Acute complications of diabetes

Diabetic ketoacidosis (DKA) is caused by increased breakdown of fat (lipolysis) to acetyl Co-A, which occurs in the absence of insulin in cells dependent on insulin for glucose uptake, such as muscle and adipose tissue. In serious cases, this is transformed in the absence of oxygen (and aerobic carbohydrate metabolism) to acetoacetate, acetone (a ketone), and β-hydroxybutyrate. The β-hydroxybutyrate is the cause of the acidosis, while the acetone accounts for the patient's breath smelling of ketones. DKA is an emergency that has a high mortality rate, and the patient needs to be admitted to hospital.

14.3.2 Long-term complications of diabetes

Sustained hyperglycaemia can cause damage to a number of organs and cells through the following mechanisms:

- non-enzymatic glycosylation of proteins and lipids
- forcing glucose through the polyol pathway
- activation of protein kinase C.

The presence of elevated glucose causes glucose to become bound to fats and proteins (called glycosylation). This can occur in red blood cells, interstitial tissues, and blood vessels, and the glycosylated proteins and fats are called advanced glycosylation end products (AGEs). The AGEs can lead to thickening of blood vessel walls, release of cytokines from inflammatory cells, inactivation of nitric

oxide (leading to loss of vasodilation), and promotion of platelet aggregation.

The polyol pathway is an alternative metabolic pathway for glucose in cells that don't require insulin for glucose transport. These include the kidney, red blood cells, blood vessels, and nerves. In the polyol pathway glucose is metabolized to sorbitol, which is slowly converted to fructose. The accumulation of sorbitol causes cell injury by drawing water into the cells due to increased osmotic pressure.

Protein kinase C is activated in tissues in the presence of hyperglycaemia. This can lead to production of cytokines, cell proliferation, and increased vascular permeability.

Thus, over time the hyperglycaemia in diabetes can result in:

- damaged nerves (diabetic neuropathy)
- damaged eyes (diabetic retinopathy)
- damage to the kidneys
- damage to small and large blood vessels.

Diabetic neuropathy can lead to loss of sensations, particularly in the peripheries (e.g. fingers and toes/feet). This means patients may not feel things that may damage their extremities (e.g. standing on sharp objects) and this can lead to untreated injuries. Sometimes patients with diabetic neuropathy experience profound pain and tingling in the area of the damaged nerves. The pain usually does not respond to conventional analgesia (see Chapter 20 for information on treating neuropathic pain).

Diabetic macrovascular disease (damaged large vessel) can lead to heart disease, stroke, and kidney disease. The vascular damage can also lead to impotence in males (because of decreased blood flow to the penis), and to ulcers on the legs and feet (compounded by the lack of sensation). Microvascular (small blood vessel) damage in the eye leads to diabetic retinopathy. This leads to vision loss and eventually blindness.

Andreas presents with one the major complications of untreated diabetes: a foot ulcer.

14.4 Diagnosis of diabetes

Patients with type II diabetes may show few early signs or symptoms, therefore blood glucose level (BGL) measurements are the most important tools used to diagnose and monitor the progression of diabetes. Diabetes is usually diagnosed when BGLs are >7.0 mmol/L for fasting patients and >11 mmol/L when taken at random. However, lower levels (e.g. random levels between 5.6 and 11 mmol/L) may not exclude diabetes and could indicate reduced glucose tolerance, which is a prediabetic state. In these cases a patient can undergo a glucose tolerance test, during which the patient takes a measured amount of glucose and their BGL is carefully monitored.

Persistent high BGLs lead to increased glycation, whereby covalent bonds are formed between glucose and proteins in the body. One such protein is haemoglobin. The glycated products survive for several weeks in the body. Elevated **glycated haemoglobin levels (HbA1c)** is the key test used to monitor long-term glycaemia control in diagnosed patients. It gives a picture of how much glucose has been in the blood for the last few months and is extremely useful to check compliance and long-term response to treatment.

> Andreas' diabetic treatment was stepped up when his HbA1c level increased above the recommended reference of 6.5–7.5. This was proof that even prior to his admission into hospital there had been too much glucose in his blood.

Sometimes the glucose that has concentrated in the blood overflows into the urine via the kidney (called **glycosuria**). In the dim past, urine tasting was used to diagnose diabetes. The urine of a patient thought to have diabetes was tasted and if it was sweet, the patient was diagnosed with diabetes. Today we can measure glucose in the urine using a simple dipstick that changes colour in response to level of glucose in the urine. However, blood glucose monitoring is becoming easier, is more accurate, and has now largely replaced urine testing.

14.5 Management of diabetes mellitus

Management of diabetes is quite complex and involves combining diet modifications with pharmacological agents. The two main groups of pharmacological agent used are insulin and the oral antidiabetic drugs. The use of insulin is compulsory for type I diabetes where the benefits of the using insulin to tightly control blood sugar levels have been shown to improve mortality and morbidity.

Oral antidiabetic drugs are usually the drugs of choice in the initial stages of type II diabetes. Insulin is usually required during the later stages when pancreatic insulin stores have become completely depleted.

Therapy for diabetes is monitored using measures of blood glucose (BGL and HbA1c). While there is still some controversy about what the target levels for patients with diabetes should be, the consensus now is that the tighter (i.e. closer to normal blood glucose) the control the better the long-term outcomes. This means usually aiming for a BGL of less than 6 mmol/L and an HbA1c of less than 7% (although less then 6.5% is recommended by some).

14.5.1 Insulin treatment

Many years ago, insulin isolated from beef (bovine) or pork (porcine) were the only forms of exogenous insulin. The porcine insulin bares the most similarity to the human insulin with a difference of only one amino acid. With advance in technology, genetically altered *Escherichia coli* is used to produce human insulin and this has almost completely replaced bovine and porcine insulin.

Insulin cannot be taken orally because it is destroyed by enzymes in the GI tract and therefore it must be given by injection. The most common method of administration is by subcutaneous injection, administered by the patient; the intravenous and intramuscular routes are used in an emergency.

Insulin preparations fall into three main groups:

- short-acting
- rapid-acting
- intermediate/long-acting.

Short-acting insulin preparations

Short-acting insulin preparations contain soluble insulin mixed with zinc (e.g. Actrapid®). This form of insulin is usually administered subcutaneously approximately 30–45 minutes before meal times or intravenously for urgent lowering of blood glucose. An insulin pump, which delivers this form of insulin through a subcutaneous needle, can also be used for patients who have difficulty controlling their blood sugar levels.

> Andreas received Actrapid® by intravenous injection on admission to quickly lower his extremely elevated blood glucose levels.

Rapid-acting insulin preparations

Two new short-acting insulins have been recently developed. They are recombinant human insulin analogues in which one amino acid is switched through genetic engineering. One is **insulin aspart**, which has a substitution of the amino acid proline by aspartic acid at position 28 on the B-chain. The other is **insulin lispro**, which has inversion of the amino acids proline and lysine at positions 28 and 29 on the B-chain.

 Ordinary soluble insulin, like Actrapid®, forms into hexamers, which must break apart into monomers to be absorbed into the bloodstream. The modifications in the side chains with insulin aspart and insulin lispro means they remain as monomers and can be absorbed quickly (Figure 14.1).

This rapid absorption means insulin aspart and insulin lispro can be given just before eating. This reduces the risks of patients forgetting to eat and suffering **hypoglycaemia** (low blood sugar levels).

Intermediate and long-acting insulins

These insulin formulations contain a mixture of insulin and other substances that modify the pharmacokinetics of the insulin. These substances are protamine, cationic proteins, or zinc ions. The addition of these results in a gradual onset and long duration of action of the insulin formulation. The onset of action of intermediate insulin could be up to 2 hours and the effect could last for up to 20 hours. The onset of action of long-acting insulin is within 4 hours, lasting up to 36 hours.

Insulin glargine and **insulin detemir** are new long-acting insulins that do not use the addition of substances such as protamine or zinc to get a prolonged action. Insulin detamir has a 14-carbon fatty acid (myristic acid) bound to the B-side chain. This addition causes it to become bound to albumin, from which it only slowly dissociates, giving it a prolonged effect. Insulin glargine, which also has changes in the side chains, is less soluble at physiological pH than ordinary insulin. Thus, when it is injected it forms microprecipitates, from which the insulin is only slowly released. This gives it the flattest (peakless) profile of all the insulins. While insulin detemir is given once or twice a day, usually insulin glargine is only given once daily, in the evening.

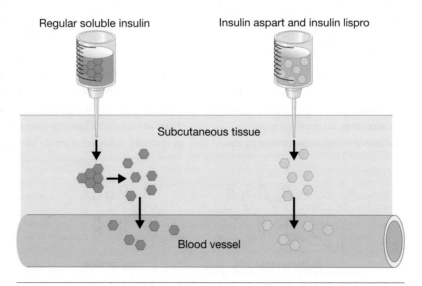

Regular soluble insulin

Insulin aspart and insulin lispro

Subcutaneous tissue

Blood vessel

Figure 14.1 Absorption of regular insulin vs insulin aspart and insulin lispro.

Adverse effects of insulin

The two most common adverse effects are local injection site effects and hypoglycaemia.

Local effects. The local effects are caused by repeated injections in the same spot and can lead to **lipodystrophy** (abnormal changes in fat distribution) and scarring. While this is not life threatening, it can look unsightly and can change how the insulin is absorbed. To avoid this, patients are instructed to rotate the injection sites.

Hypoglycaemia is a potentially life-threatening side effect. It can occur if too much insulin is given or if the patient changes their eating or exercise patterns. For mild/moderate cases drinking a sweet drink or sucking on a barley sugar will suffice. In severe cases the patient may become unconscious. This is a medical emergency. If this occurs parenteral therapy with glucagon or intravenous glucose is required.

14.5.2 Glucagon

Glucagon is a polypeptide with a similar structure to GI hormones such as gastric inhibitory polypeptide (GIP) and vasoactive intestinal peptide (VIP). It is secreted by the α-cells of the islets of Langerhans, and has the opposite effect to insulin. It attaches to a specific G-protein-coupled receptor on cells, and stimulates adenylate cyclase (a similar effect to β-adrenergic stimulation by adrenaline). It promotes glycogen breakdown, inhibits glycogen synthesis, and promotes gluconeogenesis, resulting in the release of glucose into the bloodstream. It can be given in an emergency by intramuscular or subcutaneous injection. This means that it can be administered by a carer or ambulance personnel to an unconscious patient.

14.5.3 Oral antidiabetic drugs

These have a wide-ranging mechanism of actions aimed at increasing insulin secretion, increasing tissue sensitivity to insulin, increasing glucose uptake by the muscles, or reducing glucose absorption from the gut. These agents are mostly given orally (except for exenatide) and are used only for the management of type II diabetes. Box 14.2 details the sequence in which treatment is initiated in a typical type II diabetic patient.

Sulphonylureas

Sulphonylureas are known as **secretagogues** (agents that cause the secretion of insulin). Thus, you must have some functioning B-cells for them to work. These agents are structurally related to sulphonamide antibiotics (e.g. sulfamethoxazole, see Figure 14.2) and were discovered by accident.

The main sulphonylureas used are:

- chlorpropamide
- tolbutamide
- glibenclamide
- glimepiride
- gliclazide
- glipizide.

Sulphonylureas work by attaching to a receptor on the ATP-dependent potassium channels on the β-cells in the pancreas. This causes blockage of the K_{ATP} channel, resulting in depolarization, opening of the calcium channels, influx of calcium into the β-cell, and release of insulin (Box 14.1).

Hypoglycaemia is the most common adverse effect. The risk is related to duration of action, with **chlorpropamide** having the greatest risk and **glipizide/gliclazide** having the least risk (Table 14.3).

Another significant adverse effect of sulphonylureas is weight gain. Given that obesity is a common characteristic of many people with type II diabetes, these drugs are not first choice in patients who are already overweight. Chlorpropamide has more adverse effects

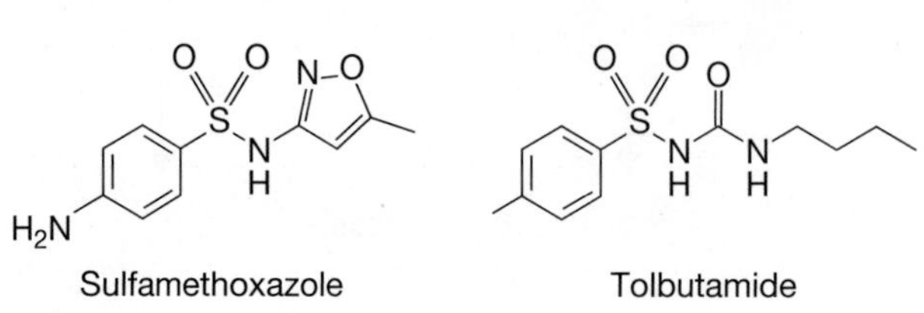

Figure 14.2 Comparison of a sulphonamide antibiotic and a sulphonylurea.

Box 14.2

Approaches to the management of type II diabetes

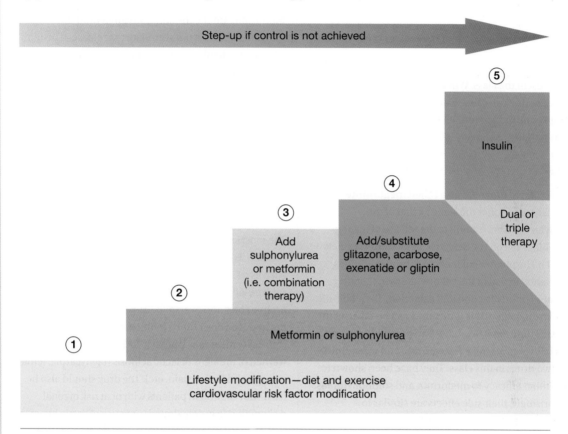

Figure b

1. Diet and exercise are a fundamental part of the management of type II diabetes. Pharmacological treatment cannot replace these treatments. Consideration should also be given to other cardiovascular risk factors, such as hypertension and hyperlipidemia.

2. Initial treatment is with either metformin or a sulphonylurea. For overweight patients the best choice is metformin. In the elderly, if metformin is not tolerated, repeglanide may be a better choice than a sulphonylurea.

3. Combination of metformin with a sulphonylurea is the next step; there is no logic in combining two sulphonylureas.

4. If patients cannot tolerate the combination of sulphonylurea and metformin, then the addition of a glitazone, exenatide, acarbose, or gliptin to either may be appropriate.

5. Triple therapy is controversial and may lead to increased risk of hypoglycaemia. Early addition (within a few months) of insulin to patients who are poorly controlled on dual or triple therapy has been shown to improve outcomes in type II diabetes. It can be given as a single daily dose of long-acting insulin, usually in the evening.

Table 14.3 Hypoglycaemic risk with sulphonylureas

Highest risk	Intermediate risk	Lowest risk
Chlorpropamide Glibenclamide	Glimepiride	Glipizide Gliclazide[a]

[a] Gliclazide only low risk in the immediate-release formulation; the sustained-release formulation has an intermediate risk of hypoglycaemia.

than the rest in the class. When taken with alcohol, chlorpropamide can cause a disulfiram-type reaction (see metronidazole in Chapter 21). For these reasons chlorpropamide has largely fallen out of favour.

Non–sulfonylurea insulin secretagogues

This new class of drugs are also called **meglitinides**. Their mechanism of action is the same as that of the sulphonylureas. They stimulate the release of insulin through blockage of ATP-sensitive potassium channels (Box 14.1). The pharmacokinetics of the meglitinides differs slightly to that of the sulfonylureas in that they have a rapid onset of action and excretion. Their half-life is 1.5 h. The benefit of this is that they can be taken with meals, affording more flexibility and possibly reducing the risk of hypoglycaemia. **Nateglinide** and **repaglinide** are the two drugs in this class. They have been shown to have a similar efficacy to metformin and sulphonylureas. Not surprisingly, their side effects are similar to sulphonylureas. However, they may cause less weight gain than sulphonylureas.

Biguanides

Metformin is currently the only surviving member of the biguanides. **Phenformin** is an older biguanide that was withdrawn after it was shown to cause fatal lactic acidosis. Although the mechanism of action of metformin is not quite fully understood, it is thought to reduce blood glucose levels through a combination of the following:

- reducing hepatic glucose production through inhibition of gluconeogenesis
- increasing cell sensitivity to insulin in the periphery, leading to increased uptake of glucose
- lowering free fatty acid levels in plasma and thereby oxidation, which could help reduce gluconeogenesis in the liver
- lowering LDL and triglyceride levels, and increasing HDL levels
- reducing glucose absorption from the GI tract.

Some of these effects are thought to be due to metformin stimulating AMP-activated protein kinase (AMPK), an enzyme involved in insulin signalling and hepatic glucose production.

Metformin, unlike the sulphonylureas and the meglitinides, does not stimulate the release of insulin, which is probably the reason for its very low risk of hypoglycaemia (when used alone). It also does not produce weight gain, probably because it causes gastric upset (anorexia and nausea). This makes it the drug of choice for overweight patients, and it is becoming the first-line therapy for most patients with type II diabetes.

> Our patient Andreas was initially commenced on gliclazide, which was later changed to metformin following the pharmacist's recommendation.

The most significant side effect of metformin is lactic acidosis. Lactic acidosis occurs in poorly perfused tissues, such as a kidney in renal impairment. In the absence of oxygen, lactate is produced during glycolysis and this accumulates and overspills, causing a drop in pH levels in the body (acidosis) and resulting in severe consequences (mortality rates can approach 70%). Patients need to be warned of the signs of lactic acidosis (tachycardia, lethargy, cramps, abdominal pain, etc). The drug should also be used with caution in patients with or at risk of renal dysfunction (e.g. dehydrated) or at risk of tissue hypoxia (e.g. a myocardial infarction or pulmonary embolism). The gastric side effects are best managed by taking the tablets with food and slowly increasing the dose.

> Andreas' metformin dose was reduced and he was advised to take his tablets with food when he complained of bloating. These measures were effective in reducing the GI effects he was experiencing.

Thiazolindiones

Similar to the sulphonylureas, the thiazolindiones (also called glitazones) were discovered by accident while trialling a new lipid-lowering drug. The first two glitazones (**troglitazone** and **ciglitazone**) unfortunately caused fatal hepatotoxicity and were withdrawn. The current glitazones (**pioglitazone** and **rosiglitazone**) are effective at lowering blood glucose levels with a much-reduced risk of hepatotoxicity.

Their mechanism of action is different from the other antidiabetic drugs. They are selective agonists at the peroxisome proliferator activator receptor gamma (PPARγ).

The PPARγ receptors are similar to steroid and thyroid receptors, and belong to the family of nuclear receptors. Following binding to the PPARγ receptor (which also becomes bound to a retinoid X receptor once activated), the glitazone–receptor complex moves to the cell nucleus and activates DNA to induce gene transcription. This has a number of effects in adipocytes (fat cells). First, there is an increase in lipoprotein lipase, fatty acid transporter protein, and glycerol kinase, among other enzymes and transporters. The effect of this on peripheral and subcutaneous fat cells is to cause them to store fatty acids, resulting in a reduction in circulating fatty acids, and reduced levels of triglycerides in liver and muscles. Second, it affects the release of hormones from adipocytes called 'adipokines'. A summary of the effects of some of these is found in Table 14.4.

The net effect is reduced insulin resistance in adipose tissue, muscle, and liver, increased use of glucose, and decreased glucose release by the liver.

The efficacy of glitazones is less than that of metformin, therefore they are recommended to be used in combination as either dual or triple therapy with metformin and sulphonylureas.

The glitazones have a number of important adverse reactions. The influence on fat cell proliferation and differentiation leads, unsurprisingly, to weight gain. However, the fat distribution favours peripheral fat over visceral fat (which is more harmful). They also affect amiloride-sensitive sodium channels in the distal collecting ducts. The activation of PPARγ results in sodium reabsorption, leading to water retention. This can result in oedema and precipitation of heart failure.

A serious, but rare, side effect is the potential to increase cardiovascular events such as myocardial infarctions. To date the association with cardiovascular events has been shown for rosiglitazone and not pioglitazone. However, more evidence is required to establish whether this is a class effect or not. Given the effects on the liver, and the fact that the two earlier glitazones were withdrawn because of hepatic toxicity, it is important to monitor liver function while on these drugs.

α-glucosidase inhibitors

To absorb sugars into the bloodstream the carbohydrates in our diets must be broken down into monosaccharide. While enzymes in the gut convert carbohydrates to oligosaccharides (usually containing three to ten sugars) and disaccharides (containing two sugars), these are further broken down in the brush border of the small intestines by the enzyme α glucosidase to monosaccharides. **Acarbose** is a reversible competitive inhibitor of this enzyme. By blocking α glucosidase it delays the absorption of glucose, resulting in a reduction in the post-prandial glucose levels, as well as a reduction in fluctuations of blood glucose levels that occur during the course of the day. It is given orally three times a day and the dose needs to be gradually increased to avoid GI complications. The main GI effects are due to unabsorbed sugars acting as substrates for GI bacteria, leading to bloating and flatulence (as gas is a by-product) and having an osmotic effect resulting in diarrhoea (see Chapter 13).

The overall effect of acarbose is modest and it is only used in combination with other oral antidiabetic medications.

Table 14.4 Effects of thiazolindiones on adipokines

Hormone	Effect of thiazolindiones	Effects in body of the hormone in relation to diabetes
Adiponectin	↑ production	Increases fat oxidation Improves insulin sensitivity Increases glucose uptake Protects the endothelium (anti-athrogenic) Anti-inflammatory
Leptin	Uncertain	Suppresses appetite Modification of inflammation Increases angiogenesis
Resistin	↓ production	Increases inflammatory cytokine production Increases insulin resistance?
TNF-α	↓ production	Promotes inflammation Phosphorylates the insulin receptor substrate-1, leading to impaired insulin signalling

TNF-α, tumour necrosis factor-alpha.

Dipeptidyl peptidase 4 inhibitors (gliptins)

Incretins are hormones produced by the GI tract. They include glucagon-like peptide-1 (GLP-1) and glucose-dependent insulinotropic polypeptide (GIP, also known as gastric inhibitory polypeptide). They are released in response to food in the GI tract and they act as an 'early warning' of impending glucose load into the bloodstream. GLP-1 has a direct effect on the pancreas, causing the release of insulin from B-cells, and inhibition of glucagon release by A-cells. The effect on B-cells is mediated through the GLP-1 receptor, which is a G-protein coupled receptor that stimulates adenylate cyclase. Other effects of GLP-1 include pancreatic B-cell proliferation, expression of the glucose transporter 2 (GLUT2) and glucokinase genes, reduced gastric emptying, and reduced appetite.

GIP was thought to primarily act by slowing gut motility and reducing the secretion of acid (hence the name gastric inhibitory polypeptide). However, now it is thought to act, like GLP-1, to promote the release of insulin from B-cells in the presence of glucose. GIP also affects adipocytes by stimulating lipoprotein lipase activity, causing increased uptake of fatty acids. While it promotes B-cell proliferation like GLP-1, it does not affect glucagon release.

The incretins have a very short duration of action in the body. For example, the half-life of GLP-1 is only 2 min. The enzyme responsible for destroying circulating incretins is called dipeptidyl peptidase 4 (DPP-4). Thus, this has become one of the latest targets for antidiabetic therapy.

Sitagliptin and **vildagliptin** are in a new class (sometimes called the 'gliptins') of drugs that competitively inhibit the DPP-4, therefore they prolong the action of the endogenous incretins. Sitagliptin has been on the market the longest and is given as an oral tablet once a day. Although there is some data supporting its use as monotherapy, the best evidence has come from trials combining it with other oral hypoglycaemic drugs. Sitagliptin is generally well tolerated, with hypoglycaemia (mainly when used with a sulphonylurea) being the major side effect. However, this class of drug is very new and long-term safety data are not available. One advantage is that there is no apparent weight gain, unlike the glitazones and sulphonylureas.

Incretin mimetics

As described above, incretins play an important role in insulin secretion. Apart from drugs to prolong the action of endogenous incretins, new drugs have been developed that mimic the endogenous incretins (incretin mimetics) and **exenatide** was the first to be marketed.

Exenatide is a synthetic form of exenedin-4, a naturally occurring analogue of GLP-1. Unlike GLP-1, it is not degraded by DPP-4 and therefore has a longer half-life (4 h) and high affinity for the receptor. Like the gliptins, there are only limited data for its use as monotherapy and it is currently recommended to be used in combination with metformin or a sulphonylurea. It is given by subcutaneous injection 1 h before eating, once or twice a day. Like the gliptins, hypoglycaemia is unlikely (unless combined with a sulphonylurea) and weight gain is not a problem. Exenatide is associated with a high incidence of GI upset (up to 50% of patients). However, this usually subsides over time. Because it slows GI emptying, the absorption of some drugs (e.g. some antibiotics) may be affected.

> Andreas was put on this drug after he gained weight on insulin.

14.6 Managing other cardiovascular risk factors

Although keeping the BGLs within the recommended target range will significantly reduce morbidity and mortality in diabetes, reducing other risk factors related to cardiovascular disease in diabetic patients leads to an even greater reduction in mortality and morbidity. There is evidence to show that keeping blood pressure below target in diabetic patients has a greater effect on outcome than maintaining BGLs within target range.

The risk factors that must be managed in diabetes are hyperlipidaemia, obesity, smoking, and hypertension.

The drugs used to manage these other risk factors are covered extensively in other chapters:

- lipid lowering drugs (Chapter 6)
- antiplatelet drugs (Chapter 4)
- antihypertensive drugs (Chapter 5)
- angiotensin receptor blockers (Chapter 5).

> All these other risk factors were initially overlooked in Andreas. However, prior to discharge, he was commenced on simvastatin, a lipid-lowering drug, as well as aspirin, an antiplatelet drug.

14.7 Obesity

Obesity is a medical condition in which the patient has accumulated so much body fat that it could have a negative effect on their health. The cause of obesity is usually a combination of excessive eating resulting from poor appetite control and a decreased metabolism. Basically, obese individuals consume more calories than they burn.

Around the world obesity is reaching epidemic proportions. Currently 1 in 4 adults and 1 in 3 children in the UK are obese. Similar numbers are reported in Australia and Canada, while in the USA over 1 in 3 of the adult population is obese.

Currently the best way to diagnose obesity is by measuring the body mass index (BMI) of the individual. The BMI is the weight divided by the square of the height. The formulas below are used to calculate BMI:

$$\text{BMI (kg/m}^2) = \frac{\text{Weight in pounds}}{(\text{Height in inches})^2} \times 703$$

$$\text{BMI (kg/m}^2) = \frac{\text{Weight in kg}}{(\text{Height in metres})^2}$$

The BMI level is a useful tool to help choose the right treatment for obesity. It is also used to monitor how effective the treatment is. However, as BMI may not accurately reflect abdominal obesity, an important risk factor, often waist measurements are used in combination with the BMI.

14.7.1 When should obesity be treated?

The factors to be considered before the decision is taken to initiate weight loss treatment in obesity are BMI, waist circumference, and other risk factors of cardiovascular disease that individuals might have. Most guidelines recommend that weight loss treatment should be initiated in patients who are overweight and have an increased waist circumference as well as two or more cardiovascular risk factors.

Table 14.5 summarizes the recommendations from the National Institute of Clinical Excellence (NICE) in the UK on when and how to initiate treatment for obese patients.

> Andreas was prescribed medication to treat his obesity because not only was he overweight, he also had three other risk factors for cardiovascular disease: diabetes, hyperlipidaemia, and hypertension.

14.7.2 Why should obesity be treated?

There are many reasons why obesity should be treated. Being obese is associated with significant morbidity and mortality. Physical illnesses associated with obesity

Table 14.5 NICE treatment guidelines based on BMI and waist measurements

BMI classification BMI unit	Waist circumference[1]			Co-morbidities present[2]
	Low	High	Very high	
Overweight (BMI = 25–29.9kg/m^2)				
Obese I (BMI = 30–34.9 kg/m^2)				
Obese II (BMI = 35–39.9 kg/m^2)				
Obese III (BMI > 40 kg/m^2)				

1. Less than 94 cm is low, 94–102 cm is high, and more than102 cm is very high for men; less than 80 cm is low, 80–88 cm is high, and more than 88 cm is very high for women.
2. Co-morbidities include hypertension, diabetes, etc.

Key to Table 14.5

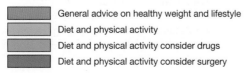

General advice on healthy weight and lifestyle
Diet and physical activity
Diet and physical activity consider drugs
Diet and physical activity consider surgery

include diabetes mellitus type II, respiratory impairment, gallbladder disease, cancers, gout, osteoarthritis, hypertension, cardiovascular disorders, infertility, and dermatological disorders. Obesity is a risk factor for cardiovascular disease and treating it will significantly reduce mortality from all causes. Obese patients will also often suffer from psychiatric illnesses such as depression, low self-esteem, and anxiety disorders, therefore tackling obesity will significantly reduce the incidence of these physical and mental illnesses, and their associated costs, morbidity, and mortality.

14.8 Management of obesity

Obesity is a chronic illness requiring long-term management. In order for the management to be effective, the patient needs to be motivated and committed to losing weight.

There are three main ways to manage obesity:

- lifestyle changes (e.g. diet and exercise)
- pharmacologically with drugs
- surgery.

Of all these, lifestyle changes are probably the most important. They are necessary for all patients and should be an integral part of the management with either pharmacological agents or through surgery. Failure to make lifestyle changes will almost certainly end up with people regaining whatever weight they have lost.

Using medication to treat obesity is only recommended as a last resort. Pharmacological treatment is usually only recommended for patients with a BMI >30 or a BMI >27 and risk factors.

The four types of medication that could theoretically be used to lose weight are:

- drugs that reduce overall calorie intake (e.g. appetite suppressants)
- drugs that increase overall calorie expenditure
- drugs that reduce fat absorption (e.g. lipase inhibitors)
- drugs that stimulate fat metabolism/expenditure.

However only two of these (appetite suppressants and lipase inhibitors) are considered safe and have a license to be used for obesity.

14.8.1 Lipase inhibitors

Of the three main fuel sources eaten by humans (carbohydrates, proteins, and fats), the fats have the greatest concentration of calories per gram. Each gram of fat contains approximately nine calories, compared with only four calories per gram for carbohydrates and proteins. Thus, reducing our fat intake is likely to have a significant effect in getting the balance between calories in and calories out right. Most of the fat in our diets is made up of triglycerides. These comprise a glycerol molecule with three fatty acids on each of the OH groups. To be absorbed they need to be hydrolysed into free fatty acids, which is done by lipases produced by the pancreas and intestines. The lipases combine with colipase, a protein co-factor that is required for its activity.

Orlistat is the only pancreatic lipase inhibitor that is licensed in most countries to be used for obesity. It is derived from hydrogenating lipstatin, which is a natural lipase inhibitor produced by *Streptomyces toxytricini*, a gram-negative bacterium. Orlistat works locally in the intestines and blocks approximately 30% of dietary fat from being absorbed. Because it has no effect on the central nervous system, unlike appetite suppressants, it is relatively safer than the other weight loss medications. This has allowed it to be sold without prescription in many countries.

However, stopping fat being absorbed can lead to several embarrassing and inconvenient GI side effects, for example loose and oily stools, flatulence associated with discharge, faecal incontinence, urgency and frequency, as well as bloating and cramps. An important adverse effect of orlistat is that it reduces the absorption of fat-soluble vitamins such as vitamin A, D, K, and E. Patients should be prescribed vitamin preparations containing these vitamins. Orlistat has been found to improve the effect of other drugs, such as insulin and pravastatin, with patients requiring a dose reduction when orlistat is used with these drugs.

> After Andreas was commenced on orlistat, his insulin dose had to be reduced because his blood sugar levels dropped.

14.8.2 Appetite suppressants

Another approach to weight loss is to reduce the intake of all kinds of food. To do this we need to modify our appetite, i.e. our desire for food. The control of appetite is a complex process involving hormones, and the central and autonomic nervous systems (Figure 14.3). The hypothalamus, in particular regions including the arcuate nucleus, the paraventricular nucleus, the ventromedial hypothalamic nucleus, and the dorsomedial hypothalamic nucleus, are central to appetite control. Importantly these regions are readily accessible to circulating hormones and are innervated by nerves, including the nucleus of the solitary tract, which receives input from the vagal nerves.

Ghrelin, insulin, cholecystokinin (CCK), glucagon-like peptide-1 (GLP-1), and leptin are important hormones secreted by the gut, pancreas, and adipose tissue. Ghrelin is a peptide released primarily by cells in the stomach and levels are increased while fasting and decreased when food is taken in. It acts at the ARC and causes an increase in neuropeptide Y (NPY) and agouti-related protein (AgRP). This results in an increase in appetite and thus promotes food intake. Leptin, a hormone produced by adipose tissue, has the opposite effect to ghrelin, and results in down-regulation of appetite. Leptin does this by reducing NPY and AgRP, and increasing pro-opiomelanocortin (POMC). The POMC causes release of α-melanocyte-stimulating hormone, which inhibits feeding. Insulin also reduces NPY and has an inhibitory effect on appetite. Thus, leptin and insulin contribute to energy homeostasis by reducing your eating if you already have large fat stores (adipose tissue) or have glucose in the bloodstream from eating (high insulin). Similarly, CCK and GLP-1, released from the gut in response to eating, also suppresses appetite in the hypothalamus, therefore in an ideal world these two systems of hormones (ghrelin and leptin/insulin/CCK/GLP-1) work in harmony to keep your basal weight and metabolism in check. However, a number of theories have been proposed to explain why patients become overweight and obese. These include becoming insensitive to hormones such as leptin, and loss of suppression of ghrelin release post-prandially.

Apart from, and in concert with, the hormonal control of appetite, a number of non-peptide transmitters are also involved. These include serotonin, noradrenaline, dopamine, and histamine. A range of endogenous peptides, including opioids and cannabinoids, also affect appetite. The effects of peptide and non-peptide transmitters in appetite control are outlined in Table 14.6.

Currently the neurotransmitters are the main targets of pharmacological interventions for appetite control. However, investigations are under way to modulate the hormones involved in feeding and satiety, including leptin and neuropeptide Y.

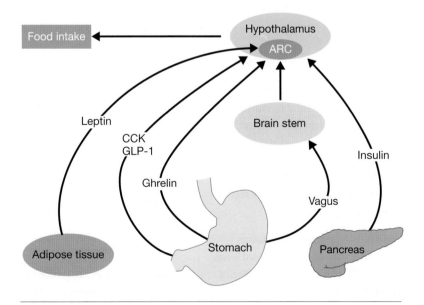

Figure 14.3 Inputs into the regulation of appetite.

ARC, arcuate nucleus; CCK, cholecystokinin; GLP-1, glucagon-like protein-1.

Table 14.6 Hormones and neurotransmitters involved in appetite

Neurotransmitter/hormone	Receptor/mode of action	Affect on appetite
Ghrelin	↑ NPY ↑ AgRP ↑ vagus	↑
Leptin	↓ NPY ↓ AgRP ↑ POMC	↓
Insulin	↓ NPY	↓
CCK	↓ vagus (CCK_A receptors) CCK_B receptors in VMH and PVN	↓
GLP-1	↓ NPY Induces upper GI motility Delays gastric emptying Stimulates insulin release	↓
Serotonin	$5\text{-}HT_{1B}$ $5\text{-}HT_{2C}$	↓
Dopamine	D_2	↓
Noradrenaline	PVN α_1	↓
	PVN α_2	↑
	LHA β_2	↓
Histamine	H_1	↓
Endogenous opiates (e.g. endorphins)	μ δ κ	↑
Endocannabinoids (e.g. anandamide)	CB_1	↑

5-HT, 5-hydroxytryptamine receptor; D_2, dopamine-2 receptor; H_1, histamine-1 receptor; NPY, neuropeptide; μ, mu opioid receptor; δ, delta opioid receptor, κ, kappa opioid receptor; AgRP, agouti-related protein; POMC, pro-opiomelanocortin; CCK, cholecystokinin; VMH, ventromedial hypothalamic nucleus; PVN, paraventricular nucleus; GLP-1, glucagon-like peptide-1; GI, gastrointestinal; LHA, lateral hypothalamic area; CB_1, endogenous cannabinoid receptor.

14.8.3 Serotonin/noradrenaline reuptake inhibitors

As noted in Table 14.6, both serotonin and noradrenaline have an important role in appetite regulation. The effect of noradrenaline has been long understood and is part of the 'fight or flight' reaction (after all, when in stressful situations or scared the last thing you want to be thinking about is being hungry). The role of 5-HT is a more recent advance in appetite control.

Sibutramine is a selective serotonin and noradrenaline reuptake inhibitor that is used in obesity. The increased levels of these neurotransmitters in the brain lead to stimulation of the $5\text{-}HT_{1B}$ and $5\text{-}HT_{2C}$ (serotonin), and α_1- and β_2-adrenoreceptors. Sibutramine also increases glucose usage in the body by stimulating brown adipose tissue breakdown with the help of the sympathetic nervous system.

Because of its CNS activity, sibutramine has more adverse drug reactions than orlistat. These include headache, dry mouth, constipation, irritability, excitation, insomnia, and increase in pulse and blood pressure. Sibutramine should not be used in patients taking other CNS drugs, such as monoamine oxidase inhibitors, phentermine, and amphetamines. It can also contribute to the development of serotonin syndrome, and therefore should not be used with SSRIs.

Amphetamines

Amphetamines have been used for weight reduction since 1950. Their mechanism of action is through an increase in dopamine and noradrenaline release from nerve endings in the feeding centre in the hyphothalamus, resulting in reduction in the appetite.

They are not recommended in most countries anymore because of the potential for drug abuse and the euphoria they produce. This is caused by the release of dopamine in the reward centres of the brain. They can also cause lethargy, rebound depression, and binge eating.

Other sympathomimetics

Over-the-counter weight-loss tablets containing ephedrine and phenylpropanolamine used to be very popular before they were found to increase the risk of stroke and death. Both ephedrine and phenylpropanolamine are sympathomimetics. Ephedrine stimulates α- and β-adrenoceptors in the feeding centre in the hyphothalamus, resulting in reduced appetite. Phenylpropanolamine, on the other hand, stimulates the release of noradrenaline and dopamine in the feeding centre, resulting in satiety and weight loss. Neither phenylpropanolamine nor ephedrine are used anymore in weight loss medications because of their potential for abuse (ephedrine) and side effects (haemorrhagic stroke with phenylpropanolamine).

Phentermine is an older prescription sympathomymetic. It acts similarly to dexamphetamine, causing the release of noradrenaline and dopamine. It was given in combination with the serotonin-releasing agent fenfluramine. However, fenfluramine was taken off the market when it was found to be associated with an increased risk of heart valve disorders. Phentermine alone is still available in some countries and it is given as sustained-release capsules, with the phenteramine bound to an ion-exchange resin.

14.8.4 Cannabinoid receptor antagonists

The cannabinoid receptor (CB1) is a relatively new target for treating obesity. The CB1 is G-protein coupled receptor that inhibits the formation of cyclic AMP (cAMP). It also blocks pre-synaptic calcium channels and activate potassium channels. Most of the CB1 receptors are found in the hypothalamus and they are involved in promotion of appetite, as well as the mesolimbic dopamine pathway, called the 'reward' centre.

Rimonabant is a CB1 receptor antagonist that is given as a single oral dose each day. Blockage of the CB1 centrally reduces appetite, while peripherally it increases insulin sensitivity and fatty acid oxidation in muscles and the liver.

Rimonabant causes a range of side effects, including nausea and vomiting, and, of greater concern, psychiatric effects, including depression and suicidal ideation. For this reason it is contraindicated in patients suffering major depression or on antidepressant treatment.

SUMMARY OF DRUGS USED FOR DIABETES

Therapeutic class	Drugs	Mechanism of action	Common clinical uses	Common comments	Examples of adverse drug reactions
Insulins	Short acting: actrapid	Stimulate intracellular insulin receptor, leading to phosphorylation of tyrosine kinase, leading to activation of serine/threonine kinases, causing translocation of glucose transporters to cell membrane, allowing glucose uptake	Type I diabetes	Injected 30–45 minutes before meals. Used in infusion for some type I patients	Hypoglycaemia Lipodystrophy weight gain Allergic reactions, local reactions (egerythema itching)
	Rapid acting: insulin aspart insulin lispro		Type II diabetes	More flexible because of quick absorption therefore can be given immediately after food	
	Intermediate acting: insulin mixtard (different strengths)			Onset of action could be up to2 hours and the effect could last for up to 20 hours	
	Long acting: insulin glargine insulin determir			The onset of action of long-acting insulin is within 4 hours, lasting up to 36 hours. Glargine has a peakless profile and is given once daily.	
Sulphonylureas	Chlorpropamide Tolbutamide Glibenclamide Glimepiride Gliclazide Glipizide	Attaches to a receptor on the ATP-dependent potassium channels on β-cells pancreatic cell, causing blockage of the K_{ATP} channel resulting in depolarization, opening of the calcium channels, influx of calcium into the β-cell, and release of insulin	Type II diabetes	Chlorpropamide: highest risk of hypoglycaemia Chlorpropamide also causes disulfiram-type reaction with alcohol Chlorpropamide rarely used because of above Gliclazide and glipizide: lowest risk of hypoglycaemia	Hypoglycaemia Weight gain Nausea Diarrhoea
Non–sulfonylurea insulin secretagogues. Meglitinides	Nateglinide Repaglinide	Same as sulphonylureas: stimulate the release of insulin through blockage of ATP-sensitive potassium channels		Rapid onset and elimination Better flexibility because can be taken immediately after food	
Biguanide	Metformin	Theories: 1) stimulates AMP-activated protein kinase, an enzyme involved in insulin signalling 2) reduces hepatic glucose production through inhibition of gluconeogenesis 3) increases cell sensitivity to insulin in the periphery, leading to increased uptake of glucose 4) lowers free fatty acid levels in plasma and thereby oxidation, which could help reduce gluconeogenesis in the liver 5) reduces glucose absorption from the gastrointestinal tract	Type II diabetes	Causes weight reduction First-line agent Contraindicated in renal impairment	Gastrointestinal (nausea, vomiting, anorexia, diarrhoea) malabsorption of vitamin B12, lactic acidosis

Therapeutic class	Drugs	Mechanism of action	Common clinical uses	Common comments	Examples of adverse drug reactions
Thiazolindiones (also called glitazones)	Pioglitazone Rosiglitazone	Binds to the PPARγ receptor (which also becomes bound to a retinoid X receptor once activated), the glitazone–receptor complex moves to the cell nucleus and activates DNA to induce gene transcription, leading to: 1) an increase in lipoprotein lipase, fatty acid transporter protein, and glycerol kinase, among other enzymes and transporters, causing peripheral and subcutaneous fat cells to store fatty acids, resulting in a reduction in circulating fatty acids and reduced levels of triglycerides in liver and muscles 2) an effect on the release of hormones from adipocytes called 'adipokines'	Type II diabetes	First two were withdrawn because of hepatotoxicity Liver function needs monitoring Contraindicated post-myocardial infarct and in left ventricular heart failure	Peripheral oedema Weight gain Headache dizziness Rosiglitazone: myocardial infarcts and increase in LDL and HDL
α-glucosidase inhibitors	Acarbose	Reversibly inhibits glucosidase, the enzyme that breaks down carbohydrates (disaccharides) to monosaccharides, delaying absorption of glucose	Type II diabetes (theoretically should be effective in type I, but not used)	Used in combination with others	Bloating Flatulence diarrhoea
Dipeptidyl peptidase 4 inhibitors (gliptins)	Sitagliptin Vildagliptin	Inhibit dipeptidyl, the enzyme responsible for destroying circulating incretins, leading to longer duration of action of incretins	Type II diabetes	Relatively new class	Hypoglycaemia headache Nausea Infections
Incretin mimetics	Exenatide	Mimics the action of GLP-1, which has a direct effect on the pancreas, causing the release of insulin from β-cells and inhibition of glucagon release by α-cells. The effect on β-cells is mediated through the GLP-1 receptor, which is a G-protein coupled receptor that stimulates adenylate cyclase Other effects of GLP-1 include pancreatic β-cell proliferation, expression of the glucose transporter 2 and glucokinase genes, reduced gastric emptying, and reduced appetite	Type II diabetes	Useful in obese patients and those unable to take insulin	Nausea Vomiting Diarrhoea Dyspepsia Abdominal pain
Glucagon	Glucagon	Opposite action to insulin Attaches to a specific G-protein-coupled receptor on cells and stimulates adenylate cyclase Promotes glycogen breakdown, inhibits glycogen synthesis, and promotes gluconeogenesis, resulting in the release of glucose into the bloodstream	Hypoglycaemia	Can be given in an emergency by intramuscular or subcutaneous injection, which means that it can be administered by a carer or ambulance personnel to an unconscious patient.	Nausea Vomiting Hypokalaemia

SUMMARY OF DRUGS USED FOR OBESITY

Therapeutic class	Drugs	Mechanism of action	Common clinical uses	Comments	Common adverse drug reactions
Lipase inhibitor	Orlistat	Blocks the action of lipase, the enzyme that breaks fat down for absorbtion	Obesity	Only drug in this class	Loose and fatty stools Flatulence Bloating and cramps
Appetite suppressants	Serotonin/ noradrenaline reuptake inhibitors Sibutramine	1) Reduces uptake of serotonin and noradrenaline neurotransmitters, regulating appetite reuptake Increased levels of these neurotransmitters in the brain lead to stimulation of the 5-HT_{1B} and 5-HT_{2C} (serotonin), and α_1 and β_2 adrenergic receptors 2) Increases glucose usage in the body by stimulating brown adipose tissue breakdown with the help of the sympathetic nervous system	Obesity		Headache Dry mouth Constipation Irritability Excitation Sibutramine with drawn in the UK in January 2010 because its cardiovascular risks were found to outweigh its benefits.
Amphetamines		Increases dopamine and noradrenaline release from nerve endings in the feeding centre in the hypothalamus, resulting in reduction in the appetite	Not recommended	Not recommended for use in most countries	Lethargy Rebound depression Binge eating
Other sympathomimetics	Ephedrine	Stimulates α and β adrenergic receptors in the feeding centre in the hypothalamus, resulting in reduced appetite	Not currently used		Stroke Hypertension Death
	Phenylpropanolamine	Stimulates the release of noradrenaline and dopamine in the feeding centre, resulting in satiety and weight loss			
	Phentermine	Noradrenaline and dopamine	Still used in some countries		Stroke Hypertension
Cannabinoid receptor antagonists	Rimonabant	1) Inhibits CB_1, a G-protein coupled receptor involved in promotion of appetite as well as the mesolimbic dopamine pathway called the 'reward' centre, leading to inhibition of the formation of cyclic AMP 2) Blocks pre-synaptic calcium channels and activate potassium channels	Obesity	The cannabinoid receptor (CB_1) is a relatively new target for treating obesity Licensed withdrawn in the United Kingdom due to concerns of suicidal ideation	Nausea Vomiting Depression Suicidal ideation

PPARγ, peroxisome proliferator activator receptor gamma; LDL, low-density lipoprotein; HDL, high-density lipoprotein; GLP-1, glucagon-like peptide-1; 5-HT, 5-hydroxytryptamine

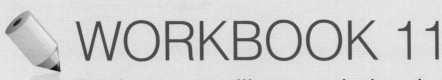

WORKBOOK 11
Diabetes mellitus and obesity

Andreas Kaiser: a simplified case history

After 3 hours of waiting, Andreas was finally seen by the consultant and two other doctors. Andreas had been admitted directly to hospital after a third visit to his GP regarding the ulcer on his left little toe that would not heal. He had made an emergency appointment although he had a routine appointment for the next day because he felt very lethargic. After taking his blood pressure and temperature, the GP rang the hospital for his blood results. The GP had sent him straight to hospital as soon as he found out the results.

His wife Monique was at his bedside, she had dropped off the twins at her mum's and came straight to hospital as soon as possible.

The consultant had Andreas' clinical notes, which detailed his clerking.

A table of clinical clerking abbreviations is given on page xi.

CLINICAL CLERKING FOR ANDREAS KAISER AT A&E DEPARTMENT

Age: 38 years

PC: Worsening ulcer on left little toe and general lethargic feeling and increased thirst and urinary frequency

HPC: Admitted via GP following aggravation of toe ulcer. Found to have pyrexia during emergency visit and blood results indicated elevated random blood glucose of 30 mmol/L and elevated white cell count.

> *Andreas' random blood glucose level (BGL) was a lot higher than the normal range of 3.5–10 mmol/l. Random BGLs >11.1 or fasting BGLs >6.1 are used to diagnose diabetes.*

> *Elevated white cell count indicates infection, probably from his ulcerated toe. The ulcer is probably due to diabetes, resulting in increased glucose, leading to cell damage through several mechanisms.*

PMH: Hypertension; hypertensive crisis 2004

> *Andreas was diagnosed with hypertension and had a life-threatening hypertensive crisis last year.*

DH: Losartan, Bendroflumethiazide

> *Andreas has been taking these two drugs for his blood pressure.*

> *Losartan is an angiotensin receptor blocker(ARB) which was commenced after he developed a dry cough with Isiropril, an ACE inhibitor.*

> *Bendroflumethiazide is a thiazide-like diuretic.*

SH: Lives with wife and twin daughters. Smokes 10 cigarettes a day. Weight = 90 kg (overweight). Mother is diabetic.

O/E:

1) Ulcer is warm and pus filled.

2) Pedal pulses are absent.

3) Absent pinprick sensation.

4) Patient seems extremely lethargic.

5) Temperature: 38.9°C (reference < 36.7°C)

6) BP = 140/80 mm Hg

> Andreas' ulcer was a result of ischaemia (lack of blood flow) to his toes because of diabetes. Absent pulses, when the doctor feels for blood flow, prove this.
>
> His nerves have been damaged (neuropathy) as a result of diabetes and he cannot feel it when the doctor pricks his feet with a pin.
>
> His temperature is elevated as a result of infection

Biochemistry:

1) Random BGL 38 mmol/L (reference 3.5–10.0 mmol/L)

2) Glycosylated haemoglobin = 11% (reference 5.5–8.5%)

3) White cell count (WCC) =16 x 10^9 (reference = 4–11 x 10^9)

Urine testing:

1) Ketones: negative

2) Glucose: positive

1) Random BGL is elevated. This is a very high level and this shows Andreas has diabetes. This is called the random level as opposed to the fasting glucose level, which is taken after the patient has been made to fast.

2) Glycosylated haemoglobin (HbA1c) is elevated. HbA1c is the name that is given to a subfraction of haemoglobin to which glucose binds irreversibly and persists throughout the life of the red blood cell. It is used to assess glucose levels over the preceding 6 to 8 weeks. Andreas' HbA1c shows that his glucose level has been high for at least the last 6–8 weeks and is useful to confirm diagnosis.

3) White cell count. His elevated white cell count is proof of infection in his toe.

4) Urinary ketones. This results from the breakdown of amino and fatty acids to synthesise ATP in the absence of glucose, in cells in which glucose entry is dependent on insulin, e.g. muscles, but also in the liver. This could lead to muscle wasting and, more seriously, life-threatening diabetic ketoacidosis. This is more common in type I diabetes. Andreas' urine ketone level is not elevated.

5) Urinary glucose. This happens because of glucose spilling into the urine when BGLs are too high. This results in loss of water through increased urinary frequency due to the osmotic effect of the glucose (draws in water).

Diagnosis: Type 2 diabetes mellitus, infected ulcerated toe

Type I or type II diabetes mellitus?

Sometimes difficult to classify patients as having type I or II. Generally:

type I:

* *younger than 30 years*

* *lean*

* *presence of ketonuria*

* *signs and symptoms coupled with elevated fasting BGL*

type II:

* *>30 years old*

* *obese*

* *family history of diabetes*

* *ketonuria less likely*

* *signs and symptoms coupled with elevated fasting BGL.*

Plan:

Send swabs and blood cultures of site of ulcer to microbiology for culture and sensitivity

X-ray left foot to exclude osteomyelitis

Intravenous antibiotics to treat infection

Start oral antidiabetic drug

Start insulin Actrapid® infusion until

BM < 11 mmol/L.

> *BM: This stands for Boehringer Mannheim (now Roche), which was the first company to make test strips to check blood glucose levels. These are still commonly referred to as BM levels but are more accurately capillary blood glucose levels.*

The doctor explains to Andreas that he has had undiagnosed diabetes for a while. This has already led to long-term complications like the ulcer, as well as immediate complications.

1a) Explain the meaning of the following:

Glycaemia

....

....

....

Glycosuria

Ketonuria

1b) What happens to blood glucose in diabetes (increase or decrease)?

2a) What is the name of the hormone that controls the transportation of glucose in some tissues?

2b) Which main type of cells in the body require insulin for glucose transport?

3) What is diabetes mellitus?

After 2 days on the insulin infusion, Andreas is fed up and wonders when it will be discontinued. He finds the infusion a nuisance because the nurses keep taking blood samples from him to check his BGLs. After each test they fiddle with the infusion setting. The doctor explains to him that he has been put on insulin although he was a newly diagnosed type II patient because his BGL was extremely high and he had a temperature. In such a case, the only way to maintain correct control of his blood glucose is through insulin infusion, which can be adjusted according to his BGLs. This is why the nurses keep taking bloods for test. The doctor promises that after the blood glucose has stabilized, the insulin will be stopped.

4a) In which body organ is insulin synthesised? What percentage of this organ is endocrine?

4b) In which cells of this organ is insulin synthesised?

5a) How many chains make up the insulin molecule?

6a) Elaborate on the steps by which glucose enters the insulin-secreting cells, leading to the release of insulin.

6b) List two other stimuli of insulin secretion besides glucose.

7) What type of receptor is the insulin receptor?

8) What is the effect of insulin on the following?

Carbohydrate metabolism

Fat metabolism

_____

_____

_____

9) In which body organs do the above take place?

_____

_____

_____

10) List two other pancreatic hormones besides insulin.

_____

_____

_____

> The doctor explains to Andreas that his increased thirst and urinary frequency were as a result of his diabetes. Excess glucose in his kidneys had spilled into his urine. Water followed the glucose leak, increasing his urinary frequency, which in turn made him very thirsty.

11a) What is the name of the glucose metabolite that is implicated in most tissue damage in cells that are not dependent on insulin for glucose take up, in diabetic patients, resulting from glucose accumulation?

_____

_____

_____

11b) Name two chronic complications of diabetes that result from the accumulation of glucose metabolites and/or advanced glycosylation end-products.

_____

_____

_____

> Andreas asks to see the doctor because he is worried about a severe complication he has heard could occur in diabetic patients called diabetic ketoacidosis. The doctor explains to Andreas that because he has type II diabetes as opposed to type I, he is less likely to suffer from this. The doctor explains that this usually happens in certain body cells where, instead of glucose being broken down to provide energy, other substances are broken down instead due to complete lack of insulin. However, he cautions Andreas that he will need to take his treatment seriously to prevent this and other complications.

12a) Which substance was the doctor referring to that is broken down in type 1 diabetes instead of glucose in certain cells?

12b) What is the name of the complication that results from this? What are the consequences?

On day 3 the doctor comes to talk to Andreas about the plans for his treatment. The insulin has been stopped and his BGL is now 9 mmol/L. The antibiotic has been altered to oral. The doctor tells Andreas that he will have to take medication for his diabetes. Initially it will be tablets but eventually he might need insulin. Andreas seems worried and tells the doctor that he hates injections. He says that although his mother uses tablets for her diabetes, his ex-girlfriend had to use injections for her diabetes. He says his ex-girlfriend's life was complicated by it so he would prefer the tablets if he had a choice. The doctor explains that his ex-girlfriend probably had type I diabetes.

13a) What is type I diabetes? At what age do type I diabetics normally develop symptoms?

13b) What is the only possible treatment for type I diabetes?

14a) Insulin is divided into three main groups according to its speed of onset of action and duration of action. What are the three main groups?

14b) To which of these groups does insulin to be taken immediately before meals belong to? For what purpose is it given?

The doctor explains to Andreas that luckily he probably has type II diabetes, which can be controlled only with tablets at the moment.

15a) What is type II diabetes?

15b) At what stage of life does type II diabetes most commonly develop? What size are the patients usually (thin or obese)?

The doctor warns Andreas that although he might not need insulin now, he could need insulin for control of his diabetes eventually. Patients may ultimately require insulin when stores of insulin become almost or completely depleted.

Andreas has commenced the oral anti- diabetic called gliclazide. This belongs to the class of anti-diabetics called sulphonylureas.

16) What is the mechanism of action of sulphonylureas?

Andreas is told that he will have to stay in hospital for a couple more days.

The doctor tells Andreas that his gliclazide will be changed to another tablet called metformin belonging to the class called biguanides because the pharmacist and diabetic nurse have both advised that metformin is more suitable for him.

17) What disadvantage/side effect of the sulphonylureas makes them unsuitable for Andreas?

Hint: Andreas weights 90 kg.

18a) What are the possible mechanisms of action of biguanides?

18b) List three advantages of biguanides over the other classes.

Andreas complains to Sunita, his wife's pharmacist friend, who comes to visit, that he feels very bloated and wonders if it could be the metformin.

Sunita asks him if he takes it with food. He says he does not because no one told him to. She explains that he needs to take it with food to prevent bloating.

Andreas keeps taking his metformin with food and realizes that he does not feel bloated any more.

Three days later, Andreas is discharged because his BGL has been within the desired range for 3 days and his ulcer is much improved.

He is discharged on the following medication:

- Bendroflumethiazide

- metformin

- Losartan

- flucloxacillin for 4 more days.

He is advised to see his surgery diabetic nurse regularly for advice and follow up. He is also encouraged to try to lose some weight. The discharge letter advises that his blood pressure and cholesterol levels should be checked.

Andreas misses all his surgery appointments.

Six months later Andreas collapses, unconscious. He comes round in a hospital bed, hooked up to monitors, with 10 pairs of eyes staring at him. He enquires about where he is. One of the owners of the eyes introduces herself as the senior registrar and the rest are students.

She tells Andreas that he passed out and was brought in by ambulance. His BGL had been too high (40 mmol/L) and he had a blood infection. The doctor tells him he has had a narrow escape. She wishes to discuss his blood results, amongst others, with him.

CLERKING FOR ANDREAS, ADMITTED WITH HYPERGLYCAEMIA

Age: 39 years

PC: Weakness, nausea, vomiting, confusion, and collapse

HPC: Wife rang ambulance after she could not rouse him. Started when he noticed pus-filled ulcer in leg 1 week ago. GP prescribed analgesia that caused diarrhoea. Felt unwell and progressively got worse over 2 days. He became increasingly feverish and lethargic. He stopped taking the medication.

PMH:

1) Hypertension; hypertensive crisis 2004.

2) Diabetes mellitus type II diagnosed 6 months ago.

DH:

Losartan

Bendroflumethiazide

Metformin

Gliclazide

Orlistat

SH: Lives with wife and twin daughters. Smokes 10 cigarettes a day. Weight = 98 kg (overweight). BMI = 31 kg/m². Mother is diabetic.

O/E:

1) Ulcer is warm and pus filled.

2) Pedal pulses are absent.

3) Absent pinprick sensation.

4) Patient seems extremely lethargic.

5) Temperature: 39.9°C (reference < 36.7°C).

6) BP = 159/80 mmHg.

Biochemistry:

1) Random blood glucose = 40 mmol/L (3.5–10.0 mmol/L).

2) Glycosylated haemoglobin = 9.5% (5.5–8.5%).

3) White cell count = 16 x 109 (4 to 11 x 109).

4) Total cholesterol = 6.9

Urine testing:

1) Ketones: negative

2) Glucose: positive

Diagnosis: Hyperglycaemic episode caused by infection and diarrhoea.

> The doctor tells him he is currently on an insulin infusion to quickly bring down his BGLs. He has also been put on four new tablets she will explain about when he is better.
>
> The next day the doctor comes and tells him one of the new tablets is called pioglitazone, which is another oral antidiabetic from a class called thiozolidinediones.

19a) On what type of receptors do thiazolidinediones bind and what is the consequence of this binding?

19b) Despite the theoretical merits of thiazolidinediones, guidelines recommend that they should only be used in combination with either a sulphonylurea or a biguanide. What is the reason for this recommendation?

> Two weeks later Andreas' BGLs seem to have actually gone up. The doctor and diabetic nurse tell Andreas he might need insulin. He is adamant he does not want insulin because he does not like needles. He wants to know what other oral medications are available.

20) List two other classes of oral antidiabetics not already mentioned.

> The doctor decides to increase the dose of his metformin instead. Andreas enquires about the other three medications he was started on. The doctor tells him one is called orlistat and it works to reduce obesity.

21a) Describe the mechanism of action of orlistat.

21b) What are the adverse drug reactions of orlistat?

....

....

....

21c) What is another drug that could be used for the same indication as orlistat? How does it work?

....

....

....

22) Explain why Andreas was put on simvastatin and aspirin.

....

....

....

Andreas is discharges home eventually on the following:

- metformin

- gliclazide

- pioglitazone

- simvastatin

- aspirin

- ramipril

- indapamide

- vitamin D and ergocalciferol.

His blood pressure is well controlled and he is committed to losing weight. The diabetic nurse and pharmacist have been to counsel him about the details of proper diabetes management.

23) Explain why Andreas was given vitamin D supplementation?

....

....

....

Six months later Andreas is admitted to hospital with a heart attack. He is stabilized and when the doctor comes to talk to him, they discuss the following concerns they both have:

• Andreas' HbA1c levels are still quite high

• Andreas' BMI has gone up to 45 kg/m^2

• Andreas' is on amitiptyline for neuropathic pain.

Although Andreas is worried about needles, he finally agrees to use insulin. His gliclazide and pioglitazone are replaced with insulin to be used three times a day. The doctor switches the amitriptyline to gabapentin, which is safer after a heart attack.

Andreas is discharged 1 week later.

Three months later he returns and appears to have gained even more weight. The doctor decides to switch his insulin to exenatide.

Chapter 15
The thyroid and contraception

Although she has been ignoring all the symptoms that she has been experiencing, Sunita finally starts panicking when she realizes that the front of her neck is actually protruding. The necklace that a year ago was her anniversary present, and a perfect fit, can now only go half-way round her neck. She panics as she imagines what she will look like in a couple of months if her neck keeps growing at this current rate. What makes it even more confusing is the fact that she has lost a lot of weight and has missed her period, even though the pregnancy test she did was negative. Although she is unaware of this, the symptoms Sunita is experiencing are typical of an over-active thyroid (hyperthyroid disease). These symptoms are almost the reverse of those of hypothyroid disease, which include bradycardia, weight gain, and sluggishness amongst others.

Hyper- and hypothyroid diseases result from excess or inadequate secretion of thyroid hormone, respectively. The thyroid gland has the very important role of facilitating growth by optimizing metabolism all over the body. Because the thyroid hormones affect almost every key function of the body, understanding the anatomy of the thyroid glands as well as the biosynthesis and functions of the thyroid hormones and how they are used to treat thyroid disease is extremely important.

Whilst undergoing treatment for thyroid disease, Sunita is prescribed medication to prevent pregnancy. The second half of this chapter looks at the hormonal changes that occur during the menstrual cycle and how they can be controlled. The chapter also covers contraception and the mechanism of action of contraceptive pills.

15.1 Thyroid hormones

The thyroid plays a key role in metabolic processes in the body by regulating the rate at which energy is used by the body. This is achieved through the action of the thyroid hormones—**thyroxine** and **triiodothyronine**—which are secreted by the thyroid glands. These hormones control the metabolism and growth rate, as well as the functioning of other body systems. This is achieved predominantly by controlling the action of most key metabolic hormones, such as insulin and glucagon. The thyroid hormones also control the sensitivity of the body to these hormones. The thyroid also releases calcitonin, another hormone that regulates calcium in the body. Thyroxine and triiodothyronine are released following activation of the thyroid glands by thyrotrophin (thyroid-stimulating hormone, TSH) released by the pituitary gland after activation by thyrotrophin-releasing hormones (TRH) released by the hypothalamus. This is illustrated in Figure 15.1.

15.1.1 Anatomy of the thyroid glands

The thyroid weighs about 30 g and is one of the largest endocrine glands. The gland consists of two lobes situated on either side of the trachea and joined together by thyroid tissue (isthmus). It lies in the lower neck in the region commonly referred to as the Adam's apple in men. The thyroid gland is made up of follicles consisting of a lumen that contains a homogenous colloid of **thyroglobulin**, a large peptide that consists of tyrosine molecules attached to proteins. These follicles are surrounded by a single layer of cells called follicular cells.

The follicles in Sunita's thyroid glands grew bigger when the gland became overactive.

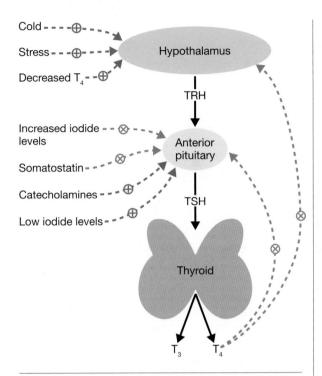

Figure 15.1 Control of the release of thyroid hormones.
TRH, thyrotropin-releasing hormone; TSH, thyroid-stimulating
hormone; T3, triiodothyronine; T4, tetraiodothyronine
(thyroxine); ⊕, increases release; ⊗, decreases release.

15.1.2 Synthesis and transport of thyroid hormones

Thyroxine (T_4) and triiodothyronine (T_3) are the main
thyroid hormones. They are produced by a coupling of
iodide with tyrosine, which eventually then forms the two
thyroid hormones (Box 15.1). Once produced the
hormones are stored in the follicular cells bound to
thyroglobulin until they are released.

Once released they are transported reversibly bound to a
range of proteins:

- thyroxine-binding globulin
- thyroxine-binding pre-albumin
- albumin.

Very little of the T_4 or T_3 is unbound (T_4 0.03% and T_3
0.3%). However, only the unbound hormone has activity.

15.1.3 The functions of thyroid hormones

The thyroid hormones are responsible for controlling the
rate of energy-utilizing chemical processes within the
cells, whilst at rest. These processes are referred to as

basal metabolism, during which thyroid hormones
stimulate the consumption of oxygen by the cells, whilst
regulating their energy production, leading to an increase
in energy turnover. Because of this control of basal
metabolic processes, the thyroid hormones influence
almost all processes within the body.

Of the two thyroid hormones, T_3 is the 'active' one, and
it exerts the effect on the cells. T_4 is considered a
prodrug and is converted to T_3 through the action of
enzymes called deiodinases. The thyroid hormones, like
steroid hormones, act through nuclear receptors. There
are four variants of the thyroid receptor: TRα_1, TRα_2,
TRβ_1, and TRβ_2. Unlike steroid receptors, thyroid
receptors are bound to DNA in the absence of the
hormone. When unoccupied the receptors act to
repress gene expression by forming heterodimers with
the retinoid X receptor (RXR). This then forms a
complex with a group of coreprocessor molecules
(proteins that reduce gene expression). However, when
T_3 binds to the receptor it causes a conformational
change that stops the coreprocessor complex and
causes activation of transcription, leading to protein
synthesis.

The functions of the thyroid hormones are complicated
and interwoven. They stimulate metabolism, leading to
depleted reserves of glycogen and fat. Thyroid
hormones control protein levels and thereby the
growth and development of many organs all over the
body. High levels lead to reduced protein synthesis,
whilst low levels lead to increased protein synthesis.
These proteins are involved in cardiac, muscular,
neurologic, hepatic and cardiovascular functioning,
and growth.

Thyroid hormones enhance β-adrenoceptor stimulation.
They increase the effect of insulin, leading to increased
uptake of glucose by the cells and increased
gluconeogenesis. On the other hand, T_3 leads to a
degradation of insulin. T_3 also increases the lipolytic
effects of catecholamines and glucagon. These effects are
summarized in Table 15.1.

This overarching effect of the thyroid hormones explains
why Sunita experienced so many different symptoms
because of hyperthyroidism. These ranged from cardiac
(heart rate) to neurological (insomnia) to weight loss
(overall metabolism) and missed periods (reproductive
system).

Box 15.1

Synthesis and release of thyroid hormones

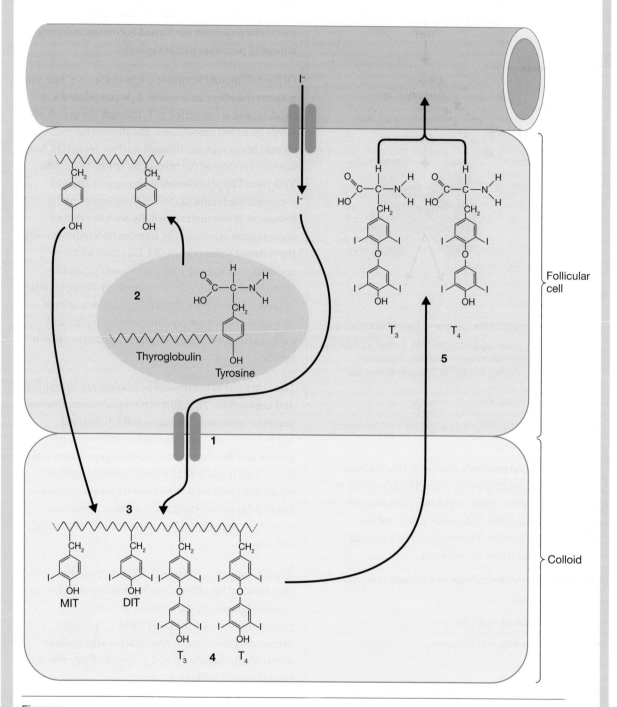

Figure a

1. Iodide is transferred from the blood via specific transporters. These are the sodium/iodide symporter (NIS, an ATPase-dependent transporter on the basolateral membrane) and pedrin (an iodide/chloride transporter on the luminal membrane). This concentrates iodine in the colloid and is referred to as the 'iodide trap'. The transcription of the genes for these transporters is up-regulated by thyroid stimulating hormone (TSH).

Box 15.1 Synthesis and release of thyroid hormones

2. Thyroglobulin, a large glycoprotein, is produced by the endoplasmic reticulum. During its synthesis tyrosine molecules are incorporated. It then moves into the colloid.

3. Iodide interacts with the tyrosine molecules on the thyroglobulin. To do this it is oxidized via thyroperoxidase in the presence of hydrogen peroxide (H_2O_2). This enzyme complex removes an electron from the iodide (producing an iodide free radical) and an electron from the tyrosine (giving a tyrosine radical). These two radicals then interact to produce monoiodotyrosine (MIT) and diiodotyrosine (DIT). This process is referred to as the *organification* of iodide. **This is the site of action for thioureylenes (e.g. carbimazole and propylthiouracil).**

4. The DIT and MIT combine to produce triiodthyronine (T_3) and tetraiodothyronine (T_4, thyroxine).

5. The thyroglobulin–T_3/T_4 complex enters the follicular cell, where it is broken down by proteolytic enzymes in lysosomes and T_3/T_4 are released.

DIT, diiodotyrosine; MIT, monoiodotyrosine; T_3, triiodothyronine; T_4, tetraiodothyronine (thyroxine).

Table 15.1 Effects of thyroid hormones

Effects on metabolism	
• Lipids	Stimulates fat mobilization Increased cholesterol and triglycerides levels in the blood
• Carbohydrate	Increase insulin-dependent glucose uptake into cells Increased gluconeogenesis and glycogenolysis
Effects on growth	In combination with growth hormone is needed for growth in young children
Effects on development	Needed for normal development of foetal and neonatal brain
Other effects	
• Cardiovascular	Increase heart rate, cardiac contractility, and cardiac output Promotes vasodilatation
• Central nervous system	Low levels lead to loss of mental alertness High levels lead to anxiety and nervousness
• Reproductive	Low levels associated with infertility

15.2 Hyperthyroidism

Hyperthyroidism, which is also called thyrotoxicosis, refers to excessive production and release of thyroxine and triiodothyronine from the thyroid glands. This leads to an increase of basal metabolism, resulting in a range of symptoms, including weight loss, increased heart rate, anxiety, insomnia, sweating, fatigue, and nervousness.

Hyperthyroidism can be either immunologic mediated or non-immunologic mediated.

15.2.1 Immunologic hyperthyroidism

This type of hyperthyroidism is characterized by a diffused enlargement of the thyroid glands. **Graves' disease** (also called Graves Basedow or Morbus Basedow in other countries) is the most common form, affecting one to two people per 1000 each year, and represents 60–70% of all cases of hyperthyroidism. It is an autoimmune condition whereby IgG binds to TSH receptors on the thyroid cells, leading to enhanced and sustained stimulation of the thyroid glands by increasing cAMP levels. This leads to increased thyroid hormone production.

T4 and T3 are produced even when TSH levels are low, as was the case with Sunita.

Graves' disease patients also have associated ocular conditions, in particular **exophthalmus** (bulging of the eyeballs) resulting from swelling caused by immune mediated inflammatory responses in the ocular fat and muscle.

Hashimoto's thyroiditis is another autoimmune disease, which is characterized by destruction of the thyroid cells. Although this can lead to an initial increase in thyroid hormone levels, as the hormones 'leak' from damaged thyrocytes, eventually it leads to hypothyroidism.

15.2.2 Non-immunologic hyperthyroidism

The non-immunologic forms of hyperthyroidism are usually tumor-like growths within the thyroid glands, which do not respond to hypothalamic control.

Examples of these are **toxic multinodular goiter** and **toxic nodules** (benign thyroid adenomas), as well as different types of thyroiditis (inflammation of the thyroid). A toxic multinodular goiter results from autonomously functioning nodules in the thyroid gland. Also called Plummers disease, it is the second most common cause of hyperthyroidism. Other causes of non-immune hyperthyroidism include drugs that contain iodine (e.g. amiodarone) and excessive use of exogenous thyroxine.

15.3 Management of hyperthyroidism

Hyperthyroidism is managed through either decreasing the synthesis/release of thyroid hormones or blunting the effect of the thyroid hormones. This could be achieved using one of the following ways or a combination:

- removal of part or the entire thyroid through surgery or destruction using radioactive iodine
- inhibition of T_4 and T_3 synthesis with thioureylenes
- blunting of the effects of T_4 and T_3 with β-adrenoceptor blockers
- blocking the release of the hormones using iodide.

15.3.1 Radioactive iodide

Radioactive iodide is very effective and is used as first-line treatment of choice for hyperthyroidism in the USA. It is used commonly for malignant thyroid tumors, in sulphur-intolerant patients (a problem with thioureylenes, see later), in patients non-responsive to thioureylenes, or in those for whom surgery is contraindicated.

The isotope of iodide that is used is ^{131}I. This is taken up into the thyroid in the place where iodide releases β- and γ-rays. The γ-rays just pass through the body, but the β-rays destroy the follicles and this leads to a reduction in thyroid hormones. Although this treatment is very effective and has few local side effects, its use is still minimal in some countries because of a legal requirement to protect the population from the radiation released by treated patients. Another disadvantage is the long time it takes to be effective (3–4 months), therefore patients often require additional treatment with thioureylenes (see later) to reduce their symptoms.

Radioactive iodide is given orally as a single dose and is generally well tolerated. In most patients hypothyroidism will occur, but this can be managed with thyroxine supplementation (see later under hypothyroidism).

15.3.2 Thioureylenes

The thioureylenes (also called thionamides in different countries), which include **carbimazole** and **propylthiouracil**, are the mainstay of treatment for hyperthyroidism. They are structurally similar, with both having a thiocarbamide group (S–C–N) in common (Figure 15.2). Carbimazole is the most commonly used thioureylene. It is a pro-drug that is converted to methimazole in the body.

Thioureylenes prevent the biosynthesis of T_4 and T_3 by acting as a substrate for, and therefore blocking, the thyroperoxidase enzyme. This prevents the oxidation of iodide and binding of the iodide to tyrosine (Box 15.1). Propylthiouracil also prevents the transformation of T_4 (less active) to T_3 (most active) in the periphery by blocking the enzyme thyroxine peroxidase, and therefore may have a quicker onset of action. The resultant effect of this is a reduction in T_4 and T_3 levels in the thyroid glands and ultimately the blood. This process happens over 4–12

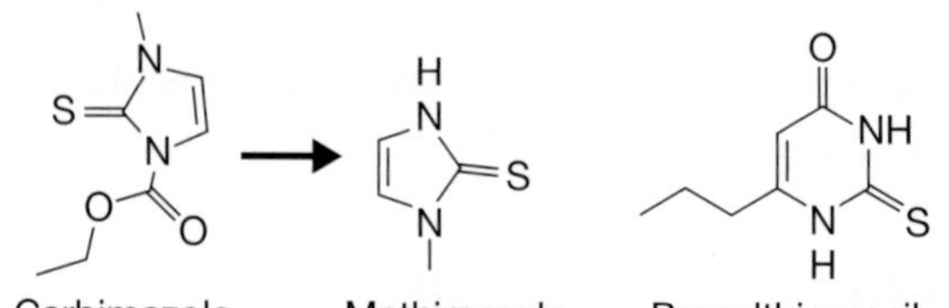

Carbimazole   Methimazole   Propylthiouracil

Figure 15.2 Commonly used thioureylenes.

weeks because existing thyroglobulin stores need to be depleted first, and circulating T_4 has a long half-life (approximately 7 days). The thioureylenes are also thought to have a suppressive effect on the immune system, which is desirable in patients with Graves' disease.

Both drugs can be given once daily, despite their short half-lives, because they are concentrated in the thyroid. The important adverse drug reactions include bone marrow suppression (agranulocytosis and neutropenia), gastrointestinal upset, and allergic reactions. The incidence of agranuloctosis and neutropenia is rare. However, given the potential seriousness of this reaction patients should be warned to report any sudden severe sore throat associated with fever because these are the common signs of bone marrow suppression. The effects on the bone marrow are reversible on stopping the treatment.

> Sunita experienced bone marrow suppression on carbimazole and she had to be taken off it and commenced on propylthiouracil.

15.3.3 Iodide ions

The release of thyroid hormone can be transiently decreased by iodide either as a side effect when iodide-containing medication is used (e.g. older cough mixtures that contain **potassium iodide**) or when intentionally used to manage hyperthyroidism. High doses of iodide in the form of iodine dissolved a solution with potassium iodide (**Lugol's iodine**) are commonly used prior to surgery to correct hyperthyroidism or in hyperthyroid crises (excessive levels of thyroid hormone that can be life threatening) to reduce levels of T_4 and T_3. After ingestion, the iodine is converted in the body to iodide. The iodide blocks thyroid hormone release by inhibiting iodine organification (see Box 15.1). This is called the Wolff–Chaikoff effect, and it is only temporary as eventually hormone synthesis continues. The effect is to cause thyroglobulin to accumulate and to reduce the number of blood vessels in the thyroid gland. This makes the gland firmer and easier to operate on. This effect is seen after 10–15 days of continuous use of the solution.

Adverse effects include angio-odema (an allergic reaction that results in rapid swelling of the skin and mucous membranes, which can be life threatening), skin irritation, conjuctivitis, bronchitis pain, and cold symptoms.

15.3.4 β-adrenoceptor antagonists (β-blockers)

Some of the symptoms experienced by hyperthyroid patients are similar to those resulting from agonism at the β-adrenoceptor. These symptoms include high pulse rate (tachycardia), tremor, and nervousness. Thyroid hormones are also thought to increase the sensitivity of sympathomimetic neurotransmitters such as adrenaline and noradrenaline by increasing the number of adrenoceptors. The β-adrenoceptor antagonists are therefore used to reduce those sympathomimetic-like effects of hyperthyroidism, even though they have no direct effect on thyroid hormone levels. Their mechanism of action is illustrated in Chapter 5. They are used in the initial period to quickly reduce hyperthyroid symptoms whilst the thioureylenes, which require longer, take effect.

> Sunita was prescribed the β-blocker propranolol initially and it contributed to reducing her symptoms of palpitations, tremor, and anxiety. The carbimazole and propylthiouracil reduced other symptoms, such as the goiter.

15.3.5 Glucocorticosteroids

Glucocorticosteroids are used for exophthalmia, which is non-responsive to other treatment, although they have no direct effect on thyroid hormone levels. Their potent anti-inflammatory effects (see Chapter 9) reduce the corneal inflammation characteristic of Graves' disease.

> Glucocorticosteroids were used in Sunita and they improved the exophthalmia, which was such a relief for her. She had been so scared she would have to live her life with bulging eyes.

15.4 Hypothyroidism

Hyopthyroidism is more common than hyperthyroidism and affects 2–5% of the population. Autoimmune thyroiditis is the most common cause of hypothyroidism. It is caused by destruction of the thyroid gland by the

body's own immune system, for example in Hashimoto's thyroiditis. Hypothyroidism can also result from other physical damage to the thyroid. Physical damage could be caused, for example, by goiter removal surgery or by medication such as amiodarone or radioiodide therapy. Other causes of secondary hypothyroidism are defects in hypothalamic or pituitary secretion of TSH due to cancers or irradiation of the brain.

Symptoms of hypothyroidism are more or less the opposite of those described for hyperthyroidism. They include weight gain, over sensitivity to cold, lethargy, menorrhagia (heavy prolonged menstrual cycle), constipation, mental slowness, dry skin, corse and brittle hair, and bradycardia. Severe hypothyroidism can lead to coma (called myxodema coma) or permanent underdevelopment in a newborn.

15.5 Treatment of hypothyroidism

Treatment of hypothyroidism is usually with thyroid hormone replacement therapy using synthetic T_4 or T_3. Iodide is used in cases where there is iodide deficiency.

15.5.1 Thyroxine (T_4)

Thyroxine, also known as levothyroxine, is the most widely used treatment for hypothyroidism. This is because it has a very long elimination half-life of 7 days, which leads to minimal fluctuation of levels if doses are missed. The long life is a result of plasma protein binding, which increases the amount of thyroxine in circulation and reduces the clearance of thyroxine. The main disadvantage of this long half-life is the extremely long time required to get to steady state (approximately 30 days), which significantly delays the time needed to achieve therapeutic effect.

Adverse drug reactions include atrial fibrillation and a worsening of angina.

Thyroxine is a pro-drug and is converted to T_3 through the action of deiodinases in the tissues.

15.5.2 Liothyronine (T_3)

Liothyronine is less bound to plasma proteins, leading to more rapid onset of action than thyroxine. The disadvantage of this is that it has a much shorter half-life and has to be taken or administered twice daily.

Liothyronine has the clinical advantage of being available as an injection, which is useful for critical patients unable to take tablets (i.e. those in a myxoedema coma, see above).

15.6 Contraception

Contraception, also called birth control, is the term used to refer to the different methods used to prevent a pregnancy. The most effective form of contraception is abstinence. However, this is difficult to maintain long term. A variety of barrier methods (e.g. condoms) and using 'safe' times in the menstrual cycle (e.g. the rhythm method) are also useful. However, of the non-abstinence methods of contraception, the most reliable are pharmacological interventions that use hormones based on endogenous female sex hormones.

15.6.1 The female reproductive hormones

Several hormones control the neurohormonal processes involved in the female reproductive system. These include the sex hormones **oestrogens** and **progestagens**, as well as the pituitary hormones **follicle stimulating hormone** (FSH) and **luteinising hormone** (LH), which control the release of the oestrogens and progestagens.

The sex hormones are steroid hormones derived from cholesterol, as illustrated in Figure 15.3.

Oestrogens

The main endogenous oestrogens are **oestradiol**, **oestrone** and **oestriol**. Oestradiol is the most potent oestrogen, and is secreted by the ovary. Oestriol and oestrone are about one tenth as potent, and oestriol is mainly secreted during pregnancy by the placenta.

Their mechanism of action is similar to that of other steroids. After binding to the intracellular type-4 nuclear receptor, the oestrogen–receptor complex moves to the nucleus, where it either induces or suppresses gene transcription. There are at least two types of oestrogen receptor: ERα and ERβ.

Oestrogens have a number of effects, including:

- development of the reproductive organs
- development of secondary sexual characteristics, e.g. breasts

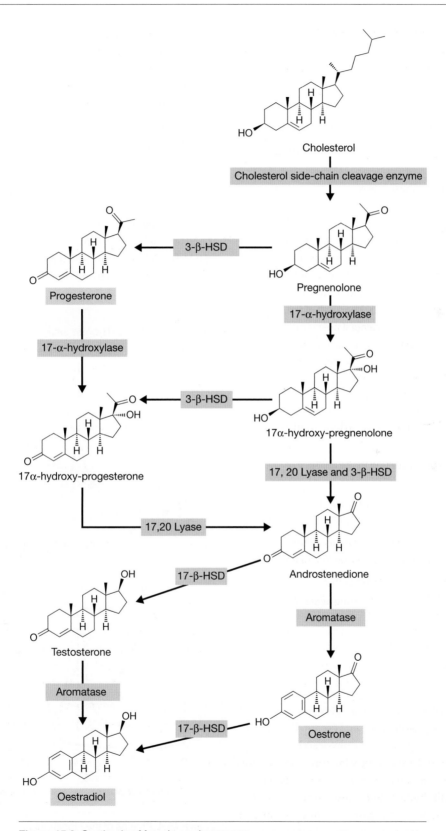

Figure 15.3 Synthesis of female sex hormones.

HSD, hydroxysteroid dehydrogenase; blue highlighted hormones are the main female sex hormones.

- increased growth and epiphysis closure, terminating growth of long bones
- control of menstrual cycle
- increase vaginal lubrication
- stimulate endothelial growth
- retention of sodium and water
- increase levels of high density lipoprotein, the good cholesterol
- increase platelet adhesiveness.

Progestogens

Progestogens are the other class of female sex hormones. Unlike oestrogens, there is only one endogenous progestogen, **progesterone**. It is also a steroid hormone produced from cholesterol. Progesterone is produced by the corpus luteum during the second half of the menstrual cycle or by the placenta if pregnancy occurs. Like oestrogens, progesterone acts through nuclear receptors in cells. The expression of progestagen receptors is controlled by oestrogens.

The effects of progesterone include:

- preparation and maintenance of the endometrium for pregnancy
- stimulation of menstruation in the absence of pregnancy
- inhibiting ovulation during the second half of the menstrual circle by inhibiting gonadotropin synthesis.
- sustaining pregnancy by maintenance of the endometrium and reducing contraction of the uterus
- inhibiting lactation during pregnancy
- increasing core temperature during ovulation (used as a method of contraception)
- normalizing blood clotting.

15.6.2 When and how are these hormones released: the menstrual cycle

Between the ages of 10 and 14 years, girls undergo several physical and biological changes, and eventually achieve fertility. This is called puberty. The physical changes they undergo include sudden growth, which precedes closure of the epiphyses (the ends of long bones converge and stop growing). The biological changes they undergo are maturation of reproductive organs and expression of secondary sexual characteristics (breasts and pubic hair). These changes are controlled by the increased release of hormones by the hypothalamus and pituitary glands (FSH and LH), which leads to release of the female sex

hormones (oestrogens and progestogens). The release of these hormones is controlled through a series of complex negative and positive feedback reactions and interactions, and controls the cyclic female reproductive processes called the menstrual cycle.

The menstrual cycle lasts between 28 and 30 days and has three key stages controlled by the actions of various hormones, as illustrated in Figure 15.4.

Menstruation (desquamation and reparation phase)

This is the first stage of the menstrual cycle, starting at day 1 and lasting 3–4 days. During menstruation, the uterus sheds the endometrium, which will have proliferated and become highly vascularized. This proliferation is in

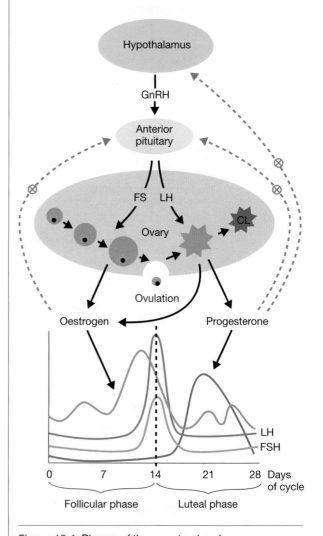

Figure 15.4 Phases of the menstrual cycle.

GnRH, gonadotrophin-releasing hormone; FSH, follicle-stimulating hormone; LH, luteinizing hormone; CL, corpus luteum.

preparation for possible implantation of the fertilized ovum during the proliferative (follicular) and secretory (luteal) stages (see later).

The endometrial shedding is brought on by increased prostaglandin levels released following regression of the **corpus luteum** (the collection of cells left after rupture of the follicle) and decreased levels of oestrogen and progesterone during days 26 and 27 of the cycle. This only happens if no fertilization occurs. The prostaglandins cause the endometrial vessels to contract and reduce blood flow to the endometrium, resulting in ischaemia, which damages the endometrium. Further contractions cause blood to leak out of the vessels. This blood, mixed with damaged endometrium, is what is released during menstruation as menses. At the end of menstruation, the 'wound' starts healing and the epithelium repairs itself.

Proliferative (follicular) phase

During this stage the endometrium proliferates and become thicker and highly vascularized. This phase is mostly controlled by oestrogens released by the ovary under the influence of FSH and LH. These hormones cause the ovaries to produce several follicles that contain one ovum each. One of the ovum, called the **Graafian follicle** (GF), develops extremely fast whilst the others degenerate. This degeneration is thought to be due to a deficiency of GnRH receptors on these follicles The GF matures and becomes filled with fluid and ovum surrounded by thecal and granulosa cells. During this maturation process, FSH and LH cause the granulose cells of the GF to produce and release oestradiol. The released oestrogen, along with low progesterone levels, sends a negative feedback to the hypothalamus, resulting in reduced release of FSH and LH. Some granulosa cells in the GF become luteal cells, which respond to LH and produce progesterone. The increasing oestrogen levels during the mid and late follicular phase switches the negative feedback to the hypothalamus and pituitary to positive.

This results in increased FSH and LH levels mid-cycle (day 14–15). The LH induces the action of cytokines, prostaglandins, histamines, and plasminogen activators, which dissolve the thecal wall and cause contraction of the GF. The contraction causes the GF to rupture and release the ovum (egg) in what is called ovulation. During the mid-cycle period the cervical cells also secrete mucous with a pH of 8–9, which is less viscous than usual and more favorable to spermatozoa. In the presence of spermatozoa, fertilization is likely to occur. If pregnancy

does occur, the sequence of events is different, and is controlled by the human chorion gonatrophin hormone initially and later on by oestrogens and progesterones produced by the placenta. However, if no fertilization occurs, the cycle continues into the luteal phase.

Secretory (luteal) phase

In the absence of pregnancy, this phase lasts 14–15 days and is predominantly controlled by progesterone. After the release of the ovum, the shell of ruptured GF turns into the corpus luteum. The corpus luteum produces progesterone and oestrogen, which initially leads to further proliferation of the endometrium. Increased progesterone levels send a negative feedback, causing the LH and FSH levels to drop. After 10 days (day 25) the corpus luteum degenerates and levels of progesterone and oestrogen reduce further, whilst prostaglandin levels increase. This initiates contraction of the endometrial vessels and eventually leads to menstruation.

15.6.3 Pharmacological methods of contraception

The most common form of pharmacologic contraception is oral using contraceptive pills. There are two main types of pills: combinations of synthetic oestrogens and progestogens, and progestogen only. Other forms of pharmacological contraception include:

- parenteral progesterone derivatives
- intrauterine progesterone devices
- transdermal patches.

The most commonly used synthetic oestrogen is **ethinyl oestradiol** (EE). It is structurally related to oestradiol (Figure 15.5) and has a similar pharmacological effect. Because of the alterations to the oestradiol structure it has better bioavailability compared to oestradiol as it avoids first-pass metabolism. The other synthetic oestrogen is **mestranol**. This is the 3-methyl ester of EE and is a pro-drug that must be converted in the liver to EE. Given that about 70% of mestranol is converted to EE, 50 µg of mestranol is equivalent to 35 µg of EE.

Synthetic oestrogens are metabolized by cytochrome P450 in the liver and eliminated in the bile as sulphates and glucuronides. Once in the gut the EE metabolites are converted back into EE by gut bacteria and the EE is reabsorbed. This is referred to as enterohepatic circulation, and it causes two peaks in the pharmaokinetic profile of EE (one for the initial

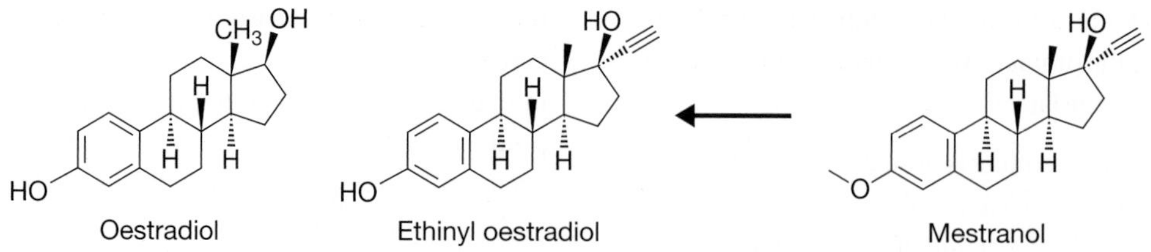

Figure 15.5 Commonly used synthetic oestrogens.

absorption and the second because of enterohepatic circulation). This is also a source of one of the potential drug interactions between combined oral contraceptives (COCs) and broad-spectrum antibiotics. When a women takes broad-spectrum antibiotics (e.g. amoxicillin, doxycycline, etc.) they get rid of the normal intestinal flora. This can interrupt the enterohepatic circulation, resulting in lower levels of oestrogens, which can lead to contraceptive failure.

A number of synthetic progestogens are used. They can be roughly divided into five groups: progesterone analogues, older testosterone analogues, newer testosterone analogues, spironolactone analogues, and anti-androgens (Table 15.2).

The newer progestogens desogestrel, drospirenone, cyproterone, and gestodene have less androgenic activity and are reserved for patients who suffer adverse drug reactions such as acne, depression, and weight gain with older progestogens.

The mechanisms by which these synthetic oestrogens and progestogens lead to contraception is by modifying or inhibiting the processes of the menstrual cycle described in Figure 15.4. These include:

- suppressing the release of FSH (oestrogens)
- inhibiting the surge of LH, which would normally lead to ovulation, and thereby preventing ovulation (progesterone)

- adaptation of the endometrial structure and conditions to make them less favourable for implantation of the fetus (progesterone and oestrogens)
- decreasing motility of the fallopian tube, which slows down the rate of transportation of the fertilized ovum (progesterone)
- thickening of the mucous produced by the cervix, making it more difficult for sperm to penetrate (progesterone).

Combined oral contraceptive pills

Combined oral contraceptive pills contain a combination of synthetic oestrogens and progestogens. The COCs are often referred to as first, second, or third generation based on the quantity and type of oestrogen or progestogen they contain. First-generation pills used high doses of oestrogen (up to 100 µg of EE equivalent) and were withdrawn in the 1970s because of links with thrombosis and pulmonary embolism (see later). The second-generation pills comprised 35–50 µg of EE-equivalent in combination with older testosterone analogues (e.g. levonorgestrel). The third-generation pills combine estrogens (sometimes with doses as low as 20 µg of EE) with new, less-androgenic progestogens (e.g. desogestrel).

The COCs can also be classified as mono-, bi-, or triphasic based on whether the hormone quantity is fixed or variable. Monophasic pills contain the same amount of

Table 15.2 Commonly used progestogens

Progesterone analogues	Older testosterone analogues	Newer testosterone analogues	Spironolactone analogues	Anti-androgens
Dydrogesterone Medroxyprogesterone	Norethisterone Norgestrel Levonorgestrel	Desogestrel Norgestimate Gestodene Etonogestrel	Drospirenone	Cyproterone

oestrogen and progesterone in all of the active pills in a pack. Biphasic and triphasic pills contain different dosages of progesterone or oestrogen throughout the pill pack. Compared with monophasics, these pills reduce the total hormone dosage a woman receives, and are thought to better match the body's natural menstrual cycle.

The COC is taken once a day at about the same time. However, unlike the progestogen-only pills (see later), if a woman forgets to take it but remembers and takes it within 12–24 hours, she will still be covered. The advantages of using a COC include their high efficacy and a decrease in the incidences of menstrual bleeding, premenstrual tension, irregular periods, anaemia, uterine fibroids, and ovarian cysts. The main disadvantage is an increased risk of the combined side effects of oestrogens and progestogens. The common side effects include nausea, vomiting, weight gain, acne, breast tenderness, and breakthrough bleeding. Most of these can be addressed by changing the pill to one with a different (usually lower) concentration of oestrogen and/or to one of the newer progestogens. The major concerns with COCs are cardiovascular events (thrombosis), breast cancer, and cervical cancer. The increase in the risk of thrombosis depends on the oestrogen dose, the type of progestogen, and having existing risk factors. The risk appears lowest with low doses of EE in combination with older progestogens (e.g. norethisterone or levonorgestrel). The highest risk is with high-dose (50 µg EE) oestrogens, followed by the combinations using newer progestagens (e.g. cyproterone). COCs may be associated with a small increased risk of cervical cancer, which increases the longer you take the COC, therefore patients are advised to have regular cervical smears. The association with an increased risk of breast cancer is still unclear and probably small.

Apart from the interaction with broad-spectrum antibiotics (see above), a number of other drugs interact with, and reduce the efficacy of, COCs. These are drugs that increase the activity (inducers) of the cytochrome P450 3A4 isozyme, and include phenytoin, phenobarbitone, St Johns Wort, rifampicin, and some antiretroviral drugs.

Progestogen-only pill

The progestogen-only pill (POP) (also called the minipill) contains either norethisterone, levonorgestrel, or ethynodiol alone. The POP works by changing cervical mucous to make it unreceptive to sperm and by altering the lining of the endometrium, making implantation less likely.

POPs have the advantage that they do not affect breast-feeding (oestrogens inhibit milk production) and therefore they are useful in the post-partum (after birth) period. They are also useful in patients who cannot tolerate oestrogens. However, the efficacy of POPs, even when used properly, is much less than that of COCs. The POP has to be taken continuously (i.e. every day) and at the same time (within 3 hours of the same time) each day. If a person forgets, even by a few hours, the efficacy is completely lost and other (e.g. barrier) methods must be used.

Changes in the menstrual cycle and increased or decreased bleeding at menstruation are the most common side effects. However, the long-term effects are less clear as POPs have not been used as long as COCs.

Parenteral progesterone-only contraception

Progesterone derivatives can be administered either intramuscularly or subcutaneously (as an implant) as contraceptives. Examples include medroxyprogesterone and etonogestrel. They provide contraception for 12 weeks (medroxyprogesterone) to 3 years (etonogestrel). They are more effective than POPs, but have adverse effects similar to those of the progestogens.

Intrauterine progesterone-only devices

These are implanted in the uterus and slowly release progesterone, which leads to contraception for a period of up to 5 years. Local irritation and other local effects are the most common adverse reactions.

Transdermal patch

This is a combination of oestrogen and progesterone in a patch applied once a week for three of the four weeks of the menstrual cycle. Adverse effects, apart from those of the COC, are generally local irritation due to the adhesive of the patch.

Postcoital or emergency contraception

This is also referred to as the 'morning after pill', although this is misnomer as it can be taken up to 72 hours after unprotected sex (although the sooner you take it the more effective it is). This pill contains a very high dose of levonorgestrel, which if administered within 72 hours will prevent pregnancy in 75% of cases. It works by similar mechanisms to regular POPs in that it inhibits LH secretion, makes the cervical mucous thick and uninviting to sperm, changes the structure of the endometrium to make implantation less likely, and slows the motility of the fallopian tube, reducing the movement of the ovum if an egg is released. It can be taken either as two tablets taken 12 hours apart (i.e. 750 µg levonorgestrel twice a day) or as a single dose (i.e. 1500 µg levonorgestrel). Nausea and vomiting are the most common side effects, and more likely with the single 1500 µg dose. If vomiting occurs within 2 hours of taking the tablet(s), then a replacement dose is needed.

SUMMARY OF DRUGS USED FOR THYROID

Therapeutic class	Drugs	Mechanism of action	Clinical uses	Comments	Examples of adverse drug reactions
Thyroid hormones	Levothyroxine (T_4 or thyroxine) Liothyronine (T_3 or tri-iodothyronine)	T_4 converted to T_3, which binds to thyroid receptor, causing a conformational change that stops the coreprocessor complex and cause activation of transcription, leading to protein synthesis	Hypothyroidism	The functions of the thyroid hormones are complicated and interwoven	Diarrhoea Vomiting Arrhythmia (usually excessive dosage)
Radioactive iodide	^{131}I	Taken up into the thyroid in place of iodide, where it releases β- and γ-rays. The γ-rays just pass through the body, but the β-rays destroy the follicles and this leads to a reduction in thyroid hormones	Hyperthyroidism	Very effective Used for: malignant thyroid tumors in sulphur-intolerant patients in patients non-responsive to thioureylenes when surgery is contraindicated Has long half-life and takes 3–4 months for effect therefore sometimes co-prescribed with thioureylenes	Hypothyroidism
Thioureylenes	Carbimazole Propylthiouracil	Prevent the biosynthesis of T_4 and T_3 by acting as substrate for, and therefore blocking, the thyroperoxidase enzyme, preventing the oxidation of iodide and the binding of the iodide to the tyrosine	Hyperthyroidism	Mainstay of treatment for hyperthyroidism Used with propranolol in acute cases	Marrow suppression (agranulocytosis and neutropenia) Gastrointestinal upset Allergic reactions
Iodide ions	Lugol's iodine	Blocks release of thyroid hormone by inhibiting iodine organification, leading to thyroglobulin accumulation and a reduction in the number of blood vessels in the thyroid gland	Hyperthyroidism, hyperthyroid crises	Commonly used prior to surgery because it makes the gland firmer and easier to operate on	Angio-odema

Chapter 15 The thyroid and contraception

Therapeutic class	Drugs	Mechanism of action	Clinical uses	Comments	Examples of adverse drug reactions
β-adrenoceptor antagonists (β-blockers)	Propranolol	Thyroid hormones are also thought to increase sensitivity of sympathomimetic neurotransmitters like adrenaline and noradrenaline by increasing the number of adrenoceptors The β-adrenoceptor antagonists are therefore used to reduce those sympathomimetic-like-effects of hyperthyroidism, even though they have no direct effect on the thyroid hormone levels	Hyperthyroid crises	Used to control symptoms of hyperthyroidism	See Drug summary table in Chapter 5

SUMMARY OF DRUGS USED FOR CONTRACEPTION

Therapeutic class	Drugs	Mechanism of action	Clinical uses	Comments	Examples of adverse drug reactions
Oestrogens	Ethinylestradiol Mestranol	After binding to the intracellular type-4 nuclear receptor, the oestrogen-receptor complex moves to the nucleus, where it either induces or suppresses gene transcription	Contraception Hormone replacement therapy	In combination with progesterone as combined oral contraceptive pill	Hypertension Oedema Weight gain VTE
Progesterones	Progesterone analogues: dydrogesterone medroxyprogesterone Older testosterone analogues: norethisterone norgestrel levonorgestrel Newer testosterone analogues: desogestrel norgestimate gestodene etonogestrel Spironolactone analogues: drospirenone Anti-androgens: cyproterone	Modifies or inhibits the processes of the menstrual cycle described in Figure 15.4	Contraception	Either in combination as combined oral contraceptive pill or alone as: a) progesterone mini pill b) injection Desogestrel, drospirenone, cyproterone and gestodene have less androgenic activity and are reserved for patients who suffer adverse drug reactions such as acne, depression, and weight gain	Menstrual disturbances Premenstrual-like symptoms

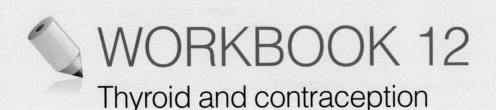

WORKBOOK 12
Thyroid and contraception

Sunita: a simplified case history

Sunita finally gave in to Eoin, her husband of 12 blissful months, and agreed to be taken to the private hospital. A year ago they had become man and wife during an extravagant ceremony in the Caribbean after a whirlwind romance. Sunita has lost a lot of weight recently and has been complaining of palpitations and insomnia. She is also quite irritable. She has missed her period for 2 months now, although several pregnancy tests have been negative. Last night the palpitations got worse and being a pharmacist she knew it was time to admit that there was something not quite right.

A table of clinical clerking abbreviations is given on page xi.

CLINICAL CLERKING FOR SUNITA KAISER

Age: 27 years

PC: Severe palpitations, fatigue, and minor swallowing difficulties. Throat protruding and eyes bulging.

HPC: She has been experiencing the above symptoms for 2 months now and they have gradually got worse. She has also lost weight and missed two periods.

PMH: Nil significant

   Sunita has been very healthy all her life until recently.

DH: Oral contraceptives

SH: Married, lives with husband, no children

O/E:

Flushed moist skin, tremor and nervousness, muscle weakness, thinning of hair, exophthalmus and mild goitre.

Pulse = 120 beats per minute. (reference: <70)

   Although non-specific, Sunita's symptoms of palpitation, tremor, nervousness, weight loss, amenorrhea, insomnia, flushed skin, hair thinning, exophthalmus, and goitre are consistent with the symptoms of hyperthyroidism.

   Her swallowing difficulties are a result of the mild goiter (swelling in the neck due to the enlarged thyroid gland).

   Exophthalmus is protrusion of the eyes, which is one of the eye signs of hyperthyroidism.

   The doctor decides to admit her and check out her thyroid function tests.

Biochemistry:

1) Thyroxine (T$_4$) = 180 nmol/L   (reference: 64–154)

2) Triiodothyronine (T$_3$) = 4 nmol/L   (reference: 1.1–2.0)

3) Thyroid-stimulating hormone (TSH) = 0.1 mIU/L   (reference: 0.5–4.7)

> *Sunita's laboratory findings are consistent with hyperthyroidism. Note that T$_4$ and T$_3$ are elevated, while TSH is low.*

Diagnosis: Hyperthyroidism (probably Graves' disease).

Plan:

Administer Lugol solution

Commence propranolol and carbimazole

> The doctor explains to Sunita that she has a type of hyperthyroidism called Graves' disease. He explains that thyrotoxicosis is caused by excessive activity of the thyroid hormones, which increases metabolic rate. (The doctor uses technical terms because he knows Sunita is a pharmacist.)

1a) What are the two thyroid hormones called?

1b) What is thyroglobulin and where is it found in the thyroid gland?

2) Elaborate on the main steps in the synthesis, storage, and secretion of thyroid hormones.

3a) List the two hormones secreted by the hypothalamus and pituitary, respectively, which regulate the function of the thyroid gland.

3b) List one aspect of thyroid hormone synthesis controlled by TSH.

4a) Why is T$_4$ regarded as a pro-hormone?

4b) How does thyroid hormone interact on its receptor?

5a) What are the two main types of hyperthyroidism and how do they differ?

5b) What happens in thyrotoxicosis?

5c) What is the cause of Graves' disease?

5d) Why were Sunita's TSH levels so low?

The doctor explains to Sunita that three drugs would be used initially to manage her hyperthyroidism and the resulting symptoms. He explains that she may eventually need surgery if the drugs fail to reduce her symptoms.

6) List three treatment options of hyperthyroidism.

7) To which group does the drug carbimazole belong and what is the action of this group of drugs?

8a) Why would propranolol be used in hyperthyroidism even though it has no direct effect on the thyroid?

After her second blood test, Sunita is readmitted to hospital because she is complaining of a sore throat and cough, and her blood tests indicate that her neutrophil count is extremely low.

8b) What is the most probable cause of Sunita's low neutrophil count?

Dr Knight, the senior doctor on the medical team, comes to see Sunita. She explains to Sunita the cause of the low blood cell count.

She changes Sunita's medication from carbimazole to propylthiouracil. Sunita seems to tolerate this better. She is discharged home after one week.

However after four months, during her follow up, the doctors decide that her symptoms are not improving as hoped. It is decided that she needs either surgery or radioactive iodine therapy. Sunita and Eoin decide that surgery is preferable because Sunita was warned that she should not become pregnant for up to four months following radioactive iodine therapy. The radioactive therapy would also take longer than surgery because it is repeated in cycles of six months. They do not want to wait any longer than necessary to start a family.

Her surgery is scheduled for two weeks later.

Following surgery, blood tests reveal that Sunita's thyroid hormone levels are lower than normal. She is also experiencing some symptoms of hypothyroidism, like lethargy and weight gain. The doctor explains to her that hypothyroidism is a possible risk of hyperthyroid surgery.

The doctor tells Sunita she will need to be started on replacement tablets.

9a) What tablets was the doctor referring to?

9b) What are the actions of these tablets?

10) What are the signs and symptoms of hypothyroidism?

Sunita is commenced on levothyroxine tablets and discharged 2 days later.

One year later, Sunita is still taking contraceptive pills. She was put on them because it was not advisable to get pregnant whilst undergoing iodide treatment. She takes them every single day and there are 28 tablets in a pack. She knows that only 21 of these are active and the other seven are just inactive tablets to increase compliance.

Since she started taking them her menstrual cycle has altered and her periods are shorter and regular.

11a) How many days constitute a normal menstrual cycle?

11b) What are the three main phases of the menstrual cycle?

12) Explain what happens during the early follicular phase.

13a) List four hormones that control the various stages of the menstrual cycle.

13b) What roles do LH and progesterone play in the menstrual cycle and in which phase?

14a) At what stage of the follicular phase do oestrogen levels peak and what is the effect of this on LH and FSH levels?

14b) What is the name of the cells that secret oestradiol?

15) What happens in the absence of pregnancy during the luteal phase (days 25-28)? What is this commonly called?

16) What are the two main types of oral contraceptive?

17a) Explain the following:

monophasic combined pill

biphasic/triphasic combined pill

_____

_____

_____

17b) What is the mechanism of action of the combined pill?

_____

_____

18) List drugs that interact with oral contraceptive drugs and explain how they interact.

_____

_____

_____

19) What is the mechanism of action of the progesterone-only pill?

_____

_____

_____

Sunita decides she would rather not use any hormonal contraception because her friend Monique tells her she suffered a severe adverse drug reaction whilst on the pill and was put on warfarin to treat it.

20) What adverse drug reaction was Monique referring to?

_____

_____

_____

Sunita decides they will just use condoms as contraception because:

• pills containing the newer progesterones, which are used when patients have adverse drug reactions to older pills, could increase the risk of thromboembolism

• if she takes the progesterone-only pill, she will have to ensure a missed pill is taken within 3 hours; this is too risky considering her forgetfulness

• her body mass index is now too high, which is a contraindication for combined oral contraceptives

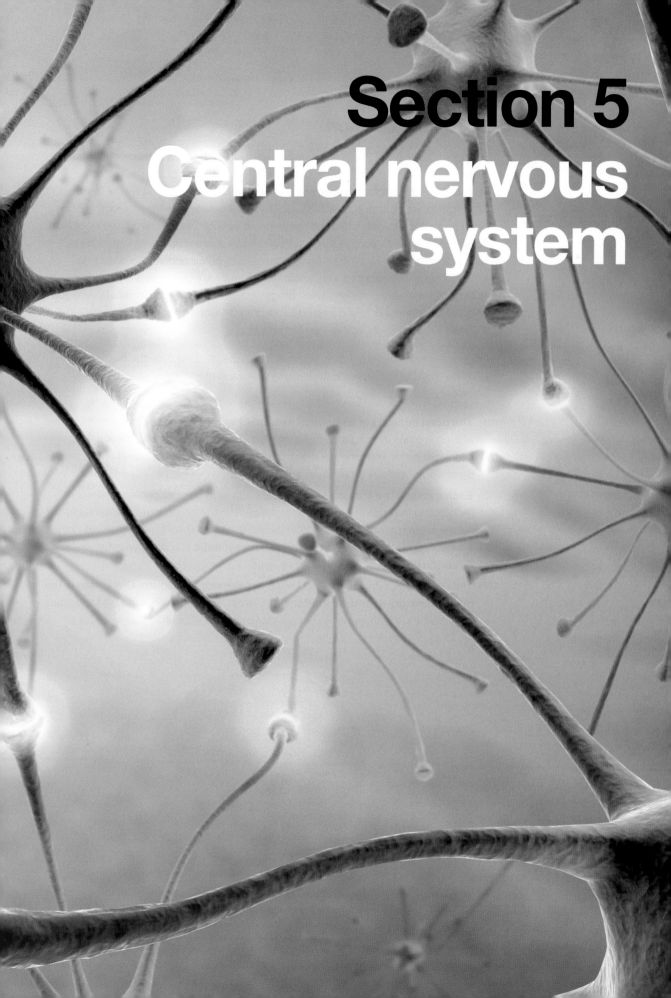

Section 5
Central nervous system

S5.1 Introduction

Suppose you were told that in an exam you will have to answer a question on the molecular biology of insanity, or the cellular basis of Parkinson's disease, or the neurobiology of epileptic seizures, or the molecular basis for relieving severe depression. You might think that is an impossible task for you to contemplate—it's too complex, you'll never understand it. Well, when you have worked through this section you will be able to do all these things. It's not that it's easy, it's just that it is possible. It's not that then you'll fully understand these subjects—no one does—but you will understand enough to explain a great deal about yourself and patients, and you'll understand a great deal about how some very commonly used drugs work to bring therapeutic benefit. And you will have the framework to understand future drug developments. It is challenging, but we hope you'll find it interesting—we certainly do.

Of course a more basic question you might be asked is: how does the brain work? Don't be afraid of this question. It's easy to make a start in a way that immediately helps us understand drug action.

1) **The brain consists of a neuronal network.** Neurons connect to and communicate with each other, forming a complex network. This is mainly by release of a neurotransmitter from one cell which then reaches and changes another cell at a synapse, as with any other neuronal system.

2) **Each synapse is a little computer.** When cells form synaptic contacts with other cells (and in the brain they may form and receive many thousands) these contacts are not like two wires meeting in an electrical circuit: each point of contact receives both excitatory and modulatory influences, both **presynaptic** and **postsynaptic**, which determine the output from the synapse.

3) The neuronal activity is kept alive by the **accelerator** in the brain. **Glutamate is the main excitatory neurotransmitter in the brain.** Most brain neurons are stimulated by glutamate, which forms the accelerator pedal of the brain.

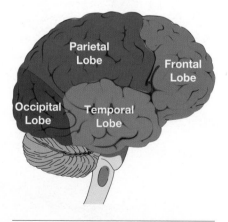

Figure S5.1 The human brain. The external surface of the brain labelled with the major divisions of the cortex.

4) Neuronal activity is controlled and dampened down by the **brake** in the brain. **Gamma-aminobutyric acid (GABA) is the main inhibitory neurotransmitter in the brain**, and it forms the brake pedal.

5) **Hundreds of other modulatory neurotransmitters** also act on the neurons, refining and directing neuronal activity. Some are capable of stimulating on their own, but mostly they mould and change the neuronal activity set up by the action of glutamate within neuronal networks.

So glutamate pushes activity up, GABA pushes it down, and hundreds of other events occur at the same time. Can we translate this into useful information for understanding treatment of disease in the brain? We can make a start: in epilepsy waves of excitation pass, out of control, through neural networks; the glutamate activity dominates over weak opposition from GABA. Put simply, GABA is too low, so we want drugs that increase the GABA influence, and that is exactly what we have in the treatment of epilepsy, as explained in Chapter 16. Also in that chapter the account of glutamate and GABA as accelerator and brake respectively are developed in Box 16.1.

So we have immediately got a grasp of brain function in a way that enables us to understand an element of drug therapy. To develop this further we might look back at the basic biology of the neuron, and forward to the introduction of regions of the brain which that we will mention later in this section.

S5.2 The brain is mostly glial cells, not neurons

Before we move on to that, let's think about one curious aspect of brain function. We talk about neurons, how they project, how they interact, receiving and sending signals to each other in a complex neuronal net that forms the basis for our thinking and feeling, for what we are. Perhaps there are 100 billion neurons in the adult brain. So is the brain mainly made up of neurons? Well, the answer is no, most of the cells in the brain are glial cells. These are conventionally thought of as a sort of housekeeping system, keeping the neurons supplied and healthy so they can do their complex job. There are several types of glial cells, the most abundant being astrocytes, and after that oligodendroglial cells. There is no doubt that glial cells play a supportive role in neuronal activity, but they also play a role in neurotransmission. For example, astrocytes are involved in the removal (taking up and destroying) of some of the neurotransmitters, terminating their action. But despite the numerical superiority of glial cells, the story of 'drugs and the brain' is still, as far as we know, mainly about neurons and the mystery of their webs and networks.

S5.3 The biology of the neuron

There are fundamental aspects which are the same for brain neurons as for neurons in the autonomic nervous system. Most important for us here are:

1) excitation of the neuron by neurotransmitter (e.g. glutamate) receptors at the cell body setting up the action potential, and its modulation by other neurotransmitters

2) the role of fast Na⁺ channels in the passage of the action potential down the axon, leading to depolarization of the nerve terminal.

3) the role of depolarization-sensitive Ca^{2+} channels at the nerve terminal in allowing Ca^{2+} into the terminal

4) the Ca^{2+}-stimulated release of neurotransmitters from storage in the vesicles into the synaptic cleft and its modulation by stimulation of receptors at the nerve terminal (**presynaptic receptors**)

5) the stimulation by the released neurotransmitter of receptors on the innervated cells (**postsynaptic receptors**)

6) removal of released neurotransmitter by breakdown (enzymes) and by active uptake, sucking the neurotransmitter back into the nerve terminal or into neighbouring cells.

Each of these stages is modified by the drugs used to treat brain disorders and described in this section. Of course there is a vast amount of additional information about brain neurons and circuits which that could be discussed, but to understand what follows it is perhaps more useful to introduce some brain regions we will encounter in this section.

S5.4 Organization of the brain into regions

Brain anatomy can become shrouded in a confusion of terminology derived from the names of long-dead anatomists, or their whimsical imaginings when looking at parts of the brain, mixed in with overlapping, often obsolete, conceptions of connections and systems which neither connect nor are systematic. Don't be put off. Here we simply introduce some of the parts of the brain which that are mentioned later.

When you look at the human brain you see a surface covered with deep convolutions (Figure S5.2A). This is the **cortex** (which makes sense since the word cortex means the outer layer). If we were to take a fresh brain and push the cortex apart and to one side (this is easily done,—it is very soft) we would see below clearly visible regions, almost as clearly as we can see organs in the abdomen when it is opened. These are the subcortical regions, and some are shown diagrammatically in Figure S5.2B.

We are used to the notion that the higher intellectual functions of the brain occur in the cortex—it is worth noting that the cortex is in intimate and two-way contact with the subcortical regions of the brain, and that the 'higher functions' are profoundly influenced by these subcortical regions. A good example is the **hippocampus** and its involvement in memory recall—disturbance of hippocampal function may occur in Alzheimer's disease, and this may contribute to memory deficits. The **limbic system** incorporates several regions, including the hippocampus, **amygdala**, **hypothalamus**, and **nucleus accumbens**, and is conventionally associated with emotions and diverse advanced mental functions. We encounter these limbic regions particularly in the schizophrenia story. The hypothalamus also plays a major role in assembling information from various parts of the brain into an action plan for the endocrine system—note its closeness, at the base of the brain, to the pituitary. There is a term

A.

B.

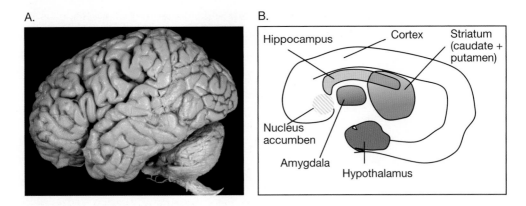

Figure S5.2 A photograph of the intact human brain (A) and a diagram showing some of the large subcortical regions (B).

The photograph in A shows the surface dominated by the convoluted cortex. The area at the bottom on the left is the cerebellum, and beneath this can be seen the beginnings of the spinal cord where it was torn off. In B the cortex is illustrated and beneath this the presence of some of the larger subcortical regions referred to later in this section.

'**basal ganglia**' that cannot be entirely ignored—it incorporates fairly large structures lying beneath the cortex, which includes parts called the **caudate** and **putamen**, which together form the **striatum**. This collection of connected regions is involved in the planning of physical movement of the body, and degeneration of a set of neurons here is the central cause of Parkinson's disease.

S5.5 Regions are overlaid with different neurotransmitters

The regions of the brain are all complex networks in which neurons may be intrinsic (beginning and ending in a single region) or connecting (beginning in one region and ending in others). These neurons are characterized by their principal neurotransmitters. In addition to glutamate and GABA, there are neurons using the diverse modulatory neurotransmitters mentioned above. When we consider that the number of different neurotransmitters is counted in hundreds, and many (most) interact with several receptor subtypes, then the number of different synaptic contacts defined by the neurotransmitter-receptor pair alone is enormous, contributing to the extraordinary complexity of brain neuronal networks. Many of these neurotransmitters—their synthesis, storage, release, removal, and particularly their receptors—are the targets of drugs used in neurology and psychiatry. We shall now enter this exciting world of brain disorders, pain, unhappiness, and insanity.

Chapter 16
Epilepsy

The most common conception of epilepsy is of a disease that results in fits (or seizures) consisting of gross movements of the whole body, with uncontrolled contractions of the limbs and facial muscles. But what about someone who has repeated episodes of staring, in which mental activity and engagement with the outside world seem to have departed? Such 'absence' seizures are a common manifestation of epilepsy. Recurrent episodes of memory recollections which overwhelm and occupy the entire mind could also be due to an epileptic fit (or seizure). What these and other seizures have in common is that they are caused by a transient period of uncontrolled excitation, with disordered waves of activity disrupting normal function in a part, or all, of the brain. Seizures may be rare and mild, or major and disruptive to normal life, and in extreme form they can be life threatening. They may remain or develop over a lifetime or they may subside as years pass. They may be banished by drugs or have their impact moderated by drugs or they may be drug resistant.

With this diversity in clinical features we will also see below a diversity of drugs available, with their pattern of use largely governed by clinical experience rather than by an understanding of drug action. Nevertheless, in this area we can see how the dysfunction in epilepsy is a failure to control neuronal excitability in the brain, and we can see how the different cellular and molecular actions of antiepileptic drugs moderate this dysfunction in different ways. In this way we can more effectively understand patients' responses, or lack of responses, and the logic of different drug combinations. Some of the complexities of managing this condition are illustrated by the patient Ambreen in the workbook at the end of this chapter.

16.1 What is epilepsy? Seizures and convulsions: prevalence, types, and causes

Epilepsy is diagnosed when patients suffer repeated epileptic seizures. These seizures are sudden episodes of abnormal bursts of excitatory brain activity, leading to transient motor, autonomic, psychic, or sensory dysfunction. Seizures can be convulsive, as with gross uncontrolled physical movements, or non-convulsive, as in periods of blank, staring behaviour (absence seizures). Epilepsy (particularly as absence seizures) commonly presents in childhood.

It should be noted that there are other causes of seizures, such as childhood febrile convulsions, caused by fever. Ambreen, our patient in the workbook at the end of this chapter, has a medical history which includes childhood febrile convulsions and 'absences'. She presented with tonic-clonic convulsions (see below) at the age of 23. This was treated as a first, unexplained, appearance of epilepsy. Her childhood experiences were not thought to be epilepsy. While convulsions are always of concern and require medical intervention, childhood febrile convulsions are not grounds for diagnosing epilepsy.

Young people with epilepsy will often grow out of it, eventually being able to give up antiepileptic drugs (AEDs) forever. This is worth noting when counselling patients and their relatives.

Some events that are not seizures at all offer potential for confusion. For example **syncope** is a term used to describe fainting, which can be mistaken for a seizure.

16.1.1 Prevalence

Epilepsy is one of the most common neurological conditions encountered in children and adults. In the UK about 1 person in 30 will develop epilepsy during their lifetime. The prevalence of epilepsy is estimated at about 0.1%, although in Denmark a recent study reveals that about 1% of the population are being prescribed **AEDs**, most commonly for epilepsy itself (AEDs are also used to treat a variety of other disorders). Frequency of prescribing increases with age—a study in the USA found that 11% of elderly nursing home residents were being prescribed AEDs, again mostly for epilepsy. Around 50–100 million people worldwide may suffer from epilepsy. The condition remains difficult to treat despite the introduction of various new drugs in the last 15 years; 30–40% of patients continue to have fits despite drugs and surgery. It is also worth noting that the objective of drug therapy is to prevent the symptoms (seizures) and not to tackle the underlying disorder.

16.1.2 Classification of epilepsies is by type and pattern of seizures

The term epilepsy covers a variety of conditions that are recognized as diverse in terms of:

- causes
- cellular and molecular dysfunction providing the conditions in which seizures can emerge
- localization of abnormal neuronal activity within the central nervous system
- clinical manifestation of the seizures.

In clinical practice the decision as to which type of epilepsy is present is based on the type of seizure observed and whether this is localized in origin (**partial**), or involves all of the brain from the outset (**primary generalized**), as set out in Figure 16.1. Superimposed upon these categories are the terms **simple** (meaning no loss of consciousness) and **complex** (with some loss of consciousness).

The use of drugs is then grouped according to which of these categories of seizure activity they are useful in reducing.

Partial seizures

The term partial (or focal) refers to how the seizure begins, meaning localized to a region of the brain at the outset. The activity may (a) remain localized, (b) spread to adjacent regions of the brain, or (c) spread throughout the cerebrum. The latter cases are then described as **secondarily generalized tonic–clonic seizures** (see below).

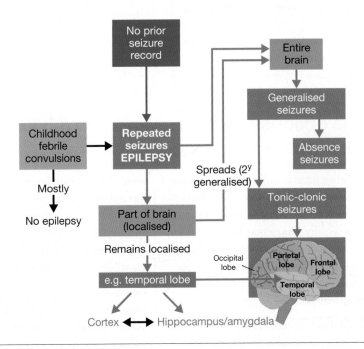

Figure 16.1 Scheme of types of seizure activity commonly seen in eplilepsy.

On the left febrile convulsions are placed separately—these are not epilepsy. Epilsepsy is characterized by repeated seizure activity, either localized or affecting the entire brain (generalized).

16.1 What is epilepsy? Seizures and convulsions: prevalence, types, and causes

419

An example is **temporal lobe epilepsy**, which is both common and difficult to control with drugs. It may remain localized, or it may spread.

Simple partial seizure The temporal lobe is itself divided into discrete regions with clearly different functions, including the region of the cortex (neocortex), which falls within the temporal lobe, and the regions beneath, namely the hippocampus and the closely associated amygdala. Simple partial seizures remain very localized to their origin, only affecting a part of the temporal lobe. This may be only the cortex, for example, or the subcortical structures (hippocampus/amygdala). The result is a range of seizure experience, which may be no less disabling for being intriguing. These may include experiences of smells, emotions, recall of past events, loss of memory, religious experience, and sensation of feelings localized to regions of the body.

Complex partial seizures Temporal lobe epilepsy means that the abnormal neuronal activity spreads to encompass the entire temporal lobe, but not beyond, causing a loss of ability to function that may manifest as a limited loss of consciousness with inability to respond to others and bizarre mental experiences and behaviours.

Secondarily generalized tonic–clonic seizures Secondarily generalized tonic–clonic seizures occur when the activity spreads widely throughout the brain. The features of generalized tonic–clonic seizures are described below. It is of interest to note here that a patient may describe a set of experiences (the aura) as preceding a full epileptic fit. This is the experience of a simple/complex partial seizure activity (the aura) preceding the spread to a generalized tonic–clonic phase (the fit).

Primary generalized seizuress

These are seizures with activity widely spread throughout the brain from the outset. We can divide these into several subcategories. Some main ones useful for understanding drug action are:

Primary generalized tonic–clonic seizures, which involve widespread gross muscular activity in the limbs, face, and elsewhere. A severe attack will typically have the following features:

- The short **tonic phase** (usually less than 30–40 seconds) comprises contracted muscles, with extended head and neck, open eyes, limbs straight. The patient falls to the ground with a loud cry as breathing muscles spasmodically contract, the body stiffens, and there is cessation of breathing, perhaps with incontinence.

- The more sustained **clonic phase** may last for 30 minutes, but is usually much shorter. There are rhythmic contractions and relaxations of muscles generating gross uncontrolled body movements (e.g. of face and limbs), resulting in widespread convulsions. Coordination of respiratory muscle contraction is lost, which with the prior cessation of breathing during the clonic phase results in cyanosis (blue coloration of the skin due to low oxygen saturation of the blood).

Absence seizures commonly involve widespread excitation from the outset, giving a period of blank staring and unresponsiveness of short duration (commonly 10 s or less). There is no accompanying movement of face and limbs, and posture is retained. Absence seizures often present in childhood and can be frequent.

Myoclonic seizures are relatively rare, involving a very brief spasmodic contraction of muscles, resulting in a jerky movement.

Continuous seizures

Seizures as described above are episodic, meaning that they are of short duration (e.g. less than 5 minutes, usually a lot less than this) with a gap (very variable, perhaps minutes, perhaps weeks) before the onset of the next. With **status epilepticus** the seizure activity is of long duration. If convulsive, this is a medical emergency, potentially life threatening.

There are some drugs that are used to prevent all classes of seizure activity and some that are only useful against particular types, as described in section 16.4.

The role of electroencephalograms

Electroencephalograms (EEGs) are recordings of brain electrical activity taken from surface electrodes placed on the head. Electroencephalography is a central tool used in the diagnosis of eplilepsy. It provides information for the neurologist which contributes to the diagnosis of epilepsy and to an understanding of the type of seizure activity (e.g. if partial, where the origin lies). Interictal EEGs refers to recordings made on patients between seizures. These can show abnormalities and so may be a useful aid to diagnosis. Rapid, repetitive, and synchronized discharges, clearly seen on an EEG trace as large repetitive waves, are characteristic of epileptic seizures and may help to distinguish between different types of seizure. Interestingly, large repetitive waves are characteristically seen with absence seizures, confirming that a pattern of uncontrolled excitation occurs in both these classes of event.

It is of importance to note, however, that EEGs from some non-epileptic patients show abnormal patterns and some epileptic patients do not have EEGs that are characteristic of epilepsy. Despite this, EEGs remain a valuable aid to diagnosis, in conjunction with a full medical history, good witness accounts of seizures, and observations of signs and symptoms.

16.1.3 Causes of epilepsy: most cases are idiopathic

We can divide the causes of epilepsy into three areas:

- An inherited component—primary generalized epilepsy may often be familial, but in a complex way. This may make the its origins unclear. Nevertheless, if both parents have epilepsy then there is an increased probability of offspring being affected.

- Non-structural metabolic causes—where identified these may, for example, be related to alcohol abuse or hypoglycaemia.

- Physical damage to part of the brain, possibly caused by trauma, ischaemia (brain cell death due to inadequate oxygen supply as in stroke), or tumours.

However, in reality most cases of epilepsy must be called *idiopathic*, meaning of no known cause. These may well fall into the first category above, genetic in cause, but if so the genetic cause remains unknown.

Our fictional patient Nora develops generalised tonic-clonic seizures at the age of 23, with no known precipitating factors. The cause is unknown—perhaps she had a genetic predisposition which emerged at a particular stage in development or in response to a particular set of precipitating circumstances or environmental insults.

It is tempting to think that we will be able to attach a cause to epilepsy that is related to the biological basis discussed in the next section. This cellular and molecular level of thinking about epilepsy is mostly in terms of the influence of excitatory and inhibitory neurotransmitters. A future genetic model of epilepsy may well explain the *cause* of the neurotransmitter imbalance that lies at the heart of epilepsy, but possibly this will reveal a more fundamental change in brain biochemistry, which leads to changes in neurotransmitters.

16.2 The biological basis of epilepsy: brakes and accelerators

In Box 16.1 you will find an overview of the role of the major excitatory and inhibitory neurotransmitter systems in the brain, with some comments on how this relates to experimental epilepsy (where seizure activity is intentionally generated in animals as a tool to understanding human epilepsy). Here we note that, as described in the introduction to this section, in the brain there is a single principle excitatory neurotransmitter (glutamate) and a single main inhibitory neurotransmitter (γ-aminobutyric acid, GABA).

16.2.1 Glutamate

Glutamate is released from glutamatergic nerve terminals throughout the brain. It acts on two main classes of receptors (Box 16.1). Here we can focus on one of these classes, the ion channel receptors, which have an intrinsic ion channel opened when the receptor binds glutamate. The ion channels let in Na^+ and Ca^{2+}, as set out in Box 16.1, which depolarizes the cells—this glutamate/ion channel system then is always excitatory. There are three classes of glutamate ion channel receptor: NMDA, AMPA, and kainate receptors, as explained in Box 16.1.

These glutamate ionotropic receptors are very widespread in brain neurons and provide the major excitatory input to maintain brain activity. We can regard these receptors, then, as **the accelerator pedal of the brain** (Box 16.1).

Unopposed, this extensive network of stimulation would become uncontrolled, leading to waves of dysfunctional activity, as in seizures. Fortunately, in most of us the glutamate excitation is moderated by GABA inhibition.

16.2.2 γ-aminobutyric acid

γ-Aminobutyric acid is released from extensive networks of GABAergic neurons. It acts on two types of receptors (Box 16.1). $GABA_A$ receptors are intrinsic ion channel receptors that allow Cl^- currents. This hyperpolarizes cells, leading to inhibition of neuronal excitability. $GABA_B$ is a 7-transmembrane G protein coupled receptor (Box 16.1), which exerts a modulatory influence.

Both these GABA receptor types are widespread in the brain and both are implicated in the action of some AEDs, as explained below. The extensive $GABA_A$ receptors exert an inhibitory influence to restrain the glutamate-based

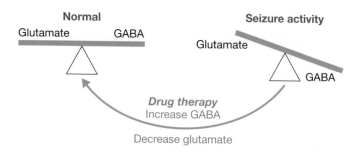

Figure 16.2 Imbalance between glutamate and GABA influences
in the brain results in unrestrained glutamate excitatory influences.
Drugs may then restore the balance by increasing the GABA influence
(e.g. tiagabine, vigabatrin, and benzodiazepines) or reducing
glutamate (e.g. topiramate and felbamate). Note that many AEDs mix
these and other actions. For example, topiramate both increases the
GABA influence and blocks Na$^+$ channels. Blockade of voltage-
sensitive sodium channels and/or calcium channels is common to
many AEDs, and this may itself reduce release of neurotransmitters,
particularly glutamate, thus indirectly reducing the glutamate influence.

excitations in the brain, and it is these which we can
regard as **the brake pedal of the brain** (Box 16.1).

Given the above it is no surprise that seizure activity, being an
unrestrained disorganized excitation, is associated with an
imbalance in the glutamate/GABA system (Figure 16.2).

16.2.3 Voltage-sensitive Na$^+$ channels

Voltage-sensitive Na$^+$ channel opening is necessary for
the formation of seizure activity. The start of excitation is
mostly glutamate mediated, but for repeated waves of
excitation to spread rapidly through the neural network
requires abnormally high frequencies of action potential
firing in the glutamatergic neurons that form part of the
network. This in turn requires rapid and repeated
opening of fast voltage-sensitive Na$^+$ channels. Box 16.2
reminds us that following opening, these Na$^+$ channels
close, (contributing to the downward depolarizing
phase) and that at this time they are for a moment not
able to be opened (they are refractory). The faster the
firing rate of cells, the more flow there is through this
refractory state. Drugs which bind selectively to this
refractory state will cause the accumulation of channels
that are unavailable for opening, and as explained in Box
16.2 such drugs will have a selective effect on very fast
firing neurons, leaving normal firing rates unaffected.
Some AEDs do this and so the biology of the voltage-
sensitive Na$^+$ channels helps us to understand the action
of some very useful drugs.

16.2.4 Voltage-sensitive Ca^{2+} channels

Voltage-sensitive Ca^{2+} channels are involved in the
propagation of rapid periodic bursts of excitation. These
channels are located at the cell surface, and so their
opening when the membrane depolarizes allows Ca^{2+} to
flow into the cell down its concentration gradient. Two
effects are:

- a contribution to depolarization and so action potential
  firing
- when located at the nerve terminal, depolarization is
  coupled to neurotransmitter release, including release
  of glutamate, and thus to stimulation of the next cells in
  the neural network.

There are a number of different types of voltage-gated
Ca^{2+} channels, namely **L-, N-, P/Q-, R-, and T-types**; this
is important to us because different AEDs interact with
different types of Ca^{2+} channels. T-type channels have a
number of subtypes, and serve a number of neuronal
functions. They open with very small depolarizations (e.g.
to –60 mV) which are not sufficient to open the other Ca^{2+}
channel subtypes, and have in particular been associated
with the early initiation of bursting activity in neurons. The
other Ca^{2+} channel types (L-, N-, P/Q-, and R-types) open
only with larger depolarizations (e.g. around –40 mV),
and some of them have been particularly associated with
Ca^{2+} entry in terminals and thus with stimulated
neurotransmitter release.

Box 16.1

Accelerators and brakes in the brain: the molecular substrates of epilepsy

Glutamate, acting on its ion-channel receptors, is the major excitatory influence keeping brain activity going (the accelerator pedal). Balancing this is γ-aminobutyric acid (GABA), the major brake in the brain. Interestingly, these two compounds are closely related—glutamate is an amino acid with a second carboxylic acid (–COOH) group and GABA is formed when one of these is removed by a single enzyme, glutamic acid decarboxylase.

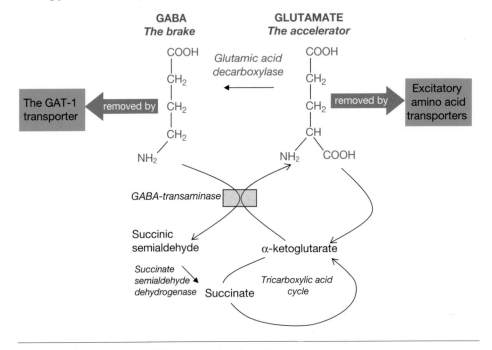

Figure a Glutamate and GABA are very closely related.

Some of the interconversions between these two key brain neurotransmitters are shown in Figure a. GABA breakdown by GABA-transaminase and GABA removal from the synapse by uptake into nerve terminals and glial cells by the GABA transporter GAT-1 are both targets for antiepileptic drugs (AEDs). There is also the suggestion that the links to the tricarboxylic acid cycle are affected by AEDs, such as inhibition of succinate semialdehyde by valproic acid. The connection of these links to the therapeutic response is, however, speculative.

Glutamate receptors The glutamate receptors can be divided into four categories: the three subtypes of ionotropic receptors and the family of metabotropic receptors. We are only concerned here with ionotropic receptors.

Ionotropic receptors are where the receptor and channel are the same, being composed of several transmembrane units which form mono- or hetero-multimeric structures creating ligand-gated ion channels. As well as glutamate receptors other examples are $GABA_A$ receptors (see below) and nicotinic aceylcholine receptors (Chapter 2).

Ionotropic glutamate receptors are subdivided into **NMDA**, AMPA, and kainate receptors. The ion channel is opened when glutamate acts at its receptor binding site. Other conditions may also be required. For example, glycine acts as a co-transmitter with glutamate at the NMDA receptor illustrated in Figure b—both glycine and glutamate must bind to their separate sites on the receptor for the channel to open. We see the requirement for glycine exploited in the development of new antipsychotic drugs in Chapter 18 (Box 18.3). In this novel strategy for antipsychotic medication the objective is to increase activity at NMDA receptors, in contrast to antiepileptic therapy, where the objective is to decrease the influence of glutamate relative to GABA.

All these ionoptropic glutamate receptors have ion channels for Na^+ and/or Ca^{2+}. On binding glutamate Na^+ and Ca^{2+} then flow down their concentration gradients into the cell. This depolarizes the cell. *So glutamate action is always excitatory.* These glutamate receptors are widespread.

GABA receptors $GABA_A$ recetors have an intrinsic ion channel (ionoptropic) but in this case the ion channel is for Cl^-, which enters the cell down its gradient and depolarizes the cell membrane. $GABA_B$ receptors are 7-transmembrane G protein-coupled receptors (Chapter 2), which lead to the inhibition of adenylyl cyclase, lowering cyclic AMP. This occurs at both presynaptic sites (decreasing release of other neurotransmitters) and postsynaptically (leading indirectly to an increase in K^+ permeability and a dampening down of excitability. *So GABA action is always inhibitory.* GABA receptors are widespread within the brain.

The correct level of activity at GABA receptors in the brain is essential to prevent seizure activity is not in doubt. This is shown by the following observations:

- administration of the $GABA_A$ antagonists picrotoxin and biculline cause seizures,
- knockout mice for one of the $GABA_B$ subunits ($GABA_{B1}$) have major epileptic activity.

In addition to binding GABA the GABA receptors also have binding sites for benzodiazepines, which act as allosteric regulators at this site, enhancing the inhibitory effect of GABA.

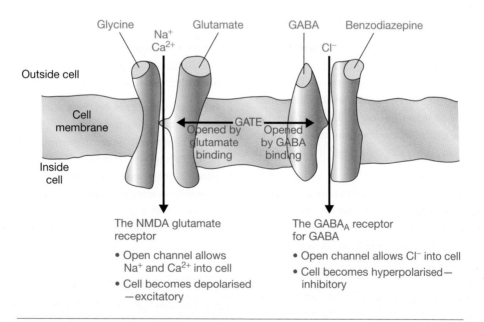

Figure b Glutamate NMDA receptors and GABA receptors have a lot in common but have opposite effects on neuronal excitability.

Box 16.2

The use-dependent Na⁺ channel-blocking action of some AEDs

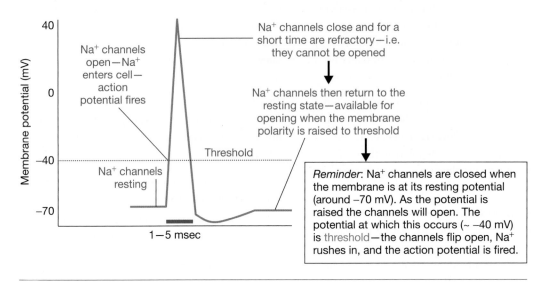

Na⁺ channels open—Na⁺ enters cell—action potential fires

Na⁺ channels close and for a short time are refractory—i.e. they cannot be opened

Na⁺ channels then return to the resting state—available for opening when the membrane polarity is raised to threshold

Threshold

Na⁺ channels resting

Reminder: Na⁺ channels are closed when the membrane is at its resting potential (around −70 mV). As the potential is raised the channels will open. The potential at which this occurs (~ −40 mV) is threshold—the channels flip open, Na⁺ rushes in, and the action potential is fired.

1—5 msec

Figure C A typical neuronal action potential.

The membrane potential is negative inside in the resting cell, becomes transiently positive, and then returns to negative.

Figure c illustrates the progression of voltage-sensitive Na⁺ channels from the resting state to open. This happens when the membrane polarity is raised from its baseline of –70 mV (or below) to about –40 mV. At this polarity (the 'threshold') the resting channels are opened and Na⁺ enters the cell as the action potential is fired. The channel then closes, but at this point it is transiently in a refractory state, when it is not available for opening.

A use-dependent Na⁺ channel-blocking AED binds preferentially to this refractory state. Figure d shows a neuron firing action potential with a very high frequency, as may occur in an epileptic seizure. The introduction of an AED (red bar) delays the return of refractory channels to the resting state, so delaying the availability of sufficient Na⁺ channels to support the high firing rate. Consequently the rate of firing falls.

However, when the cell is firing at a normal rate to begin with (bottom panel) then there is sufficient time for the channels to return to the resting state even with the delay imposed by the drug, and so there is no effect on firing rate. Consequently, a use-dependent drug will not interfere with normal patterns of neuronal activity in the brain, but will calm down neurons firing with abnormally high frequency.

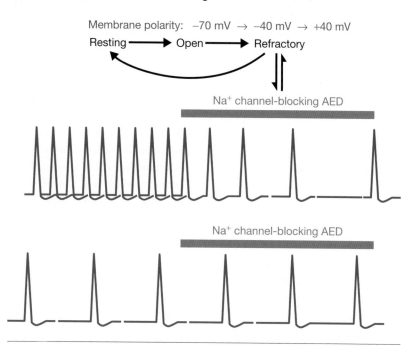

Figure d AEDs may selectively bind to the refractory state of the channel.

After opening the channels transiently go into a refractory state—they are closed but cannot open even when in a depolarized (e.g. +40 mV) membrane. These use-dependent Na+ channel blockers will then selectively bind to and 'delay' the channels in this state. This shift in equilibrium will have most effect on rapidly firing neurons (upper trace) and less effect on slowly firing neurons (lower trace), when even with the 'delay' there will be sufficient time for the refractory channels to return to the resting state (available for opening)

We have encountered some of these channels before, notably L-type channels, when considering the cardiovascular system in Section II. We recall that there are many clinically available L-type channel blockers, and it is instructive to note that none of these are AED, even though L-channel inhibition is considered one of the mechanisms of action of some AEDs (see below). This either means that L-channel inhibition is not connected with the way these AEDs work or that this inhibition contributes to the antiepileptic effect when it occurs combined with other mechanisms of action.

16.2.5 The biological basis of epilepsy: do we have a GABA hypothesis?

When we propose a biological theory for a complex disorder it may be considered useful even if we know it does not encompass all, or even most, aspects of the disorder. This is true, for example, of the dopamine hypothesis for schizophrenia, which we will see in Chapter 18 has been very useful to understand drug action despite its limitations. We can therefore consider a simple GABA hypothesis for epilepsy.

Hypothesis: Epilepsy is caused by a global or regional inadequacy in GABA influence on brain function, due either to deficient GABA influence or elevated glutamate influence.

This hypothesis, either explicitly stated or assumed, has driven much drug discovery, resulting in new AEDs useful for many patients, and can therefore be considered a useful starting point when thinking about the biological basis of epilepsy.

16.3 Three mechanisms in the drug treatment of epilepsy

The objective of taking AEDs is to prevent the occurrence of seizures while minimizing unwanted effects. The target in this area of clinical pharmacology is clear and simple: the elimination of seizures. At the end of this section we discuss the strategy in treating epilepsy, noting that the goal is to achieve this target with just one drug, while recognizing that this is not always possible. The issue of unwanted effects and drug interactions is serious with AEDs, and one reason for striving to use only one drug is to minimize these. Single therapy is also likely to improve compliance, another important issue with AEDs.

AEDs are a frustrating subject for those seeking a rational science-based understanding of prescribing because the action of drugs is complex, involving many different cellular mechanisms, often combined in one drug. It is perhaps the multiple cellular sites of actions that are essential for an effective clinical response, and so in this area it is not productive to seek a single mechanism of action for each drug, just as it is probably not a good strategy for a drug company to seek new drugs that have only one molecular target.

Furthermore, the mechanism of action of AEDs that is responsible for the clinical effect is often unknown. This is true of newer drugs as well as first-generation drugs. Despite these issues we can introduce some of the known actions of AEDs by considering three broad types of cellular mechanism:

- decreased sustained high frequency firing of action potentials *Na+ channel.*
- increased GABA influence
- blockage of T-type Ca^{2+} channels.

16.3.1 Decreased sustained high frequency firing of action potentials

As described above, epileptic activity is characterized by very high frequency of action potentials in neurons within the affected regions. Three actions of AEDs target these rapidly firing neurons:

- Delaying recovery of Na^+ channels by selective binding of drugs to the refractory state has been referred to in section 16.2.3 above, and this type of use-dependent drug action is further explored in Box 16.2. The objective is to dampen down the activity of the rapidly

firing neurons while leaving normal activity unaffected.

- AEDs acting as antagonists at AMPA and NMDA glutamate receptors reduce the propagation of the activity through the neural network.
- AEDs acting to block L-, N-, P/Q-, and R-type voltage-sensitive Ca^{2+} channels may reduce the excitability of neurons and evoked release of neurotransmitters, including glutamate. Note that T-type blockade is discussed as a separate mechanism, see section 16.3.3.

AEDs acting in these various ways to reduce high frequency neuronal discharges include carbamazepine, gabapentin, lamotrigine, phenytoin, topiramate, and possibly sodium valproate.

16.3.2 Increased GABA influence

From an experimental point of view it is of interest to note that the convulsant drugs picrotoxin and bicuculline have their effect by blocking $GABA_A$ receptors, down-regulating the inhibitory GABA influence on neuronal excitability. These drugs have no clinical use. From a clinical point of view it is not surprising that drugs that enhance the GABA influence are often anticonvulsant, and we will discuss examples below. Two classes of mechanisms for raising the GABA influence can be identified:

1) Increase GABA levels in the synapse. This is done with AEDs by at least two mechanisms:

   a. inhibit uptake from the synapse by blocking the GABA transporter called GAT-1

   b. inhibit GABA breakdown by inhibiting GABA transaminase.

2) Enhance GABA receptor function, for example benzodiazepines act on a binding site in the $GABA_A$ receptor (see Figure b in Box 16.1).

The consequences of these two types of drug effect are not the same. The first, increasing GABA levels at the synapse, will stimulate both $GABA_A$ and $GABA_B$ receptors. The second, the action of benzodiazepines, will enhance the influence of $GABA_A$ receptors only. This may have profound clinical consequences, for confusing the issue here is the important observation that some GABA-enhancing drugs used to treat epilepsy can precipitate certain seizure types, and this may relate to actions at the different GABA receptors. These issues are considered in Box 16.3.

Box 16.3
Pro-epileptic effects of antiepilepsy drugs

It is recognized that some AEDs precipitate or exacerbate certain types of seizure. Understanding this presents a challenge to our understanding of epilepsy and of normal brain function. However, it must be said that we have only an imperfect understanding of this issue and this is probably limited to the exacerbation of absence seizures by certain AEDs.

The most common observation is that absence seizures can be elicited by GABA-enhancing drugs. How can a pathology that is due to uncontrolled excitation be made worse by increasing the main inhibitory influence in the brain? The simple explanation is that a drug that inhibits an inhibitory pathway will be excitatory, as set out in Figure e.

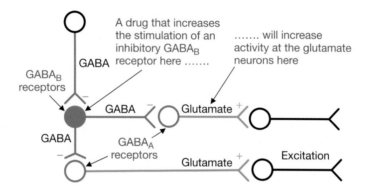

Figure e Hypothetical scheme indicating how GABA$_B$-receptor agonists may enhance excitability in an imaginary neuronal network.

GABAergic (i.e. GABA releasing) neurons are shown with red axons and terminals; glutamatergic (i.e. glutamate releasing) are shown with green axons and terminals. Cell bodies with GABA receptors are shown in red: when this is the GABA$_A$ receptor, open circle; GABA$_B$ receptor, solid circle. With this hypothetical scheme we can see that an agonist at an inhibitory GABA$_B$ receptor, such as those found in the hippocampus (within the temporal lobe) may reduce the inhibitory influence of GABA$_A$ receptors on glutamate release, leading to excitation which may precipitate epileptiform activity.

AEDs may increase GABA influence by increasing GABA concentrations at the synapse, resulting in increased activity at GABA$_A$ and GABA$_B$ receptors, or acting at the GABA$_A$ receptor selectively. It has been noted that absence seizures may be precipitated by the non-specific GABA-enhancing drugs (e.g. vigabatin and tiagabine). Benzodiazepines, which bind and enhance the GABA$_A$ receptor/Cl$^-$ channel and lack effect at the GABA$_B$ receptors, do not worsen absence seizures and may be used (e.g. clonazepam) in their management. This leads to the suggestion that

it is the GABA$_B$ stimulatory effect specifically that presents a problem with absence seizures. This has been incorporated into the model in Figure e. This is a complex area.

1. We know, for example, that in the hippocampus GABA$_B$ receptors can inhibit glutamate release from some neurons and GABA release from others. However, the overall role of GABA in the brain as essential to prevent seizure activity is not in doubt (see Box 16.1).

Box 16.3 **Pro-epileptic effects of antiepilepsy drugs**

2. An important complicating issue is that the effect of manipulating GABA at its different receptors will depend on the brain region involved. This may be true of both GABA$_A$ and GABA$_B$ activity.

3. There is a prospect of regional selectivity for AEDs in the future, for example there are four isoforms of human GABA$_{B1}$ subunits and these have a specific regional distribution in the brain. If at some time in the future drugs selective for these isoforms could be found then the issues of pro-and antiepileptic activity of AEDs may be able to be resolved.

The issue of enhancement of absence seizures with AEDs is not limited to the GABA-enhancing drugs. It has also been associated with one of the other main AED mechanisms of action, which is the inhibition of rapidly firing Na$^+$ channels (Box 16.3). This means that carbamazepine, for example, may precipitate absence seizures.

The outcome at the present time for clinical use is that ethosuximide and sodium valproate are used for absence seizures—both act, at least in part, by blocking T-type Ca^{2+} channels.

But just when you thought you had reached the end of this set of complexities, it is important to note that proepileptic effects are not limited to absence seizures: there is concern that using ethosuximide alone in patients with both absence and tonic–clonic seizures may risk increasing the frequency of generalized tonic–clonic seizures.

Drugs acting mainly through these mechanisms include the benzodiazepines, tiagabine, topiramate, vigabatrin, and valproate.

16.3.3 Blockage of T-types Ca^{2+} channels

This is placed in a separate category because ethosuximide, which is believed to derive its therapeutic effect mainly from T-type Ca^{2+} channel blockade, has a separate profile of clinical use (see below), which is used for absence seizures. This leads to the possibility that T-type channel inhibition prevents absence seizures.

In addition to ethosuximide it is notable that valproic acid also acts in part by T-type channel blockade.

16.4 Drugs used in the treatment of epilepsy

An orderly classification of AEDs on the basis of the mechanism of action at the cellular and molecular level cannot be made because so many drugs have multiple actions and for many (or perhaps most) it is not clear how they work. Knowing which drugs are most useful against which types of seizures is obviously important, but not satisfying as a basis for classification because many drugs have diverse clinical applications. Here then we divide drugs into older first-generation drugs and newer second-generation drugs, and provide brief comments about mechanism of action and clinical use for the major drugs in each category. Not all AEDs are mentioned. In the following section (16.5) we provide some comments on the strategy for treating epilepsy with drugs.

16.4.1 First-generation AEDs

These are likely to be the first drugs tried in most cases.

Sodium valproate

Valproate is one of the drugs available as first-line medication for all seizure types, and is particularly favoured as a first drug for primarily generalized seizures. It is also used in migraine and as a mood stabilizer—as an alternative to lithium for bipolar disorder, see Chapter 19.

There is no adequate account of valproate's mechanism of antiepileptic action. As with other AEDs its therapeutic response is likely to be the result of several mechanisms acting in concert, including:

- enhanced GABA influence—inhibition of GABA transaminase
- decreased glutamate influence by moderation of NMDA receptors
- T-type Ca^{2+} channel block.

Adverse effects include liver toxicity, especially with young children.

Carbamazepine

This is a drug of choice for partial and primarily generalized tonic–clonic seizures. The principle mechanism of action is probably use-dependent Na^+ channel block (Box 16.2); like other drugs with this action it may exacerbate absence seizures (Box 16.3). In addition carbamazepine may have actions which enhance GABA and block L-type Ca^{2+} channels. Like valproate, it is also used for other conditions, including pain disorders, particularly trigeminal neuralgia, and bipolar disorder.

Phenytoin

Like carbamazepine this drug is a first-choice drug for partial and primarily generalized tonic–clonic seizures, but is not used for absence seizures. Its main action is thought to be at Na^+ channels. Plasma drug level monitoring is important in aiding dosage with phenytoin.

Benzodiazepines

Not commonly first-line drugs for epilepsy, benzodiazepines (see also Chapter 19) are of interest because of the mechanisms by which they interact with the GABA receptor/Cl^- channel (see Figure b in Box 16.1):

- increased affinity of the $GABA_A$ receptor for GABA
- increased current carried by the $GABA_A$ receptor Cl^- channel.

This results in a selective enhancement of GABA influence at this receptor type (see Boxes 16.1 and 16.2). **Clonazepam** is available to treat all forms of epilepsy, but its use may be limited by its tendency to produce drowsiness. Diazepam, along with clonazepam and midazolam, is used to treat status epilepticus.

Ethosuximide

Unusual among AEDs this is a drug limited in use to essentially one seizure type, absence seizures. It is also unusual in that its molecular mode of action is also relatively selective as a T-type Ca^{2+} channel blocker. Ethosuximide or sodium valproate are the drugs of choice for absence

seizures. Adverse effects have been reported to include the possibility of exacerbation of tonic–clinic seizures in some patients with mixed (absence/tonic–clonic) epilepsy. In approximately 50% of patients with absence seizures who also suffer from tonic–clinic seizures ethosuximide would leave the tonic clinic aspect untreated—valproate remains a sensible option to treat both seizure types.

16.4.2 Second-generation AEDs

The last 15 years or so have seen the introduction of a bewildering variety of AEDs, some developed with specific cellular/molecular targets, most commonly at mechanisms to enhance GABA influences. Some of these drugs are introduced here.

Lamotrigine

This is a drug of choice for partial seizures (including secondary generalized) and primary generalized tonic–clonic seizures. It may be first line or second line after valproate or carbamazepine have failed. It may be used alone or with another drug. It is believed to act mainly as a Na^+ channel blocker (Box 16.3) and in common with other such drugs it is not used to treat absence seizures.

Topiramate

This can be used alone or in combination for partial and primary generalized tonic–clonic seizures. This drug is now more widely prescribed for non-epileptic conditions (migraine and bipolar disorders). Its combines several mechanisms, including:

- Na^+ channel blocker
- enhanced $GABA_A$ receptor function
- inhibited glutamate function at the receptor level
- blockade of L-type Ca^{2+} channels.

Gabapentin

This is an AED designed to interact directly with the GABA receptor as a GABA-mimetic. Curiously, it did not do this, but was found to have antiepileptic properties nevertheless. Used mainly for partial seizures, either alone or more commonly as an add-on therapy, it is also has other widespread uses, e.g. neuropathic pain. Its mechanisms of action may include interaction with voltage-sensitive Ca^{2+} channels.

Vigabatrin

Vigabatrin is used as an add-on drug to treat partial seizures when monotherapy has failed. This drug is an irreversible inhibitor of GABA transaminase, increasing GABA concentration in the synapse. It suffers from common and serious visual field-disturbance side effects, and therefore should only be used as a last resort.

Tiagabine

This is another drug available as an add-on in the prevention of partial seizures. Tiagabine inhibits neuronal and glial uptake of GABA by the GAT-1 transporter, increasing and prolonging GABA influence at the synapse.

Oxcarbazepine

This is a Na^+ channel blocker drug (Box 16.3) that may be used as adjunct therapy in the treatment of partial and generalized seizures.

16.5 Strategy and side effects in the drug treatment of epilepsy

Strategy starts with the objective in each patient of eliminating seizures with only one drug. The initial drug tried should be a first-generation AED. The exact first drug chosen will depend on the individual patient, particularly with respect to age (children are more often treatable with only one drug), nature of seizures, co-morbidities, and interactions with drugs other than AEDs. Drug interactions are particularly important with AEDs, and guidance from an appropriate reference should be sought. Many of the antiepileptics (e.g. carbamazepine, phenytoin, oxcarbazepine, barbiturates, and topiramate) are inducers of hepatic enzymes and this can lead to reduced effectiveness of several drugs. Of importance is the oral contraceptive, and patients may be better to use non-hormonal contraceptive methods (e.g. barrier methods) instead.

All epileptic drugs have a limited window for effective treatment with minimum adverse effects, meaning that dosage is very important and that it may be necessary, when possible, to monitor plasma levels of the drug. For example, phenytoin plasma levels are considered important, while valproate plasma levels are less so. Target plasma concentrations may be obtained from a reference source.

If a single drug is not effective or not acceptable due to side effects (see below) then its use should be tapered off and a second drug introduced and used alone. This pursuit of monotherapy may then be abandoned if a single drug at maximal doses without unacceptable side effects brings benefit but does not deliver adequate control. Such a drug may be continued and a further drug, an add-on (adjunct therapy), considered. However, before combination therapy is considered, it is important to ensure that monotherapy failure is not due to poor compliance (a common problem).

A selection of drug combinations for AED polytherapy is likely to be based on clinical considerations, but it is of interest to note that combination selection based on mechanism of action has been reported to be useful. It has been suggested, for example, that combining a sodium channel blocker with a drug-enhancing GABA influence may be particularly advantageous, for example carbamazepine/vigabatrin. Importantly, however, these mechanistic strategies are unlikely to dominate in an area as complex as epilepsy.

Side effects. Potential side effects will influence the choice of initial drug. For example, adolescents may be particularly troubled by possible side effects of phenytoin: gum hypertrophy, hirsutism (unwanted hair growth, particularly difficult in a female), and acne. The common unwanted effects of AEDs are drowsiness and movement problems such as nystagmus (a disorder of eye movement), slurring of speech, and poor control of limb movement. These effects are reduced by careful and slow increase in dose, with the objective always of achieving the lowest dose possible to give seizure control. All AEDs present problems in pregnancy, and a reference guide should be consulted to exclude certain drugs and achieve an acceptable degree of seizure control while minimizing risks (remembering the significant risk that uncontrolled epilepsy has on the unborn child). Some aspects of this are developed in Workbook 13. It is now recognized that AEDs present a small risk of increased suicidal thoughts and behaviour, and patients should be monitored and counselled with this in mind.

There is a theme of proepileptic effects in some AEDs that should be considered. These are discussed in Box 16.3.

Anticonvulsant therapy is usually continued for years. Where a patient becomes seizure free over 2–3 years then gradual withdrawal can be considered. For some patients, lifelong drug therapy is needed.

SUMMARY OF DRUGS USED FOR EPILEPSY

Therapeutic class	Drugs	Mechanism of action	Common clinical uses	Comments	Examples of adverse drug reactions
First-generation antiepileptic drugs	Sodium valproate	1) Inhibits GABA transaminase 2) Decreases glutamate influence by moderation of NMDA receptors 3) Blocks T-type Ca²⁺ channel	Primary generalized seizures Migraine Mood stabilizer—an alternative to lithium for bipolar disorder	Fewer drug–drug interactions than other antiepileptic drugs	Nausea Vomiting Weight gain Tremor (dose-related) Drowsiness Elevated liver transaminase
	Carbamazepine	Prevents repetitive firing of sodium-dependent action potentials in depolarized neurons and blocks voltage-dependent blockade of sodium channels	Epilepsy—generalized tonic–clonic and partial seizures Trigeminal neuralgia prophylaxis of manic-depressive psychoses	Not effective in petit mal and myoclonus Metabolized by cytochrome P450 3A4 enzyme, leading to interaction with several drugs	Drowsiness Blurred vision Diplopia Headache (all dose-related) Rash Dry mouth Gastrointestinal Thrombocytopenia Raised liver function test
	Phenytoin Fosphenytoin	Theories: 1) reduces sodium conductance, enhances active sodium extrusion, blocks repetitive firing, and reduces post-tetanic potentiation 2) enhances gaba-mediated inhibition and reduces excitatory synaptic transmission post synaptically 3) pre-synaptic actions to reduces calcium entry and blocks release of neurotransmitters pre-synaptically	Epilepsy (particularly grand mal, focal and partial seizures (focal, including temporal lobe)) Trigeminal neuralgia	Not effective for absence (petit mal) seizures Non-linear pharmakokinetics Fosphenytoin is a prodrug of phenytoin and can be given intramuscularly.	Nausea Vomiting Gingival hypertrophy Acne Hirsutism
	Benzodiazepines: clonazepam clobazam diazepam midazolam	1) Increases the affinity of the GABA_A receptor for GABA 2) Increases the current carried by the GABA_A receptor Cl⁻ channel	Epilepsy Diazepam, clonazepam, and midazolam are used to treat status epilepticus Clonazepam is used for all forms of epilepsy Anxiety	Usually reserved for second-line use in epilepsy	Drowsiness Dependence
	Ethosuximide	Selectively blocks T-type Ca²⁺ channel	Epilepsy (particularly absence seizures)		Anorexia Nausea Vomiting Epigastric pain Weight loss

Therapeutic class	Drugs	Mechanism of action	Common clinical uses	Comments	Examples of adverse drug reactions
	Oxcarbazepine	Blockade of voltage-sensitive sodium channels	Epilepsy (particularly partial seizures)	Patients should seek help if signs of blood hepatic or skin disorders	Gastrointestinal Acne Alopecia Fatigue Headache Agitation Confusion Blurred vision
	Primidone	Thought to alter ionic fluxes, thereby affecting the neuronal membrane	Epilepsy (all forms except absence seizures)		Hepatitis Hypotension Respiratory depression Nausea Visual disturbances
	Phenobarbital	Mimics GABA	Epilepsy (all forms except absence seizures)		Hepatitis Hypotension Respiratory depression
Second-generation antiepileptic drugs	Lamotrigine	Blocks Na$^+$ channel	Epilepsy (particularly partial seizures)	Not used for absence seizures	Rash Hypersensitivity Hepatotoxicity Serious skin reactions (especially in children)
	Topiramate	1) Blocks Na$^+$ channel 2) Enhances GABA$_A$ receptor function 3) Inhibits glutamate function at the receptor level 4) Blocks L-type Ca^{2+} channels	Epilepsy (partial and primary generalized tonic-clonic seizures) Migraine Bipolar disorder		Somnolence Fatigue Headache Dizziness Weight loss Depression
	Gabapentin	Mimics GABA on GABA receptors Interacts with voltage-sensitive Ca^{2+} channels	Epilepsy (particularly partial seizures) Neuropathic pain	Avoid abrupt withdrawal	Fatigue Sedation Dizziness Tremor Abnormal thinking Hypertension Dry mouth Weight gain

Therapeutic class	Drugs	Mechanism of action	Common clinical uses	Comments	Examples of adverse drug reactions
	Pregabalin	Binds to an auxiliary subunit (α2-δ protein) of voltage-gated calcium channels in the central nervous system, displacing [3H]-gabapentin	Epilepsy (particularly partial seizures) Generalized anxiety disorder Neuropathic pain		Drowsiness Visual disturbance Fatigue Sedation Headache Memory impairment Abnormal thinking Insomnia Ataxia Lethargy
	Vigabatrin	Irreversibly inhibits GABA transaminase, increasing GABA concentration in the synapse	Epilepsy (partial seizures)	Reserved as last resort because of ADR	Disturbance of visual fields Diplopia Fatigue Sedation Memory impairment
	Tiagabine	Inhibits neuronal and glial uptake of GABA by the GAT-1 transporter, increasing and prolonging GABA influence at the synapse.	Epilepsy (partial seizures)	Avoid in acute porphyria	Diarrhoea Dizziness Tiredness
	Lacosamide	1) Selectively enhances slow inactivation of voltage-gated sodium channels, resulting in stabilization of hyperexcitable neuronal membranes 2) Binds to collapsin response mediator protein 2 (CRMP2), a phosphoprotein mainly expressed in the nervous system and involved in neuronal differentiation and axonal outgrowth.	Epilepsy (partial seizures)		Dizziness Headache Diplopia Nausea

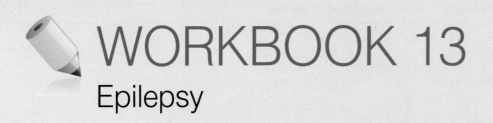

WORKBOOK 13
Epilepsy

Ambreen, a patient with a first tonic–clonic seizure at age 23

Ambreen: a simplified case history

It happened when they were strolling along the half-deserted beach. Life was never the same from that moment on. Ambreen and Pavitar had been having another lazy day, snorkelling and birdwatching on the beach on North Stradbroke Island, off the coast from Brisbane. They originally met in his pharmacy on the island 2 years ago. She was also a pharmacist, having trained in England and now working in Brisbane. They planned to get married and run the local pharmacy in this small community together.

Ambreen stopped. Turning back to her Pavitar noticed she looked strange—stiff and upright, with her neck and arms straightened, she made a strange sound, like a large exhale, and then was on the ground, writhing with a shaking movement involving her entire body, especially her legs, which seemed to have a life of their own. Pavitar stared down at her, startled and afraid. For a moment it looked as though he would do nothing. Then his medical training kicked in; without conscious thought he knew she was having a tonic–clonic epileptic seizure. He knelt beside her, turned her partly on her side and firmly placed his hand under her chin, applying firm upward pressure to keep her airways open. Leaving her legs to thrash around he kept her lying safely on the soft sand, talking gently to her all the while. It was with alarm that he realized that she was not breathing properly, and holding one of her hands still he saw that her fingers had a bluish tinge. His fear returned, but within about 3 minutes her movements stopped, her breathing became orderly, and she lay still. Using his mobile phone the island's ambulance was there within a few minutes and they went straight to the dock, where the Stradbroke Flyer had been held up to take them to the mainland. Ambreen by now was conscious again, but confused, holding her head and complaining of pains. Once on the mainland the long ambulance ride to the hospital in Brisbane was a nightmare—Ambreen had two more fits in the ambulance, with only minutes between them. With a shiver of alarm the term 'status epilepticus' crept into Pavitar's mind.

A table of clinical clerking abbreviations is given on page xi.

CLINICAL CLERKING FOR AMBREEN

Age: 23 years

PC: Convulsive episodes

HPC: Had two episodes of febrile convulsions as a child. Three years ago she started having episodes that she now describes as staring, which she thought was daydreaming. Has since had no further episodes.

PMH:

Two febrile convulsions as a child

Episodes of absence

Otherwise healthy

Ambreen has been completely healthy apart from contracting the usual childhood viruses. During two such viral infections her temperature got so high that she had convulsions. Although most children who suffer from febrile convulsions do not become epileptic, a small percentage do. Her staring episodes could be due to absence epilepsy.

DH: Microgynon (oral contraceptive)

The only medication Ambreen currently takes is oral contraceptives.

Because she had two further seizures close together while in the ambulance on the way to the hospital, Ambreen was treated with a diazepam suppository (rectal tubule).

Diazepam (rectally) is a benzodiazepine used for treating status epilepticus (seizures persisting for 30 min or more) or when two discrete seizures are not separated by complete recovery of consciousness, as was the case with Ambreen. Intravenous diazepam may be used instead of rectal.

SH: Recent pharmacy graduate, lives alone

O/E: Normal

Unlike most illnesses, epilepsy is episodic. Patients may appear perfectly normal between seizures, showing no signs of illness with a routine medical examination.

Biochemistry:

1) Urea and electrolytes (Us & Es) = normal

2) Full blood count (FBC) = normal

3) Toxicology and alcohol screen = normal

4) Glucose levels = normal

The above tests are all normal, ruling out the following other possible causes of seizures: infection, hypoglycaemia, or intoxication. Also, she has not been subjected to flashing lights, which could also precipitate seizures.

Investigations:

1) Brain imaging scans

2) Electroencephalography (EEG)

3) Magnetic resonance imaging (MRI)

EEG is the most common examination for suspected epilepsy. EEG detects electrical activity in the brain and can be used to reveal any abnormalities in brain activity. EEG is the key test in diagnosing and pinpointing the epileptic focus, the brain region where seizures originate which shows abnormal electrical activity.

However, EEG can be unreliable in diagnosing epilepsy, with at least 50% of sufferers showing no abnormalities. Conversely, 20% of unaffected people exhibit minor EEG abnormalities and 1–3% show frankly epileptic discharges. Similarly, a small number of people without epilepsy show photosensitive reactions (i.e. seizure induced by flashing lights) on their EEG traces.

To prevent a misdiagnosis, an MRI scan was also ordered.

MRI uses magnetic fields and radio waves to generate a three-dimensional picture of the inside of the body. MRI can be useful in determining the cause of epilepsy by detecting possible structural abnormalities (e.g. tumour or scar tissue) in the brain.

However, Ambreen's MRI scans revealed no structural abnormalities that could explain her seizures, as is often the case with epilepsy.

It is often difficult to confidently diagnose epilepsy. For example, misdiagnosis is common with up to 10% of teenagers with epilepsy actually experiencing nothing more serious than syncopal attacks (i.e. 'fainting' due to a temporary decrease in blood flow to the brain). The best diagnostic tool is often an independent witness to the attacks.

In Ambreen's case Pavitar and the paramedics were witnesses and their account was invaluable.

The diagnosis must also be accurate as a diagnosis of epilepsy may stigmatize the patient and can have other life-changing implications (e.g. driving), as treatment often needs to be continued for years. Brain imaging is therefore now commonly used to aid diagnosis.

While in hospital, Ambreen suffers from two more seizures accompanied by incontinence.

Diagnosis: Epilepsy: generalized tonic–clonic seizures with absence seizures

Plan:

Commence sodium valproate

The aim of pharmacologic treatment is to control seizures without affecting normal function or inducing side effects. To minimize adverse drug reactions, treatment should be initiated with a single drug at the lowest possible dose, therefore optimizing its use.

Established (i.e. 'first-generation') antiepileptic drugs should be used first line.

The choice of drug used can depend on several factors, including:

* *seizure type*

* *personal history of the patient (e.g. concurrent drugs, pregnancy, etc.)*

Sodium valproate is effective for treating epilepsy in which both generalized tonic–clonic seizures and absence seizures occur.

1) What is epilepsy? Describe what occurs in neurons during a seizure.

2) List three possible causes of epilepsy.

3) What possible changes in neuronal excitability may occur in epilepsy?

4) List the major seizure categories, including two seizure types from each.

5) What is the main aim of treatment in epilepsy?

6) Describe the nature of the duration of treatment for epilepsy.

7) List the three primary mechanisms of action of antiepileptic drugs.

8) When is diazepam commonly used in the treatment of epilepsy?

---

9) What are the proposed mechanisms of action of sodium valproate?

---

10) Describe one mechanism of action by which sodium valproate can reduce seizures without affecting normal neurophysiological function.

Ambreen stays in hospital for 2 weeks and during this time she suffers from two more episodes. After her drug dose is doubled, she remains seizure-free and is therefore discharged home after 2 weeks.

Meanwhile Ambreen's parents have arrived from England to look after her. Pavitar must return to his business—it has been struggling with emergency pharmacist cover, but he must stay open, since it is the only pharmacy on the island. When he gets back he studies the latest reports on the drug treatment of epilepsy, and realizes that there have been some new drugs since he qualified, but that the fundamental landscape of epilepsy treatment has not changed.

However, Ambreen starts having more seizures at home. She visits her family doctor twice and despite further increases in dose, she still has one seizure a week. Her neurologist decides to admit her to hospital because she is now prescribed the maximum dose for her medication. The doctor had prescribed the maximum dose on the neurologist's advice since Ambreen was not responding and was apparently not suffering from side effects.

The neurologist decides that while she is in hospital they will observe her patterns of seizures before further dose increases or changes to her medication. On the second day in hospital, Ambreen develops encephalopathy (brain dysfunction often caused by metabolic abnormalities). An urgent plasma level is carried out and her sodium valproate levels are extremely elevated at 1280 µmol/L (normal range: 700 µmol/L maximum).

Note that plasma levels of sodium valproate are not an index of drug efficacy, although they may be useful for indicating toxicity.

The neurologist is confused because despite the elevated levels of drug, Ambreen is still fitting and yet is side effect-free at home. He convinces Ambreen to be truthful about her compliance. Ambreen admits that she had not been taking her medication due to side effects and her doctor had thus kept increasing the dose. In hospital she had to take the dose because the nurse was watching. Exposure to such a high dose lead to intoxication.

11) What are the side effects of sodium valproate?

Following further investigation, the neurologist realizes that because Ambreen is a pharmacist she had not been properly counselled by the prescribing pharmacist about her medication during her previous admission. Ambreen has not been in a fit state to think clearly about her own condition, and anyway has never felt confident about her understanding of antiepileptic drugs.

It is vital that a patient with epilepsy agrees with treatment goals. The expected outcomes of treatment and potential side effects and management should be discussed with the patient. Every patient should be empowered to be involved during the decision-making process because this will lead to better adherence and clinical management.

The patient must be made to understand the following:

• the aims and implications of treatment

• the importance of regular medication.

Without these, treatment may fail.

The pharmacist has an important role in the management of epilepsy:

• contributing to ensure that the best choice of drug is made

• contributing to drug monitoring by applying pharmacokinetic knowledge, including monitoring side effects and drug–drug interactions

• preparing medication (e.g. intravenous diazepam)

• contributing to health monitoring of patients

• contributing to discharge arrangements (e.g. dose titration plans)

• contributing to compliance by carefully counselling patients about their medicines.

Ambreen phones Pavitar, who wants to tell her that as a pharmacist she should have known better, but also he feels guilty himself—he should have been there to keep an eye on things.

The neurologist decides that because of the side effects Ambreen is suffering, the sodium valproate should be changed to another drug. The ideal new drug should be another antiepileptic effective for treating both generalized tonic–clonic and absence seizures. Otherwise sodium valproate may have to be replaced with two drugs.

12) Which other drugs are effective for treating tonic–clonic seizures?

---

13) Of these drugs, would any also be beneficial in treating absence seizures?

_____

_____

_____

> The neurologist discusses the options with Ambreen. He talks to her about phenytoin, which he says is an older drug very effective for various forms of seizures.

14) What are the mechanisms of action of phenytoin?

_____

_____

_____

> The neurologist tells Ambreen that despite being effective there are reasons why he is reluctant for her to use phenytoin. These include certain side effects that could be distressing to a young woman.

15) What are the side effects of phenytoin?

_____

_____

_____

16) Which of these could lead to non-compliance in a young woman?

_____

_____

_____

> He also tells her that she will have to go to her family doctor every so often for her blood level of phenytoin to be checked.
>
> The neurologist and Ambreen decide against phenytoin after careful consideration. They then discuss carbamazepine.

17) What similarities in the mechanisms of action exist between phenytoin and carbamazepine?

_____

_____

The doctor tells Ambreen that her oral contraceptive pills will be affected by carbamazepine.

They decide against carbamazepine. The neurologist tells Ambreen that there is a newer antiepileptic drug that has a similar mode of action as phenytoin and carbamazepine. The drug also has certain advantages, particularly in women of childbearing age:

1) It does not interact with oral contraceptives.

2) It can be used in pregnancy.

Preliminary results from the UK Epilepsy and Pregnancy Register, a prospective study of the outcome of pregnancies in women presenting with epilepsy in 2002, suggest that the risk of congenital malformations in the infants of women taking the following drugs is as follows:

carbamazepine 2.3%

sodium valproate 7%

lamotrigine 3%

As a result, the Committee on Safety of Medicines (CSM) has advised that women of childbearing age should not be prescribed sodium valproate without specialist neurological advice.

The interaction between carbamazepine and the oral contraceptive pill has led to concern that this drug may also not be ideal for women of childbearing age.

Lamotrigine may be considered as a first-line drug for use in women of childbearing age with generalized epilepsy, although the lowest possible therapeutic dose should be used during pregnancy. Lamotrigine also decreases the enzyme dihydrofolic acid reductase, resulting in lower folic acid levels. Folic acid supplements are therefore advised, particularly in pregnancy or in women attempting to conceive. As an alternative approach recommended in some areas, for example in Australia, there is no 'drug of choice' in pregnancy, and all but valporate should be considered.

Lamotrigine is also suitable for the treatment of seizures if the patient wishes to take the oral contraception as it is not a hepatic enzyme-inducing drug.

Lamotrigine is commenced at a very low dose, as sodium valproate inhibits its metabolism and could therefore increase the risk of side effects. Once an appropriate dose is reached, sodium valproate is slowly withdrawn. Withdrawal is carried out incrementally when switching anti-epileptic drugs in order to avoid withdrawal seizures. The withdrawal process typically takes 2–3 months but because of the severity of the side effects Ambreen suffered, this rate is accelerated.

Lamotrigine is commenced and the dose is increased slowly in order to avoid the previous issue with non-compliance caused by the side effects that Ambreen had. The neurologist and pharmacist monitor Ambreen very carefully.

18) How would you counsel a patient starting lamotrigine for the first time?

....

....

....

19) How would you switch from one antiepileptic drug to another?

In general, the following should be monitored with all anti-convulsants:

• _Clinical efficacy: seizure control should be monitored._

• _Adverse drug reactions: slow initiation often reduces the risk._

• _Therapeutic drug monitoring (TDM): measuring serum drug levels and their pharmacokinetic interpretation is integral in the management of patients on carbamazepine and phenytoin (it is less useful with the other antiepileptic drugs)._

TDM should be used:

• _at the onset of therapy_

• _if seizure control is poor or sudden changes in seizure control occur_

• _to monitor drug–drug interactions or if toxicity is suspected_

• _if poor or non-compliance is suspected_

• _when changing antiepileptic drug._

While TDM in stabilized patients occurs only once or twice annually, patients in any of the above categories need more regular TDM.

After three further seizure-free weeks in hospital, Ambreen is discharged on 100 mg daily of lamotrigine.

Before her discharge, she would like to know what other drugs are available should the lamotrigine fail. The neurologist tells her that there are several newer antiepileptic drugs available as second-line or adjunctive therapy if initial treatment fails.

Examples of these include tiagabine, topiramate, vigabatrin, and gabapentin. There are also older drugs that could be used, such as clonazepam, although these are often associated with certain side effects.

20) What are the mechanisms of action of topiramate?

21) Would topiramate be a suitable choice for Ambreen if required? Why?

22) List three antiepileptic drugs that act by enhancing GABA transmission in a different way and describe their mechanism of action in detail.

_____

_____

_____

Six months later, Ambreen is examined in the clinic. She has been seizure-free except for one episode of absence. She is worried about the absence seizure. The neurologist tells her there is one drug that could be added to her lamotrigine that would probably control absence seizures. However, taking the drug has the risk of potentiating tonic–clonic seizures. In view of this and the fact that it was just a single episode of absence, the neurologist would prefer to wait another 6 months. They agree that if Ambreen has any more absence seizures then they will discuss adding this drug or a newer one.

Ambreen has not returned to Stradbroke Island in all this time—she is nervous about not being close to the hospital. However, at this time she feels stable enough to leave Brisbane, and decides to stay with Pavitar and help him with his pharmacy. She and he agree that the more peaceful life away from the city might also do her good and so they settle down together.

23) Which drug used for treating absence seizures is the neurologist referring to and what is its mechanism of action?

_____

_____

_____

After 4 years on lamotrigine Ambreen is seizure-free and she plans to discuss discontinuing her medication with her doctor.

24) Can antiepileptic drug treatment be discontinued? How?

_____

_____

_____

Pavitar and Ambreen stay together during this time, enjoying island life. One thing troubles Ambreen—she wants to have children but is afraid that there may be a chance she will pass her epilepsy on to them. She thinks that perhaps her problems reside in her genes. Pavitar tells her there is nothing to worry about, there is no danger that epilepsy can be passed on to her children.

25) Has Pavitar given her the right information? What would you say if you were her pharmacist?

_____

_____

_____

_____

Ambreen is also anxious about the dangers to the developing child when taking antiepileptic medication during pregnancy.

26) How would you counsel Ambreen if you were her pharmacist?

_____

_____

_____

Chapter 17
Degeneration in the brain: Parkinson's disease and Alzheimer's disease

Gerald is a smartly dressed 75-year-old man sitting in his front room. He tries to get up when you enter. It is clear getting out of his chair unaided would be a struggle, so you gesture to him to remain seated. He talks quietly, in a monotone, and you move closer to hear what he has to say. His facial expression is rigid—no movement, little attempt at eye contact. He makes small ineffectual waving movements with his arms. You hand him his medication, and he stiffly, slowly, takes his pill, and just manages to swallow it down with some water. You wonder how he manages to keep his life together.

A while later he speaks, now clearly, with strength and intonation in his voice, turning to look at you with a positive and lively expression on his face. He says: 'I think I can try and get up now'. Pushing himself from the chair with his hands he is perhaps a little stiff, but he quickly stands, straightens, and smiles. You see now that he is a tall slender man, looking almost athletic despite his age. A moment's hesitation and he takes several steps forward, each more fluent than the last. 'I think I can turn.' He makes a waving movement with one arm, as if to get himself going, turns on the spot to face you, steps forward, and reaches out to shake your hand. His handshake is firm, and he squeezes very hard. When you flinch he makes a small laugh, as if to say, 'See, I still have strength, I am OK.'

Looking at Gerald you have to remind yourself that this is the same person who a short while ago was almost immobilized in his chair. You know that a particular cluster of cells in his brain have died off, they will never come back, meaning (as explained below) that he is lacking sufficient dopamine in part of his brain required for movement control. You know that when he took his pill he was getting a compound into his brain that would be turned into dopamine, restoring for a while dopamine levels, restoring his control of movement. As you talk he tells you of what will happen to him in the hours ahead, how he has a period of normality, then with the drug effect reaching its peak how he will start to have movements he doesn't want—some bobbing and ducking and waving—then how as the drug effect wears off his immobility and stiffness will return, and once again he will be the disabled man you saw sitting in his chair when you entered.

This man has Parkinson's disease (PD), which is the second most common neurodegenerative disorder—the most common is Alzheimer's disease. PD is mainly a disease of the elderly. Our patient Gerald described above is typical, but about 5% of cases are under 50 at diagnosis, such as the patient in Workbook 14. PD is a progressive disorder, meaning cells continue to die, the patient's condition deteriorates, and the response to therapy becomes less and less satisfactory. On average, however, life expectancy is normal—onset of the disease is usually late, and patients generally die with PD rather than as a result of PD. You will already have gathered that the drug treatments have a truly enormous beneficial effect in maintaining and restoring function and quality of life, but that as the years go by they are, for so many patients, deeply inadequate. This is an example of therapy where there will be a sequence of drug use, with potentially bewildering combinations that change over the years. Understanding how these drugs work and the science underlying therapeutic strategies will help us to help these patients to live relatively normal lives.

In this chapter we consider both Parkinson's and Alzheimer's disease—both neurodegenerative disorders, both mainly but not exclusively diseases of the elderly, and both named after long-dead physicians: James Parkinson was English, writing in 1817, and Alois Alzheimer was German, writing in 1907. Only a very small amount of the chapter is spent on Alzheimer's. This does

not reflect the significance of the disease, the suffering it causes and the challenge it poses to healthcare— Alzheimer's imposes an enormous and increasing burden on families, society, and the provision and distribution of medical resources. The way different societies handle this burgeoning challenge will be one of their defining characteristics in the future. The reason we spend so little of this chapter on Alzheimer's is simply because its drug treatment is very limited and so the pharmacological basis of Alzheimer's therapy is not an extensive subject.

17.1 Symptoms and diagnosis of Parkinson's disease

A diagnosis of PD is based on presenting symptoms and is supported by a characteristic response to medication. Core symptoms can be put into four categories:

- tremor (particularly of the hands when rested on a support)
- rigidity (in limbs, overall posture and face)
- bradykinesia (slow or limited movement)
- posture—assuming a bent/hunched/stooped position when standing *and* postural instability (as when walking, leading to danger of falling).

Diagnosis may be confirmed and progression of disease monitored by functional imaging (e.g. positron emission tomography (PET) scans). This means a brain scan is

done that is able to assess the functional state of the dopaminergic systems in the brain, monitor the decline in this aspect of brain function as time passes, and perhaps monitor changes in response to treatment.

Diagnosis may also be confirmed with a positive response to a dose of drugs (e.g. L-dopa, see below) that restores dopamine activity to the brain.

Non-motor symptoms. These are symptoms other than difficulties with movement, for example issues such as **depression**, **sleep problems** and **cognitive deficits**. Cognitive deficits means lack of understanding or difficulty in making sense of day-to-day occurrences. Some further discussion of non-motor symptoms is given in Box 17.1.

17.2 Neurodegeneration: selective death of brain neurons

The dopamine pathways in the brain are illustrated in Figure 18.3. In schizophrenia we consider the notion that the problem is an inappropriately high level of dopamine influence in the cortico-limbic brain regions, which are parts of the brain related to higher function and emotion. In PD we know that there is a major loss of dopaminergic influence in the striatum (caudate/putamen) and that this part of the brain is concerned with the control of movement.

17.2.1 Parkinson's disease is associated with the death of nigrostriatal dopamine neurons

The nigrostratal pathway comprises a very dense collection of cell bodies in a small part of the brain called the substantia nigra, with axons ascending to provide a massive

innervation of the much larger striatum. This comprises the nigrostriatal pathway. These are dopaminergic neurons. On post mortem, when the brain is sectioned the dopamine oxidizes to a very dark colour, hence the term substantia nigra (meaning black body). Post-mortem observation of PD brains early on showed the loss of this dark patch of tissue. The central pathology of PD is that these neurons die off (Figure 17.1). As a result there is a progressive loss of dopaminergic terminals, and of released dopamine, in the striatum. The evidence is that over half of these nigrostriatal neurons will have died by the time a patient is diagnosed with the disease. It is likely that in most cases the degeneration will have go on for several years before that, and that the loss will continue, giving greater movement problems and poorer response to medication.

Box 17.1

Lewy bodies and the involvement of brain systems other than the nigrostriatal system in non-movement symptoms of PD

Nigrostriatal neuronal loss is the cardinal feature, with associated loss of dopamine in the striatum, resulting in the main symptoms of movement disorder. It is important to note, however, that the situation is more complex in at least two ways, both of which may contribute to the spectrum of symptoms seen in PD:

- Dopaminergic neurons of the substantia nigra mainly project to the striatum and related basal ganglia areas, but they also contribute in a relatively minor way to dopamine input to some cortical areas, and this input will also be down-regulated in PD.

- Non-dopaminergic neurons are also affected, with variable evidence of ascending degeneration.

Both of these are likely to be associated with the non-movement symptoms of PD, which are typically prominent at the later stages of disease progression. The involvement of non-dopaminergic neurons is seen in the progressive appearance of Lewy bodies. These are spherical aggregates of intracellular proteins that are found in the cell bodies of the substantial nigra in PD—their accumulation is thought to cause cell death. While they are associated with the substantia nigra, prior to this they appear in the olfactory bulb and lower brain stem, regions associated with the sense of smell and sleep patterns, which are sometimes lost in advance of the onset of classic PD symptoms.

In established PD the major non-movement disorder conditions are depression, sleep problems, and cognitive deficits, as well as peripheral effects associated with autonomic nervous system dysregulation (e.g. sweating, gastrointestinal, and sexual problems). While some conditions, for example depression, could be exacerbated by the effects of the movement disorder, it is thought that the major source of these symptoms is neurodegeneration beyond the substantia nigra. This includes the death of cholinergic, noradrenergic, and 5-hyroxytryptaminergic (serotoninergic) neurons. Symptomatic treatment of these manifestations of disease is very much on an individual basis, with drugs often able to provide a degree of relief.

The presence of non-dopaminergic neurodegeneration provides some guidance as to the true nature, and origins, of PD. The reasons why these neurons die remain to be established, but an emerging understanding of some of the mechanisms of cell death should lead to advances in neuroprotective drugs that will slow or halt the progression of the disease.

17.2.2 Other brain systems are also important in Parkinson's disease

The movement disorder symptoms of PD are as a result of degeneration of the nigrostriatal dopaminergic projection, but it is apparent that neurons may also die in other brain systems (e.g. serotoninergic (5-hyroxytryptamine, 5-HT) neurons). This may contribute to the spectrum of non-movement disorder symptoms seen in many cases of PD. This is explored further in Box 17.1.

17.2.3 A cholinergic–dopaminergic balance in the striatum is lost in Parkinson's disease

It remains the case that the dominant pathology is death of nigrostriatal neurons, leading to a deficit in dopaminergic control over the striatum. For correct control of movement disorders the striatum must maintain a balance between the influence of cholinergic and dopaminergic neurons. In PD the increasing loss of dopamine input reaches the point

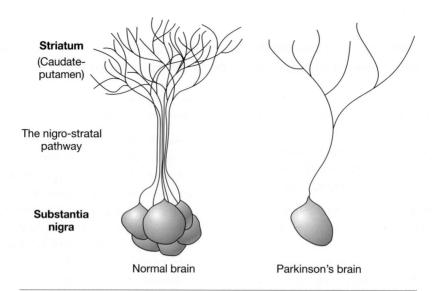

Figure 17.1 Schematic representation of the loss of nigrostriatal neurons in the brain of Parkinson's patients.

The number of dopaminergic neurons in the substantia nigra of a normal human brain will in reality number many thousands on each side, and over half (perhaps up to 90%) will be lost in PD. The diagram shows the loss of axons in the ascending pathway, and the consequent loss of the extensive branching from the axons, which results in loss of terminals. The majority of dopamine in the striatum is located in storage vesicles within these terminals, and so the result is a critical reduction in the dopamine available for release, and a down-regulation of the dopaminergic influence that can be exerted on striatal function. This imbalance results in the lack of control of movement seen in PD.

where the striatum is so imbalanced, the cholinergic influence is too dominant, that movement control is lost. So it is possible to regard the main symptoms of PD as being due to an over-dominant cholinergic system within the striatum (Figure 17.2).

17.3 Drug treatment of Parkinson's disease

Figure 17.2 shows that the cholinergic–dopaminergic imbalance in the striatum could be corrected by anticholinergic therapy or increasing the dopaminergic influence. Essentially all treatments for PD are dopamine-enhancing drugs, but there is a small role for anticholinergics. In addition to restoring motor function by restoring dopamine influence, there is also considerable interest in drugs which may slow or halt the loss of neurons—this is largely a hope for future drug treatment.

17.3.1 Anticholinergic drugs in the treatment of movement dysfunction

Figure 17.2 shows that the cholinergic–dopaminergic imbalance could be corrected by drugs which decrease the cholinergic influence in the brain. As expected the receptors for acetylcholine here are muscarinic cholinergic receptors, and so a muscarinic acetycholine receptor antagonist such as atropine would be expected to be effective. Such drugs as **benztropine** and **procyclidine** are effective against tremor and rigidity, but not against the paucity of movement (e.g. bradykinesia) that characterizes PD, and so overall are less effective than the dopamine-enhancing drugs. This, along with unwanted side effects, means that they are not usually used to treat PD but are available to reverse movement dysfunction produced by antipsychotic medication, as seen with patient Shaun in Chapter 18. However, this does not include tardive dyskinesia, which is not reduced by these antimuscarinic drugs.

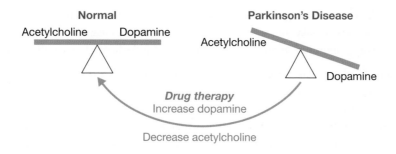

Figure 17.2 Loss of dopaminergic–cholinergic balance in the striatum.
A fall in dopaminergic input following the death of nigrostriatal neurons
(Figure 17.2) leads to acetycholine having a disproportionately large
influence. That this imbalance contributes to the symptoms of movement
disorders is suggested by the observation that both dopamine-enhancing
and anticholinergic drugs (e.g. atropine) reduce symptoms in PD patients.

17.3.2 Dopaminergic drugs in the treatment of movement dysfunction

Strategies for increasing dopamine influence in the striatum involve:

- directly stimulating the receptor with an agonist drug
- increasing synthesis of dopamine in the brain by supplying the precursor as a drug
- decreasing breakdown by inhibiting one of the two enzymes responsible, catechol O-methyl transferase (COMT) and monoamine oxidase B (MAO-B)
- enhancing dopamine release.

In reality it is commonplace for these different approaches to be used in combination, meaning that most patients will take more than one drug.

Furthermore, this is a progressing disease, and consequently the response to drugs will change with time. In particular, medication that is effective early is likely to be less satisfactory later, drug doses and combinations will change, unwanted effects will intrude, and clinical management will be a changing practice over the years.

The limitations and complications of drug therapy have been alluded to at the beginning of this chapter with the patient Gerald, and appear again with Andreas in the workbook at the end of this chapter. We will mention here two commonly encountered problems: **peak-dose effects**, as the dose taken orally reaches its maximum effect it creates involuntary movements, and **wearing off**, where immobility can reoccur as the effect of one dose declines before the next dose is effective. In addition, the 'on–off' phenomenon can result in a rapid switch to immobility, a severely compromising situation.

Direct-acting dopamine agonists

Direct-acting dopamine agonists bind to and stimulate the striatal dopamine receptors. These may be desirable for first-line treatment, particularly in less elderly patients. They have the potential to improve motor performance with less unwanted movement effects than L-dopa (see below). Their initial use in younger patients means that L-dopa therapy can be kept back for later, which given the limited number of years in which L-dopa gives maximum benefit may be a considerable advantage. However, as the disease progresses they are seen to be less effective than L-dopa, and the direct-acting agonists also carry an enhanced risk of neuropsychiatric side effects (see section 17.3.4).

Some, particularly earlier, direct dopamine agonists fall into a particular chemical class called ergots. These have the unfortunate risk of fibrotic side effects, e.g. in the lungs and heart, requiring monitoring. These drugs include **bromocryptine, pergolide, lisurgide**, and **cabergoline**.

Apomorphine is a direct acting D2–dopamine receptor agonist that is only used in difficult cases, such as when the patient can't swallow pills or with severe 'on–off' phenomena, when the drug is given by subcutaneous injection. Apomorphine is a strong emetic (i.e. it makes you vomit) and so must be preceded by the antiemetic D2 antagonist **domperidone**. It might be wondered why domperidone is able to counteract the emetic effect of apomorphine without interfering with the anti-PD effect, given that both these drugs act at D2 receptors in the brain. The answer is that while apomorphine distributes freely around the brain, domperidone cannot pass the blood–brain barrier and so cannot reach the striatum.

However, it can get to the chemoreceptor trigger zone, where the blood–brain barrier is very leaky, and so selectively blocks the effect of apomorphine there.

There is a view that the periodic stimulation of striatal dopamine receptors by short-acting direct agonists contributes to the risk of unwanted movement effects—longer-lasting drugs may therefore decrease **peak-dose** and **on–off** effects. This has lead to the development of both long half-life drugs and sustained release preparations. **Pramipexole** and **ropinirole** are examples of long half-life drugs intended to provide continuous dopaminergic stimulation. **Rotigotine** is a dopamine agonist that can be delivered slowly via a transdermal patch.

Unwanted movement effects with L-dopa therapy (see below) are often more troublesome with young patients and so in the workbook Andreas, who has early-onset PD, is given pramipexole. This works well for him for 3 years, but after this his symptoms re-emerge and he is eventually prescribed L-dopa to be taken concomitantly.

Provision of dopamine precursor L-dopa

The reasons why L-dopa is the optimal choice for dopamine precursor treatment are based on a simple neurochemical basis.

The pathway for dopamine synthesis is:

$$\text{L-tyrosine} \xrightarrow{\textit{Tyrosine hydroxylase}} \text{L-dihydroxyphenylalanine}$$

$$\text{(\textbf{L-dopa})} \xrightarrow{\textit{Dopa decarboxylase}} \text{Dopamine}$$

The **tyrosine hydroxylase** step is rate limiting. The **dopa-decarboxylase** step is not—there is a lot of this (or equivalent) enzyme around. So if you give L-dopa it will freely be converted to dopamine, bypassing the rate-limiting step, and substantially increasing dopamine availability at its receptors in the brain.

L-dopa is always administered with a peripheral decarboxylase inhibitor. If L-dopa (also called **levodopa**) is swallowed, the majority is metabolized in the gut wall and very little (less than 1%) will get to the brain. The peripheral metabolism to dopamine is also responsible for some unwanted side effects, such as nausea and hypotension, so L-dopa is given with a peripheral inhibitor of decarboxylase (peripheral means one that distributes around the body but does not enter the brain). **Carbidopa** and **benserazide** are available, combined with L-dopa into a single tablet (**co-beneldopa** and **co-careldopa**, respectively). This delivers more drug to the brain, meaning dosages are reduced, and results in less dopamine in the periphery, meaning that some side effects are lessened. It is this

combination of drugs which produced such an extraordinary (albeit temporary) alteration in Gerald's condition, and it is this which is the bedrock of anti-PD treatment.

Co-beneldopa or co-careldopa is the tablet our patient Gerald would have taken, to such dramatic effect, at the beginning of this Chapter. The patient Andreas in the workbook is treated with co-beneldopa, in both immediate-release and modified-release preparations. However, in his case this is not without serious unwanted side effects, both movement disorder and psychiatric.

With L-dopa, a short half-life drug, there is a fluctuating stimulation of dopamine receptors in the brain as the concentration of L-dopa rises to a peak following drug administration and then falls away. As with the direct-acting dopamine agonists described above, this may contribute to serious adverse effects. Strategies to flatten these fluctuations include the use with L-dopa of COMT and MAO-B inhibitors (see below), to further reduce peripheral L-dopa metabolism (thus delivering more to the brain) and slow the rate of clearance of brain dopamine produced following L-dopa. Both co-careldopa and co-beneldopa are available in modified release form, which, as with the long-acting direct agonists, is intended to reduce peak dose and end of dose wearing-off effects.

MAO-B and COMT inhibitors

One strategy to increase neurotransmitter availability in the synapse, where it can act on receptors, is to inhibit the enzymes responsible for its metabolism. In the brain, released dopamine is broken down by two enzymes, MAO-B and COMT, and drugs which are inhibitors of both these enzymes will modify dopamine availability in the brain (see Box 17.2) and have consequently assumed a significant role in the management of PD.

Monoamine oxidase enzymes and their inhibitors are discussed further in Chapter 19, and in particular in Box 19.1, introducing the two forms, MAO-A and MAO-B. Both forms break down dopamine, but MAO-B is the most effective target in the treatment of PD. In the context of this disease, with the loss of 70–80% of dopamine in the striatum, inhibitors of COMT and MAO-B can be seen as making the most of the dopamine that is left. COMT will metabolize both L-dopa and dopamine, and is found throughout the body, particularly in liver, thereby playing a role in the first-pass metabolism which limits availability of L-dopa in the brain. MAO is also found in the liver (and elsewhere) but it does not metabolize L-dopa, and so the contribution of peripheral effects to therapy of PD is probably limited.

Box 17.2

Inhibition of MAO-B and COMT in the manipulation of brain dopamine levels

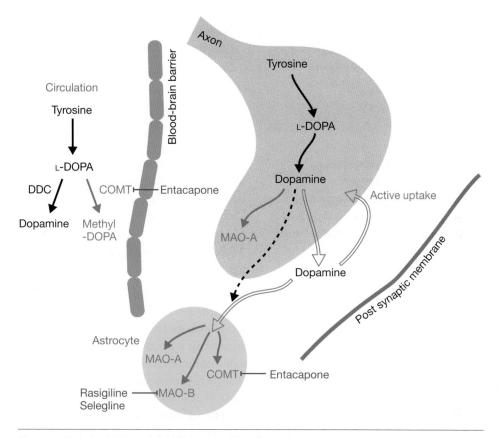

Figure a Role for MAO and COMT in controlling dopamine.

On the left the blood–brain barrier is shown at the microvasculature endothelial cells. The breakdown of L-dopa in the circulation is by dopa-decarboxylase (DDC) and COMT. In the therapeutic use of L-dopa DDC is inhibited by a peripheral decarboxylase inhibitor that does not enter the brain (e.g. carbidopa), while a COMT inhibitor (e.g. entacapone) may further reduce the peripheral breakdown of L-dopa. Entacapone will have a further effect in reducing the breakdown of extracellular dopamine released from the nerve terminal by inhibiting COMT within the brain in the high population of astrocytes. Similarly inhibition by selegiline or rasagiline of MAO-B found in the astrocytes will reduce extracellular dopamine breakdown.

The role of monoamine oxidase and its two forms, monoamine oxidase A (MAO-A) and monoamine oxidase B (MAO-B), are discussed more extensively in Chapter 19 and Box 19.1. Monoamine oxidase B (MAO-B) and catechol O-methyltransferase (COMT) are both involved in the metabolism of dopamine in the brain (see Figure a). Two differences between them help to explain the different effects of inhibitory drugs:

- While both COMT and MAO-B are found in the brain, both are also found in other tissues. Of particular importance here, COMT has high levels in the liver.
- COMT metabolizes both dopamine and L-dopa (see figure a).

This accounts for the consequences of inhibition of these enzymes.

MAO-B inhibitors available for PD (**rasagiline** and **selegiline**) may be used alone in the treatment of early PD, when movement dysfunction is modest and cognitive impairment is absent. Presumably at this early stage there is significant residual dopamine input into the striatum to be enhanced; this means that L-dopa treatment may not be necessary for a while. It is logical, however, that as more neurons die and there is less and less dopamine that this strategy serves to delay the use of L-dopa, rather than avoid it. It is also logical that when L-dopa is used MAO-B inhibitors will be a useful adjunct therapy, enhancing availably of dopamine, and reducing end-of-dose problems.

A curious issue with selegiline is that it is metabolized to an amphetamine, therefore it is advisable to take this drug in the morning to avoid this stimulating effect at night. Another issue with MAO-B inhibitors is that they cannot be given with selective serotonin reuptake inhibitors such as fluoxetine (see Chapter 19 and Workbook 14 at the end of this chapter). The reason is that both enhance, by different mechanisms, the availability of 5-HT at its receptors, and that the combined effect presents increased risk of hypertension and CNS excitation.

COMT inhibitors. The benefits of L-dopa therapy can be enhanced by COMT inhibitors such as **entacopone**, mainly given with L-dopa to help resolve end-of-dose problems by inhibiting peripheral metabolism. Another COMT inhibitor, **tolcapone**, is also available, but as this has a risk of liver damage it is only used in severe cases unresponsive to other therapy, and then with liver function monitoring. Both these drugs commonly cause diarrhea.

Dopamine release

A drug causing release of dopamine from its storage vesicles in the nerve terminals will deliver dopamine to the synapse, and therefore to the dopamine receptors in the striatum and

elsewhere. **Amantidine** is the only drug available for the treatment of PD which is believed to act in this manner, although the mechanism of action is not entirely clear; it is also a weak direct agonist at dopamine receptors.

17.3.4 Dopaminergic drugs and psychotic illness

We will establish in the next chapter (Chapter 18, Schizophrenia) that excessive stimulation of dopamine receptors in the brain is associated with schizophrenia and that the major drug therapies for this condition reduce the influence of dopamine in the brain. This is thought to be due to dopamine in the cortico-limbic areas, and not the striatum. However, when dopamine receptor-stimulating drugs are given in PD the effect is widespread in the brain, and will include an enhancement of dopamine stimulation in cortico-limbic areas of the brain. It is not surprising, therefore, that it is not unknown for PD patients on L-dopa and associated therapy to develop psychotic symptoms. (The converse is also true,—as discussed in Chapter 18 common side effects of antipsychotic medication (dopamine receptor antagonists) are movement disorders. What is needed in both cases is drugs specifically targeted at the appropriate brain regions.)

In Workbook 14 Andreas develops psychotic symptoms as a consequence of the drugs used to treat his PD. He is given clozapine, and antipsychotic dopamine antagonist. It might seem odd—his one set of drugs are used to stimulate dopamine receptors in the brain, and then as well he is given a drug to antagonist those receptors. The answer lies in the dopamine receptor subtypes: clozapine is a poor antagonist at the D2-dopamine receptors which we aim to stimulate in the treatment of PD, while being effective at other receptors which bring about the antipsychotic effect. Another antipsychotic such as haloperidol which is a very potent D2 antagonist would not be suitable in Andreas's case.

17.3.3 Strategy in the drug treatment of Parkinson's disease

The severity of initial presenting symptoms, age and general health of the patient, and the progression of the disease with time all mean that there is no single strategy to be applied to the management of PD. As indicated at the beginning of this chapter a drug approach that is effective at first can be expected to become less satisfactory with time with respect to both controlling symptoms and unwanted effects, some of which have been indicated. However, as a general guide to an initial approach to drug therapy we might consider the following generalizations based on the presenting symptoms:

- Modest movement disorder, no cognitive problems: start on MAO-B inhibitor.
- Mid-range movement disorders, no cognitive problems: direct-acting dopamine agonist.
- Severe movement disorder with cognitive problems, and older (70+): L-dopa with peripheral decarboxylase inhibitor.

The notion of the evolving pattern of drug use that would be expected to develop can be gained from reading Workbook 14.

17.4 Symptoms and diagnosis of Alzheimer's disease: a brief comment

Alzheimer's is a progressive physical and selective degeneration of the brain tissue resulting in a variety of mental symptoms that accumulate and get worse over a number of years. It is mainly a condition of the elderly (about 5% of the population over 65 years old, much more for the over 80-year-olds), explaining its increasing prevalence in the ageing populations of the developed world. However, from the start it has been recognized that there are cases of early onset and it is now recognized that the neuropathological changes seen in early onset cases is of the same pattern as that older patients (see below) and so the disease is considered to be the same one.

There is a clear contribution from inheritance in some families (familial), while in other cases this does not seem to be the case (sporadic).

Early symptoms are characteristically reduced memory for recent events, with variable difficulties in concentration and some disorientation, depression, aggression, self-care, and ability to interact with those

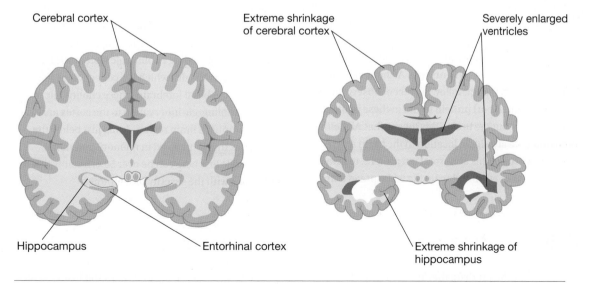

Figure 17.3 Drawing derived from a cross-section of a normal human brain (left) and an Alzheimer's brain (right). Taken from Wikipedia.

closest. There is progressive impairment of cognitive and functional capacities: global memory impairment, loss of recognition of relatives and everyday objects, loss of purposeful movements and planning activities, loss of judgment, and disintegration of personality, leading to a gross loss of ordered mental activity, with increasing incapacity.

These symptomatic changes are a result of neuropathological changes seen at post mortem (even in younger patients), which characteristically include tissue shrinkage, with larger gyri (surface spaces between the tissue of the cortex) and enlarged ventricles (the fluid-filled spaces deep within the brain). In particular there is loss of frontal and temporal lobes. The hippocampus, a region associated with memory recall, may also show signs of degeneration. Some of these gross changes are illustrated in Figure 17.3.

Plaques and tangles are bodies seen as histological markers at post mortem in Alzheimer's. Plaques accumulate in the cortex as part of the normal ageing process, but to a much greater extent in Alzheimer's brains (Figure 17.4).

The relationship of plaques and tangles to neuronal loss and loss of brain function has been the subject of an enormous amount of research in recent times. It is beyond the remit of this text to enter into this fascinating world. However, it is worth noting that both the plaques and tangles are thought to play a role in destroying brain function, and that future drugs may target both. For example, plaque proteins (amyloids) and their processing are the subject of hopeful strategies to develop new drugs which may halt or slow progression of the disease. Tangles, which are intracellular bodies found at post mortem in brains from patients with Alzheimer's, are also likely to get in on the act, following recent observations that an abnormal (tau) protein found in these bodies can spread throughout the brain. This means that Alzheimer's could originate at a single location in the brain and then spread, by virtue of this abnormal tau protein, to invade to adjacent regions, eventually causing widespread damage

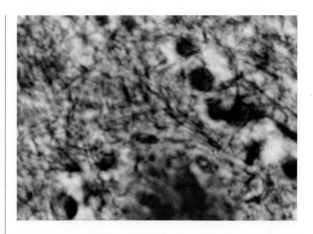

Figure 17.4 A histological section of cerebral cortex from a patient with presenile dementia showing the accumulation of plaques, seen here as densely staining bodies.
From Wikipedia.

and loss of brain function. This picture of a progressive disease is important because it may reveal opportunities for future drugs to interfere with its spread, reducing brain damage.

We have discussed that some well-known neurotransmitter systems have clusters of cell bodies in subcortical regions lower down in the brain which send their axons to branch and terminate within higher regions. In PD we have seen that these systems degenerate, providing an example of an ascending neurodegenerative disorder. There is evidence of cell loss from ascending neuronal systems in Alzheimer's as well. These include 5-HT (serotonin) and noradrenaline containing neurons. But of particular importance for us here is the loss of acetylcholine-containing neurons forming the ascending cholinergic system with its origins in the nucleus basalis, which is a collection of cell bodies located in the basal forebrain. These cholinergic neurons provide cholinergic innervation to the cortex and the hippocampus (a brain region sitting just below the neocortex that is involved in memory functions). Cholinergic loss here can be over 50%; notably this loss correlates with the severity of symptoms.

17.5 Drug treatment of Alzheimer's disease

The most significant drug therapy for Alzheimer's is based on restoring a degree of cholinergic function in the brain. This is introduced below. In addition there is a different drug approach based on the

glutamatergic excitatory system in the brain. This drug acts as an NMDA antagonist. The gluamate/NMDA system in the brain is discussed briefly in Chapter 18, Box 18.2.

Drug treatment for Alzheimer's should be initiated by an experienced specialist within an appropriate monitoring framework, with the option of continuing care by GPs.

17.5.1 Acetycholinesterase inhibitors in the treatment of Alzheimer's disease

It has been understood for a long while that acetylcholine released from neurons in the brain and elsewhere is rapidly removed by aceylcholinesterases, which are widespread enzymes that split acetylcholine into two fragments. Inhibition of acetycholinesterases will therefore increase the availability of acetylcholine at its receptors in the brain. The main drugs available are **donepezil, galantamine**, and **rivastigmine**.

17.5.2 NMDA antagonism in the treatment of Alzheimer's disease

Glutamate is the principle excitatory neurotransmitter within the brain (see Chapter 16, Box 16.1). Over-stimulation with glutamate can lead to cell death due to excessive calcium entry into the cell. A main route for glutamine-stimulated calcium entry is the NMDA receptor.

Memantine is a competitive NMDA antagonist that will reduce this route for the flow of calcium into cells, and this drug has been used for the management of moderate-to-severe Alzheimer's disease. Its role in treating Alzheimer's is not yet settled.

SUMMARY OF COMMON DRUGS USED FOR PARKINSON'S AND ALZHEIMER'S DISEASE

Therapeutic class	Drug	Mechanism of action	Common clinical uses	Comments	Examples of adverse drug reactions
Dopamine receptor agonists	Apomorphine Pramipexole Rotigotine	Stimulates dopamine receptors	Parkinson's disease Parkinsonism	Treatment should be increased slowly Causes fewer motor complications than levodopa Has more neuropsychiatric side effects that levodopa Apomorphine used in advanced disease	Excessive daytime sleepiness Hypotensive reactions
	Ergot-derived dopamine receptor agonists: bromocriptine cabergoline pergolide_			Patient's erythrocyte sedimentation rate, creatinine levels, and chest X-ray should be obtained before starting treatment	Gastrointestinal Drowsiness Hallucinations Impulse control disorder (e.g. pathological gambling) Cardiac fibrosis
Anticholinergics	Benzhexol (trihexyphenidyl) Benztropine Biperiden Orphenadrine Procyclidine	Blocks muscarinic actions of acetylcholine to produce a wide range of effects, including the reduction of excess cholinergic activity present in dopamine deficiency in Parkinson's disease	Drug-induced Parkinsonism Parkinson's disease	Generally not used in idiopathic Parkinson's disease because they are less effective than dopaminergic drugs and could cause cognitive impairment	Constipation Dry mouth Nausea Vomiting Tachycardia
Drugs containing levodopa	Levodopa with benserazide (co-beneldopa) Levodopa with carbidopa (co-careldopa)	Levodopa is converted in the brain and periphery to dopamine and replenishes depleted striatal dopamine The peripheral dopa decarboxylase inhibitors (benserazide or carbidopa) reduce peripheral dopamine production	Parkinson's disease	Peripheral decarboxylation would reduce the therapeutic effectiveness of levodopa but is responsible for many of its side effects, hence levodopa is usually administered together with peripheral decarboxylase inhibitors such as carbidopa and benserazide so that lower doses may be given to achieve the same therapeutic effect.	Nausea Taste disturbances Dry mouth Dementia Arrhythmias Psychoses Depression Excessive daytime sleepiness

Therapeutic class	Drug	Mechanism of action	Common clinical uses	Comments	Examples of adverse drug reactions
Monoamine oxidase-B inhibitors	Rasagiline Selegiline	1) Reduces breakdown of dopamine by irreversibly inhibiting monoamine oxidase type B 2) Blocks dopamine reuptake	Parkinson's disease	Patients should avoid taking with seretonine reuptake inhibitors and dopamine because concomitant usage has led to reactions leading to delirium and death	Nausea Constipation Diarrhoea Vertigo Insomnia Hallucinations
Catechol-O-methyltransferase inhibitors	Entacapone Tolcapone	Prevent breakdown of levodopa in the periphery by inhibiting the enzyme catechol-O-methyl transferase, allowing more levodopa to reach brain	Parkinson's disease	Patients on tolcapone should be monitored because it is hepatotoxic	Gastrointestinal Urine discolouration Dry mouth Confusion
Other drugs for Parkinson's disease	Amantadine	Increases dopamine release and blocks cholinergic receptors acts as an NMDA antagonist in the glutamatergic pathway from subthalamic nucleus to globus pallidus	Parkinson's disease	Improves bradykinesia, tremor and rigidity	Anorexia Nervousness Inability to concentrate Insomnia
Aceylcholinesterase inhibitors	Donepezil Galantamine Rivastigmine	Decrease breakdown of acetylcholine, reducing the apparent deficiency of cholinergic neurotransmitter activity in Alzheimer's disease	Alzheimer's disease	Rivastigmine is available as a patch	Gastrointestinal Dyspepsia Insomnia Vivid dreams Depression Fatigue Drowsiness Weight loss Urinary incontinence Hypertension
NMDA antagonism	Memantine	NMDA antagonist, which may reduce glutamate-induced neuronal degradation	Alzheimer's disease	Glutamate is associated with Alzheimer's disease	Constipation Hypertension Headache Dizziness

NMDA, N-methyl-D-aspartate

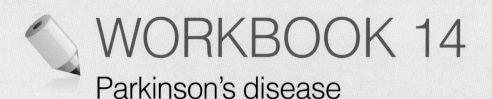

WORKBOOK 14
Parkinson's disease

Andreas, a case of early-onset Parkinson's disease: benefits and limitations of drug therapy

Andreas, a simplified case history

Andreas, the hypertensive patient from Workbook 2, wonders how to break the news to his lovely girls. He thought he had it all: the perfect wife Monique and his lovely twin daughters. Monique, whom we encountered in Workbook 1 when she had a deep vein thrombosis, used to work as his secretary in the pharmaceutical company where he was the senior quality control pharmacist for orphan drugs. After completing a 3-year course Monique is now a medicine management technician at the local hospital whilst Andreas has been promoted to director.

Recently it all started going wrong. He realized he found it difficult getting out of a chair. His GP diagnosed this as stiffness caused by a sports injury.

Then his daughter remarked that his hand was trembling when he put it on the table. After several more GP visits complaining of various mild diverse symptoms, such as tightness in his arms and legs, shaking of his hand, inability to relax his grip on his cutlery after eating, and memory loss, he has been referred to the neurology clinic.

He had had several visits to the clinic and has somehow managed to keep it secret. Initially he decided not to tell Monique because he did not want to worry her. He keeps replaying the clinic visits over and over in his head, especially the most recent one when the diagnosis was confirmed.

A table of clinical clerking abbreviations is given on page xi.

CLINICAL CLERKING FOR ANDREAS AT FOUR OUTPATIENT APPOINTMENTS

Age: 45 years

> *The average age of onset of Parkinson's disease (PD) is 55 years, and the incidence rises significantly with increasing age. However, about 5–10% of people with PD have 'early-onset' disease that begins before the age of 50. Early-onset forms of the disease are often inherited and some have been linked to specific gene mutations.*

PC: Inability to relax grip of his cutlery after eating, memory loss, slight shaking of hand, and a slight limp

HPC: Referred to neurologist by GP following visits with the above symptoms which developed over the past 18 months. Was diagnosed with depression by GP after one such consultation.

PMH: Hypertension, depression, hypertensive crises 8 years ago, recently, gastroenteritis. Diabetes, ischaemic heart disease.

> *He suffers from hypertension.*

> *GP recently diagnosed depression.*

DH:

1) Fluoxetine, *for depression*

2) Bendroflumethiazide, *for hypertension*

3) metformin, *for diabetes*

4) simvastatin, *lipid lowering, for heart disease*

5) aspirin, *antiplatelet, for heart disease*

6) losartan, *for hypertension*

> 1. *Fluoxetine is used for depression, which he was diagnosed with recently. Psychiatric disturbances like depression are very common (30%) in PD.*

> 2. *Bendroflumethiazide is for hypertension, which he has been taking since he had the hypertensive crises 8 years ago.*

Recently took non-prescribed metoclopramide for nausea due to gastroenteritis.

SH: Lives with wife and two daughters.

O/E:

1) Blood pressure = 138/85 mm Hg (reference: <140/90 mm Hg)

2) Pulse = 60/min (normal)

> *Blood pressure and pulse are both normal.*

O/O:

Well-nourished and strong-looking man with following signs:

- slight tremor of left hand at rest
- reduced blink rate
- monotonous voice
- slight difficulty initiating walking
- muscle rigidity
- sweating.

Andreas' symptoms are very slight and barely detectable by an untrained eye.

They will get worse if it is PD.

Tremor, rigidity, bradykinesia, and postural disturbances are the four classic features of PD.

- *Tremor. The tremor associated with PD has a characteristic appearance. Typically, the tremor takes the form of a rhythmic back-and-forth motion at a rate of 4–6 beats per second. It may involve the thumb and forefinger, and appear as a 'pill-rolling' tremor. Tremor often begins in a hand, although sometimes a foot or the jaw is affected first. It is unilateral on presentation. The voice escapes the tremor. It is most obvious when the hand is at rest or when a person is under stress. For example, the shaking may become more pronounced a few seconds after the hands are rested on a table. Tremor usually disappears during sleep or improves with intentional movement.*

- *Rigidity. Rigidity, or a resistance to movement, affects most people with PD. A major principle of body movement is that all muscles have an opposing muscle. Movement is possible not just because one muscle becomes more active, but because the opposing muscle relaxes. In PD, rigidity comes about when, in response to signals from the brain, the delicate balance of opposing muscles is disturbed. The muscles remain constantly tensed and contracted so that the person aches or feels stiff or weak. The rigidity becomes obvious when another person tries to move the patient's arm, which will move only in ratchet-like or short, jerky movements known as 'cogwheel' rigidity.*

- *Bradykinesia. Bradykinesia, or the slowing down and loss of spontaneous and automatic movement, is particularly frustrating because it may make simple tasks somewhat difficult. Patients find it difficult to start walking: the gait becomes shuffling with short steps and the arms are held flexed to the waist. The person cannot rapidly perform routine movements. Activities once performed quickly and easily—such as washing or dressing—may take several hours.*

- *Postural instability. Postural instability, or impaired balance, causes patients to fall easily. Affected people also may develop a stooped posture in which the head is bowed and the shoulders are drooped.*

A number of other symptoms could accompany PD. Those related to Andreas are:

- *Facial expression and blink rate: The face becomes mask-like, with mouth open and diminished blinking, which may be confused with depression.*

- *Voice: Speech becomes hypophonic (a weak voice), with a characteristic monotonous, stuttering dysarthria (a disorder of the movement required for production of speech).*

- *Sweating: This is a sign of autonomic nervous system disorder.*

- *Depression. This is a common problem and may appear early in the course of the disease, even before other symptoms are noticed.*

FH: Grandfather suffered from PD

Early-onset forms of PD are often inherited, and some have been linked to specific gene mutations. People with one or more close relatives who have PD have an increased risk of developing the disease themselves.

Differential diagnosis:

Parkinson's disease

Drug-induced parkinsonism

Toxin-induced parkinsonism

Arteriosclerotic parkinsonism

Lewy body dementia

Although the neurologist thinks Andreas has got PD because of his symptoms, age, and family history, he still considers the likelihood that it could be one of the following:

- **Drug-induced parkinsonism.** A reversible form of parkinsonism sometimes results from use of certain drugs, such as chlorpromazine and haloperidol, which are prescribed for patients with psychiatric disorders. Some drugs used for gastrointestinal disorders (metoclopramide), high blood pressure (reserpine), and epilepsy (valproate) may also produce parkinsonian symptoms. Andreas recently took metoclopamide for nausea after contacting a stomach virus. (He took it from his grandmother and knows he should not have!! A pharmacist should know not to borrow medication!)

- **Toxin-induced parkinsonism.** Some toxins and chemicals can cause parkinsonism. Investigators discovered this reaction when heroin addicts who had taken an illicit street drug began to develop severe parkinsonism. Andreas works with chemicals and could have been exposed.

- **Arteriosclerotic parkinsonism.** Sometimes known as pseudoparkinsonism, vascular parkinsonism, or atherosclerotic parkinsonism, arteriosclerotic parkinsonism involves damage to the brain due to multiple small strokes. Andreas suffers from hypertension; non-compliance with his medication could have resulted in cerebrovascular episodes.

Investigations: Positron emission tomography (PET) scan

Normally, establishing the diagnosis of Parkinson's disease is based on clinical symptoms. However due to Andreas' young age, the decision was taken to confirm the diagnosis with a PET scan.

It is extremely important to get the correct diagnosis because treatment is lifelong.

PET scan: PET imaging or a PET scan is a diagnostic examination that involves the acquisition of physiologic images based on the detection of radiation from the emission of positrons. Positrons are tiny particles emitted from a radioactive substance administered to the patient. The subsequent images of the human body developed with this technique are used to evaluate a variety of diseases.

Because PET allows study of body function, it can help physicians detect alterations in biochemical processes that suggest disease before changes in anatomy are apparent with other imaging tests, such as computerized tomography (CT) or magnetic resonance imaging (MRI). CT and MRI brain scans of people with PD usually appear normal.

Diagnosis: Parkinson's disease. (stage 1)

Although it is impossible to predict what course PD will take for an individual person, one commonly used system is the Hoehn and Yahr scale.

Stage 1: Symptoms on one side of the body only.

Stage 2: Symptoms on both sides of the body. No impairment of balance.

Stage 3: Balance impairment. Mild to moderate disease. Physically independent.

Stage 4: Severe disability, but still able to walk or stand unassisted.

Stage 5: Wheelchair-bound or bedridden unless assisted.

Plan: Commence pramipexole

Although there is no general consensus on when to initiate symptomatic treatment, generally, treatment is started when the patient begins to experience functional impairment as defined by:

- *employment status*
- *whether the dominant side is affected*
- *bradykinesia or rigidity.*

Andreas' dominant side is affected and his symptoms are affecting his job.

Pramipexole, a non-ergot dopamine agonist, is chosen predominantly because of his age.

Eventually, he will need L-dopa (also called levodopa) and possibly other drugs. The doctor wants to postpone using them because of their side effects and short length of expected period of effectiveness.

1a) List three clinical conditions resulting from the death of neurons in the brain.

1b) What is the critical and common factor in these conditions?

2a) What is Parkinson's disease?

2b) What part of the brain is affected in PD? Abnormal cystoplasmic bodies are found in the brain tissue post mortem. What are they called and where in the brain are they found?

3a) Which neurotransmitters are predominantly affected?

3b) How are they affected?

4a) List four symptoms of PD experienced by Andreas.

4b) Non-movement disorder symptoms are associated with PD. Give examples and indicate how common they are.

4c) Try to identify which neurotransmitter systems in the brain might be responsible for these different non-motor symptoms, and with this in mind try to suggest drug therapies that might alleviate these symptoms.

Andreas finally tells Monique about his diagnosis. She is distraught and he consoles her by explaining the following, which he was told and vaguely recollects from his pharmacology.

PD is not by itself a fatal disease, but it does get worse with time.

The average life expectancy of a PD patient is generally the same as for people who do not have the disease. The progression of symptoms in PD may take 20 years or more.

There are many treatment options available for people with PD.

He explains that he has been prescribed a drug called pramipexole, a dopamine agonist. Although she is a medicine management technician, she has never come across the drug because the patients in her hospital are predominantly cardiac, respiratory, or surgical patients.

Andreas explains to her about the drug, which he has read up on. He explains that the two main classes of drug used as first-line for Parkinson's are direct-acting dopamine agonists or L-dopa (levodopa) with a peripheral decarboxylase inhibitor.

5a) List the two main classes of dopamine agonists used in the management of PD.

5b) Explain the mechanism by which dopamine agonists relieve the symptoms of PD.

Andreas asks the doctor why the dopamine agonist was chosen over the L-dopa in his case although it is more expensive. The doctor explains that dopamine agonists, although expensive, are the preferred option in younger patients. Their advantages include:

- -they do not compete with circulating amino acids for absorption and transportation into the brain
- -they have a longer half-life than L-dopa and need fewer daily doses, making compliance easier for the patient.

6a) What other advantage has dopamine agonist got over L-dopa?

6b) What is the advantage of non-ergot dopamine agonist over ergot dopamine agonist?

7) Why might longer-lasting agonists, such as pramipexole, be advantageous in reducing certain unwanted side effects?

Andreas' symptoms improve with pramipexole for 3 years, after which his symptoms start resurfacing.

- almost all patients will eventually require L-dopa because it is the mainstay of management of PD
- this is because the disease results from absence of dopamine in the brain
- by replenishing the dopamine the patient gets better
- he cannot put off levodopa anymore.

Andreas is prescribed co-beneldopa (a combination of levodopa and a dopa-decarboylase inhibitor) to take alongside his pramipexole.

8) What is the evidence that supports the theory that dopamine deficit is the cause of PD?

9a) Why can you not just give dopamine instead of levodopa?

9b) What percentage of levodopa do you think gets to the brain after oral administration?

9c) What happens to the rest (explain the roles of both decarboxylase and catechol O-methy transferase (COMT))?

10a) What is the other drug in co-beneldopa besides levodopa?

10b) What is its use?

10c) What is the effect of a COMT inhibitor on delivery of oral levodopa to the brain? Explain the mechanism.

After 1 year on co-beneldopa Andreas' symptoms change in presentation.

He finds he feels very stiff and can barely move before his morning dose.

11a) What in your opinion is happening?

11b) What measure would improve this?

The doctor adds in an extra dose of controlled-release co-beneldopa to be taken at bedtime. This helps to alleviate the morning symptoms.

Three months later Andreas starts experiencing strange reactions 1 to 2 h after his doses of medication. These include grimacing, lip smacking, and protruding tongue.

12) List four side effects of levodopa.

....

....

....

The doctor decides to reduce the doses of all of Andreas' parkinson's medication and change all the co-beneldopa doses to modified release.

Besides the neurologists, Andreas is also looked after by several other professionals.

The pharmacist plays the following role:

- ensures he understands the role of his drugs in the symptomatic treatment of PD and possible adverse effects

- ensures Andreas and his carers understand the importance of compliance and timing of drug doses

- anticipates problems and advises

- advises on methods of improving and maintaining compliance as the disease progresses and drugs are added.

A psychotherapist is there to talk to and help emotionally. Andreas also gets support from the Parkinson's Disease Society.

Andreas starts feeling more depressed and his GP decides to increase the dose of fluoxetine.

After a couple of months Andreas starts behaving strangely and is diagnosed with schizophrenia secondary to levodopa. He is prescribed clozapine.

13) Why did the psychiatrist choose clozapine instead of, for example, haloperidol to treat the psychotic symptoms? (See Chapter 18 for more on these drugs.)

....

....

....

Andreas' schizophrenia is controlled with the clozapine and his motor reactions improve with the dose reduction and switch to control release.

One year later, he experiences prolonged periods when he is unable to move. The effect of his drugs also seems to be wearing off after 3 h maximum.

The doctor decides to replace the pramipexole with entacapone.

14a) To what class of drug does entacapone belong?

14b) What is entacapone's mechanism of action?

14c) What are the adverse effects of this class of drugs?

Andreas improves following this switch. He is, however, worried about his options if and when the effects of his current medication wear out.

He discusses his concerns with his consultant, who reassures him that, although not ideal, there are other options to be tried, including selegiline, rasagaline, amantadine, apomorphine, and antimuscarinics.

Andreas recalls from his pharmacology lectures that anticholinergics are used more commonly in drug-induced parkinsonism.

15) Which class of drugs are commonly implicated as causing parkinsonism? How does this come about?

16a) Which symptoms of Parkinson's disease will anticholinergics improve?

16b) Explain in detail how anticholinergics work to alleviate certain symptoms of PD.

17) What are the side effects of anticholinergics?

Andreas asked the doctor to give him some more information about the other drugs selegiline and rasagiline, which he mentioned are also good for end-of-dose deterioration. They discuss selegiline as a possible drug for Andreas. One issue the doctor mentions is that if he were to be given selegiline he would have to be taken off fluoxetine.

18) Describe the mechanism of action of selegiline in PD.

19) Why should selegiline be taken in the morning?

20) Why should selegiline not be taken with fluoxetine? Set out the mechanisms and consequences of this drug interaction. (Refer to Chapter 19 for more on this.)

Amantadine and apomorphine are other options for Andreas.

21a) What are the suggested mechanisms of action of amantadine in PD?

21b) What is the mechanism of action for apomorphine? When is it commonly used?

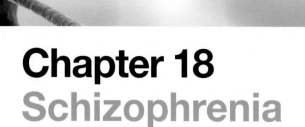

Chapter 18
Schizophrenia

The onset of a schizophrenic episode is often a confusing, distressing, and anxiety-provoking time, particularly if this is the first such experience. Schizophrenia commonly presents in young adults, and so the primary symptoms, and the disorientation which follows, may be superimposed on adolescent insecurities and lack of confidence. The individual may not, in such circumstances, be well placed to assess and choose between the various support services and therapeutic options on offer. The families of young adults presenting with schizophrenia may share in this distress and anxiety; parents may be horrified at the suffering of their offspring, fearful for the future and experience feelings of guilt relating to ideas about being bad parents and passing on bad genes.

In the workbook in this chapter we meet Shaun, who is a seriously distressed young man with bizarre and disruptive behaviours. Despite medical intervention he continues to have episodes of psychotic behaviour, which continue over a number of years. He tries a number of different antipsychotic drugs until a solution is reached for him that largely controls his symptoms and does not present with unacceptable unwanted effects. However, over the period of a few years for which we follow his story he seems unable to remain symptom-free without his antipsychotic medication. His troubles are not uncharacteristic of such patients. As for his long-term prospects—well, schizophrenia is a chronic condition. However, there is every reason for optimism that with continued medication the burden of schizophrenia will

be reduced—and it is always possible that he may be one of those who, given time, is able to quit his drug therapy and remain symptom-free.

In schizophrenia the cause, severity, and symptoms vary between patients. The long-term outcome, also variable, is likely to depend on many factors. These include the broader issues of non-pharmacological treatments and support services that are offered to the patient. Non-drug treatment is likely to play a major part in the management of the condition—the balance between drug and non-drug therapies will vary with the patient and with the doctor/therapist.

Here we focus on drug treatment and particularly on the notion that drug treatment of schizophrenia is best understood at the cellular and molecular level. At their best these drugs restore a working balance between different neurotransmitter systems in the brain; which neurotransmitters, and how they are affected, depends on the individual drug being used. Our understanding of these issues is imperfect, but we can begin to place the clinical use of different classes of antipsychotic drugs within a scientific framework. Even the incomplete knowledge we have of drug action provides the foundations for a rational approach to therapy. In addition, the focus on cellular events in the brain, the neurotransmitter approach, enables us to briefly consider the prospects for fundamentally new drugs in the treatment of this destructive disorder.

18.1 What is schizophrenia? Symptoms, diagnosis, and causes

Schizophrenia varies between individuals, but common to all is a pattern of disordered thinking. This may be

observed as clusters of symptoms, which may be classified and described in a variety of ways.

18.1 What is schizophrenia? Symptoms, diagnosis, and causes

471

18.1.1 Symptoms of schizophrenia

The disordered thinking of schizophrenia can be organized into different groups (Figure 18.1):

- **Disorder of form**, apparent as an incoherent speech pattern, jumbled words or disorganized sentences, reflecting a disordered stream of thought.

- **Disorder of content**. For example, a patient may believe that his/her thoughts are being broadcast and can be heard by others, or that thoughts are being directly inserted into their head by other people or inanimate objects. The patient may suffer from delusions, such as of inflated importance or power, and exhibit delusional behaviour.

Symptoms may include:

- **Hallucinations**, principally auditory, such as hearing voices. The voices may be telling the patient what to do, including self-harm or harming others.

- **Flattening of affect** refers to a withdrawn individual not showing normal responses to the good and bad things of everyday life, perhaps resulting in poor personal care. The patient may appear to lack normal emotional responses.

- **Motor behaviour disorders.** Movement may be lowered (sitting in a stupor), raised (excitable), or dysfunctional (e.g. aimless or clumsy movements).

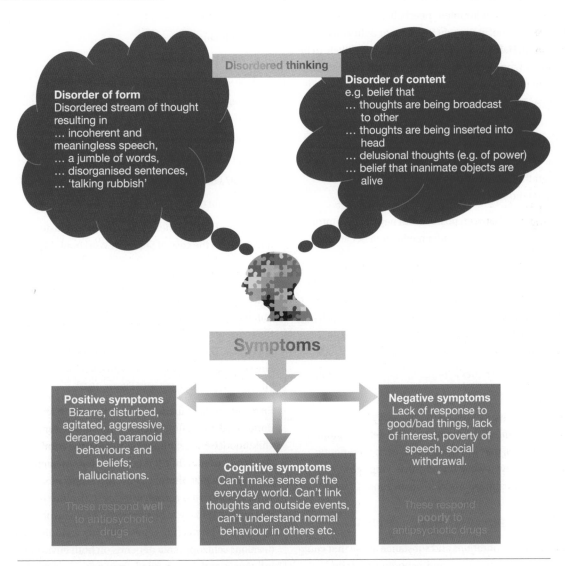

Figure 18.1 Disordered thinking in schizophrenia generates a spectrum of symptoms.

Patients vary considerably in the balance between these symptoms.

On top of this, the drugs used to treat schizophrenia may themselves cause motor dysfunction.

- **Avolition** is an inability to initiate and sustain goal-directed activities.

Some people may continue an apparently undisrupted everyday life despite suffering from a cluster of these characteristics. However, for other individuals the consequences may include an inability to make sense of the world, bizarre and disruptive behaviours, leading to social withdrawal, fearful and angry responses, and failure to attend to work or educational needs.

The symptoms above may be divided into:

- **positive symptoms**, which are those associated with madness, such as jumbled speech, hearing voices, paranoia, belief in thought insertion or delusions of grandeur. Hallucinations, when present, are likely to be auditory (contrasting with the visual hallucinations caused by hallucinogens such as LSD).
- **negative symptoms**, such as lack of affect, lack of interest in everyday life, and apparent lack of emotion
- **cognitive symptoms**, which derive from poor concentration and memory, and difficulty in integrating thoughts, resulting in a difficulty in understanding events and people.

The distinction between positive and negative symptoms is important when we consider medication because:

- negative symptoms are generally hard to treat compared to positive symptoms
- while it is positive symptoms that often result in hospitalization, resistance negative symptoms, which may persist on discharge from hospital with antipsychotics, may significantly impair ability to function
- some drugs are better at reducing negative symptoms than others.

Notably, negative symptoms in some patients may worsen with time. It is possible that this deterioration, when it occurs, may be reduced with early therapeutic intervention, even when the negative symptoms themselves are unresponsive to medication.

18.1.2 Diagnosis of schizophrenia

Other medical conditions and substance abuse that could account for the behaviours and symptoms must be excluded early in the investigation. In the workbook we see that Shaun has blood tests done. These are to exclude other conditions—there is no blood test for schizophrenia.

Schizophrenia varies a lot from one patient to another, making consistent diagnosis difficult. Criteria for diagnosing schizophrenia come from the Diagnostic and Statistical Manual of Mental Disorders (version DSM-IV-TR) and the International Statistical Classification of Diseases and Related Health Problems (ICD-10).

Diagnostic schemes are likely to require all of the following three to be present:

1) The presence of a minimum of two symptoms from a list such as:
   a. delusions
   b. hallucinations
   c. disorganized speech
   d. grossly disorganized catatonic behaviour
   e. negative symptoms (poverty of speech, absence of emotions)
   f. avolition (i.e. inability to initiate and sustain goal-directed activities)
2) social/work/school disruption
3) a duration of at least 6 months.

Elements of each of these three symptom clusters are illustrated in the case of Shaun in Workbook 14.

18.1.3 Causes of schizophrenia

The origins of schizophrenia have been the subject of much research and are still unclear, and mostly beyond the scope of this text. However, some brief observations are useful. There are multiple causes of schizophrenia. The simplest way to divide the causes is into environmental and genetic (Figure 18.2).

Environmental influences start in the womb and are dominated by the functioning of the family during childhood. Genetic influences involve the combination of genes inherited. While it is possible that research will discover a 'schizophrenia' gene, this seems most unlikely. What you inherit is a *propensity* for schizophrenia, and this in itself is likely to be polygenic, i.e. to involve an *ensemble* of interacting genes. Whether an individual develops schizophrenia depends on both environmental influences and the inherited propensity to develop schizophrenia. The significance of an inherited

18.1 What is schizophrenia? Symptoms, diagnosis, and causes

473

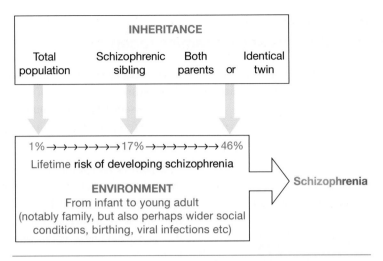

Figure 18.2 The interplay between inheritance and environment in the causes of schizophrenia.

component can be seen in the **prevalence of schizophrenia**. This is about 1% (lifetime risk) in the general population, about 17% if there is a schizophrenic brother or sister, and about 46% if in addition both parents suffer from the condition (Figure 18.2). Of course siblings and parents mostly live within the same family and so we must assume that the common environmental influences contribute to these family clusters. However, the comparison of identical and non-identical twins is helpful. If one is schizophrenic then in identical twins (where the genetic makeup is identical) there is a 46% risk of the other twin developing the condition, compared to about 17% for non-identical twins (the same as for non-twin brothers or sisters). These and many other types of studies have established the view that the causes of schizophrenia include a complex interaction of inheritance and environmental/developmental influences.

18.1.4 A biological basis for schizophrenia?

These issues (genetic *vs* environmental) have an influence on the way we view the treatment of schizophrenia with drugs. If a patient has an inherited developmental deficit this may lead to an abnormal structure, neural network, or neurotransmitter balance in the brain that we can define with a biological theory for schizophrenia. The most influential biological theory relates to an overactive

dopaminergic influence in specific brain regions. It is the ventral tegmental/corticolimbic system (system 3 in Figure 18.3) that is most important in schizophrenia. The dopamine pathways and receptors in the brain are further described in Box 18.1, and in Box 18.2 the dopamine hypothesis for schizophrenia is discussed, together with the glutamate theory. We note that there are other GABAergic, cholinergic, and serotoninergic (see section 18.2.2) theories relating to schizophrenia, and also that there are theories derived from structural and functional studies that are not related to a particular neurotransmitter. With our focus on drug action the neurotransmitter-based theories are most helpful, since we can then try to correct this neurotransmitter imbalance with targeted drugs and have some expectation of success in terms of clinical benefit.

If we reject the notion of a biological cause it is not necessary to reject the benefits of drug therapy or of the importance of developing better drugs, but expectations of resolving the difficulties of schizophrenic individuals with drug therapy will be lower. What the summary of drug actions below tells us is that any biological answer is unlikely to be simple, that advances in drug discovery are of enormous importance to improving the prospects for schizophrenic individuals, and that drug treatments also offer disturbing pitfalls and reverses, as illustrated in the case of Shaun in the workbook.

Box 18.1

Brain dopamine pathways and dopamine receptors

The central feature which all antipsychotic drugs have in common is that they act as antagonists of dopamine receptors. For this and other reasons it has been suggested that the symptoms of schizophrenia may be caused by dopamine over-activity in certain parts of the brain (see Box 18.2).

There are two main ascending dopamine pathways in the brain and one short projection. These are illustrated in Figure 18.3.

The nigrostriatal system is the most dense dopamine system in the brain. The substantia nigra comprises a compact collection of cell bodies that send a large number of axons up into the areas designated as the striatum (also called the caudate and putamen) and the globus pallidus. Here the densely packed dopaminergic terminals contain the highest concentration of dopamine in the brain. These terminals form synapses with a variety of cell bodies, including those of intrinsic cholinergic neurons.

The other main ascending system, the corticolimbic system, has cell bodies in the ventral tegmental area that send their axons upwards to the limbic and cortical areas, which are associated with emotions, reward, and other higher brain functions. Not surprisingly this is the system implicated in schizophrenia.

In addition to these two major ascending systems there is a short projection within the hypothalamus, located at the base of the brain near the pituitary. This projection is sometimes called the tuberoinfundibular system'. The cell bodies are located in the arcuate nucleus (the tuberal region) and send short axons down to the median eminence (the infundibular region) at the base of the hypothalamus. The dopamine released here acts to inhibit the release of prolactin from the anterior pituitary.

Dopamine receptors

Dopamine acts on a family of receptors designated D_1–D_5. These are all coupled via heterotrimeric G-proteins to enzymes and ion channels, which together regulate neuronal function. To understand the evolving characteristics of the antipsychotic drugs it is necessary to have some understanding of this family of receptors and their location within different brain regions.

D_1 dopamine receptors are very abundant in all main dopamine projection areas. Dopamine acting on these receptors results in the stimulation of cyclic AMP synthesis, among other actions. D_1 receptors are the main dopamine receptors within the prefrontal cortex.

D_2 dopamine receptors are also abundant in the main dopamine projection areas—they are particularly important for the action of antipsychotic drugs, both with respect to wanted and unwanted outcomes.

D_3 and D_4 dopamine receptors are overall much less abundant than the D_1 and D_2 receptors, and are preferentially located within the ventral tegmental to corticolimbic projection areas, not in the nigrostriatal areas. This is a potentially important difference for the action of antipsychotic drugs since it suggests the possibility of specific regulation of corticolimbic functions independent of nigrostriatal movement control. D_3 receptors are particularly abundant in the prefrontal cortex.

D_5 dopamine receptors show similarities to the D_1 receptors, but are of lower abundance with some concentration within corticolimbic areas.

D_1-like and D_2-like families. It is possible to cluster the D_2–D_4 dopamine receptors into a D_2-like family. They are all linked to the inhibition of cyclic AMP synthesis, the activation of potassium channels and the inhibition of calcium channels, all of which can be summarized as dampening down neuronal activities. D_1 and D_5 receptors may then be grouped together as D_1-like, both of these being coupled to an increase in cyclic AMP synthesis.

Implications for antipsychotic drug therapy. The following comments can be considered with those set out in section 18.2.8.

- In the search for drugs treating both negative and positive symptoms of schizophrenia it is tempting to imagine that the objective is a highly selective drug at either D_3 or D_4 receptors, since these should be devoid of significant nigrostriatal effects and thus free of extrapyramidal side effects.

- More selective D_4 antagonists have indeed been made, but this has not led to the predicted improved outcome.

- Selective D_3 antagonists are being developed.

- While D_3 and D_4 receptors have mainly corticolimbic distribution, even here D_1 and D_2 receptors are more abundant, suggesting that D_3/D_4 manipulation will only offer a small part of the potential for control of dopamine influences in these brain regions.

- It is now understood that a degree of agonist activity at certain receptors subtypes may be characteristic of currently used drugs and may contribute to the therapeutic response.

In summary it is likely that D_2 antagonism will remain the cornerstone of antipsychotic therapy in the context of improved drugs which act at other dopamine receptor subtypes and receptors for other neurotransmitters (e.g. serotonin). While we can see some of the features of this landscape, there are still too many unknowns to be able to make the therapy an exact science. Hence the trial-and-error aspect to the prescribing of antipsychotic drugs, as illustrated by the management of Shaun's illness in Workbook 15.

18.2 Drugs in clinical use for the treatment of schizophrenia

Over 20 different drugs are currently available for the routine treatment of schizophrenia. Each varies in effectiveness against particular categories of symptom and in the likelihood of unwanted effect. These differences include:

- a sedative effect—positive with agitated patients, unwanted in some others

- attenuation of positive symptoms—of widespread value for schizophrenic patients, both in the short term for those with acute exacerbations and in long-term maintenance

- effectiveness in treating negative symptoms—of widespread importance, but many antipsychotic drugs are ineffective in treating negative symptoms

- a risk of producing adverse movement effects—often referred to as **extrapyramidal[1] side effects**

- **antimuscarinic effects**, with some drugs being potent muscarinic acetylcholine antagonists.

To some degree these variations in clinical outcome can be understood in terms of the different interactions with receptors found in the brain. The starting point for such considerations is the interaction of drugs with the dopamine receptors.

18.2.1 Antipsychotic drugs are dopamine antagonists

All antipsychotic drugs in clinical use are antagonists at dopamine receptors, an action that is important for their therapeutic effect. There are five main dopamine receptor subtypes, and three main sets of dopamine neurons, within the brain. The location of the neuronal systems and their receptors in the human brain are outlined in Figure 18.1 and Box 18.1. A broad appreciation of the functions served by the

---

1. You will frequently encounter the term 'extrapyramidal' in accounts of the unwanted movement effects of antipsychotic drugs. Movement instructions from the cortex pass through the 'pyramids' in the brainstem on their way down to the spinal cord and the motor neurons. The extrapyramidal system, which modulates and plans movement control, does not pass through these brainstem 'pyramids', but it does pass through the striatum (caudate/putamen). This extrapyramidal system depends on a suitable dopamine

input from the substantia nigra to the striatum to function properly, and it is this which is disturbed in Parkinson's disease and by the dopamine antagonists used to treat schizophrenia.

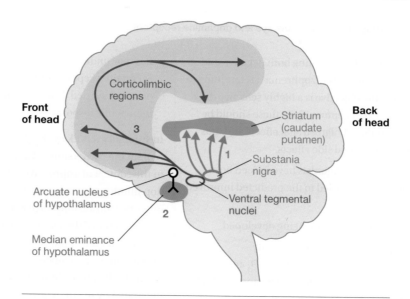

Figure 18.3 Three dopamine neuronal system in the brain.

1, The nigrostriatal system involved in movement planning an Parkinson's disease; 2, the hypothalamic system involved in endocrine control; 3, the ventral tegmental–corticolimbic system, which is implicated in schizophrenia.

three neuronal systems (which are simply illustrated in Figure 18.3), and the subtypes of receptors which they interact with, is necessary to understand how the different drugs produce their different spectrum of wanted and unwanted effects.

The dopamine cell bodies form clusters that send projections to major areas of the brain where neuronal function is influenced by the dopamine released from their nerve terminals. The three main systems are illustrated in Figure 18.3.

- The cell bodies densely packed into the substantia nigra send axons to terminate in the basal ganglia (striatum: caudate/putamen, globus pallidus). This pathway is essential for movement control; as discussed in Chapter 17 its degeneration is the central pathology in Parkinson's disease. Its disruption by antipsychotic drugs results in the movement disorder side effects discussed below and illustrated in Workbook 15.

- The shortest pathway is a population of dopamine-releasing neurons in the hypothalamus. The dopamine released here inhibits prolactin release from the pituitary into the bloodstream, explaining a further unwanted effect of dopamine antagonist (antipsychotic drug) therapy, elevated blood prolactin (hyperprolactinaemia), which may result in conditions such as male breast enlargement (gynaecomastia), a recognized possible side effect of antipsychotic drug therapy.

- The longest pathway is from clusters of cell bodies in the ventral tegmental system not far from the substantia nigra, which sends axons all the way up to the cortex and limbic systems, including the frontal lobes, nucleus accumbens, amygdale, and hippocampus. These areas are involved in higher mental functions, emotional responses, memory, selective attention, and appropriate responding to positive and negative events. It is not surprising, therefore, that of the three dopamine systems, it is this one that has been associated with schizophrenia and the therapeutic response to antipsychotic medication.

In Box 18.1 the five main dopamine receptor subtypes (D_1 to D_5) are described, and it has been indicated that while D_1 and D_2 are widespread throughout the brain it is of particular interest when considering antipsychotic drugs that D_3 and D_4 receptors are relatively selectively localized in the corticolimbic projection areas. It is their relative paucity in the caudate/putamen that makes them of interest in antipsychotic drug development, providing the possibility of a drug that acts with partial selectivity at the corticolimbic areas. There has been a focus of attention on D_4 receptors because of the clinical value of clozapine (see below), an effective antipsychotic with relative selectivity for D_4 receptors. More recently there has been interest in D_3 receptor antagonists as effective

Box 18.2
Dopamine, glutamate and the biological basis of schizophrenia

Our knowledge of the biology of schizophrenia has been the subject of intense research over the years. Fascinating advances have been made from both molecular and developmental approaches. That this has not resulted in a unified comprehensible theory that stands the test of time and directs clinical practice is not surprising, given that we have only a very crude understanding of the way the brain works in terms of higher mental functions. Given the diversity of the pathology across individual patients it is quite possible that such a unified theory will never be forthcoming. Here we shall only introduce two of the mainstream concepts:

- **the dopamine hypothesis**, which has proved the most durable and the most influential in terms of understanding drug therapy
- **the glutamate hypothesis**, which is relatively new and is proposed as the most promising route for entirely novel antipsychotic drugs.

The dopamine hypothesis

At its simplest the dopamine hypothesis states: **Schizophrenia is a result of an overactive dopamine system in the corticolimbic regions of the brain**. There are many variations on this simple expression of the theory, but they all include an element of dopamine over-activity in part of the brain or at certain dopamine receptor subtypes (see Box 18.1).

Some of the evidence for the dopamine hypothesis that has stood the test of time is listed below:

1. All antipsychotic drugs are dopamine antagonists. (But the clinical antipsychotic effect is delayed, while dopamine antagonism is very rapid, which weakens the support this offers for a simple dopamine over-activity hypothesis).

2. Amphetamine, which increases dopamine availability in the synapse, may produce a psychosis-like state. (This is not as good a mimic of a schizophrenic psychotic episode as is seen with phencyclidine, see below).

3. Post-mortem studies—there are many findings in the literature that have not proved reproducible. In some, but not all, studies D_2 density was greater in post-mortem schizophrenic brains than in matched controls.

4. Imaging studies in live patients (e.g. by positron emission tomography):
   a. Dopamine receptor occupancy by endogenous dopamine is greater in schizophrenic patients,
   b. The synaptic level of dopamine is higher in schizophrenic patients.
   c. Amphetamine gives a higher release of dopamine in schizophrenic patients (i.e. more dopamine is available for release in the dopaminergic terminals of schizophrenic patients than in matched controls).

While the evidence base for dopamine dysregulation being the cause of schizophrenia may seem modest, it has retained a dominant position over many years, perhaps in part because it sits alongside the dopaminergic theory for the action of antipsychotic drugs.

The dopamine hypothesis refined: overactivity at D_2 (corticolimbic) and underactivity in D_1 (prefrontal cortex)

Many refinements of the dopamine hypothesis have been proposed. An influential example is the hypothesis of opposite influences of D_1 and D_2 receptors. It is clear that the negative symptoms are resistant to D_2 antagonism and that activation of D_1 receptors in the frontal cortex is required for normal function. This leads to the suggestion of over-active D_2 receptors (corticolimbic areas) as the cause of positive symptoms and a deficit in dopamine stimulation of D_1 receptors (prefrontal cortex) as contributing to negative and cognitive symptoms.

The glutamate hypothesis

More recently the glutamate hypothesis has focused on the role of the NMDA glutamate receptor. Glutamate is the major excitatory neurotransmitter in the brain (see Chapter 16, Box 16.1). It is activation of glutamate receptors, found on essentially all brain neurons, that provides the driving force for neuronal activity in the brain. It is this system that we have encountered when considering the action of certain anti-epileptic drugs in Chapter 16.

Glutamate receptors include a class called NMDA receptors. These are ion channel receptors, i.e. they cross the cell membrane (Figure b, Box 16.1) and contain an intrinsic ion channel for calcium and sodium ions. When activated they open these two ions enter the cell (they are at a higher concentration outside the cell than inside) and therefore they have an excitatory effect (i.e. they depolarize the cell).

A glutamate hypothesis was first suggested following a report in 1980 of reduced cerebrospinal fluid in schizophrenia patients. Despite the fact that there has been difficulty in replicating this finding, a glutamate hypothesis has gained ground, supported by other evidence indicated below. The glutamate hypothesis at its simplest is: **schizophrenia is a result of under-activity at the NMDA glutamate receptors in the brain**.

Some of the evidence that has given rise to this hypothesis is listed below. (It should be noted that not all these findings have been replicated in every study undertaken).

1. The abuse drug phencyclidine (PCP) can induce a psychosis-like state that is a good mimic of schizophrenic psychosis on acute admission to hospital.

2. PCP is an antagonist at NMDA receptors. Other NMDA antagonists acting at other sites can also give rise to psychosis-like symptoms.

3. Neuropathological evidence:
   a. reduced gene expression of messenger RNA for NMDA receptors
   b. reduced glutamate in the spinal cord
   c. reduced glutamate uptake sites (a presynaptic marker for glutaminergic terminals) on autopsy (post mortem tissue).

4. Drugs enhancing NMDA function (e.g. glycine, see below) may reduce negative symptoms.

The last item on this list implies a route for novel antipsychotic drug development. In addition to glutamate acting at its binding site, a requirement for NMDA receptor activation is that glycine occupies its own separate binding site on the NMDA receptor complex (see Figure a). Glycine therefore acts as an excitatory co-transmitter in the brain.

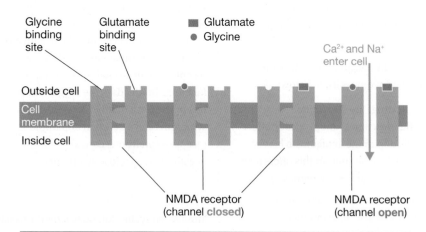

Figure a Both glycine and glutamate must bind to their binding sites on the NMDA receptor for the channel to open.

While activation of glutamate receptors by a glutamate-mimetic drug would have widespread undesirable effects in the brain, increasing NMDA receptor activity by increasing glycine at its site has been considered a possible therapeutic approach, giving rise to two strategies for drug development:

1. Administration of glycine agonists. These include glycine, D-serine, and D-cycloserine. Clinical trials have indicated a therapeutic effect when these are used as adjunct therapy with established neuroleptics. On a cautious note, not all studies have shown a beneficial outcome.

2. Administration of glycine uptake inhibitors. Glycine is removed from the synapse by an active uptake mechanism, the glycine transporter, which is found on nerve terminals and astrocytes. This effective removal system results in a subsaturating level of glycine in the vicinity of NMDA receptors. Inhibition of this transporter increases the glycine concentration at these receptors, enhancing glutamate neurotransmission at the NMDA receptor.

Both these strategies are being actively pursued, although whether these glycine-enhancing drugs will ever achieve routine clinical use remains to be seen.

---

antipsychotic agents which treat cognitive and negative symptoms of schizophrenia without unwanted movement effects.

In addition to action at dopamine receptors the antipsychotic drugs are antagonists at a variety of other neurotransmitter receptors, notably including muscarinic acetylcholine receptors and 5-hydroxytryptamine (serotonin) receptors. These additional actions have a significant impact on their use in the clinic and will be considered later. But why is the dopamine receptor antagonism assumed to be the cause of the central antipsychotic effect? There are a number of pieces of evidence connecting dopamine activity and schizophrenia—some are discussed in Box 18.2—but a salient example is a paper published in 1976 reporting affinity at dopamine D_2 receptors and clinical dose for a wide range of antipsychotic drugs (Figure 18.4). This showed a good correlation between the two, providing sound support for the notion that the D_2 antagonism contributes to the clinical benefit.

18.2.2 Most antipsychotic drugs are serotonin (5-HT$_2$) antagonists

Not all antipsychotic drugs are effective antagonists at 5-HT$_2$ receptors (**sulpiride**, for example), but the majority are. The main interest here is in the subtype 5-HT$_2$A receptors. With some drugs (e.g. **risperidone**) 5-HT$_2$

antagonism has been thought of as central to the antipsychotic effect. With many others (e.g. **clozapine**) it is suggested that this antagonism is a contributor, alongside dopamine receptor blockade, to the therapeutic response. It is also well established that serotonin antagonism reduces unwanted movement effects. Models of serotonin–dopamine interaction have been produced which that may partially explain the beneficial effects of 5-HT antagonism. The limited direct evidence for serotonin dysfunction in schizophrenia has discouraged the development of a serotonin- hypothesis.

18.2.3 Movement disorder side effects (extrapyramidal symptoms)

The earliest of modern antipsychotic drugs (which were often called major tranquillisers, or neuroleptics) include drugs still commonly in use, and are referred to as **typical antipsychotics**. These first-generation drugs and their derivatives have a powerful antipsychotic effect, but they also exhibit a high incidence of movement disorders (extrapyramidal side effects). The movement disorders produced by antipsychotic drugs have adversely affected many schizophrenic patients and severely limited the usefulness of these drugs. Indeed it is in part this unwanted effect that motivated the search for different drugs which that resulted in the development of the newer **atypical antipsychotics.**

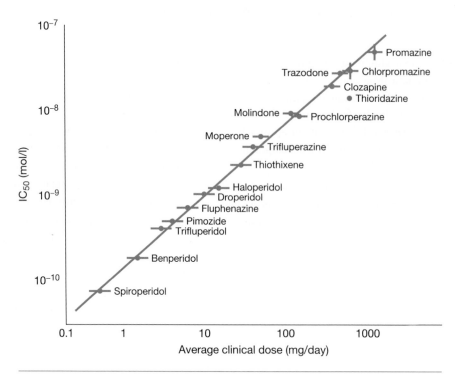

Figure 18.4 An early study showing correlation between affinity for dopamine D_2 receptors (IC_{50}) and average clinical dose for a variety of antipsychotic drugs.

Despite certain caveats, such as the influence of degree of penetration of the blood–brain barrier on the extent to which clinical dose correlates with concentrations in the brain, this is a compelling illustration of the relationship between dopamine D_2 receptors and the response to antipsychotic medication. From Seeman *et al.*, Nature 361: 717 (1976).

Extrapyramidal side effects will be considered here in three categories:

- **Acute dystonic reaction** (occulogyric crisis)—immediate to short-term onset (see Workbook 15).

- **Parkinsonian symptoms** include many of the broad features we have seen in Parkinson's disease, including tremor, rigidity, and abnormal posture. Given that Parkinson's disease is characterized by a loss of dopaminergic innervation to the striatum, it is understandable that a drug which that diminishes the dopaminergic influence in the striatum by acting as an antagonist at the dopamine D_2 receptors could have similar outcome. May occur from onset of taking medication.

- **Tardive dyskinesias** are a distressing and disabling set of involuntary movements of the tongue, jaw, and lips which sometimes follow long-term drug use.

The starkest difference between these movement disorders for patient welfare is that, while parkinsonian symptoms disappear on withdrawal of the drug, tardive dyskinesias may persist as a permanent disability.

If we recall the treatment of Parkinson's disease in Chapter 17 we will note that symptoms can be relieved not only by increasing the dopaminergic input (L-DOPA therapy) but also by diminishing the cholinergic influence in the striatum (Figure 17.2). This is important when trying to understand drugs and schizophrenia in two respects. Firstly, many antipsychotic drugs act as antagonists at muscarinic acetylcholine receptors as well as at dopamine receptors. This anticholinergic effect at the striatum may reduce the tendency to produce movement effects, i.e. all other things being equal drugs with strong anticholinergic effects may have less pronounced extrapyramidal effects. Secondly, short-term relief from acute dystonias (movement and posture dysfunction) may be achieved by using an antagonist at the muscarinic acetylcholine receptor which acts at the striatum, helping restore the cholinergic–dopaminergic balance. This was done in the workbook for Shaun when he had an occulogyric crisis.

Importantly, though with respect to these unwanted movement side effects there is considerable variation in both patients and drugs. Not all patients are equally susceptible to parkinsonian symptoms, and even among the typical antipyschotics the drugs vary in the incidence of these extrapyramidal effects. Notably the atypical antipsychotics have a lowered tendency to generate movement disorders; the reason for this varies, but generally it is explained by differences in the way they bind to the different dopamine receptor subtypes, and the extent to which they act as antagonists at other receptors, such as those for acetycholine (as indicated above) and serotonin. The atypical antipsychotics (e.g. olanzapine) may cause unacceptable weight gain and metabolic effects.

18.2.4 Other side effects

The **antimuscarinic effects** include dry mouth, blurred vision and disordered control of urination. Antimuscarinic effects originating in the brain may include confusion. The **sedative effects** are important—wanted in agitated patients for short short-term effects, largely unwanted in long-term maintenance—and varies considerably between different drugs. In addition some patients may experience other side effects, such as gynaecomastia and other related symptoms as indicated above. This is as a result of dopamine D_2 receptor blockade in hypothalamic pathways, leading to endocrine imbalances such as increased prolactin secretion.

Of rare occurrence but of some importance is the increased risk of cardiac ventricular arrhythmias with some extremely rare cases of sudden cardiac death. Causes are likely to include an effect of the drug on specific cardiac K^+ channels.

18.2.5 Typical antipsychotic drugs

The introduction of the first modern antipsychotic drugs into psychiatric practice in the early 1950s had a major impact, enabling large reductions in the number of chronically hospitalisedhospitalized mental patients. The broad characteristics of typical antipsychotic drugs are effectiveness against positive symptoms, poor response of negative symptoms, and significant problems with adverse effects, most notably movement disorders. These common characteristics vary between individual drugs and individual patients.

Pharmacology of typical antipsychotics

Phenothiazines are a chemically defined group of drugs. Included is **chlorpromazine** (structure in Figure 19.1), the drug which had such a major impact on psychiatric practice following its introduction in 1952. For the first time it was possible to reduce the positive symptoms of schizophrenia, with a dose-related sedative effect, without concurrent clouding of consciousness. A variety of phenothiazines have been developed, and these may usefully be classified into three types according to their risk of sedative, anticholinergic, and extrapyramidal effects (Table 18.1).

The **butyrophenones** are a different chemical class of antipsychotics which includes **haloperidol** and benperidol. Haloperidol is a widely prescribed drug with low propensity for sedative and antimuscarinic effects, but importantly the use of these compounds is restricted by their high risk of extrapyramidal effects.

Chlorpromazine and haloperidol are the archetypal typical antipsychotics. Other typical antipsychotics which that are neither phenothiazines nor butyrophenones include **pimozide**, **flupentixol**, and **zucopenthixol**. These drugs tend to have a clinical pharmacology like Group 3 phenothiazines, namely low sedative and anticholinergic propensity and high risk of extrapyramidal effects. It is this critical tendency to produce movement disorders in drugs which otherwise have a very desirable clinical pharmacology that lead towards the drugs classed as

Table 18.1 Classifying the phenothiazine antipsychotics.

	Sedative	Antimuscarinic	Extrapyramidal	Examples
Group 1	High	Moderate	Moderate	Chlorpromazine, levopromazine, promazine
Group 2	Moderate	High	Low	Pericyazine, pipotiazine.
Group 3	Moderate	Moderate/low	High	Fluphenazine, prochlorperazine, perphenazine, trifluoperazine

Table 18.2 Some typical antipsychotics and neurotransmitter receptors

Drug	Antagonist at receptors (affinity)				
	D_1	D_2	mACh	5-HT_2	Histamine H_1
Chlorpromazine	++	+++	++	++	++
Haloperidol	+	+++	--	+	--
Flupentixol	++	+++	--	+++	++
Sulpiride	--	+++	--	--	--

The number of + signs indicates the relative affinity of the drug for the receptor.

atypical antipyschotics. However, before we discuss these drugs it is of interest that **sulpiride** is a drug that may be classified as a typical antipsychotic which that has low risk of sedative, antimuscarinic, and extrapyramidal effects.

The receptor pharmacology of four typical antipsychotics is outlined in Table 18.2.

18.2.6 Atypical antipsychotics

The newer antipsychotic drugs are a very mixed group, in terms of their pharmacology and their clinical effects.

Pharmacology of atypical antipsychotics

The newer antipsychotic drugs have in common with the older drugs that they are antagonists at dopamine receptors, but differ in the selectivity they show for subtypes of dopamine receptors. They may also differ from typical antipsychotics in the potency with which they bind to dopamine receptors. Both these characteristics can be used to explain why atypical antipsychotics may have less effects on dopamine in the striatum while effectively inhibiting dopamine in the cortico-limbic areas.

- The drugs are competitive antagonists at dopamine receptors. A lower potency drug may be ineffective at the dopamine receptors in the striatum, where the synaptic dopamine concentration is very high, and effective when in competition with the much lower dopamine levels at the receptors within the cortico-limbic areas.
- The differential distribution of D_3 and D_4 receptors, with a preferential prevalence in cortico-limbic areas (Box 18.1), may mean that a drug selective for these receptor subtypes may exhibit some selectivity for these areas of the brain.

- Both typical and atypical antipsychotic drugs are 'dirty' drugs in that they act as antagonists at receptors for a variety of neurotransmitters. It is likely that the combination of antagonist affects of some atypical drugs helps with some patients. In particular, antagonism at the serotonin 5-HT_2 receptor may improve the clinical outcome with some atypical drugs.

Major atypical antipsychotic drugs include **amisulpiride** (a longer acting derivative of suplride), **aripiprazole**, **olanzapine**, **quetiapine**, **risperidone**, and **clozapine**. Risperidone, clozapine, and olanzapine are notable for their high ratio of block of 5-HT_{2A} receptors to dopamine receptors. Generally these drugs have the characteristics indicated above for atypical antipsychotics of increased effectiveness (compared to typical antipsychotics) against negative symptoms with a reduced propensity for extrapyramidal movement side effects. Clozapine is an important drug in that it is a very effective antipsychotic agent, targeting D_4 receptors with a degree of selectivity. However, it must be used with caution since it has a propensity to cause the dangerous condition of agranulocytosis (lowered white blood cells, namely neutrophils) necessitating regular (e.g. weekly) monitoring of blood counts. For this reason clozapine use is restricted to certain categories of patients who have failed to respond to two other antipsychotics.

There are other situations when atypical drugs may carry certain additional risks in some patients, e.g. the recognized increased risk of stroke in elderly patients with dementia which that indicates that olanzapine and risperidone should not be used in the management of dementia in elderly patients (see also discussion of Alzheimer's dementia in Chapter 17).

The receptor pharmacology of some atypical antipsychotics is outlined in Table 18.3.

Aripiprazole is an interesting drug in that its partial agonist (see Chapter 2) action at D_2-receptors combined with its high affinity for these receptors means that in the striatum it will reduce the effect of endogenous dopamine but provides a weak stimulation of its own. So there will still be a degree of D_2 stimulation in the striatum, perhaps explaining the low tendency to give movement effects. The therapeutic benefit is likely to come from reduced D_2 influence elsewhere in the brain combined with reduced 5-HT receptor influence.

Table 18.3 Atypical antipsychotics and neurotransmitter receptors

Drug	Antagonist at receptors (affinity)					
	D_1	D_2	D_4	mACh	5-HT$_2$	Histamine H$_1$
Risperidone	--	++	+++	++	+++	++
Olanzepine	+	+++	+	+	+++	+
Clozapine[a]	++	++	+++	++	+++	++
Aripiprazole[b]	--	+++	+	--	++	+

The number of + signs indicates the relative affinity of the drug for the receptor.
[a] Clozapine may have some agonist activity at 5-HT$_{1A}$ receptors, D_1 dopamine receptors, and M$_4$ muscarinic acetycholine receptors in some brain areas.
[b] Aripiprazole is a partial agonist at dopamine D_2 and 5-HT$_{1A}$ receptors and an antagonist at 5-HT$_{2A}$ receptors.

18.2.7 Strategy in the drug treatment of schizophrenia

It should be noted that there is considerable dispute as to the relative merits of atypical vs typical antipsychotics. Combined with the great variation in individual patient response, both with respect to clinical benefit and unwanted effects, this means that a single strategy for drug treatment of schizophrenia is unlikely to be found which is consistent over time and across different countries. In Workbook 15 Shaun is started on a typical neuroleptic (haloperidol) and only commences an atypical drug when this is not effective. The first atypical drug used was olanzapine, but he eventually settled with the use of clozapine as the most effective for him. His story illustrates some persistent themes:

- it is likely that a patient may have to try several drugs, sequentially, before the best solution for that individual is found

- only one antipsychotic drug is taken at any one time

- anxiolytics in the form of benzodiazepines may be used in combination with antipsychotic drugs to quieten agitated patients, reducing the need for sedative doses of antipsychotic drugs in acute phases of treatment

- clozapine, an effective drug with significant side effects, is according to some guidelines restricted to patients who have tried two other antipsychotic drugs, one of which should be an atypical drug, without satisfactory outcome.

It should also be noted, however, that the treatment of Shaun in Workbook 15 does not follow a further recommendation found in some guidelines that a newly diagnosed patient should be prescribed atypical antipsychotic drugs as a first-line treatment. This illustrates that treatment must be individually tailored, and will vary considerably from one patient (and one psychiatric practice) to the next.

Here we are concerned with drug treatment, but as in many other clinical fields it must be remembered that non-drug aspects of therapy are of crucial significance—this is mentioned for our imaginary patient Shaun when the initial plan is for medication combined with de-escalation (see Workbook 15).

18.2.8 The future for antipsychotic drug therapy

It is likely that dopamine D_2-family receptor antagonists, in one form or the other, will remain the cornerstone of antipsychotic drug therapy. Here we mention two areas for development which that are likely to impact on the drugs used:

- The further development of drugs with targeting at specific combinations of dopamine receptor subtypes combined with action at other (mainly biogenic amine) neurotransmitter receptors. It is becoming increasing clear that specific agonist activities, as well as the D_2-family antagonism, may play a role in the therapeutic response.

- The development of drugs enhancing activity at the glycine site of the NMDA receptor to up-regulate this aspect of glutamate neurotransmission (Box 18.2). Evidence suggests that such drugs may assume a place as *adjuncts* to dopamine antagonists, rather than replace them.

More dopamine antagonists (and agonists)?

These developments all have dopamine receptor antagonism central to the putative antipsychotic effect, in some cases with effects at other neurotransmitter receptors.

- **D_3 dopamine receptor antagonists.** We have already mentioned above (section 18.2.1) that antagonists at the D_3 dopamine receptor are of interest for generating a drug effective against negative symptoms and relatively free of movement disorders.

- **D_2 antagonist/D_1 agonist.** The Chinese herb *Stephania* has given rise to the drug stepholidine, which is a combined D_1 agonist and D_2 antagonist shown to be active in the prefrontal cortex, nucleus accumbens, and ventral tegmental area. This becomes a very interesting possible drug given the theory of D_2 hyperactivity and D_1 underactivity described in Box 18.2, and the significance of these areas for schizophrenia.

- **Asenapine** is a novel compound with D_2 antagonism, but more potent antagonism for D_3 and a variety of 5-HT receptors. There are positive signs for its potential as a future antipsychotic drug.

One of the themes that candidate antipsychotic drugs such as stepholidine and asenapine illustrate is that a clean drug, acting at only one receptor, is probably not the best approach. What is wanted is a drug targeting multiple specified receptors, and lacking effect at others which produce unwanted effects. It is likely that different patients will respond to different combinations of receptor activity.

More glutamate and less dopamine?

A central theme of antipsychotic drugs is their antagonism at the dopamine receptors in the brain.

However, recently a new approach apparently independent of dopamine antagonism has evolved which just possibly may result in entirely novel drugs. A close relative of the anaesthetic ketamine, phencyclidine (PCP) is a drug of abuse which that produces a very faithful psychosis-like episode in certain individuals. Both positive and negative symptoms are mimicked. Phencyclidine is an antagonist at receptors for the excitatory neurotransmitter glutamate called NMDA receptors, which we have encountered before in Chapter 16 (Figure b, Box 16.1). This has lead to the hypothesis that a *reduction* of glutamate activity in the brain may contribute to the generation of symptoms of schizophrenia (Box 18.2), and that drugs that *increase* activity at NMDA receptors may help resolve symptoms. However, glutamate or similar agonists acting at all glutamate receptors are cytotoxic, and so cannot be used.

In Box 18.2 it is explained that glycine acts as a co-agonist at the NMDA receptor. This means that glycine *and* glutamate binding to their respective site is necessary for receptor activation (see Figure 1b, Box 18.2). This has lead to some interesting drug development strategies to achieve this, in particular the use of glycine agonists and the development of inhibitors of glycine uptake as potential antipsychotic drugs. These ideas are developed a little further in Box 18.2; the approach shows how the attention of pharmacologists may offer fundamentally novel help for those suffering from this devastating disorder. On a cautious note, however, it is likely that if NMDA-enhancing antipsychotic drugs do become available, they will act as adjunct therapy to the D_2-antagonist medications, perhaps targeting negative symptoms, rather that being used as stand-alone therapy.

SUMMARY OF COMMON DRUGS USED FOR SCHIZOPHRENIA

Therapeutic Group	Class/Drugs	Mechanism of action	Common clinical uses	Comments	Examples of adverse drug reactions
Phenothiazines	Group 1 Chlorpromazine, Levopromazine Promazine	Antagonist at D_1 and D_2 receptor	Psychosis Schizophrenia Anxiety Hiccups Nausea	High sedative, moderate antimuscarinic and extrapyramidal side effects	**See comments** **Extrapyramidal side effects** Dystonia Akathisia Parkinsonism Tardive dyskinesia Neuroleptic malignant syndrome **Antimuscarinic side effects** Dry mouth Urinary retention Sedative effects
	Group 2 Pericyazine pipotiazine			Moderate sedative, high antimuscarinic and low extrapyramidal side effects	
	Group 3 Fluphenazine, prochlorperazine perphenazine, trifluoperazine			Moderate sedative, moderate/low antimuscarinic and high extrapyramidal side effects	
Butyrophenones	Benperidol haloperidol	Antagonist at D_2 and D_1 receptor	**Haloperidol** Psychosis Schizophrenia Anxiety Hiccups Tourette's syndrome **Benperidol** Control of deviant anti-social sexual behaviour	Low antimuscarinic and high extrapyramidal effect	
Other typical antipsychotics	**Diphenylbutylpiperidines** Pimozide	1) Antagonist at D_2 receptor 2) Blocks voltage-operated calcium channels 3) Thought to be antagonist at opiate receptors	Schizophrenia Tourette's syndrome	Low sedative and anticholinergic propensity and high risk of extrapyramidal effect	
	Thioxanthenes Flupenthixol Zuclopenthixol	Antagonist at D1 and D2 dopamine receptors	Psychosis Schizophrenia		
	Substituted benzamides Sulpiride amisulpiride	Antagonist at D_2 receptor		Low risk of sedative, antimuscarinic and extrapyramidal effects.	

Therapeutic Group	Class/Drugs	Mechanism of action	Common clinical uses	Comments	Examples of adverse drug reactions
Atypical antipsychotic drugs	Olanzapine, quetiapine, Risperidone Paliperidone (Metabolite of risperidone) Sertindole zotepine	Block both dopamine and $5HT_{2A}$ receptors but with more affinity at $5HT_{2A}$ than dopamine receptors	Schizophrenia Mania Psychoses		Weight gain Dizziness Postural Hypotension Sleep disturbances Agitation Anxiety
	Aripiprazole	Partial agonist activity at D_2 and 5-HT1a receptors and antagonist at 5-HT2a receptors	Schizophrenia Mania	Metabolised by hepatic CYP3A4 and CYP2D6 enzymes leading to interactions	Akathisia Tremor Dizziness Somnolence Sedation Headache Blurred vision
	Clozapine	Weak antagonist at t D_1, D_2, D_3, and D_5 receptors, and high potency at D_4 receptors. Antagonist at alpha-adrenergic, cholinergic, histaminergic, and serotonergic receptors	Schizophrenia	Reserved for third line use Patients need close monitoring of FBC	Agranulocytosis Myocarditis Myopathy GI obstruction

WORKBOOK 15
Failure and success in long-term drug treatment

Shaun develops a serious mental illness as a young man

The patient: a simplified case history

Tom, the warden of the university hall of residence, breathes a sign of relief as he opens the door to let in the police. He had finally decided to call them after Billy, Shaun's flatmate, had rung him to tell him what Shaun had done this time round. Although it was January and the temperature was less than zero outside, Shaun was roaming about in nothing but his ripped boxers and sandals. Earlier, after smashing his computer because ET, his alien friend, had told him to do so, he had jumped out of the window from the second floor because 'they' were after him. Tom and Billy's attempts to get him inside had been futile; Shaun had become more aggressive and pushed them away. Then he had run off shouting that 'they' would kill him if he was found.

After a short search, Shaun was found in the student restaurant telling anyone who would listen that the aliens had finally invaded the earth and that he, Shaun, was going to be king of the new planet. When he saw Billy and his warden he accused them of being foreign spies sent by the high priest.

After a bit of a struggle, Shaun calmed down and agreed to be taken to the psychiatric hospital at the request of a psychiatrist contacted by the police.

Billy agreed to be interviewed about recent changes in Shaun's personality.

A table of clinical clerking abbreviations is given on page xi.

CLINICAL CLERKING FOR SHAUN SLATER AT PSYCHIATRIC ADMISSIONS WARD

Age and gender: 23-year-old male student

PC: Frightened and aggressive young man who jumped from second floor, running around half-naked in January cold, talking about aliens and foreign spies in incoherent sentences

HPC: He had completely changed from being a well-groomed 'life and soul of the party' on campus to becoming an isolated and antisocial unkempt person. After initially missing a few lectures he had finally stopped attending all of them, claiming the lecturers were trying to brainwash him. He spent most days locked in his room 'working' on his computer. His new passions were theology and astrophysics and he spent all day on chat rooms discussing the meaning of life and where the universe was heading. He had thrown his TV away saying that the voice kept giving him instructions. He told all his friends to stay away, claiming that his only mate was ET, an alien, who had moved into the attic whilst waiting for the 'others'. He refused to talk to his flatmate, who had become very worried about him. He had also broken up with his girlfriend, saying she had been told by 'them' to destroy him.

PMH: Nil significant

Mental status examination

Appearance: Unkempt young man with poor hygiene. Agitated and somewhat frightened expression.

Speech: Shaun's speech is of a fast rate and he jumps from topic to topic within a single sentence. He says, for example, during interview, 'ET will get my shoes, you are reading my mind, listen they will destroy you.' Shaun is unable to accurately answer simple questions; instead his responses are long-winded and loosely connected to the question asked. In response to being asked why he jumped out of a window, Shaun replies 'windows are the aperture between the sun and the worlds, connecting all souls to the system.'

Thought process: Shaun firmly believes that others sent by a higher power are out to kill him. Shaun also believes that his thoughts are being stolen directly from his mind and being replaced by evil instructions.

Delusions: Shaun thinks he will be king of the new world and everyone is out to get him.

Hallucinations: He apparently sees and talks to aliens and hears voices from his TV talking directly to him and asking him to do certain things.

Insight and judgment: Shaun is refusing to admit that he is unwell, which shows lack of insight. Running around unkempt and half-naked in the winter shows poor judgment.

Negative symptoms: He is unable to concentrate in class and his speech is now brief and lacks spontaneity.

Social/occupational dysfunction: Shaun does not socialize anymore and he quit his part-time job and broke off with his girlfriend for no good reason.

Duration: This has been going on for over 7 months, possibly longer.

Exclusion of schizoaffective and mood disorder: From his history, the patient interview and his flatmate's interview, depression and mania can be excluded by the psychiatrist.

Substance abuse/general medical condition exclusion: Urine screen: Negative for cannabis

Relation to a pervasive development disorder: Excluded: Shaun has no history of any developmental disorder

> *Mental status examination based on two systems of classification is used most commonly to diagnose suspected schizophrenia. These systems are:*
>
> * *The Diagnostic and Statistical Manual of the American Psychiatric Association, text revision (DSM-IV-TR)*
>
> * *The International classification of diseases from the World Health Organization 10 (ICD 10 WHO).*
>
> *By using the criteria adapted from these systems, psychiatrists are less likely to misdiagnose schizophrenia. This is because they are prompted to take the whole clinical course, and not just the presenting symptoms, into account.*

Overview of diagnostic criteria

1) Characteristic symptoms: minimum two present for 1 month

Delusions, hallucinations, disorganized speech, grossly disorganized behaviour, negative symptoms (poverty of speech, absence of emotions, avolition (i.e. inability to initiate and sustain goal-directed activities)).

Shaun has exhibited more than two of these symptoms for over a month.

2) Social/occupational dysfunction

Positive if dysfunction is present over a significant period in at least one of the areas of work, interpersonal relationships, or self-care and is of such severity that it is significantly below the level before onset of symptoms.

Shaun's level for all the above is below what it was before the symptoms started.

3) Duration: continuous signs persist for more than 6 months.

Shaun has had his symptoms for more than 7 months.

4) Schizoaffective and mood disorder exclusion

Rule out major depressive, manic, or mixed manic episodes as cause of symptoms.

The psychiatrist ruled these out for Shaun.

5) Substance/general medical condition exclusion

Rule out drug/medication abuse.

Rule out medical condition.

Shaun's urine test was negative for cannabis, so this can be ruled out as a possible cause.

A positive test would have complicated the diagnosis for the following reasons:

a) Cannabis use could cause psychotic episodes that could have the following characteristics:

• euphoria

• fragmented thoughts

• paranoid ideation

• hallucination and hyperacusia (abnormal acute hearing).

b) Cannabis improves the negative symptoms of schizophrenia and is sometimes used illegally as self-medication by schizophrenics. therefore for a patient testing positive it is plausible that they started using it after the onset of symptoms because it made them feel better.

c) Studies have failed to show distinguishing symptoms between the two.

6) Relation to a pervasive development disorder: Does the patient has a history of a disorder such as autism?

The psychiatrist ruled these out for Shaun.

Full blood count: Nil significant

A full blood count involves a blood sample being taken from the patient. The sample is sent to the laboratory and the concentration of key components are measured and compared to standard levels expected. These include:

- *haemoglobin*

- *mean cell volume (MCV)*

- *red blood cells (RBC)*

- *white blood cells (WBC) (neutrophils,monocytes,lymphocyte)*

- *coagulation (prothombin time)*

Abnormalities could mean that Shaun's symptoms could be due to a physical illness. It is important to exclude this possibility.

Shaun's test showed nothing of significance, so it can be concluded that he is physically healthy.

Thyroid function test: Nil significant

Liver function test: Nil significant

Neurologic examination: Unremarkable

Psychosocial history: After investigation the team found out that Shaun had been brought up by his gran. His mum had left him when Shaun was a baby and Shaun's dad had recurrent psychotic episodes and therefore was unable to look after Shaun.

Differential diagnosis: Schizophrenia

Shaun has most of the classic symptoms of schizophrenia:

- *auditory hallucinations (hearing voices from the television)*

- *delusions (he is going to be king and his flatmate is a foreign spy)*

- *gradual loss of social skills (no girlfriend or friends anymore)*

- *suspiciousness*

- *loosening of associations (confused thought and incoherent speech)*

- *poor hygiene*

- *impaired insight and judgment.*

These symptoms will be utilized to assess and monitor his response to treatment.

Problems with diagnosing schizophrenia

Although the criteria above are used in diagnosis, it is still very controversial whether a patient diagnosed with schizophrenia actually has only one single underlying disorder. This controversy and uncertainty about diagnosing schizophrenia leads to the following problems for patients, their families, and their carers.

1) *Some doctors in both primary and secondary care are reluctant to make the diagnosis and could as a consequence delay treatment.*

2) *Some patients and their families are reluctant to accept the diagnosis or the fact that it is compulsory for it to be treated.*

3) *Schizophrenia is associated with a high degree of stigma, which is perceived by certain people to be a high price to pay considering the diagnostic uncertainties.*

Shaun is refusing to accept treatment and to stay in hospital. The team decide to admit him under section 2 of the Mental Health Act 1983.

Mental Health Act 1983

Section 2 is an order for involuntary admission for assessment for a maximum of 28 days. It is used when an individual is thought to suffer from mental disorder and is thought to present a risk to themselves or others and refuses to come or stay in hospital voluntarily, when admission is thought to be the best option. Two medical recommendations are required and one must be from an accredited psychiatrist. Both medical recommendations then have to be agreed to by an approved social worker, who then makes an application for the section.

These details of compulsory admission apply to the UK only, but many other countries have a similar system.

Plan:

1) De-escalation and medication

De-escalation is related to structured reassurance and support in a tranquil environment. It is used to treat sufferers in acute crisis before and in conjunction with drug treatments. In extreme situations where a patient is so distressed as to pose an immediate risk of harm to himself or others, physical restraint techniques and controlled seclusion environments can be used in conjunction with rapid tranquillization under strict guidelines and monitoring by trained staff.

2) Medication for rapid tranquillization:

- *haloperidol to be administered immediately*

- *lorazepam four times a day as required*

Shaun refused oral treatment—intramuscural administration is used in a non-cooperative patient refusing to swallow tablets.

3) Others

- *ECG (electrocardiogram – see Chapter 7)*

- *Blood pressure (see Chapter 5)*

- *Admit until stable*

- *Repeat urine test weekly*

For review at a multidisciplinary team meeting the following morning.

The multidisciplinary team consists of doctors, nurses, pharmacists, and social workers or any other healthcare worker involved in the care of that particular patient. They meet and discuss how best to treat the patient and take into consideration each other's perspectives and opinions.

Haloperidol is a high potency drug available for intramuscular use that has a rapid calming and sedative effect (contrasting with the slow onset of the selective antipsychotic effect). The policy/ good practice is to give one single dose only, although more could be prescribed for continued agitation in the acute phase only if attempts to calm patients with psychotherapy or a benzodiazepine (e.g. lorazepam, see Chapter 19 for discussion of benzodiazepines) are unsuccessful. Haloperidol is less sedative than some other typical antipsychotics—benzodiazepines may be used in agitated patients if sedation is required. Benzodiazepines are safer than antipsychotics for long-term sedation.

Shaun has a complex illness requiring personalized long-term treatment. Try to understand the condition and the trail of success and failure in his treatment over the years.

1a) What is psychosis?

1b) What is schizophrenia?

2) List four positive symptoms of schizophrenia.

3) List three negative symptoms (using their clinical name) of schizophrenia experienced by Shaun.

4) What are the two factors thought to play a role in the development of schizophrenia?

Hint: Shaun's dad had psychotic episodes.

5a) Dopamine in the brain is thought to play a central role in the pathogenesis of schizophrenia and the action of antipsychotic drugs.

Using the figure below, which is a cartoon of the human brain, draw in the two major dopaminergic pathways. Indicate where the cell bodies and the major projection areas are, using in your labelling

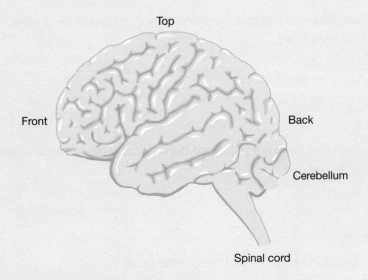

Top

Front

Back

Cerebellum

Spinal cord

the terms substantia nigra, striatum, ventral tegmental nuclei, limbic and mesocorticl areas, olfactory tubercle, nucleus accumbens prefrontal cortex, and cingulated cortex.

5b) Of these two major projections indicate in a single sentence the main functions they control and a common medical condition associated with each.

6) What came first—the treatment of schizophrenia with dopamine antagonists or the dopamine neurochemical theory for schizphrenia? Explain.

7a) State in a single sentence the dopamine hypothesis for schizophrenia.

7b) State in a single sentence the dopamine receptor theory for the therapeutic action of antipsychotic drugs.

8a) Indicate the five dopamine receptor types and the way these can be grouped into two main families of dopamine receptors.

....

....

....

8b) Which dopamine receptor(s) are implicated in the action of most older antipsychotics?

....

....

....

9a) What are the two main categories of antipsychotic drugs?

....

....

....

9b) Explain how the distinction is made between the two categories.

....

....

....

....

The ward manager comes in early and gets handover from the junior nurse who looked after Shaun at night. The junior nurse says the lorazepam and haloperidol seem to be working because Shaun is quiet, but that during the night the junior doctor had administered a further dose of intramuscular haloperidol. They go to rouse Shaun and get him ready for the ward round and find him lying in a weird posture with his eyes fixed to the ceiling. The student nurse screams but sister calmly asks her to get the senior doctor, who administers a muscarinic acetylcholine receptor antagonist called procyclidine. Shaun's posture rapidly returns to normal. The doctor explains to Shaun that he has just suffered a type of acute dystonic reaction (abnormal face and body movements) called an oculogiric crisis (eyes rolling back into head), which is a side effect of haloperidol.

Procyclidine is a drug that can be used to treat parkinsonian symptoms. It is an anticholinergic drug that counters the effect of haloperidol on the control of movement (see Chapter 17 and Figure 17.1 for a discussion of anticholinergic drugs in the control of movement disorders).

10a) What is meant by the term 'extrapyramidal side effects'?

....

....

....

10b) Name three main categories of extrapyramidal side effects.

11a) Referring back to question 5 and the two main dopaminergic projection regions, where is haloperidol acting to produce its beneficial therapeutic effect and where is it acting to produce its unwanted movement effects?

11b) Try to concisely explain why extrapyramidal side effects come about when dopamine antagonists are added.

> Amongst all extrapyramidal symptoms, acute dystonia has the earliest onset, with most cases occurring after the first few hours or days after treatment commencement or dose increase. It is characterized by:
>
> • prolonged muscle contraction
>
> • abnormal postures, including tongue protrusion
>
> • oculogyric crisis
>
> • torsion of the neck.
>
> Young age, male gender, and a high dosage of high-potency typical antipsychotics and a past history are risk factors. Shaun had three of these risk factors.

12) What is the mechanism by which procyclidine works to treat acute dystonias and other extrapyramidal side effects?

> During the multidisciplinary ward round the team discuss the patient in his absence, after which he is brought in. During their discussion, they agree that an error was made by the junior doctor in prescribing and administering further haloperidol and the pharmacist pointed out that intramuscular doses of haloperidol should be lower than oral doses because of the absence of first-pass metabolism in the liver. The team agree to stop haloperidol and try olanzapine for Shaun. Lorazepam should be used as required if he gets agitated again. Olanzapine is an atypical antipsychotic.

They apologise to Shaun when he is brought in and propose the new drug to him. They tell him his new drug is newer, more expensive, and better, and will not cause the reaction he experienced. Shaun agrees to try it.

13) What is thought to be the mechanism of action of olanzapine which makes it different from typical antipsychotic drugs?

_____

_____

_____

14a) What are the common side effects of the atypicals that are different from the typical antipsychotics?

_____

_____

_____

14b) Explain the theory behind the cause of these side effects.

_____

_____

_____

After 3 weeks, Shaun has improved slightly, although he still has some symptoms. His positive symptoms have improved more than the negative ones. Despite this, he is thought to be safe to go back to university under the care of a community psychiatric nurse.

Six months later Shaun is back in hospital for the second time since he was discharged. Both admissions were because he had an aggressive psychotic episodes. His olanzapine dose was doubled after the last admission. On day two of this admission, the nurse finds Shaun's medication under his mattress.

During the ward round Shaun admits that he has not been taking his medication. The reason he says is because he has been putting on weight, and he blames the drug for this. They explain to him that this is possible—weight gain is a recognized side effect of olanzapine. Shaun has decided that because he gets side effects each time he will not take any more medication.

15) How would you counter Shaun's argument that he does not want further antipsychotic drug therapy because he does not want to put up with side effects?

_____

_____

_____

Shaun's concerns about side effects have led him to do some research. He asks about tardive dyskinesia, which he has read about. He wants to know if he is likely to get that.

16a) What is tardive dyskinesia?

16b) Consider the different drugs mentioned for Shaun and explain whether you think Shaun is right to be concerned about the possibility of developing tardive dyskinesias.

16c) Would it to be right to advise Shaun that there is no need for concern when using atypical antipsychotic drugs?

16d) Would it to be right to advise Shaun that there is no need for concern because if tardive dyskinesia occurs he would simply be taken off the drug and the problem would go away?

After 2 months Shaun seems to be having more symptoms, although they seem to be more of the negative symptoms. The team decide to put him on clozapine.

17a) In what way is the clinical outcome likely/possibly better with clozapine?

17b) Explain this by reference to the mechanism of action of clozapine.

17c) Why might clozapine not be recommended as a first-line drug?

_____

_____

Shaun is put on the clozapine register and has to have blood tests very often.

18) What is the reason for a clozapine register? What does it mean?

_____

_____

_____

Shaun seems stable on the clozapine and is almost symptom free 1 year later. He is now back with his girlfriend and will graduate at the end of the year. He wants to know from his community psychiatric nurse when he can stop the drug. He is given an appointment to see the psychiatrist. The doctor advises him to slowly taper and then stop the drug if no symptoms re-emerge.

Two years later Shaun is back on the clozapine because his symptoms resurfaced when he tried to quit. However, he now has a job and also got married. Together with his wife they decide not to have children but would like to adopt.

19a) What percentage of patients get to lead a normal life after being diagnosed with schizophrenia? What do you think might be the factors influencing whether this occurs?

_____

_____

_____

19b) Shaun asks his family doctor whether he should avoid having children, given that there is an inherited component to the risk of getting the disease. If you were that doctor what questions might you ask and what advice might you give?

_____

_____

_____

Chapter 19
Depression and anxiety

The odd thing about depression and anxiety as medical conditions requiring treatment is that we all experience the features of these conditions as part of the ups and downs of our lives. Most of us feel unhappy, fed up, or sad from time to time. It is 'normal' to feel such things. On the other extreme, if I have a complete lack of interest in life, am overwhelmed by feelings of meaningless or hopelessness or just nothing, feel so down that I fail to function (work, family, etc.) and perhaps have suicidal thoughts—if I have any combination of these for any length of time then it may be obvious to all that I 'need help', that I should go and see my doctor, that I am ill. Similarly with anxiety—most of us worry and fret about normal things in life, but if we are disabled or made very unhappy by worry, rational or otherwise, then therapy may be justified. So for severe forms of depression and anxiety it is perhaps beyond dispute that medical intervention is required. But what about milder conditions—do you think it is the doctor's job to try to treat common unhappiness?

In both depression and anxiety the general practice doctor and the mental health specialist have to distinguish who is in need of treatment and who is not, and, crucially, who needs urgent treatment. In depression and anxiety treatment means psychological therapies or drugs. It is clear that psychological therapies are often desirable, being as or more effective than drugs, and of course they come without the attendant unwanted effects. However, drugs are immediately available while rapid intervention with psychological therapy may not be on offer. In the minority of patients the need for rapid intervention may make immediate drug therapy important. The strength of this argument is complicated by the recognition that, as explained below, some drugs in this area take up to 2 to 3 weeks to benefit patients. For many patients a combination of psychological therapy and drugs may be the best route forward.

What if, when drugs are offered, the patient says they believe this is a psychological illness, not physical, and so do not want to take drugs. If we are considering milder depression and anxiety this may be a good question, and patient involvement in therapy may need explicit recognition of this. However, a patient with 'a psychological problem' may well benefit from drug therapy, and indeed this may be the case for the majority of prescriptions written for these conditions.

What follows in this chapter is an account of antidepressant and anti-anxiety drugs, with an example of their application in a clinical situation developed within the workbook.

Depression and anxiety often come together, and some categories of drugs are recognized to be effective against both. The patient story we have developed for the workbook first presents with anxiety, with depression developing later. Here we shall consider depression first, then consider issues relating to anxiety.

19.1 Depression

Depression is the most common mental health problem seen in general practice. We might ask whether we can make a distinction between depression as an illness and depressive symptoms in an individual that is not ill. This is explored in Table 19.1.

Table 19.1 Symptoms and illness in depression

Depressive symptoms	Depression (illness)
13–20% of population experience depressive symptoms: feelings of sadness and upset normal reactions to distressing situations or events usually pass with time	3% of population suffer clinical depression more than just feeling sad or upset intense feeling of sadness/hopelessness/guilt motor retardation symptoms vary in severity, duration, and frequency can have acute onset or take years to develop could be either chronic or short lasting

19.1.1 Diagnosing depression

Of course there is great uncertainty in this area, with mild depression in particular being poorly defined. The World Health Organization's International Criteria for Disease (ICD-10) has what is essentially a symptom-counting approach to try to recognize where depression is a clinical condition and to categorize different levels of depression (Box 19.1).

These issues are important to us, since they lead to decisions about treatment and prescribing. There are a number of depression-rating scales and patient questionnaire approaches available to diagnose and assess the severity of depression, some explicitly linking to guidelines about treatment. The popularity of these varies between different countries.

In general practice a screening strategy may have priority. It may be that depression is under-diagnosed. Patients may be resistant to using the depression word, and doctors may prefer to accept depression as 'normal' in old age rather than subject elderly patients to powerful drugs. Screening here helps the initial identification of patients who may be depressed. Screening depression questionnaires may be time and cost effective, with the simplest form being a two-question test: 'During the last few weeks have you been bothered by feeling down, depressed, or hopeless?' or 'During the last few weeks have you felt little interest or pleasure in doing things?'

19.1.2 A biological theory for depression?

Depression is probably best considered as a psychological illness that may have a biological basis to it in some or all patients. Severe major depression may be considered a purely 'organic' illness, meaning that it may be solely a physical condition of the brain, perhaps originating from a neurotransmitter imbalance. You may encounter strongly held differences of opinion on these matters. What is clear is that changing the biological function of the brain with drugs can profoundly alleviate symptoms in many patients. While this doesn't necessarily mean there was a biological 'fault' in the first place, it does encourage the question of whether or not we can identify a biological difference that contributes to some degree or other to depressive illness. There are many ideas about the biological basis of depression, but perhaps the most important for those interested in drug action relates to the biogenic amines, or monoamines, of the brain.

The monoamine hypothesis (also called **the biogenic amine hypothesis**) for depression in its simplest form is that a low level of monoamine function in the brain leads to depressive symptoms. The main monoamines (or biogenic amines) are serotonin (5-hydroxytryptamine, 5-HT), noradrenaline, and dopamine (see Box 19.2). That antidepressant drugs interfere with the lifecycle of these neurotransmitters in the brain is beyond doubt. This may take the form of an increase in the levels of noradrenaline/serotonin in the synapse. Whether or not this tells us that the problem in the first place was an imbalance in monoamine function is in doubt. It may be wise to conclude that we have a credible monoamine theory for drug action, but perhaps not for depression itself. Regardless of this, the monoamine/biogenic amine hypothesis is important for antidepressant drug prescribing, and so is further explored in Box 19.3.

Box 19.1

Diagnosis and rating of depression

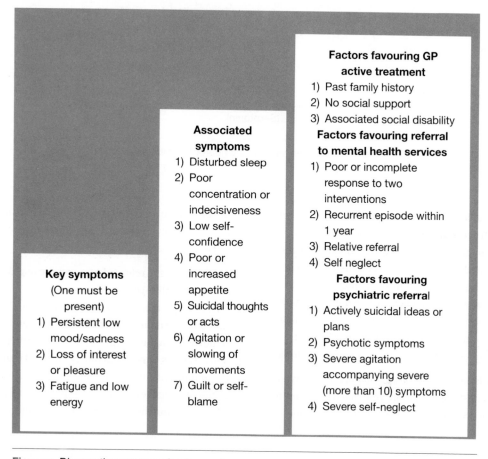

Factors favouring GP active treatment
1) Past family history
2) No social support
3) Associated social disability

Factors favouring referral to mental health services
1) Poor or incomplete response to two interventions
2) Recurrent episode within 1 year
3) Relative referral
4) Self neglect

Factors favouring psychiatric referral
1) Actively suicidal ideas or plans
2) Psychotic symptoms
3) Severe agitation accompanying severe (more than 10) symptoms
4) Severe self-neglect

Associated symptoms
1) Disturbed sleep
2) Poor concentration or indecisiveness
3) Low self-confidence
4) Poor or increased appetite
5) Suicidal thoughts or acts
6) Agitation or slowing of movements
7) Guilt or self-blame

Key symptoms
(One must be present)
1) Persistent low mood/sadness
2) Loss of interest or pleasure
3) Fatigue and low energy

Figure a Diagnostic symptoms for depression.

Diagnosing depression The International Criteria for Disease (ICD-10) of the World Health Organization (WHO) and the Diagnostic and Statistical Manual of Mental Disorders (DSM-IV) are used to guide the diagnosis and classification of mental health disorders in Europe and America, respectively.

The diagnostic symptoms are divided into key and associated symptoms (Figure a). There are also other factors to be considered.

ICD-10 definitions of depression

Not depressed: fewer than four symptoms

Mild depression: four symptoms

Moderate depression: five or six symptoms

Severe depression: more than seven symptoms, with or without psychotic features

Symptoms should be present for more than 1 month and present most of every day.

Box 19.2

Monoamine oxidase and its inhibition

Figure b The three main brain monoamine neurotransmitters.

Most antidepressant drugs are thought to act at synapses of brain neurons, which release the monoamines (also called biogenic amines). The term monoamine means a compound that has a singe amine group (this is an $-NH_2$). The most important brain monoamines for antidepressant drug action are 5-hydroxytryptamine (5-HT, also known as serotonin) and noradrenaline (also known as norepinephrine). Dopamine is also a monoamine, and it is affected by some antidepressants.

These three monoamines, and others such as tyramine, are all substrates for the enzyme called monoamine oxidase (MAO) found in many cell types and located on the outer mitochondrial membrane, able to metabolize substrates located in the cytoplasm. Under most circumstances this secures a very low cytoplasmic concentration of noradrenaline, 5-HT, and dopamine.

Release of biogenic amines is mainly vesicular, but may also be from the cytosol 'Release' of a neurotransmitter refers to how it gets out of the nerve terminal into the extracellular part of the synapse, where it may stimulate receptors. It is the released neurotransmitter that is active at any one moment of time. The monoamines at the nerve terminal are stored at a very high concentration in membrane-bound vesicles. When the nerve terminal is activated by depolarization and Ca^{2+} entry, the vesicle fuses with presynaptic membrane, releasing its monoamines into the synaptic cleft. This is the normal manner of neurotransmission across a synapse. However, in addition monoamines are found in the cytoplasm of the terminal—here they

are broken down by MAO. Under certain conditions some of this cytoplasmic neurotransmitter can leak out of the synapse and into the cleft.

In both cases the released monoamine (e.g. 5-HT or noradrenaline) can stimulate receptors on the post-synaptic membrane. It is important for brain function that neurotransmitters are efficiently removed from the synaptic cleft. For noradrenaline and 5-HT this is mainly achieved by rapid reuptake: the neurotransmitters are transported back into the terminal by active uptake using specific transporter proteins within the nerve terminal membrane.

Most antidepressant drugs act by increasing the amount of noradrenaline or 5-HT within the synaptic cleft. They do so either by inhibiting MAO or by inhibiting uptake.

There are two forms of MAO Monoamine oxidase is found in two forms in the human brain: MAO-A and MAO-B. MAO-A is involved in metabolizing 5-HT, while both forms of enzyme are effective against dopamine, noradrenaline, and adrenaline, as indicated in Table B19.1.

Where are these two monoamine oxidase types found in the brain? It might seem a simple question to ask which of the two enzymes is found in which regions of the human brain. Since selective inhibitors are clinically available this is an important question. However, the picture is not clear. For example, it is reported that MAO-B is the main form found in human basal ganglia (including striatum)

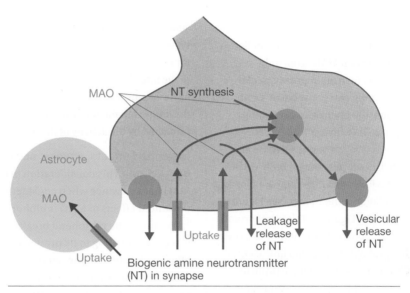

Figure c Both monoamine oxidase and active uptake reduce monoamine neurotransmitter availably in the synapse.

The classic vesicular release is shown. This occurs in response to action potential reaching the nerve terminal. In addition 'leakage' across the membrane is shown. MAO is involved in the removal of neurotransmitters such as 5-HT, noradrenaline, and dopamine from the cytosol and (by enzymes in the astrocytes) from the extracellular space. Biogenic amine neurotransmitters in the synaptic cleft itself are mainly removed by specific active uptake. MAO reduces the availability of neurotransmitter for vesicular release, and prevents accumulation of biogenic amine neurotransmitter in the cytosol of the nerve terminal, preventing 'leakage' release. Inhibition of MAO will increase the amount of neurotransmitter available for vesicular release and permit the build-up of amine in the terminal, allowing for 'leakage' release. Further illustration of the role of MAO, and the role of catechol O-methy transferase, is shown in Box 17.2 Figure a. NT, neurotransmitter; MAO, monoamine oxidase.

Table B19.1 Substrate specificity and clinically available selective inhibitors of MAO-A and MAO-B

	Preferred substrates	Selective inhibitors	Main clinical target
MAO-A	5-HT, noradrenaline, dopamine	Moclobemide	Depression
MAO-B	Noradrenaline, dopamine	Selegiline Radsagiline	Parkinson's disease

Note that most MAO inhibitors are non-selective; these are available to treat depression.

and it might seem that this provides a logical basis for the use of the selective MAO-B inhibitor selegiline in the treatment of Parkinson's disease (Chapter 17). However, there are also reports that the MAO located specifically within the *nerve terminals* in striatum of human brain is MAO-A, somewhat confusing the issue.

◥

Brain MAO is found in astrocytes as well as neurons It may be that the answer lies in recognizing that the brain MAO is not only neuronal, it is also present in brain microvascular endothelial cells (forming part of the blood–brain barrier and protecting the brain from circulating amines) and in glial cells (which considerably outnumber the neurons in the brain). Of these glial cells it is known that astrocytes contain both MAO-A and MAO-B, and it is likely that these play a major role in removing extracellular monoamines (see Figure c and Chapter 17, Box 17.2 Figure a). This is important for understanding the action of MAO inhibitors, since it tells us that they probably have their clinical effect by both increasing non-vesicular release (from the cytosol) and decreasing the removal of extracellular monoamine. In the case of dopamine in the striatum, it seems possible that the former effect, within the nerve terminal, is mainly by MAO-A, while the latter effect at the astrocytes is by the combined presence of both MAO-A and MAO-B. The use of the selective MAO-B inhibitor selegiline is, according to this model, likely to have its clinical effect (Chapter 17) by reducing the astrocyte-mediated removal of extracellular dopamine, rather than by inhibiting cytosolic breakdown.

Constructing a similar hypothesis for 5-HT and noradrenaline of relevance to the use of antidepressants is perhaps too speculative for this text. However, recognition of the complexities of MAO inhibition in the brain does help us understand some of the different clinical responses to MAO inhibitors and monoamine uptake inhibitors (see Box 19.3 and the main text).

Monoamine oxidase found outside the brain may be important for unwanted effects The functions of MAO are not limited to the brain. Activity is high in intestines, liver, lungs, and placenta. One role is to protect the body from exogenous amines, such as those from the diet. So if you eat high tyramine-containing foods, notably cheese but also, for example, yeast extracts, then breakdown will occur in the intestinal wall and liver (first-pass metabolism), any escaping into the circulation will be destroyed in the lungs, and the unborn child will be doubly protected by the activity in the placenta.

Unwanted effects, cheese, and drug interactions This consideration of extracerebral MAO has relevance when considering the unwanted effects of MAO inhibitors. Not surprisingly the peripheral breakdown of tyramine is reduced, leading to its presence in the blood. The effect of tyramine in the nerve terminal is also enhanced, since it is normally broken down by neuronal MAO. This can result in a hypertensive crisis, as the tyramine displaces noradrenaline from sympathetic nerve terminals, leading to cardiac and vascular stimulation. Both MAO-A and MAO-B are involved in the breakdown of tryramine, so not surprisingly drugs selective for either one (see Table B19.1) are less likely to give this unwanted response than are the non-selective MAO inhibitors.

Similar considerations may help to explain why MAO inhibitors should not be given with antidepressant uptake inhibitors. The combination can have very serious, potentially fatal, consequences. Drugs such as the tricyclic antidepressants, selective serotonin reuptake inhibitors (SSRIs) and serotonin and noradrenaline reuptake inhibitors (SNRIs) (see the main text 19.2.2 and 19.2.3 Box 19.3) act to inhibit uptake of biogenic amines and it may be that the combined effect of reducing clearance by uptake and by breakdown results in the adverse effects that may be seen. To prevent this occurring a considerable drug-free period (minimum of 2 weeks, sometimes up to 5 weeks) should occur when switching between MAO inhibitors and these other drug classes.

Box 19.3

The biogenic amine theory for depression

Antidepressant drug action converges on the biogenic monoamines, in each case raising the availability of serotonin (5-HT) and/or noradrenaline at the receptors in the synapse, and thereby (in the short term) increasing neurotransmission at the synapse. They do this in a variety of ways:

1. they inhibit the uptake mechanism that clears biogenic amines released in the synapse (e.g. tricyclic antidepressants, SSRIs, and SNRIs)

2. they inhibit enzymes that breakdown the biogenic amines (MAO inhibitors)

3. they enhance release of biogenic amines from the nerve terminal (mirtazepine).

It is striking that each class of drugs uses a different strategy to the same end. It seems likely from this that the antidepressant action of the drugs does follow in some way from this common enhancement of biogenic amine availability at the synapse. It is also striking that benefit seems to accrue from both serotonin effects and noradrenaline effects. These observations concerning drug action have provided a main support for the development of bigenic amine-related hypotheses for depression discussed in section 19.1.2 and illustrated in Figure d. Consideration of drug actions gives rise to the simplest (and perhaps most unsupportable, see below) hypothesis: a low level of biogenic amine function in the brain leads to depressive symptoms.

The biogenic amine hypothesis for depression has given rise to various offspring, one being the serotonin hypothesis, which at its simplest states that diminished serotonin influence plays a role in generating the symptoms of depression. This has proved of enormous importance as a scientific rationale for the use of selective serotonin uptake inhibitors as antidepressants.

One elaboration of the serotonin hypothesis says that low serotonin influence in the brain results in a secondary down-regulation of noradrenaline and dopamine influence. This is sometimes developed further by assigning particular symptom clusters to a deficit in these neurotransmitters (for example serotonin—anxiety, obsessions, compulsion; noradrenaline—lack of alertness and interest in life; dopamine—lack of attention and motivation, lacking in response to pleasure and reward).

This gives rise to the 'Russian doll' structure of interconnected hypotheses in Figure d.

While stimulating discussion about the nature of depression and the action of antidepressant drugs, there are many reasons for questioning the biogenic amine hypotheses. Even a concise assessment of the evidence for and against this idea is beyond the scope of this text, and just a couple of points will be made here. Of particular note for us is that support for the hypothesis has come from the finding that, as explained above, antidepressant drugs raise the influence of these neurotransmitters, so the story is told that they

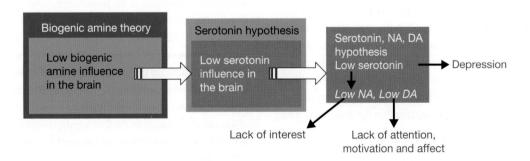

Figure d Schematic of biogenic amine—serotonin hypotheses for depression. NA, noradrenaline; DA, dopamine.

were low in the patient and that this deficit is restored by the drug. The trouble is that they have this effect quickly, while the antidepressant effect is delayed by around 1–3 weeks, during which time adaptive responses in the brain occur, such as reduced receptor function. The clinical benefit therefore correlates not with the initial enhanced biogenic amine influence, but with the adaptive responses which follow. We now know that for serotonin this may not be such a major obstacle for accepting the final 'serotonin hypothesis' version as previously thought, since, as explained in section 19.2.1, the enhancement of serotonin neurotramission may have to wait for the down-regulation of the inhibitory $5HT_{1A}$ receptors and this takes up to 3 weeks.

Other evidence weakening the biogenic amine hypothesis comes from the observation that some antidepressant drugs do not enhance biogenic amine activity—tianeptine actually enhances serotonin reuptake. There are also drugs that lower the serotonin and noradrenaline influence in the brain without creating depression.

It may be wise to conclude that the biogenic amines are involved in the therapeutic response to the drugs, but that it is not clear what this tells us about the nature of depression itself.

19.2 Antidepressant drugs

Drugs are the mainstay of treatment of depression presenting in general practice. Two general issues relating to the use of antidepressant drugs will be mentioned.

19.2.1 Overview of antidepressant drugs

Do antidepressant drugs work?

The efficacy of antidepressant drugs has been questioned. Something like half of patients will fail to respond to their first-line drugs. Some statistical analyses conclude that the drugs are not significantly more effective than placebo. This conclusion has been questioned.

Firstly, you should note that the beneficial effects of antidepressants are not rapid. Patients should not expect to experience any relief from their depression until they have been taking the drugs for 2–3 weeks. This delay, and its consequences for our understanding of how the drugs work, is raised at several points below. This delay has no bearing on the eventual benefits that the drugs may bring.

Amid the uncertainty it is clear that:

1) the benefits of antidepressant drugs are often modest and must be weighed against side effects

2) the benefits are greater in more severely depressed patients. These observations fit with some current guidelines suggesting that antidepressants should not be used as the first treatment in mild depression (NICE guidelines in the United Kingdom), but that treatment works for many or most patients with moderate or severe depression.

Are antidepressant drugs over-prescribed?

The important question here is: are drugs being prescribed to those for whom there is no significant overall benefit? If over-prescribing has occurred this is thought more likely with mild depression. One finding that has encouraged the belief that these drugs are being over-prescribed is that there has been an increase in prescribing of antidepressants around the world, even where studies shave shown no increase in depression in the population. However, rather than indicating over-prescribing now, this could reflect earlier under-prescribing. It may also reflect the improved nature of recent drugs, notably with respect to fewer unwanted effects for the same level of benefit. This enables more sustained prescribing with real benefit to patients. The important conclusion to emerge for us is that drugs may not always be appropriate as the first approach to mild depression, but that they should be used for sustained or severe depression.

Mechanism of action of antidepressants

Most antidepressants are thought to work by increasing the availability of the target biogenic amine neurotransmitter in the synaptic cleft, i.e. they increase neurotransmission at these synapses. The increase in neurotransmitter in the synaptic cleft is achieved by inhibiting its removal by uptake (as mentioned in Chapter 2, section 2.5) or breakdown by enzymes (Box 19.2, Figure c). Most antidepressants work by inhibiting uptake. Their classification partly reflects the specific neurotransmitters being affected, mainly serotonin or noradrenaline. An alternative mechanism, reducing monoamine breakdown, is the basis of action of the monoamine oxidase inhibitor group of antidepressants (Box 19.2).

19.2.2 Selective serotonin reuptake inhibitors

Widely used for both depression and anxiety, selective serotonin reuptake inhibitors (SSRIs) are the most commonly prescribed antidepressants. They are recommended as first-line drug treatments for patients with six or more symptoms on the ICD-10 checklist (Box 19.1) or milder depression that does not resolve with non-drug approaches or with those with a history of severe depression, when delay may be unwise.

Mechanism of action

The molecular target of SSRIs is the serotonin (5-HT) transporter called 5-HTT (or SERT). When serotonin is released from a nerve terminal its concentration rises in the synaptic cleft, then rapidly falls as it is removed by being drawn back into the nerve terminal (Box 19.2, Figure b). In the case of serotonin this presynaptic reuptake is the main mechanism for clearance from the synapse and termination of activity. The protein transporter that achieves this active uptake is located within the presynaptic membrane—this is the 5-HTT. When an SSRI is given it will produce a rapid block of this uptake.

It might be thought that this results in a rapid increase in serotonin availability at the postsynaptic receptors in the nerve terminal field and that this results in a rapid increase in serotoninergic transmission in the brain. However, the situation is a little more complex because the 5-HT cell bodies also release serotonin (from the dendrites) and this is cleared by uptake. This means that when an SSRI is given the serotonin level around the cell bodies increases. This gives an increased stimulation of inhibitory serotonin receptors, the $5HT_{1A}$ receptors, on the cell bodies. These reduce the firing of the neurons and serotonin release in the terminal field is reduced. Over time (10 days to 3 weeks) the $5HT_{1A}$ receptors desensitize, the firing rate of the neurons is restored, and then the full effect of SSRIs on increasing serotonin in the cortex and

limbic areas of the brain is seen. It is notable that this time course may correspond to a delay in therapeutic effect, which as noted above is characteristically around 3 weeks.

Individual variations in response to SSRIs: polymorphism in the 5-HTT gene

There is a single gene for 5-HTT—in any individual the 5-HTT protein will be the same in all tissues, notably in neurons and platelets. However, there is a polymorphic region in the gene, which results in two variants, the short version (S) with a 44 base pair deletion compared to the long version (L). The homozygous genotype (LL) shows more serotonin uptake than the LS or SS genotypes, so presumably these individuals tend to have reduced intrasynaptic serotonin. This means that there are some inherited differences in serotonin handling that may result in different psychological characteristics for the individual and also different responses to SSRIs.

Differences between SSRIs

Popular SSRIs include **citalopram**, **escitalopram**, **fluoxetine**, **paroxetine**, and **sertraline**. There is not much to choose between these SSRIs, with each having similar efficacy and long half-lives (that is around or over 24 hours, with fluoxetine being longer). Fluoxetine has been favoured in children as showing efficacy, but like other SSRIs may have a potential to increase self-harm and suicidal thoughts in young people, indicating caution.

Unwanted effects of SSRIs

The SSRIs are generally well tolerated and present fewer unwanted effects than the tricyclic antidepressants (TCAs) they have largely replaced. Of major concern is whether these drugs lead to an increase in suicidal thoughts or actions, particularly in the young, as mentioned above. This may exclude certain high-risk patients from SSRI medication and mandate careful monitoring in others.

Less critically the following adverse effects may occasionally be encountered:

- dystonia or parkinsonism (these could be treated with anticholinergics)
- insomnia usually at the beginning (take in the morning)
- nausea or diarrhoea, which usually gets better after a week
- constipation, dry mouth, and urinary retention
- sexual dysfunction.

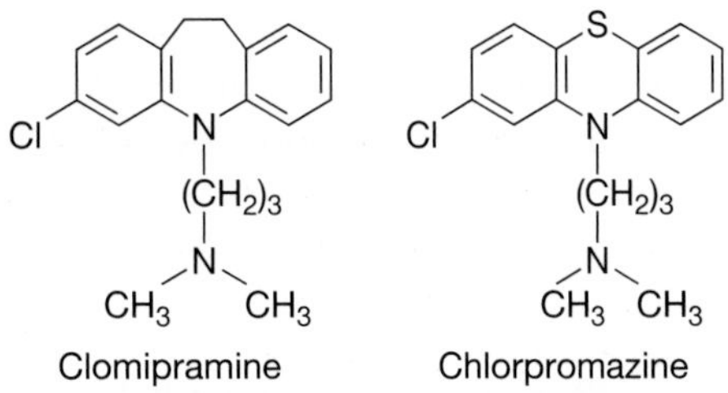

Figure 19.1 Similarity in structure between clomipramine and chlorpromazine.

Clomipramine is a tricyclic antidepressant. A simple change from C–C to –S– in the central ring turns this molecule from one which binds monoamine transporter proteins to one which binds to dopamine receptors. This converts the antidepressant clomipramine into the antipsychotic drug chlorpromazine (see Chapter 18).

SSRIs should not be taken with monoamine oxidase inhibitors

One entirely avoidable problem is the combination of SSRIs with monoamine oxidase (MAO) inhibitors (see Box 19.2 and below); this may lead to a potentially fatal central serotonin syndrome. Considering the long half-life of these drugs it is necessary to have a long (e.g. 2 weeks) drug-free period when switching between these two classes of medication.

19.2.3 Other uptake inhibitor antidepressants

These comprise an early and influential class of drug, the TCAs, and the more recent serotonin and noradrenaline reuptake inhibitor (SNRI) and selective noradrenaline reuptake inhibitor (NARI) classes. They have in common a mode of action that includes the inhibition of reuptake of noradrenaline with varying degrees of serotonin reuptake inhibition. While their beneficial effects do indeed vary, it seems that the main advantage of these two more recent classes is relatively few unwanted effects.

Tricyclic antidepressants

Tricyclic antidepressants were the most popular antidepressants before the arrival of the SSRIs. These two groups of drugs have similar efficacy, but the TCAs are more troublesome in terms of unwanted effects and toxicity on overdose (see below).

Tricyclic antidepressants include **amitryptyline**, **clomipramine**, **dosulepin**, **lofepramine**, and **imipramine**. The name for this group derives from a

characteristic three-ring structure illustrated for clomipramine in Figure 19.1. Also shown in this figure is the structure of the antipsychotic chlorpromazine (Chapter 18). It is interesting to see how a simple change in structure at the central ring (C–C in place of –S–) changes the clinical use of this compound so profoundly.

Mechanism of action. Noradrenaline, like serotonin, is cleared from the synapse by uptake (see Box 19.2, Figure c). The TCAs are non-specific biogenic amine uptake inhibitors. Their antidepressant action is mainly because they inhibit noradrenaline as well as serotonin uptake by binding to the transporter proteins in the presynaptic and glial (Box 19.2, Figure c) sites. This slows removal of the neurotransmitter, increasing neurotransmission at both these types of synapse. The TCAs have a spectrum of antagonist actions at receptors for histamine, serotonin, and noradrenaline that contribute to their unwanted effects.

Differences between TCAs include their sedative qualities. This may influence drug choice, with more sedating TCAs (e.g. clomipramine) being beneficial for agitated patients and less sedating (e.g. lofepramine) for withdrawn patients.

Adverse effects of TCAs include anticholinergic effects (i.e. they are antagonists at muscarinic acetycholine receptors): blurred vision, dry mouth, constipation, urinary retention ,and tachycardia (raised heart rate). This set of effects usually disappears over a couple of weeks. It is one reason why it may be desirable to introduce the drug at a low dose, slowly increasing. Antagonism at α_1-adrenoceptors and H_1 histamine receptors may cause hypotension and sedation, while serotoninergic effects may lead to sexual dysfunction. Toxicity on overdose is associated with cardiac conduction abnormalities.

TCA-related drugs

Mianserin is an inhibitor of noradrenaline reuptake and an antagonist at α_2-adrenoceptor receptors, resulting in increased noradrenergic neurotransmission. It has largely been superseded by other drugs. **Trazodone** is a weak inhibitor of serotonin uptake and an antagonist at 5-HT$_{2C}$ receptors, and has both antidepressant and anti-anxiety effects. It has fewer anticholinergic effects and may have fewer cardiac conduction effects on overdose.

Serotonin and noradrenaline reuptake inhibitors (SNRIs)

The main member of this class is **venlafaxine**, which has many characteristics similar to TCAs, including the broad nature of unwanted effects. However, these adverse effects are less common than with TCAs, probably because of lower affinity for noradrenaline, histamine and acetylcholine receptors. However venlafaxine, by enhancing noradrenergic neurotransmission, does have a hypertensive effect.

Duloxetine is popular in some settings for major depression – this also inhibits both serotonin and noradrenaline reuptake.

Selective noradrenaline reuptake inhibitors (NARIs)

The odd thing about this class of drugs, defined by its main mechanism, is that the older TCA, nortryptyline, has essentially the same mode of action.

However, as a class of drugs the only NARI is **reboxetine**. The inhibition of noradrenaline uptake is selective over serotonin uptake. Again the pharmacology is broadly similar to TCAs, with fewer unwanted effects, which when seen are likely to include dry mouth and insomnia.

Tianeptine

Tianeptine, available in some countries, falls into a class of its own—its actions include the *stimulation* of serotonin uptake, which makes it interesting for its contrary mode of action.

19.2.4 Noardrenergic and specific serotoninergic antidepressants (NASSAs)

Noardrenergic and specific serotoninergic antidepressants form a class of antidepressant with a fundamentally different mode of action from the others, and with only one clinically useful drug, **mirtazepine**. The actions of this drug are as an antagonist with the following characteristics:

- Blocks α_2-adrenoceptors located presynaptically on the noradrenergic nerve terminals, decreasing their inhibitory effect and increasing noradrenaline release.
- Blocks α_2-adrenoceptors located presynaptically on the serotoninergic neurons, enhancing serotonin release.

These two effects may contribute to the therapeutic effect.

- Blocking specific serotonin receptors (5-HT$_{2A}$ and 5-HT$_3$). This effect may mean that the increased serotoninergic neuroansmission can occur in the absence of nausea and headache, which may be mediated by the action of serotonin at 5-HT$_{2A}$ and 5-HT$_3$ receptors.
- Blocking histamine H$_1$ receptors. This may be responsible for the sometimes unwanted effect of sedation.

19.2.5 Monoamine oxidase inhibitors

This is an early class of drugs which were popular before the introduction of TCAs. If you inhibit the breakdown of a neurotransmitter then you may make it more available at its receptors, and this is the basis of action of MAO inhibitors. Monoamines are removed from the synapse by combined reuptake and intracellular enzymic breakdown, so with the MAO inhibitors and the uptake inhibitors (TCAs, SSRIs, etc. as described above) we have drugs for use in depression which can attack both these mechanisms. By inhibiting breakdown MAO inhibitors increase the availability of neurotransmitter for release, increasing the amount in each vesicle (i.e. increasing the quantum release) and also increasing the 'leakage' from the nerve terminal.

We encounter MAO inhibitors in two contexts: here as antidepressants and in Chapter 17 in the management of Parkinson's disease. The drugs are distinct: MAO comes in two forms, MAO-A and MAO-B (Box 19.2). The Parkinson's disease drugs are selective inhibitors of MAO-B (and target dopamine in the brain, see Chapter 17), while the antidepressants are either non-selective (**phenelzine, isocarboxazid**) or selective MAO-A inhibitors (**moclobemide**).

Some aspects of MAO and its inhibition in the synapses of the brain are explored in Box 19.2, where it is also pointed out that MAO is also found outside the brain. The main disadvantage of MAO inhibitors is the powerful and widespread interactions with both food and other drugs, which make them potentially hazardous (Box 19.2). The resultant dietary restrictions and concerns about drug interactions have meant that this class of antidepressant is mainly used for patients who do not respond effectively to SSRIs or TCAs.

Diet and the MAO inhibitors

MAO-A in the intestines and liver normally destroys dietary tyramine, but when this enzyme is inhibited then tyramine can have a profound and toxic effect on the body. This is in part because it enters noradrenergic nerve terminals of the sympathetic branch of the autonomic nervous system and releases noradrenaline, which may result in a hypertensive crisis. This is the 'cheese effect', for cheese has high tyramine content. Patients taking antidepressant MAO inhibitors must therefore have a diet low in tyramine, meaning that they must avoid cheese, yeast and yeast extracts, beer, some red wines, and some meat products (e.g. chicken liver). When it occurs, the hypertensive tyramine response usually results in an extreme headache, which may be the prelude to brain haemorrhage and so must be treated with urgency.

Irreversible and reversible inhibitors of MAO

Phenelzine and isocarboxazid are irreversible inhibitors of MAO. This means that when the drug is removed the effect of the drug lasts until the body has synthesised new enzyme. One consequence of this is that dietary restrictions must be maintained at least 2 weeks after stopping drug use. It is also important when considering the interaction of MAO inhibitors with SSRIs. The combined effect of MAO inhibitors with these uptake inhibitors is dangerous. It is important therefore to have a sustained drug-free period when switching in either direction, since SSRIs have a long half-life and most MAO inhibitors have an irreversible effect outlasting the presence of the drug.

One exception is moclobemide, which is a reversible MAO-A inhibitor, giving it a short duration of action. This means that when switching from moclobemide an SSRI can be introduced without delay, but when switching from an SSRI to moclobemide it is still important to have a sustained drug-free period.

Clinical use

MAO inhibitors should be used when responses to other antidepressants have failed or when SSRIs and TCAs cannot be used, for example because of suicidal tendencies or a pre-existing heart condition, and when patients are compliant with respect to dietary restrictions.

19.2.6 St John's wort

While guidelines may indicate that the use of St John's wort for depression is not to be actively encouraged, patients who are doing well on this self-medication may be counselled to continue. The preparation is reported to have an efficacy similar to other antidepressants for mild depression. It is a non-selective noradrenaline and serotonin uptake inhibitor. Its main advantage is fewer unwanted effects. Its main disadvantage is the variation between preparations and the interactions with other drugs. Because of the latter point it is important to know whether or not a patient is using this herbal remedy.

19.2.7 Strategy in the drug treatment of major depression

In Workbook 16 Sunita is troubled by both anxiety and major depression. She struggles to reach a suitable resolution of her depression. The notion that an SSRI is the answer to all these problems proves to be wrong. It is often the case that SSRIs will provide the help patients need, but it should always be remembered that drugs are likely to be only a part of the therapeutic strategy and may not be warranted at all in the case of mild/moderate depression. The first line, unless there are contraindications, is likely to be an SSRI, with monitoring of a therapeutic response over the following weeks. Then, as we see in the case of Sunita, if the response is not adequate then an alternative SSRI or venflaxine, reboxetine, or mirtazepine may be considered, and if these do not prove suitable or effective then an MAO inhibitor should be considered.

19.3 Bipolar illness

Mood swings from depression to mania are characteristic of bipolar (or manic-depressive) illness, and the drugs which specifically target this condition are referred to as mood stabilizers or antimanic drugs. The main treatment is lithium; in addition some drugs which we have encountered as anti-epileptic drugs in Chapter 16 may be helpful, such as valproic acid and carbamazepine.

19.3.1 Lithium in the treatment of bipolar disorder

The action of lithium is both complex and interesting, and may include changes in the excitability of brain nerve cells, their response to neurotransmitters, and their long-term survival.

The therapeutic response is mainly related to inhibiting mania, rather than diminished depression. (Confusingly, some psychiatrists will use lithium to treat major unipolar depression). Treatment is by oral administration and is long term, with benefit appearing after 2–3 weeks. The effect is to reduce the onset of manic episodes.

Lithium is a toxic compound, with a narrow therapeutic window (the levels which give benefit without toxicity) and this necessitates monitoring of plasma levels. Toxic effects include gastrointestinal and renal impairment with frequent urination, blurred vision, and CNS effects such as sedation and giddiness—the drug should be withdrawn. Major organ-system failure can follow severely toxic doses.

19.4 Anxiety

As a clinical entity anxiety comes in many forms. In every case the use of psychological therapies is important and drug therapy may not be the best option. Three common manifestations of anxiety which lead to drug treatment are panic disorder, phobic disorder, and generalized anxiety disorder (GAD). Some of the classifications of anxiety are introduced in Workbook 16; our patient Sunita has a diagnosis of GAD in the first part of this workbook, from which, over time, she progresses to develop major depressive disorder.

19.4.1 Drug treatment of generalized anxiety disorder

Immediate relief of symptoms can be provided by the use of benzodiazepines. This frequently prescribed group of drugs is described below. Since these drugs are recommended for short-term use only, the long-term drug management of anxiety requires a different approach, and this should be the use of antidepressants licensed for anxiety, such as the SSRI **paroxetine**.

Anxiety can be associated with stress and with over-activity of the sympathetic branch of the autonomic nervous system. This will result in increased stimulation of adrenoceptors, which in some cases produces symptoms that distress and add to the anxiety. These autonomic symptoms may include tachycardia and palpitations, and tremor: patients experiencing these types of symptoms may benefit from a β-adrenoceptor antagonist (β-blocker) such as propranolol or oxprenolol (see Chapter 5). Relieving the physical symptoms may help relieve the anxiety that caused them.

Benzodiazepines

This is a class of drugs which act by binding to a specific site within the GABA$_A$ receptor, resulting in a greater response to stimulation of the receptor by its agonist GABA, reducing neuronal excitability (Box 16.1). We have encountered these drugs in the treatment of epilepsy (Chapter 16) but they are most commonly prescribed for anxiety disorders and as hypnotics (i.e. they help people go to sleep).

While they have been widely over-prescribed in the past, and perhaps still are, they are very useful in the short-term treatment of anxiety.

Their main advantages are:

a) rapid onset
b) powerful antianxiety action
c) low toxicity and side effects profile.

Their main disadvantages are:

a) the occurrence of drowsiness when a reduction in anxiety is required
b) the development over a period of weeks of:
   - tolerance: the effectiveness of the medication at resolving anxiety becomes less
   - dependence: symptoms of intense anxiety, dizziness, and tremor occur when the drug is stopped.

In the workbook it is made clear that Sunita's treatment with diazepam is relieving the symptoms and not tacking the underlying disorder. In some cases this is a sufficient approach; the underlying disorder will resolve with time and the drug 'buys time' for this to happen without disruption and unhappiness in the meantime. In Sunita's case the lowest dose tablet is prescribed, which with recognition that it is only appropriate for short-term therapy will reduce the chances of dependence problems.

Different benzodiazepines have very similar pharmacological actions and are mainly chosen on the basis of their pharmacokinetic profile. **Diazepam**, **alprazolam**, **chlordiazepoxide** and **clobazam** have long half-lives. Diazepam has a long-lasting active metabolite. This means that if taken at night diazepam will continue to have an effect during the next day. This may include sedation, which may be desirable, but may be an unwanted effect. **Lorazepam** and **oxazepam** are shorter acting benzodiazepines.

SUMMARY OF COMMON DRUGS USED FOR DEPRESSION, BIPOLAR DISORDERS AND ANXIETY

Therapeutic class	Drugs	Mechanism of action	Common clinical uses	Comments	Examples of adverse drug reactions
Monoamine oxidase inhibitors	Phenelzine Tranylcypromine l	Irreversibly inhibits monoamine oxidases A and B, increasing the synaptic concentrations of adrenaline, dopamine, noradrenaline, and serotonin	Depressive illness	Could cause accumulation of amine neurotransmitters and tyramine found in certain foods, by blocking their metabolism—this could lead to a dangerous rise in blood pressure, therefore food like mature cheese, pickled herring, marmite, and other antidepressants should be avoided	Postural hypotension Dizziness Drowsiness Headache Gastrointestinal disorders Elevated liver enzymes Weight gain Drymouth Visual disturbance
Reversible monoamine oxidase inhibitors	Moclobemide	Irreversibly inhibit monoamine oxidases A	Depressive illness Social anxiety disorder	Less interaction with tyramine but patients should still avoid tyramine-rich foods	
Selective serotonin re-uptake inhibitors	Citalopram Escitalopram Fluoxetine Fluvoxamine Paroxetine Sertraline	Selectively inhibit the presynaptic reuptake of serotonin (5-hydroxytryptamine)	Major depression Anxiety disorders, e.g. panic disorder, obsessive compulsive disorder Bulimia nervosa Premenstrual dysphoric disorder	Have long half-lives Treatment with either moclobemide or a monoamine oxidase inhibitor or drugs that contribute to serotonin toxicity should be avoided for at least 2 weeks due to the risk of serotonin toxicity	Nausea Agitation Insomnia Drowsiness Anxiety, Weight gain Sexual dysfunction
Tricyclic antidepressants	Amitriptyline Clomipramine Dothiepin Doxepin Imipramine Nortriptyline Trimipramine	1) Inhibits reuptake of noradrenaline and serotonin into presynaptic junctions 2) Blocks cholinergic, histaminergic, α_1-adrenergic and serotonergic receptors	Depression Nocturnal enuresis Neuropathic pain (amitriptyline and nortriptyline) Migrane (amitryptyline) Phobic and obsessional states (clomipramine) Cataplexy–adjunct (clomipramine)	Choice is based on sedative and antimuscarinic effects Clomipramine has a greater effect on serotonin transport than other tricyclic antidepressants	Sedation Dry mouth Blurred vision Constipation Weight gain Orthostatic hypotension Sinus tachycardia Urinary hesitancy or retention Reduced gastrointestinal motility

Therapeutic class	Drugs	Mechanism of action	Common clinical uses	Comments	Examples of adverse drug reactions
Other antidepressants	Duloxetine	Inhibits serotonin and noradrenaline reuptake	Major depressive disorder Diabetic neuropathy Stress urinary incontinence	Sometimes restricted for specialist use	Nausea Drymouth Constipation Reduced appetite
	Mirtazepine	Antagonist at presynaptic α-adrenoceptor, increasing central noradrenergic and serotonergic neurotransmission	Major depression	Fewer antimuscarinic effects but causes sedation	Weight gain Oedema Sedation
	Reboxetine	Selectively inhibits noradrenaline reuptake		Caution in cardiovascular disease and epilepsy amongst others	Nausea Dry mouth Constipation Tachycardia Headache Insomnia
	Venlafaxine	Inhibits reuptake of serotonin and noradrenaline	Major depression Generalized anxiety disorder	Similar to tricyclics, both have less antimuscarinic and sedative effects	Constipation Nausea Anorexia Weight changes Diarrhoea Hypertension
	Mianserin	Tetracyclic antagonist at α_2 adrenergic, serotonergic and H_1 histaminergic receptors	Major depression	Little antimuscarinic effect	Leucopenia Agranulocytosis Jaundice Weight gain
	St John's wort	Inhibits reuptake of noradrenaline and serotonin	Depression	Affects hepatic enzymes involved in metabolism, leading to side effects Main advantage is fewer unwanted effects and main disadvantage is the variation between preparations and the interactions with other drugs	Nausea Vomiting Diarrhoea

Therapeutic class	Drugs	Mechanism of action	Common clinical uses	Comments	Examples of adverse drug reactions
Lithium salts	Lithium carbonate Lithium citrate	Inhibit dopamine release, enhance serotonin release and decrease formation of intracellular messengers	Treatment and prophylaxis of mania, bipolar disease and recurrent depression	Narrow therapeutic window Drug levels monitored to prevent toxicity and ensure therapeutic levels Long half-life	Gastrointestinal disturbances Fine tremor Renal impairment Polydipsia Leucocytosis Weight gain Oedema
Antiepileptic drugs	Carbamazepine	See Chapter 16	Prophylaxis of bipolar disease	Used second line	See Chapter 16
	Valproic acid		Treatment of manic episodes	Used second line	
Benzodiazepines	Diazepam Nitrazepam Clonazepam Alprazolam Flunitrazepam Lorazepam Oxazepam Chlordiazepoxide Clobazam	Bind to a specific site within the GABAA receptor, resulting in a greater response to stimulation of the receptor by its agonist GABA, reducing neuronal excitability	Anxiety Epilepsy Insomnia Alcohol withdrawal (chlordiazepoxide)	Diazepam, alprazolam, chlordiazepoxide and clobazam have long half-lives Diazepam has a long-lasting active metabolite so if taken at night it continues to have an effect the next day Lorazepam and oxazepam are shorter-acting benzodiazepines	See Chapter 16

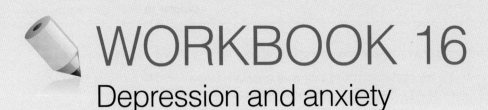

WORKBOOK 16
Depression and anxiety

SUNITA again, this time with depression and anxiety

Sunita: a simplified case history

Sunita, whom we have encountered before, developed depression and anxiety following the birth of her children. Her struggle with this, and the difficulties of helping her with drug-based therapy, illustrate some of the themes encountered in the treatment of these two conditions.

The memory of their romantic wedding on the beach puts a rare smile on Sunita's face. Sunita finds she hardly smiles anymore because she is too busy worrying that something will go wrong. She still cannot believe that despite the rocky patches she now seems to have everything she ever wished for. First she had the thyroid crises, then the pregnancy that, though difficult, led to the birth of their three bundles of joy: triplets! (We met one of the triplets earlier, Elvis, who suffers from eczema)

The triplets are now 9 months old and getting into a routine. Nursing triplets was a full-time job and she felt like the family cow at times. The situation is much improved now with the help of nannies and housekeepers. Although Sunita feels blessed most of the time, she cannot stop worrying and feeling anxious. Most nights, she finds it difficult to fall asleep. Sunita also finds it difficult to concentrate and has become a 'calamity Jane', dropping things all the time. She is even getting too scared to hold her own babies, afraid she might drop them. This has gone on for over 5 months now. More recently she has been experiencing stomach pain alongside the anxiety.

Although Sunita feels unable to tell her husband about these symptoms she has no such inhibitions with Monique, her best friend. Monique convinces her to see her GP.

A table of clinical clerking abbreviations is given on page xx.

CLINICAL CLERKING FOR SUNITA AT GENERAL PRACTITIONER'S SURGERY

Age: 31 years, weight 70 kg

PC: Trouble falling asleep, worrying. Feeling nervous and anxious, difficulty concentrating. Also has dry mouth and epigastric discomfort.

HPC: The above symptoms have been developing for over 5 months and she kept it to herself initially because she felt she should just pull herself together.

Most of Sunita's symptoms are common symptoms of both depression and anxiety disorders.

Anxiety is in itself a key characteristic of almost all psychiatric disorders. The fact that Sunita has 9-month-old babies makes a diagnosis of post-natal depression a possibility.

⇒*More information is required to enable a diagnosis.*

PMH: Hyperthyroidism three years ago. Delivered triplets 9 months ago.

DH: Nil

Anxiety disorders can be divided into:

1 Primary anxiety disorder: no associated cause.

2 Secondary anxiety disorder: medical or substance causes (e.g. medication).

3 Anxiety in response to acute stress.

4 Anxiety in association with other psychiatric disorders.

- *Sunita has had hyperthyroidism in the past, a condition associated with anxiety if thyroid hormone levels are deranged. Thyroid function tests could confirm or rule this out.*

- *Sunita is not currently on any medication. All medication, including over-the-counter drugs, should be considered as a possible cause of anxiety.*

- *Sunita has had stressful and traumatic life events which may provoke anxiety for anyone. Although this is usually self-limiting and not long lasting, some people may find it difficult to adjust.*

On observation and questioning:

1) Appearance and behaviour: Sunita is well groomed and dressed, her speech is coherent but she is fidgety.

2) Mood: Sunita is anxious and worried about everything and her worries seem exaggerated.

3) Sensorium: Sunita is oriented to person time and place.

4) Thoughts: No hallucinations.

5) Others: Sunita cannot relax, but she has not:

- got suicidal thoughts
- experienced loss of interest and pleasure in normal activities
- had appetite or weight losses
- got diurnal variation in mood and early-morning waking.

6) Her stomach pain is just a dull sensation, not sharp or severe. The pain only occurs with severe anxiety. Antacids and ranitidine bought over the counter do not make it better. It comes on when she is anxious and resolves when she isn't.

Sunita has quite a few target symptoms associated with generalized anxiety disorder (GAD):

- *excessive worrying*

- *tension, inability to relax and sleep disturbances.*

To differentiate GAD from depressive illness, patients should be questioned about symptoms such as loss of interest and pleasure, loss of appetite and weight, diurnal variation in mood and early-morning waking.

Sunita does not experience all of these other symptoms.

The stomach pain is not indicative of dyspepsia.

7) Blood pressure = 135/ 85 mm Hg (<140/90 mm Hg)

8) Pulse = 80/minute (60/minute)

Physical examinations will reveal or rule out any possible physical/medical causes:

- *Her blood pressure is not elevated.*
- *Her pulse is elevated, she is tachycardic, a common symptom of anxiety.*

SH: Lives with husband, three children, two nannies and a housekeeper. Stopped breastfeeding 1 month ago. Mother suffers from GADs.

Genetic factors have a modest role in the aetiology of GAD.

Studies indicate abnormalities in the serotonergic system.

Investigations:

1) Biochemistry

- Electrolytes

sodium: 142 mmol/L (reference 135–145)

potassium: 4.2 mmol/L (reference 3.5–5.5)

These are both within the recommended range.

- Others

3,5,3',5'-tetraiodothyronine or thyroxine (T4) = 120 nmol/L (reference 64–154)

triiodothyronine (T_3) = 1.5 nmol/L (reference 1.1–2.0)

thyroid stimulating hormone (TSH) = 0.9 mIU/L (reference 0.5–4.7)

Her thyroid function tests are normal, indicating that hyperthyroidism can be ruled out as a possible cause.

Diagnosis: Generalized anxiety disorder

The International Criteria for Disease (ICD-10) and Diagnostic and Statistical Manual of Mental Disorders (DSM-IV) distinguish between phobic anxiety disorders, where anxiety is associated with particular situations, and other anxiety disorders in which anxiety occurs in the absence of specific triggering events or circumstances.

Plan:

Commence diazepam (three times daily)

Refer for psychotherapy

Although non-drug treatments are available, these are restricted to patients with mild symptoms or when immediate symptom relief is not necessary.

Sunita needs to be treated immediately to prevent post-natal depression.

She has also been referred for psychotherapy for investigation and treatment of the primary cause of her GAD.

Sunita starts taking the tablets and feels better after a couple of days. Eoin, her husband, is relieved and finds it amazing that drugs can have such a profound influence on the brain. He asks Sunita about the human brain.

1a) Have a guess at how many neurons approximately make up an adult brain. Do you think neurons are the most numerous cell type in the brain? Name some other types of cell you may find in the brain.

1b) List two functions of the brain.

2a) What are glial cells?

2b) Give an example of a glial cell.

3a) What is the difference between a neurotransmitter and a neuromodulator?

3b) List three suggested neuroanatomical substrates of anxiety.

4a) List three amino acid neurotransmitters in the central nervous system (CNS).

4b) Which of these are excitatory and which are inhibitory? On which receptors do they work? Where predominantly do they work?

5) What are the functions associated with 5-hydroxytryptamine (5-HT; serotonin) pathways?

6) What symptoms of anxiety was Sunita experiencing?

7a) What is the evidence supporting a role for 5-HT in anxiety?

7b) What is the evidence for and neuropharmacological support for the role of noradrenaline (norepinephrin) in anxiety?

8a) List two main approaches to the treatment of anxiety.

Eoin worries because he has heard about the risk of addiction with diazepam and mentions this to Sunita.

She explains that although he is right and there is a risk of addiction, she will only use it short term (for 4 weeks) to prevent this.

She says her doctor explained to her that the drug will not cure her anxiety; it will only provide a useful short-term symptomatic treatment. She has had two sessions with her psychotherapist and hopefully together they will get to the root cause of her illness and get rid of the symptoms.

8b) Which classes of drugs are commonly used to treat anxiety?

Eoin wonders why the doctor wanted to know if Sunita was still breastfeeding. Sunita explains that it is because diazepam would be present in breast milk because of its pharmacokinetics and therefore the babies would be exposed.

9a) Describe the $GABA_A$ receptor. Is it inhibitory or excitatory?

9b) What is the difference between $GABA_A$ and $GABA_B$?

Eoin wonders why Sunita will not drink a glass of wine when they go to the pub.

Sunita explains to him that diazepam interacts with alcohol and increases the CNS depressant effect of the drug. This would make her drowsy and cause hangover symptoms. It is also because of this that she has not been driving.

10a) What are the adverse effects of benzodiazepines?

10b) How can these risks be reduced?

10c) What are the advantages of benzodiazepine over the barbiturates?

> Sunita completes her 4-week medication course and psychotherapy sessions. After 6 months, she is back to her old self and enjoying life to the full. She no longer needs the diazepam.
>
> But life is unpredictable, and Sunita's problems are not so easily resolved. Shockingly, 18 months later Sunita attempts suicide.

CLERKING IN HOSPITAL FOR SUNITA KAISER

PC: Blurred vision, dizziness, confusion, drowsiness, anxiety, agitation, and unresponsiveness, slurred speech, weakness

HPC: (Taken from her friend Monique) Following 3 months of insomnia, worrying, feeling worthless and useless, nervous, appetite loss, loss of interest in everything, Sunita finally took an overdose, resulting in above symptoms.

O/E:

1) Respiratory rate: 28 breaths per minute

2) Blood pressure: 100/60 mm Hg

3) O_2 saturation: 90%

4) Nystagmus

5) Hypotonia

6) Respiratory depression

> Sunita is experiencing most of the classic symptoms of benzodiazepine overdose.
>
> She took an overdose after months of experiencing symptoms of depression.

PMH: Hyperthyroidism 3 years ago. Generalized anxiety disorder 18 months ago.

DH: Ingested 50 diazepam tablets (bought from the internet) with alcohol.

> *Although mortality from a pure benzodiazepine overdose is rare; it could happen if benzodiazepine is taken concomitantly with alcohol or other sedative-hypnotics.*
>
> *It is especially worrying that the benzodiazepine was bought over the internet, therefore its quality could be questionable.*

SH: Lives with three children, two nannies and a housekeeper. Separated from husband 3 months ago after publicized affair. Mum suffered from depression.

Biochemistry:

1) Electrolytes

- Sodium 142 mmol/L (reference 135–145)
- Potassium 4.2 mmol/L (reference 3.5–5.5)

> *These are both within recommended range.*

2) Toxicity screen: positive for alcohol and benzodiazepine

Both urine and blood toxicology screens, testing the presence and concentration of diazepam in Sunita's body, are positive and confirm the diagnosis.

> *The screening is important because:*

- the tablets were bought over the internet and could be contaminated or too potent
- Sunita could have ingested other toxic chemicals besides the tablets found.

Diagnosis:

Benzodiazepine overdose secondary to depression

Plan:

Flumazenil

Urgent referral to psychiatrist

> *Flumazenil is a benzodiazepine antagonist that is used as an antidote in the treatment of benzodiazepine overdose.*
>
> *The onset of action is rapid and usually effects are seen within 1 to 2 minutes.*
>
> *The peak effect is seen at 6 to 10 minutes.*

After she comes round, Sunita regrets what she did and agrees to be admitted to the psychiatric assessment unit.

MEDICAL NOTES FOR SUNITA AT PSYCHIATRIC ASSESSMENT UNIT

PC: Hospital referral following overdose with diazepam

HPC: Three months of persistent low mood, loss of interest (anhedonia), fatigue, disturbed sleep, suicidal thoughts, poor appetite and low self esteem

SH: Separated from husband 3 months ago. Lives with triplets and house help. Sunita's mum suffered from depression.

Biochemistry:

Urea and electrolytes all within normal range including thyroid function tests.

> *Hypothyroidism and anaemia could lead to symptoms of depression. These are ruled out for Sunita because her blood results are all normal.*

Diagnosis:

Severe depression

> *Other descriptions used are recurrent, treatment–resistant and chronic depression.*
>
> *The likelihood that Sunita has got depression is quite high because she has:*
>
> - *two of the key symptoms*
> - *five associated symptoms present most of the day for 3 months*
> - *attempted suicide*
> - *severe self-neglect*
> - *a mum who suffered from depression (this which makes her five times more likely to suffer from depression)*
> - *experienced a stressful life event (separation from husband), physical illness, and recently had children.*

Plan:

Admit to ward

Commence antidepressant drug

The psychiatrist explains to Sunita that depression is associated with depleted levels of chemical transmitters in the mid-brain, and antidepressants may work by raising the levels of these naturally occurring chemicals.

11) List three of the chemical transmitters he was referring to.

....

....

....

12a) What is the monoamine hypothesis of depression?

12b) Elaborate on the evidence for and against the monoamine hypothesis of depression.

The doctor discusses choices of a drug for Sunita with the team, including a pharmacist.

The factors influencing choice that they discuss are:

- **Clinical presentation:** Some types of depression have a better response to certain classes of antidepressant, e.g. selective serotonin reuptake inhibitors (SSRIs) when anxiety dominant, sedative antidepressants in retardation.

  Not applicable to Sunita.

- **Contraindication:** Patients with cardiac problems should not be treated with tricyclic antidepressants (TCAs) and venlafaxine, and patients with glaucoma should not be treated with those with anticholinergic side effects.

  Not applicable to Sunita

- **Cost:** Although drug cost is a consideration, the overall cost incurred from dropouts or hospital admission for TCA overdose must be taken into consideration. (Although TCAs are cheaper and as effective as SSRIs, they are currently not recommended as a first-line option due to their greater spectrum of adverse effects.)

  Considered for Sunita.

- **Previous response:** If a patient had a good response previously to an antidepressant, it should be tried again. Similarly, if they had a poor response it should be avoided.

  Not applicable to Sunita.

13) What are the main types of antidepressants?

> They talk about monoamine oxidase (MAO) inhibitors. The doctor jokingly asks Sunita if she would give up cheese.

14) Explain the mechanism of action of MAO inhibitors.

_____

_____

_____

15a) Explain which and why certain cheeses or cheese food items could be a problem for a patient on older MAO inhibitors.

_____

_____

_____

15b) How do these older MAO inhibitors differ pharmacologically to the newer ones?

_____

_____

_____

> They then discuss TCAs.

16a) What is the mechanism of action of TCAs?

_____

_____

_____

16b) What are their disadvantages?

_____

_____

_____

> The team decide to prescribe paroxetine, an SSRI, for Sunita. The new junior doctor writes it on the drug chart to be taken at night.
>
> SSRIs are the first-line choice recommended by guidelines for depression from the National Institute of Clinical Excellence (NICE) in the UK. SSRIs are the first choice because they are as efficacious as TCAs but are less likely to be discontinued because of side effects and are safer in medically complicated patients. They are also better than TCAs for Sunita because she has already attempted suicide and could do so again.

17a) What is the mechanism of action of SSRIs?

After a week, Sunita finds she feels restless and cannot sit still at all. She also finds her anxiety symptoms have returned. She is very worried and wonders if this has been caused by the paroxetine. The doctor confirms that the restlessness could be akathisia, an extrapyramidal (EPS) side effect caused by paroxetine. The anxiety could be as a result of the activating effect of the SSRI.

17b) Explain how EPS could be caused by SSRIs.

The doctor proposes two possible solutions for the akathisia:

• reduce the dose of paroxetine

• prescribe atenolol (a β-blocker) at a low dose.

The doctor decides to reduce the dose of paroxetine. He also prescribes a low dose of diazepam. Sunita cannot understand why she is experiencing side effects although she is still feeling depressed.

The doctor explains to Sunita that:

• -it may take at least 2 weeks before she feels any better

• the full benefits may take up to 6 weeks to manifest themselves

• the side effects of antidepressants tend to be worse in the first 2 weeks and although they are very common, they are generally not serious.

18) What are other side effects of SSRIs? How can they be treated?

One day later, Sunita complains of increased insomnia. The pharmacist notices that the paroxetine was written up by the junior doctor for night-time and she changes the time of administration to morning.

After 4 weeks, Sunita's symptoms are showing no signs of improving. Moreover, although the akathisia and insomnia have improved she now suffers from severe nausea as well. Her psychiatrist admits that the paroxetine does not seem to be working for her and informs her that he will discuss her case with the multidisciplinary team (MDT) and try to find an alternative antidepressant.

The MDT discuss the advantages and disadvantages of several options that could replace the paroxetine. The choices they consider are listed below.

Drug (class)	Advantages	Disadvantages
Another SSRI	Alternative SSRI may present less suicide risk in patient with suicidal history	History of ADR and therapeutic failure with paroxetine and effective treatment required urgently
Venlafaxine (SNRI)	Other class, effective, less activating than SSRI	Risk of hypertension, cost, some ADR similar to SSRI
Mirtazapine (NaSSA)	Less nausea, headache and anxiety than SSRI	Increased appetite, weight gain, drowsiness
Reboxetine (NARI)	Better ADR profile than TCA	Dry mouth, constipation, insomnia
Moclobemide (MAO inhibitor)	Newer and better MAO inhibitor	Tyramine reaction, insomnia, nausea agitation, confusion
Lofepramine (TCA)	TCA with fewer ADRs, effective	Possible hepatotoxicity, some ADRs as for other TCAs

SSRI, selective serotonin reuptake inhibitor; ADR, adverse drug reaction; SNRI, serotonin and noradrenaline reuptake inhibitor; NaSSA, noardrenergic and specific serotoninergic antidepressant; NARI, selective noradrenaline reuptake inhibitor; TCA, tricyclic andtidepressant; MAO, monoamine oxidase.

19) How does the mechanism of action of venlafaxine an SNRI differ from that of mirtazapine, a NaSSA?

20) Describe the mechanism of reboxetine.

They decide to try mirtazapine because its side effects of cause weight gain and sedation could actually be desirable for Sunita, who is now underweight and suffers from insomnia.

The pharmacist advises switching from paroxetine to mirtazapine using a recommended regime of stepping down. This is to avoid serotonin syndrome, which could occur when combinations of serotonergic antidepressants are prescribed. Serotonin syndrome is rare but can be fatal. Features of serotonin syndrome are confusion, delirium, shivering, sweating, changes in blood pressure, and malignant hyperthermia. It is most common when SSRIS are combined with MAO inhibitors.

Eoin, who has started visiting Sunita, brings some St Johns wort that was recommended by one of his friends as a herbal, and therefore safer, antidepressant.

21a) Explain the mechanism by which St John's wort exerts its effects as an antidepressant.

Luckily, Sunita can vaguely recall that St John's wort is not a good idea for her, although she is too tired to remember why. She asks the ward pharmacist.

21b) Why should Sunita not use the St John's wort, which is herbal and therefore could be thought to be safe?

Two months later, although she is on the maximum dose of mirtazapine, Sunita is still only slightly improved. She is despondent and has given up.

Eoin is now a changed man and very supportive, and has given up racing to be with his family. Sunita has allowed him to move back into the house.

The MDT agree that the two options left are electroconvulsive therapy (ECT) or lithium alongside the mirtazapine.

Eoin is horrified because he thinks lithium is for bipolar disease only. He also cannot bear the thought of Sunita undergoing ECT.

22a) What are the mechanisms of action of lithium?

....

....

....

22b) What are the side effects of lithium?

....

....

....

The doctor explains to Eoin and Sunita that sometimes lithium is used for resistant depression. He also explains that carbamazepine and sodium valproate are other, less effective, options.

He explains that lithium levels will need to be monitored and Sunita will have to be monitored for serotonin syndrome because of the increased risk of this with lithium. He explains that despite these, lithium or ECT is the next option.

They both decide to give lithium a try.

Sunita is given information about lithium signs of toxicity and when levels are checked. She is also told which drugs lithium can interact with.

The lithium seems to do the trick and Sunita is much improved after 2 months.

One year later Sunita is back to normal and wants to come off the antidepressants.

She asks her psychiatrist if she can.

There is controversy over how long a patient should stay on an antidepressant for.

Patients should be advised to continue taking the medication for at least 4 months after the depression improves, and preferably to make a slow, supervised reduction. It is important to warn the patient about adverse effects with sudden withdrawal, which can happen with any antidepressant.

For recurrent depression, treatment should be continued for longer periods, about 2 years.

Two years later Sunita's psychiatrist agrees to try stopping the antidepressants for Sunita. He explains that the dose of the drugs should normally be gradually reduced over a 4-week period. If withdrawal symptoms are mild, the patient should be reassured. If symptoms are severe, the original antidepressant can be reintroduced at the dose that was effective (or another antidepressant with a longer half-life from the same class) and then reduced gradually while monitoring symptoms.

Sunita's doses are gradually reduced and eventually she is able to come off the drugs.

She and Eoin have had marriage counselling and Eoin realizes that life on the racing circuit had contributed to making him have the affair. He has found a coaching job and never wants to travel without his family again. They are back to being a happy family of five.

Chapter 20
Pain and its drug treatment

Pain is a very familiar concept, and yet to ask what we mean by pain raises some curious issues. If you put your hand on a hot surface in the kitchen you will feel immediate pain and very rapidly move your hand away. If no tissue damage is done then the pain will disappear. This pain has certain characteristics: it has an obvious cause, it is intense, rapid in onset, very quickly leads to a motor response without conscious control, and stops when the cause is removed. Suppose the surface is hot enough to cause a burn—tissue damage. Then pain will persist after removing the cause, the pain will be different, may subside and then get worse. What's causing this pain now? There's no hot surface to provide an explanation. Then think of getting sunburn. It may not hurt you, but afterwards at night the brushing of sheets against your skin may be painful. What is causing this pain? We may think of pain as the transmission of a message—this *hurts*—from nerve endings in the tissues (e.g. skin or viscera) rapidly to the brain, but consider a patient familiar with sharp and acute arthritic pain in a toe that occurs periodically and always goes after a minute or two. Then consider *the same pain* occurring quite unexpectedly in a patient who has never experienced it before. The second case will be perceived as much more painful than the first—it *is* more painful. Then consider the observation that stimulation of particular parts of the brain can relieve pain coming from the body—it can actually reduce the pain message coming up the spinal cord towards the brain, so it must send signals from the brain down to the spinal cord, inhibiting assembly of a '*this hurts*' package of information (the 'pain package') to be sent up to the brain. This inhibition can be activated by means other than brain stimulation, e.g. minor electrical stimuli applied to the skin can relieve pain, such as in childbirth. Try thinking of pain as something that is formed not at the site of the painful stimulus, but in the brain. It normally happens as a result of packaged information reaching it from the spinal cord, but the pain itself is formed in the brain. Then many things, such as the influence of environment and psychological state on the intensity of pain, and the action of pain-relieving medication, become easier to understand.

As we consider pain we expose a fascinating and complex world that affects us all, and which thankfully can be modified by drugs acting at various levels to reduce the perception of pain. An example is provided in Workbook 17, in which some ups and downs of treatment of Lucy for pain following a road traffic accident injury are followed. This involves medication with opioid (morphine-related) pain killers. Long-term use of opioid drugs raises issues of addiction, a concern realized in Lucy's case.

20.1 Pain perception

The introductory comments made above indicate that pain perception is not a simple process. The initiation of this process is the stimulation of nociceptive nerve endings. **Nociception** is the perception of noxious stimuli resulting in pain, and the elements of the nociceptive nerve terminal which respond to the stimuli are called nociceptors (or pain receptors). The stimuli causing acute pain are often physical trauma or heat, but this often leads to sustained pain in which the nociceptor is stimulated by chemicals released by adjacent cells. This is important since this first chemical step is a target for commonly used drugs.

20.1.1 Three levels in pain perception

The process of pain perception starts with the activation of the nociceptor (the pain nerve terminal), firing a train of action potentials in primary afferent pain fibres which synapse in the spinal cord, activating ascending spinal pathways up to the brain. At each level the process is subject to moderation by other stimuli or neuronal activity. Moderating influences may reduce or enhance the sensation of pain—many analgesic drugs[1] act by interfering with the pain-enhancing mechanisms or enhance the pain-reducing mechanisms, as described below. In Box 20.1 some of the pain perception pathway is illustrated by dividing it into three levels.

Level 1: The nociceptor

This is located at the origin of the pain, where stimuli activate the nociceptive nerve terminals. Figure a in Box 20.1 indicates the expected physical stimuli and uses bradykinin and histamine as examples of chemicals that directly stimulate the nerve terminals. Both bradykinin and histamine act on their cell surface G-protein coupled receptors, directly activating the nerve to fire action potentials. The nociceptive nerve terminals stimulate two main types of fibres in the primary pain afferent nerves which carry the action potentials to the spinal cord. These are the fast myelinated **Aδ fibres** and the slow **C fibres**.

Modulation of pain at the level of the nociceptor: prostaglandins, opioids, and the TRPV1 receptor. Importantly for the action of drugs like aspirin and ibuprofen (non-steroidal anti-inflammatories (NSAIDs), see below) these responses to the pain-eliciting stimuli are increased by prostaglandins. Stimuli which stimulate phospholipase A$_2$ (PLA$_2$, see the Introduction to Section 3) therefore cause an increased synthesis of prostaglandins in the adjacent cells. These then pass out of the cell and reach the prostaglandin receptors on the nociceptive nerve terminals. Prostaglandins do not stimulate the nerve terminals. They do, however, sensitize the pain terminal to painful stimuli. We know this because if you inject prostaglandins beneath the skin of a volunteer it does not hurt. If instead you inject bradykinin it does hurt. If you inject bradykinin with prostaglandins it hurts even more! The response has been sensitized by prostaglandins. In the example of sunburn mentioned in the introduction to this chapter the skin is sensitized in

part by UV-enhanced prostaglandin synthesis, lowering the threshold for stimulation of nociceptive terminals.

The enhanced response to a normally painful stimulus is called **hyperalgesia**. When a normally non-painful stimulus elicits pain this is called **allodynia**. Here hyperalgesia and allodynia have been introduced at the first level of pain perception, the nociceptor, but it is reasonable that contributing mechanisms occur at all levels of pain perception.

Contrary to the effects of prostaglandins, there is evidence that opioids (both endogenous and drugs such as morphine) suppress activation of nociceptors as one of the several mechanisms by which they act as analgesics (see below). The conflicting actions of prostaglandins and opioids at the nociceptor level are illustrated in Figure 20.1. Also shown is the presence of the TRPV1 receptor, which integrates signals coming into the nociceptor, modulating the output sent to the spinal cord. All of these elements are targets for analgesic drugs.

Stimulation of non-nociceptive afferent fibres can reduce the 'upward' transmission of pain. Also featured at Level 1 in Box 20.1 (Figure a) are other afferent nerve terminals which respond to a variety of stimuli but excite action potentials in non-nociceptive nerve fibres

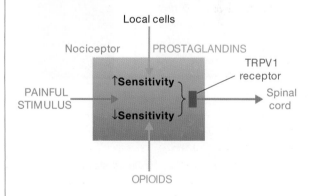

Figure 20.1 Enhancing, inhibiting, and modulating the sensitivity of the pain receptor (the nociceptor).

The nociceptor is located in the tissue at the receiving end of the painful stimulus (e.g. in skin, viscera, etc.) and is the first point at which the pain pathway is activated. This very simplified figure shows that even at this first step there are moderating influences at work. Prostaglandins, e.g. produced from stressed/damaged adjacent cells, sensitize the nociceptor (so it becomes more easily activated) while opioids desensitize the nociceptor (it becomes less easily activated). The vanilloid TRPV1 receptor plays a role in integrating painful stimuli and modulating the output of the nociceptor.

---

1. We are concerned here with systemic pain relief: local anaesthetics generally work by blocking the *transmission* of pain.

Box 20.1

Pain: how it reaches the brain—nociception and inhibitory pathways

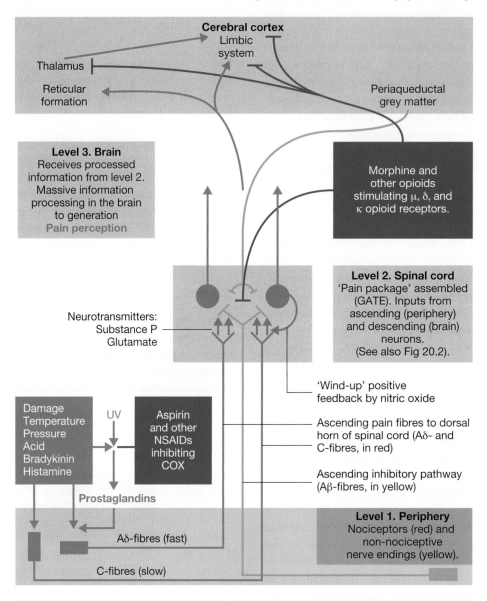

Figure a

Ascending and descending pathways in pain perception. The process starts at the bottom of the figure, with the stimulation of pain afferents (red, C-fibres and Aδ-fibres), and ascends to pain perception in the brain via the information processing interface in the spinal cord. Inhibition of pain perception is shown in the form of ascending non-pain afferents and descending inhibitory neurons from the brain, both attenuating synaptic events in the ascending pain pathway in the spinal cord

Pain perception is the end of a process which begins with stimulation of nociceptors, shown in red on the left. These are nerve endings which send axons that carry action potentials, either fast in the Aδ-fibres or slow in the C-fibres, directly to the dorsal horn of the spinal cord. Here they synapse with ascending pain neurons.

Examples of the neurotransmitters are substance P or glutamate, acting on neurokinin 1 or AMPA and NMDA receptors respectively. From here axons ascend directly to the brain. Moderation and information processing takes place from the first step at the nociceptors (see Figure 20.1) at the spinal cord (Figure 20.2), and in the brain. The *gate* occurs at the level of the spinal cord, both ascending (from non-nociceptive afferent pathways) and descending (from brain) inhibitory neurons can shut down the assembly of the 'pain package' of information before it reaches the brain. The modulation of the process at the nociceptors by non-steroidal anti-inflammatories (note they also work elsewhere) and the brain and spinal cord by opioid analgesics is shown in blue.

(Aβ fibres). These synapse in the spinal cord, influencing the processing of pain signals in Level 2.

Level 2: The dorsal horn of the spinal cord

Ascending sensory fibres (including nociceptive Aδ and C fibers and non-nociceptive Aβ fibers) synapse in the substantia gelatinosa of the dorsal horn of the spinal cord at every level of the neuraxis (i.e. from the neck to the base of the spine). There they synapse with the cell bodies of neurons (nociresponsive neurons), stimulating a train of action potentials which carry the signal up to the brain, where it may be perceived as pain. Stimulating this train of action potentials requires depolarization of the cell body of the nociresponsive neuron. The primary pain afferents release neurotransmitters which do this (i.e. act on receptors which cause depolarization). This is illustrated in Figure 20.2 by reference to substance P and glutamate, released from the terminals of the Aδ and C neurons. Substance P acts on its NK1 (named after neurokinin) and glutamate on its NMDA and AMPA receptors (see Chapters 16 and 18).

The ascending pain signal is weakened by inhibitory neurons

The transmission of information in the ascending pain pathway is regulated by a number of mechanisms at the level of the synapse in the spinal cord. An inhibitory input is provided by non-painful stimuli activating the Aβ fibres which inhibit the synapse (Figure 20.2). This pathway is activated by a variety of stimuli and may explain the pain-reducing effect of mechanostimulation such as rubbing the skin. A mechanism such as this may also contribute to the analgesic effect of small non-painful electrical stimulation of the skin by procedures such as transcutaneous electrical stimulation (**TENS**). Commonly used as an analgesics device, for example in childbirth,

TENS may activate ascending inhibitory fibres which attenuate pain signals at the level of the spinal cord synapse.

Of great importance is the descending inhibitory pathway, which has its origins in several levels of the brain. Shown in Figure 20.2 and Box 20.1 is the periaqueductal grey. This is in the midbrain. It receives and processes information from higher brain centres (e.g. limbic regions, hypothalamus, and cortex), projecting to synapse in the brainstem raphe nuclei. These are collections of serotoninergic (5-HT) neuron cell bodies that send axons down the spinal cord to an interneuron in the dorsal horn, releasing opioid neurotransmitters that inhibit the ascending pain synapse shown in Figure 20.2. The opioid peptides do this by stimulating their receptors (μ, δ, and κ opioid), and the activation of these spinal receptors is one of the mechanisms whereby drugs such as morphine bring about their analgesic effect.

It is possible to directly activate with drugs the spinal mechanisms which reduce the upward transmission of pain signals. This is called **epidural analgesia**—drugs such as opiates are directly introduced into the epidural space of the spinal cord with a catheter—which is used in childbirth or postoperatively.

Nitric oxide forms a short excitatory loop that enhances transmission of pain signals

Stimulation of the ascending pain pathway synapse in the dorsal horn of the spinal cord leads to release from the cell body of nitric oxide (NO), as illustrated in Figure 20.2. This acts as a membrane permeable retrograde neurotransmitter, i.e. it drifts out of the postsynaptic site 'back' to the presynaptic site, where it excites further neurotransmission. The result is that repeated stimulation

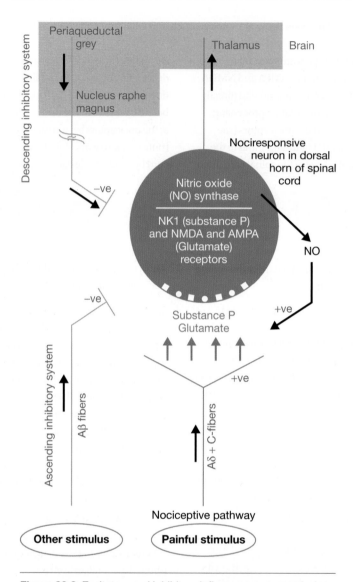

Figure 20.2 Excitatory and inhibitory influences on transmission of pain signals in the spinal cord.

This is an illustration of the processing of information which takes place at the dorsal horn of the spinal cord. Signals from the ascending pain pathway, carrying pain signals from their source up to the brain, are shown in red (with substance P and glutamate shown as examples of the excitatory neurotransmitters). On the left side (yellow) inhibitory pathways are shown both ascending from the periphery and descending from the brain. On the right retrograde transmission is shown—excitation in the cell body leads to release of nitric oxide (NO), which then acts on the synapse to enhance subsequent synaptic responses.

of the pathways leads to an augmentation of neurotransmission and an increased perception of pain despite a steady level of the original painful stimulus. This process is sometimes called 'wind up': earlier stimuli 'wind up' the responses to later stimuli. Spinal 'wind up' may not only amplify the short-term pain, but its positive feedback may cause pain signalling to the brain to persist beyond the input of pain signals to the spinal cord, so this is one possible contributor to the continuation of pain even when the painful stimulus has ended.

Level 3: The brain

The pathways in the brain responsible for the processing of pain signals and for the experience of pain are complex and poorly understood, and not separate from other cognitive and emotional functions. The latter point encourages the recognition that how much pain you experience is not just the result of the input of nociceptive signals to the brain, but is the outcome of this in the context of your expectations, confidence, fears, happiness/unhappiness, control over events, arousal, etc. On a simpler level we can say that pain inputs from the spinal cord project directly to the reticular system and the thalamus, and then on limbic and cortical systems, where our conscious experience of pain is moulded. In these processes, which probably involve the full and bewildering complex of different brain neurotransmitters and receptors, the opioid peptide neurotransmitters (e.g. enkephalins, endorphins, and dynorphin) and their receptors (μ, δ, and κ) have a major role to play. Not surprisingly, these brain opioid systems are also important for the analgesic action of morphine and the related drugs described below.

20.2 Assessment of pain

Pain can only be effectively managed if it is properly assessed and its consequences correctly evaluated.

Visual analogue and verbal rating scales are the most common tools used to determine pain severity and aid in the choice of analgesia. They provide information about the pattern, duration, location, and characterization of

20.1.2 What the spinal cord tells the brain: gate control

We can see from the discussion of Level 2 above that a great deal of information processing relating to pain signals takes place in the dorsal horn of the spinal cord. This will occur with inputs at all levels of the spine, from the bottom of the sacral vertebrae (the tail) to the top of the cervical vertebrae (up to the head). At Level 2 the pain signal inputs from the periphery can be shut down or allowed to proceed. In other words the local neural network acts as a gate, deciding which signal to let through to the brain, which to reduce, and which to shut down. This decision will be influenced by many things, including the information sent down from the higher brain centres, which we have described above as descending inhibitory influences, and the ascending inhibitory inputs of peripheral origin carried to the spinal cord by Aβ afferent neurons (Figurre 20.2). This view of pain perception is called the **gate control** theory, and has been very influential in understanding the clinical management of pain, including the use of pain-relieving drugs.

pain. Figure 20.3 provides an indication of the nature of visual/verbal scales.

These scales help the patient rate and portray the subjective feeling of pain they are experiencing. The pain severity is whatever the patient says it is and the clinician must not let personal bias interfere with choice of treatment.

20.3 Analgesic drugs

Analgesic drugs are those that are used to relieve pain. They do this by interacting with the pain perception pathways described above. In considering the biology of pain perception we note that, as expected, a number of neurotransmitters are involved in the journey of the pain signal from the stimulation of the nociceptor to the conscious experience of pain. These include those which carry the pain signals, such as substance P and glutamate in the dorsal horn of the spinal cord (Figure 20.2), and those involved in the gating mechanisms leading to attenuation of the pain signal, such as the opioid peptides. These synapses are an obvious point at which drugs might act; in clinical analgesia, however, we have no drugs acting

directly to reduce the upward glutamate- and substance P-dependent neurotransmission, nor acting on the NO-dependent retrograde neurotransmission (Figure 2.2) responsible for amplifying pain conduction in the spinal cord ('wind-up'). We do, however, have a variety of drugs which mimic the opioid component of the pain inhibitory mechanisms. These are called the **opioid analgesics**.[2] The other main class of drugs, the **non-opioid analgesics**, are dominated by the NSAIDs such as aspirin and

---

2. Opioid or opiate? The native system (receptors and peptides) is always referred to as opioid. The drugs may be called opioid (preferred by many) or opiate; since both may be encountered in the literature, both are used here.

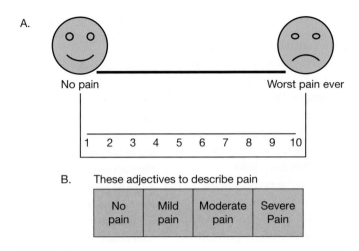

Figure 20.3

Assessment of pain. Two schemes are illustrated, which may be used together. **A,** An example of a visual analogue scale is a 10-cm long line labelled with two extremes at each end. One extreme is labelled 'no pain' and the other is labelled the 'worst pain ever'. The patient marks on the line provided. This means that the patient's experience of pain does not have to be translated into words. In **B** the patient is prompted to choose from a choice of words to indicate the nature of the painful experience. Note that in each case it is the *experience* of pain which is being expressed and assessed, not the intensity of the pain-inducing stimulus.

ibuprofen, which we have previously encountered in Section 3, and paracetamol (acetaminophen).

20.3.1 The opioid analgesics

The origin of the opioid analgesic drugs was opium collected from poppies, as indicated in Box 20.2. Morphine is the major active ingredient of opium. Despite the generation of many derivatives, morphine remains the most important analgesic in clinical use, against which the performance of other drugs is measured. Morphine is not the most powerful opioid drug. Etorphine, for example, is many times more potent than morphine but due to powerful unwanted effects cannot be used in the clinic—its main use is as an anaesthetic for elephants!

In Chapter 2 we mention several aspects of drug action at its receptors, including **affinity**, **potency** and **efficacy**:

- Affinity and potency. Firstly, think of the *concentration* of drug necessary to occupy the receptors. The lower the concentration (e.g. the amount required to **occupy half the receptors**) the greater the affinity of the drug

for the receptor. A high affinity will contribute to a high potency—the concentration required to give **half the maximal response**.

- Efficacy. Think of how strongly the drug activates a receptor once it is bound. A drug that binds and maximally activates its receptor (high efficacy) is a **full agonist**. If it binds but does not activate the receptor at all (no efficacy) then it is a pure **antagonist**—it will prevent an agonist from binding. If it binds and can only partly activate the receptor then it is a **partial agonist**. A partial agonist can both stimulate the receptor (but not fully) and act as an antagonist in the presence of a full agonist, which it may displace from the receptor.

Here, in the clinical pharmacology of the opioids, we can see the relevance of these issues to understanding safe and effective pain management—we encounter full agonists, partial agonists, and pure antagonists.

There is a further complexity, which is that there are three opioid receptors to consider. Drugs may independently vary in their potency and efficacy for these receptors,

Box 20.2
Opioid peptides, opioid receptors, and opiate drugs

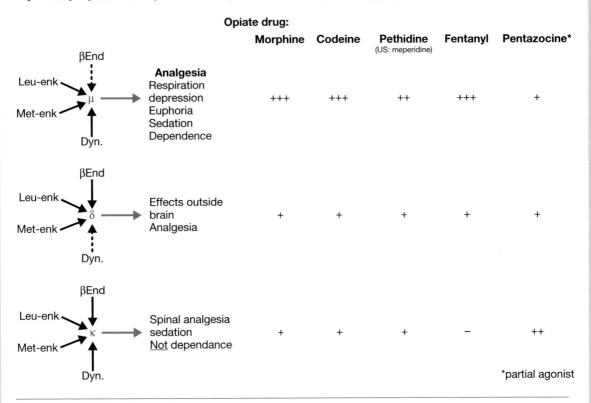

| | Opiate drug: | | | | |
	Morphine	Codeine	Pethidine (US: meperidine)	Fentanyl	Pentazocine*
Analgesia Respiration depression Euphoria Sedation Dependence	+++	+++	++	+++	+
Effects outside brain Analgesia	+	+	+	+	+
Spinal analgesia sedation Not dependance	+	+	+	−	++

*partial agonist

Figure b

Three types of opioid receptor (μ, δ, and κ). The endogenous peptides that stimulate them are shown on the left, some consequences of their stimulation are shown in the middle, and examples of the drugs that stimulate them on the right. The number of + signs indicates the extent to which each receptor type is activated by the drug to give the therapeutic response.

Certain poppies have for centuries been cultivated for the narcotic properties of opium, the crude extract which exudes from a cut poppy seed capsule. Opium contains morphine and some other active compounds, including codeine. Morphine and these other active compounds have been extracted and characterized, providing the origin of the current collection of clinically used opiate analgesic drugs. Semisynthetic derivatives have been made. This means the extracted morphine is chemically modified to create a new drug. An example is the derivative diacetylmorphine, or diamorphine, also known as heroin. The first completely synthetic opiate was pethidine (meperidine), which bears only a passing structural resemblance to morphine.

Morphine and its derivatives are now known to act in the brain and elsewhere on a specific family of cell surface G protein-coupled receptors that are part of the endogenous opioid system. The receptors are stimulated by a number (>20) of natural agonists, the opioid peptides. The prominent and widespread examples shown in Figure b are the two enkephalins, leu-enkephalin (Leu-enk) and met-enkephalin (Met-enk), β-endorphin (β-End), and dynorphin (Dyn). These are released as neurotransmitters from certain central nervous system and peripheral nerves, activating the three main receptors, designated μ, δ, and κ (kappa) opioid receptors.

Also shown in this scheme are some clinically significant drugs and the degree to which they activate the different receptors, indicated by the number of + signs. In this scheme +++ means a drug strongly binds and activates the receptor. These indications of the strength of a drug at each receptor are a consequence of both potency (affinity or binding to the receptor) and efficacy (ability to activate the receptors), as explained in Chapter 2 and section 20.3.1

of this chapter. The scheme shows clearly the different effects of drugs at different receptors, but that mostly the therapeutic analgesics are strong stimulators of the μ opioid receptor.

---

contributing to their different effects. Box 20.2 introduces the three receptors (μ, δ, and κ, as mentioned above), the clinical responses to their activation, and their pattern of stimulation by both native opioid neurotransmitters (the opioid peptides) and some clinically used opiate drugs. Notably, the most effective clinically effective analgesics are powerful stimulators of the μ opioid receptors. Indeed, the analgesic effect of therapeutic opioid drugs is thought to be principally via the μ opioid receptor. The same is true for much of the rewarding aspects of taking opiates, and with the development of tolerance and dependence. If stimulation of μ receptors makes you feel very good, but this effect gets less with repeated stimulation, then you will need increasing amounts of drug to give the same effect (tolerance), absence of the drug may leave you feeling very bad (dependence), and addiction may follow (Box 20.3).

Non-analgesic effects of opioid analgesics

There is a common pattern of non-analgesic effects, many but not all of which are unwanted.

- **Nausea** and **vomiting** are always unwanted. These are central effects.
- **Reduced gut motility** is due to action at mesenteric μ receptors. This is the basis of the treatment of **diarrhoea** with morphine (mixed with kaolin) and with **loperamide**, which is a μ receptor agonist with the enormous advantage of having no central effects. Loperamide is the active ingredient in various proprietary antidiarrhoea treatments. However, reduced gut motility resulting in **constipation** is an unwanted effect in the context of pain management with opioids.
- **Euphoria** accompanies the use of morphine and related drugs in pain management. Aspects may be desirable in some circumstances, but it is mostly undesirable and is a component of the abuse of these drugs.
- **Drowsiness** may under some circumstances be desirable.

- **Cough suppression** (antitussive effect) is common to opioid analgesics, exploited in cough-supressant preparations.
- **Miosis** is the reduction in the pupil of the eye—'pin-point' pupils—which commonly accompanies opioid use. It is not seen with pethidine (meperidine).
- At higher doses **respiratory depression** is an acute danger, leading to death in overdose.

Overdose is a concern with morphine-like drugs. Overdose causes coma, respiratory depression, and death. Miosis ('pin-point' pupils) with respiratory depression may help in the recognition of opioid overdose. The treatment of overdose is to use the pure antagonist **naloxone**. Naloxone may be given intravenously, when it will rapidly reverse opioid-induced respiratory depression, and is a life-saving treatment in this medical emergency. It is of relatively short half-life with an effective action of 2–4 hours, so repeated administration may be necessary to avoid return to a respiratory-depressed state.

Tolerance to morphine may lead to dependence. The effect of morphine will reduce with repeated administration—more drug will have to be given to have the same effect. This is called tolerance. At the same time dependence may occur. This means normal function is dependent on the presence of the drug. Tolerance and dependence can lead to addiction. This is discussed further in Box 20.3. The extent to which tolerance and dependence occur within the therapeutic setting varies enormously, depending on the drug, its dose, route of administration, clinical problem, and individual patient. It is widely accepted that such issues should not restrict the use of powerful analgesics in pain relief for terminally ill patients. However, within a drug-abuse setting repeated use of a full opiate agonist such as morphine or heroin will always lead to tolerance, dependence, and addiction. This process starts with the first use of such a drug.

Box 20.3
Tolerance, dependence, and addiction to opioids

When an opioid drug such as morphine is repeatedly administered to an experimental animal so that it is continuously present then the response to the drug will reduce with the passage of time and the animal will appear to be returning to the condition it was in before the drug was started. To get an effect it will be necessary to escalate the dose of drug given. This adaptive process in the animal will begin within a few hours of continual presence of the drug and continue to develop over days. What is happening to the animal during this period of time? Is this the same pattern of events which leads to drug abuse and drug addiction? Does the same thing happen if a drug is given to a patient?

Experimental tolerance and dependence Returning for a moment to the experimental animal, as the period of time with morphine becomes extended, the physiology of the animal changes in an attempt to restore normal function. Consider two aspects of the situation:

- The animal will no longer change in response to the next same dose of morphine. This lack of response (or reduced response) is called **tolerance**. To gain an equivalent response may require an increased dose of drug.

- If the morphine is taken away then the changed physiology of the animal will become apparent as the drug level falls and the animal will seem to be sick. Normal function is dependent on the presence of the drug. This is called **dependence**.

Tolerance begins with cellular tolerance What are the changes that occur in the experimental animal that give rise to this tolerance and dependence? We know that morphine actions starts at the three types of opioid receptor (see Box 20.2) and it is not surprising that changes begin with down-regulation of opioid receptors. Down-regulation here means that the same stimulation of the receptor by an agonist gives a reduced signal from the receptor into the cell. With opioid analgesics it is the occurrence of these events at the μ receptor (Box 20.2) that is thought to be the most important for understanding clinical issues.

Cellular tolerance can have many components:

- Reduced receptor number. Receptors are internalized and destroyed in response to agonist binding faster than they are replaced at the cell surface

- Reduced receptor coupling. The μ opioid receptors are G-protein coupled receptors (GPCRs), which are coupled through Gi/o heterotrimeric G proteins (see Chapter 2) to a variety of responses inside the cell. They become desensitized on exposure to agonists as a result of a variety of mechanisms, such as phosphorylation of the receptor and internalization. As a result they uncouple from their signalling mechanisms.

- Reduced levels of effectors proteins or changed responsiveness of effectors proteins. GPCRs often have their effect through changing the activity of enzymes and ion channels (Chapter 2).

Following this, within the cell there may be a host of cellular events downstream of the receptor, where the cell adapts and generates a smaller response to repeated stimulation with opioid drugs.

Tolerance in neuronal networks In the central nervous system processes of tolerance and dependence also occur through adaptive changes of neuronal networks and information processing. This may occur in the information processing that occurs in the spinal cord and subsequently in the brain. Putting this all in the framework provided by Box 20.2, we can envisage a process of tolerance that becomes more complex as we move from the nociceptor, through the pain pathways with their synapses, neurotransmitters and receptors, up to the brain, and ultimately the higher centres where pain perception is finally assembled.

Dependence (and addiction) may follow from tolerance This pattern of events may mean not only that the brain produces a less benevolent response to the administered drug (contributing to tolerance), but also that if the drug is removed then there will be less response to the natively released opioid peptides (contributing to dependence). This may be aversive (unpleasant, for animal or person). The collection of aversive events following removal of the drug is referred to as the **abstinence syndrome**. In an opiate-addicted person it may be severe and prolonged.

Addiction and drug-seeking behaviour To avoid or terminate the intolerable effects of absence of the drug leads to **drug-seeking behaviour**, and here we may feel we have reached an understanding of the biological basis of **addiction** to opiates (e.g. heroin addiction) in humans. In drug addicts it is the drug-seeking behaviour itself (e.g. crime and prostitution) that is most devastating for individuals and damaging for society.

Treating opiate addiction with opiates There are many approaches, and many controversies, concerning the treatment of those addicted to opiates. However, one notion is clear: if addicts have reliable access to acceptable opiate drugs then they will not need to pursue destructive drug-seeking behaviour. A strategy for withdrawal can then be pursued. This is the basis of methadone clinics. Methadone is orally available, with a long half-life, and will prevent the occurrence of an abstinence syndrome in opiate addicts. Methadone itself is addictive. The abstinence syndrome following methadone addiction is itself likely to be more prolonged than with morphine, perhaps less intense. However, a stable addict getting drugs through a methadone clinic may be better than an addict accessing street drugs through the proceeds of crime. Furthermore **replacement therapy** with methadone will often be tied to a reduction strategy, with the objective of eliminating opiate usage.

Methadone clinics are not acceptable to all societies and in many places are unavailable.

Tolerance, dependence, and addiction in the therapeutic setting Long-term analgesia with opioids must take into account issues of tolerance (may need to give increasing doses to achieve the same amount of pain relief). However, tolerance is not always seen within the therapeutic context. In addition there is the possible development of dependence. Addiction is less likely to be the outcome—very considerable individual patient variation may be encountered, with some vulnerable patients identified as at risk. Dependence may commonly be seen as a mild/moderate abstinence syndrome on abrupt withdrawal—some indicators of physiological function take over a month to return to normal. Dependence may commonly be dealt with by a slow tapered withdrawal (i.e. slowly reducing the dose over weeks).

Considerable investment has gone into trying to develop powerful opioid analgesics without addition potential. Some success has been achieved, for example the partial agonists like buprenorphine, while not free of addiction potential, are not sought by heroin addicts, but the goal of an addiction-free analgesic as effective as morphine has not been reached.

Some opioid analgesic drugs

Morphine is clinically the mainstay of opioid analgesia. Generally the various opioid drugs available have much of their pharmacology in common with morphine. This can be seen in the scheme presented in Box 20.2.

Morphine is very widely used for the relief of acute and chronic pain. It has a half-life of about 4 hours, with some metabolites having analgesic activity. It can be taken orally, when it is slowly absorbed, and so where rapid pain relief is required it is administered by intravenous or intramuscular injection. For relief of chronic pain, slow-release preparations are available. It has all the effects described above, with dependence and tolerance leading to a high addiction potential.

Diamorphine (heroin) is the acetylated derivative of morphine, with which it shares most of its pharmacology,

including highly effective pain relief. Diamorphine enters the brain more rapidly than morphine, which in some circumstances may give it some advantages in pain relief and which probably contributes to its popularity as a drug of abuse. It is not legally available in all countries.

Codeine (methylmorphine) occurs naturally (along with morphine) in crude opium. It is much less effective than morphine in pain relief, but it is suitable for the relief of mild pain. Codeine has the advantage of having less addiction potential and so is widely available. Codeine is anticough (antitussive) and causes constipation. Its derivative, **dihydrocodeine**, has similar analgesic activity.

Pethidine has been favoured for pain relief in childbirth. This is because new babies with their immature livers do not metabolize other opioids effectively, leading to more danger of respiratory depression. Pethidine has a shorter half-life in the adult and is more effectively cleared by the newborn, resulting in less respiratory depression. Constipation is less likely to be a problem than with morphine. However, pethidine has significantly less analgesic activity and with its shorter half-life it is not a good drug for control of long-term severe pain. Pethidine also has an unusual spectrum of toxic effects which have contributed to its limited use.

Fentanyl is a highly potent μ agonist requiring about 100-fold lower dose than morphine to give the same analgesic effect. This, combined with its short duration of action, makes is useful in analgesia during surgery. A number of derivatives are available for clinical use, such as **alfentanil**, which has a duration of action of just a few minutes, making it useful during certain surgical procedures. Importantly, fentanyl may be encountered in the long-term treatment of chronic pain when delivered as a transdermal patch—stuck to the skin like a large plaster this will provide steady release of a specified amount of drug in each hour of use. The very high potency of fentanyl makes it a very effective drug in the treatment of cancer pain. It is also available as a lozenge to be slowly absorbed in the mouth in the treatment of breakthrough pain.

Remifentanil is another rapid-onset, ultra short half-life drug used in infusion as anaesthesia during surgery. On cessation of infusion it has a half-life of about 4 minutes, a result of its metabolism by esterases widely present in plasma and tissues. This means that there will be no problem with drug-induced respiratory depression following surgery when this drug is used.

Pentazocine and **buprenorphine** are different because they are partial agonists: they bind to the receptors, but maximal activation is less than when morphine binds. Hence they are less effective as analgesics than morphine, more effective than codeine. Being partial agonists gives them both agonist and antagonist activity, meaning that they both deliver analgesia alone and may precipitate withdrawal symptoms in a morphine or heroin-using addict (see Box 20.3). As a result these drugs are not favoured by drug abusers.

However, the search for potent opioid analgesics which lack addiction potential does not end here, since when taken alone these drugs do have drug dependence and addiction potential. Furthermore, as well as precipitating withdrawal in addicts these drugs may also precipitate pain in patients already gaining pain relief from morphine.

Pentazocine has number of specific unwanted effects, including hallucinations, and is seldom recommended.

Buprenorphine has a number of interesting characteristics.

1) Compared to morphine it has a very high affinity for the receptor, contributing to high potency. This means that a small amount of drug is effective, e.g. 0.2–0.4 mg buprenorphine compared to 10 mg morphine.

2) It has lower efficacy (it stimulates the receptor less than morphine), so its maximal effect is less. It neatly illustrates the difference between potency and efficacy (Chapter 2 and section 20.3.1 above).

3) It has high first-pass metabolism and so is not used orally (i.e. swallowed), but may be used with transdermal (skin) patches or sublingually (i.e. absorbed from the mouth, e.g. beneath the tongue).

4) It has a very long half-life—used sublingually it is an effective analgesic for up to 8 hours for chronic pain relief.

5) It has a very high affinity for μ opioid receptors, so is not easily displaced by naloxone, the pure opioid antagonist. This affects treatment of overdose (see above).

6) It is also a partial agonist at a related class of receptor, the nociceptin/orphanin (NOP) receptor; this may be related to its proposed use to reduce alcohol consumption.

Tramadol is another interesting drug with analgesia action that is partly opioid in action (it is a weak agonist) and partly due to action at serotonin (5-hydroxytryptamine; 5-HT) and noradrenaline pathways in the brain. Because its analgesic effect is only partly opioid it gives less respiratory depression than a pure opioid analgesic. It is widely used for post-operative pain relief.

20.3.2 The non-opioid analgesics

This group includes the most commonly used drugs for the relief of mild to moderate pain: the NSAIDs (e.g. aspirin and ibuprofen) and paracetamol (acetaminophen). You will already be familiar with these drug names, but it is important to realize that these drugs are not interchangeable. There are fundamental differences between aspirin, ibuprofen, and paracetamol which should inform their optimal use, both in terms of achieving the required pain relief and in minimizing unwanted effects and dangers to the patient. These differences can be easily understood and are set out below.

The action of the NSAIDs is discussed in Section 3 when we consider the anti-inflammatory action of these drugs. The same molecular action, the inhibition of cyclooxygenase (COX, see section 9.3.1 and Box S3.1) and the consequent reduction in synthesis of prostaglandins and related compounds (prostanoids), accounts for the anti-inflammatory, analgesic (e.g. Figure 20.1) and antiplatelet (Section 2) effects of aspirin. In the treatment of many painful conditions a combined analgesic and anti-inflammatory action is beneficial, and so in these cases the NSAIDs are particularly appropriate. Their use in chronic inflammatory illnesses is covered in Chapter 9.

In addition to the desired range of effects described above, the NSAIDs are liable to cause gastric problems—inhibition of COX reduces the protection of the gut against stomach acidity—as discussed in Chapter 12. This is a major problem and reduces the use of NSAIDs in sensitive individuals.

Paracetamol (acetaminophen) has many actions in common with NSAIDs, but as it lacks anti-inflammatory effects it is less useful in some inflammation/pain conditions. It is, however, less likely to give rise to gastric problems, contributing to its widespread use.

Here we discuss pain relief by the NSAIDs and two other non-opioid analgesics, paracetamol and nefopam. Finally, the treatment of migraine, and of neuropathic pain introduces some other interesting analgesic drugs and these will be briefly mentioned.

NSAIDs in analgesia

The use of aspirin and other NSAIDs as analgesics should be considered in conjunction with their use as anti-inflammatory agents as discussed elsewhere (section 9.3.1), and here only brief comments relating to pain relief will be presented.

NSAIDs are used for mild/moderate pain, especially when associated with inflammation. It should be noted that maximal pain relief is less than with the most effective opioids. NSAIDs are particularly less effective with severe visceral pain. Hence the common uses of NSAIDs include for:

1) headache, back pain, sunburn

2) some pain associated with bone and other cancers (the tumour is likely to be releasing prostanoids)

3) injury pain such as broken bones and surgery

4) period pains (dysmenorrhea) with its increased prostanoid synthesis.

All NSAIDs have gastric irritation and erosions as potential serious side effects. Consequently, NSAIDs are not prescribed to those with a history of ulcers. The propensity to produce gastric effects varies between different NSAIDs and between patients (elderly patients are at greater risk), and these issues help to guide optimal prescribing. Enteric coating of certain preparations (the tablet does not dissolve in the acid environment of the stomach, but is soluble in the higher pH found in the intestines) is intended to reduce the gastric problems associated with these drugs.

NSAIDs should also not be prescribed to patients with advanced heart failure. The selective COX-2 inhibitors (which have a reduced propensity for gastric effects) and their associated cardiovascular risks have been discussed in Chapter 9 (section 9.2.1).

Caution should be observed in the use of NSAIDs in asthmatic patients (Chapter 11) —a minority of asthmatics are NSAID sensitive. These and other issues related to risks and drug interactions with NSAIDs are explored in Chapter 9. Here we shall make additional comments on only three NSAIDs in the context of pain relief.

Aspirin has an action that substantially outlasts its presence, since it covalently modifies and permanently inactivates both COX-1 and COX-2 (section 9.3.1). Recovery can only come, therefore, from synthesis of new COX protein from the cell. Hence the daily dose to produce analgesia will be much greater than to inhibit platelets, since the platelets have no nucleus and are therefore unable to synthesize new COX, while the prostanoid synthesizing cells contributing to pain will be able to replace their own COX protein over a number of hours.

Aspirin is mainly used for short-term muscle and joint pain, headache, period pains, and for patients with high temperature (fever, pyrexia). Its limited use is largely because of gastric problems (Chapter 12), from mild stomach upset (dyspepsia) to ulcers and gastric bleeding and erosion/perforation of the gastric lining. This problem may be reduced by taking aspirin with food or by the use of soluble aspirin tablets (which more rapidly disperse the drug) or buffered preparations (which may transiently reduce acidity in the stomach). In routine use, such as over-the-counter sales for headaches and similar commonly encountered discomforts, ibuprofen (see below) is often preferred because of its reduced gastric irritant effect. Where the anti-inflammatory effect is not required, paracetamol (see below) may be a better option.

Warfarin is an anticoagulant described in Chapter 4. It is commonly taken for months or years; many patients seeking advice on pain relief will be taking warfarin. Aspirin is not an anticoagulant drug, but it is antiplatelet (Chapter 4) and may exacerbate bleeding issues in patients taking warfarin. Paracetamol should be considered as an alternative.

Aspirin (or aspirin-containing products) should not be taken by children and young adults due to the danger of Reye's syndrome, which is a potentially fatal degradation of a number of vital organs. The exact age below which aspirin is prohibited varies between countries.

Aspirin has, however, achieved considerable popularity in its use as an antiplatelet drug, taken by the mature population and at a low daily dose, reducing the side effects issues.

Ibuprofen (and related drugs such as naproxen, which are sometimes described as propionic acid derivatives) has become a drug of first choice in the treatment of mild to moderate inflammation-associated pain because it is effective and generates fewer side effects, especially relating to the upper gastrointestinal tract. It is a non-selective COX inhibitor with only a mild short-lived antiplatelet effect. Its clinical effect lasts 4–8 hours, depending on dose. While available over the counter, the maximum daily dose is considerably less than that which may be medically prescribed.

Diclofenac is an interesting example of an NSAID. It is a very potent drug, acting as an inhibitor of COX with some selectivity for COX-2, but it is suspected that other actions may contribute to its clinical response, possibly including inhibition of lipoxygenase and phospholipase A_2 (See the Introduction to Section 3, Box S3.1) and other actions such as the use-dependent block of voltage-dependent Na^+ channels, a type of drug action explained in Chapter 16 (Box 16.2).

Paracetamol (acetaminophen)

Paracetamol and ibuprofen are the most commonly used drugs for the treatment of mild musculoskeletal pain and simple headaches. They are, however, fundamentally different drugs in that paracetamol is not anti-inflammatory,

while ibuprofen is. However, paracetamol is as effective as aspirin as an analgesic for commonplace mild pain, and it is also an effective antipyretic (meaning it lowers the temperature of a patient with fever). It is well tolerated, without the gastric problems associated with NSAIDs. It may be appropriate for short-term treatment of patients taking warfarin (NSAIDs may be inappropriate because of an antiplatelet effect, mentioned above and in Chapter 3).

The exact mechanisms by which paracetamol acts to generate its antipyretic and analgesic effects in the absence of an anti-inflammatory effect are not entirely understood. It is an inhibitor of COX enzymes and therefore has a mode of action in common with the NSAIDs. This results in inhibition of prostaglandin synthesis (but paracetamol does not effectively inhibit thromboxane synthesis in platelets). It seems likely that a spectrum of effects on different COX enzymes, combined with other mechanisms of action, account for its pattern of effects.

Paracetamol is available in preparations for children for the relief of mild pain and fever. Preparations containing codeine are commonly sold as over-the-counter drugs and they may offer some benefits for some patients over paracetamol alone. The patient in Workbook 17 is prescribed a proprietary codeine/paracetamol compound preparation, and it is noted that these preparations prevent independent titration of benefits/ unwanted effects for these two different types of analgesic. Compound preparations with dihydrocodeine are also available, whereas the once popular combination of paracetamol with the opiate dextropropoxyphene should no longer be prescribed.

Paracetamol overdose. The biggest problem with paracetamol is that it is dangerous on overdose. This can occur from taking 10 g per day or more—remember that with tablets containing 500 mg this means 20 tablets may be cause for concern. In a child think of 150 mg/kg body weight. While there may be short-term discomfort (e.g. vomiting), which may disappear over a day or so, the real danger is delayed liver damage 3–6 days later, which may be fatal. Suspected paracetamol overdose is always a case for urgent hospital treatment. It is one of the most common causes of acute liver failure and the most common form of drug overdose in many parts of the world.

Nefopam

Nefopam is a non-opioid non-NSAID analgesic used to relieve moderate acute and chronic pain. Its effectiveness as an analgesic lies between that of aspirin and morphine. It may be used as an adjunct, alongside other analgesics. Despite having being around for over 25 years its mechanisms of action is not clear. It does inhibit noradrenaline, dopamine, and serotonin (5-HT) uptake in the brain, and this may contribute to its analgesic effects.

Drugs used to treat migraine

Migraine takes the form of severe headaches lasting from 4 hours to days, often with visual disturbances which may (in classic migraine) precede the headache, and frequently accompanied by nausea and vomiting. The cause is complex, but includes increased release of serotonin (5-HT), release of mediators of inflammation in the brain, and dilation of local blood vessels. Migraine treatment is in part with the analgesics already discussed, such as paracetamol and NSAIDs, often with an anti-emetic (anti-vomiting drug), such as **domperidone** or **metoclopramide**. Preparations containing codeine are to be avoided because they slow gastrointestinal movements, which may exacerbate the gut problems associated with migraine. When the headache is unresponsive to these standard analgesics a major role has developed for an interesting group of drugs that are antagonists at $5HT_1$ receptors, which control aspects of cerebral blood flow—their block leads to reduced local blood flow. Effects on the release of inflammatory mediators in the brain may also play a part. **Sumatriptan** is the archetypal member of this drug group, the triptans.

Novel analgesics proposed for use in migraine interestingly include TRPV1 antagonists. We encountered TRPV1 as a receptor involved in integrating the nociceptor response to pain signals, and encouraging results suggest that blocking this receptor may lead to much needed new analgesics.

Drugs used to treat neuropathic pain

Neuropathic pain is pain associated with damage to the nervous system—central or peripheral—rather than originating from the stimulation of nociceptors. It responds poorly to conventional analgesics, although there may be a role for certain opioids, including methadone and tramadol. Instead certain drugs acting on the brain and developed for other purposes have been found to be useful. **Amitryptyline** is an antidepressant drug discussed in Chapter 19. However, at lower doses, and apparently independent of the relief of depression, amitryptyline also has an analgesic effect and may be the drug of choice for neuropathic pain. **Gabapentin** and **pregabalin** are both antiepileptic drugs (Chapter 16) that have also found a use in the relief of neuralgic pain. In Workbook 17 at the end of this chapter we see that the Lucy is given gabapentin for the relief of spinal injury pain. Warmth has been found to be a non-pharmacological way to relieve pain in some circumstances and this may relate to the use of **capsaicin** in topical form (i.e. as an ointment applied to the skin) in neuropathic pain relief. Capsaicin is the substance that makes chilli peppers taste hot. It acts on the TRPV1 receptor, resulting, when applied to the skin, in the sensation of heat and a reduction in the sensation of neuropathic pain. The explanation for this is probably that the TRPV1 receptor is profoundly desensitized following activation by capsaicin and that it is this desensitization which leads to its analgesic effect.

SUMMARY OF COMMON DRUGS USED FOR PAIN AND ADDICTION

Therapeutic class	Drugs	Mechanism of action	Common clinical uses	Comments	Examples of adverse drug reactions
Non-opioid analgesia	NSAIDS	Inhibits the action of cyclooxegenase			
	Non-selective Cox-inhibitors Aspirin Ibuprofen Diclofenac	Diclofenac also inhibits lipoxygenase and phospholipase A_2 and other actions such as the use-dependent block of voltage dependent Na^+ channels	Pain and inflammation Antiplatelet (aspirin) Pyrexia	Very effective in inflammation Take with or after food	Gastrointestinal irritation
	Selective COX 2 inhibitors Rofecoxib Valdecoxib		Pain and inflammation	Caution in ischaemic heart disease Reserved for second-line use	Gastrointestinal irritation
	Nefopam	Theory is that it inhibits noradrenaline, dopamine, and serotonin (5-HT) uptake in the brain	Moderate pain		Nausea nervousness Urinary retention
	Paracetamol	1) Inhibits prostaglandin synthesis in the central nervous system 2) Blocks pain-impulse generation in periphery through inhibition of prostaglandin synthesis and other substances that sensitize pain receptors to mechanical or chemical stimulation	Mild to moderate pain	First-line use as no gastrointestinal effect	Rash Blood disorders
Opioid analgesia	Morphine Diamorphine oxycodone	Mimics the opioid component of the pain inhibitory mechanisms, as agonist on the opioid receptors	Severe pain	Morphine mainstay opioid with half-life of 4 hours Diamorphine is acetylated morphine and enters the brain faster than morphine (not licensed in most countries and is drug of abuse)	Nausea and vomiting Reduced gut motility Diarrhoea Constipation Euphoria Drowsiness Cough suppression Miosis Respiratory depression

Therapeutic class	Drugs	Mechanism of action	Common clinical uses	Comments	Examples of adverse drug reactions
	Fentanyl Alfentanil Sufentanil			High potency, quick onset and short duration of fentanyl and derivatives make these useful in surgery Fentanyl used in patch and lozenges for chronic pain	
	Methadone		Pain Opioid addiction	Extremely long half-life	
	Codeine Dihydrocodeine		Mild to moderate pain Antitussive	Codeine and dihydrodeine less effective than morphine but less dependence potential	
	Pethidine		Severe pain (commonly used in childbirth)	Better metabolized by newborn baby therefore opioid of choice for birth Nasty metabolite makes it less popular	See above, also: restlessness hypothermia
	Pentazocine Buprenorphine	Mimics the opioid component of the pain inhibitory mechanisms, as partial agonist on the opioid receptors	Moderate pain Opioid addiction	Less effective than morphine Agonist and antagonist activity, meaning they could also precipitate withdrawal symptoms in an morphine or heroin-using addict, therefore these drugs are not favoured by drug abusers Buprenorphine is more potent than morphine but causes less stimulation at receptor High first-pass effect results in no oral preparations	Nausea and vomiting Reduced gut motility Diarrhoea Constipation Euphoria Drowsiness Cough suppression Miosis Itching due to the release of histamine Respiratory depression Hallucination (pentazocine)
	Tramadol	1) Partial agonist at opioid receptor 2) Inhibits norepinephrine and serotonin reuptake	Moderate pain	Less respiratory adverse drug reaction and therefore used post surgery	Constipation Nausea Vomiting Drowsiness

Therapeutic class	Drugs	Mechanism of action	Common clinical uses	Comments	Examples of adverse drug reactions
Neuropathic pain	Amitriptyline	See Chapter 19			
	Gabapentin	See Chapter 16			
	Pregabalin				
	Capsaicin	Acts on a Ca^{2+} ion channel receptor called TRPV1 resulting, when applied to the skin, in the sensation of heat and a reduction in the sensation of neuro analgesia	Neuropathic pain	Applied topically	Local irritation
Migrane pain	Sumatriptan zolmitriptan Almotriptan Eletriptan Rovatriptan Naratriptan Rizatriptan	Antagonists at $5HT_1$ receptors which control aspects of cerebral blood flow, leading to reduced local blood flow	Migrane attacks	Variable pharmakokinetics	Sensation of tingling Heat Heaviness pressure Coronary vasoconstriction

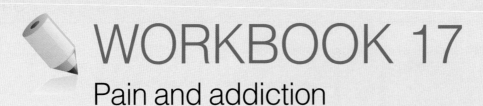

WORKBOOK 17
Pain and addiction

Lucy, the doctor with uncontrolled pain resulting in pseudoaddiction

A simplified case history

Carter has been sat next to Lucy's hospital bed for 3 hours, watching her sleep. He still cannot believe that they survived the accident. One minute he had been driving whilst reminiscing with Lucy and the next thing he remembered was waking up in an ambulance. He was told that they had been hit by another car and the other driver was at fault; he had driven right into them whilst trying to overtake. The driver of the other car had died on the spot. Lucy had sustained three fractured ribs. Carter had escaped almost unscathed with just a mild concussion. Two different ambulances had brought them into hospital, and Carter was desperately relieved when he was allowed to see Lucy and sit by her side.

Although they had been divorced for years he had never given up hope that they would one day get back together. He was delighted when she had finally agreed to go out with him for a meal. Her boyfriend, Jamie, was no competition as far as he was concerned. But instead of his hopes of a romantic evening, disaster had struck as if at random—with consequences that were to be with Lucy for a long time to come.

Lucy had been in a lot of pain when he arrived at her ward and until the registrar had, after a few tests and assessments, administered intravenous morphine. Lucy had fallen asleep shortly after. Carter was hoping the consultant would appear soon for the ward round.

A table of clinical clerking abbreviations is given on page xi.

CLINICAL CLERKING FOR LUCY KNIGHT AT A&E

Age: 33 years

PC: Severe chest pain post road traffic accident

HPC: Their car had been hit by oncoming traffic late at night. She had been slammed against the dashboard.

PMH: Asthma. Depression following divorce – 6 months off work.

The only other medication she routinely takes is the occasional pain killer for menstrual cramps.

SH: Medical doctor. Divorced and lives alone. No children or dependents.

O/E:

1) Respiratory rate = 26 breaths/minute

2) Heart rate = 108/minute

3) Blood pressure =148/90 mm Hg

> *The physiologic response pain leads to autonomic changes such as increased respiration, heart rate, and blood pressure.*

Two scales were used to assess the severity of her pain.

Assessments:

Visual analogue scales = 8

Verbal rating scale = moderate

> *See section 20.2 for explanation of these scales*

Investigations: X-ray; three broken ribs

> *Diagnostic tests are often very useful to help diagnose the source of the pain. Radiography, e.g. X-rays and other imaging procedures, are used.*

An X-ray of Lucy's chest is taken to assess the damage. It reveals broken ribs.

Neurological examination: Sensory and motor exam appear normal

Diagnosis: Severe pain resulting from three broken ribs and mild spinal injury

> *Acute pain, unlike chronic pain, is a symptom and not a diagnosis.*
>
> *Lucy's pain is acute and caused by three broken ribs.*
>
> *The neurological exam was performed to rule out spinal injury. The neurological exam consists of two types of tests:*
>
> *• sensory tests check sensitivity to temperature, pain, and pressure*
>
> *• motor tests check muscle strength and reflex functions.*
>
> *The type of spinal fracture that commonly happens after an accident is a flexion fracture whereby the vertebrae are pulled apart (distraction). This occurs when the upper body is thrown forward while the pelvis is held stable by a lap seat belt.*
>
> *Lucy seems to have escaped spinal injury despite the severe shaking she took from the accident.*

Plan:

Cocodamol

Morphine

Admit to ward

Lucy is prescribed the combination analgesia cocodamol (paracetamol and codeine) to be used regularly as well as morphine, to be used only if necessary.

She is admitted to the respiratory ward having taken only the cocodamol.

1a) What is pain?

1b) What is the purpose of pain?

2) What is the difference between acute and chronic pain?

3a) What are the two types of nociceptive afferent neurones?

3b) Describe how these two nociceptive neurones differ.

4a) What is the first stage of pain perception?

4b) List three inflammatory mediators that could trigger pain during this stage.

5a) What is the second step of pain perception?

5b) List one excitatory amino acid and one neurokinin, which act as neurotransmitters in this second step.

6a) Describe the gate control system.

6b) Name two neurotransmitters which mediate the descending inhibition of pain.

> Lucy requests morphine and her pain is assessed after a couple of hours. Her score on the visual analogue scale has now gone up to 9.

6c) What are hyperalgesia and allodynia?

> Lucy's increasing pain score indicates that her pain relief is either not adequate or she is hypersensitive.
>
> She is also complaining of nausea and has vomited once.

Possible cause of analgesia failure are:

- *-overestimation of analgesic efficacy of a drug*
- *-underestimating the analgesic requirement of a patient*
- *-prejudice against the use of analgesia, which could prevent objective therapy*
- *-patient non-compliance due to fear of addiction.*

The pharmacist remarks that because Lucy has requested morphine injection, the cocodamol (which is a combination of paracetamol and codeine phosphate) is not sufficient. She also advices that fixed dose combinations are difficult to titrate to pain and patients may suffer side effects at subtherapeutic doses without sufficient pain relief.

The doctors debate whether to use a combination of a weak opioid and another class of analgesia or to just opt for a strong opioid.

The medical student on the ward round asks how the right analgesia is chosen considering there are that many analgesic drugs available. The pharmacist explains about the analgesic ladder.

The analgesic ladder is recommended to be used to help choose the right analgesia.

The analgesic ladder has three steps:

- *non-opioid analgesia: non-steroidal anti-inflammatories (NSAIDs) and paracetamol, limited by side effects and ceiling effects (above a certain dose there is no more benefit)*
- *weak opioids, codeine, dihydrocodeine, and intermediate in strength, buprenorphine*
- *strong opioids: morphine, fentanyl, and pethidine.*

7) Set out a classification of the main analgesic drugs.

....

....

....

8a) What is the mechanism of action of NSAIDs?

....

....

....

8b) Describe how the two groups of NSAIDs differ and give the theoretical advantage of one group over the other.

....

....

....

Carter decides to go and call Lucy's parents to inform them she is in hospital.

The team decide to prescribe regular paracetamol, ibuprofen, and codeine. Significantly, morphine is also prescribed to be used when required if the other three do not alleviate the pain.

The team explain to the medical student that paracetamol, ibuprofen, and codeine provide pain relief by different mechanisms of action and so it is reasonable to use all three simultaneously for their additive effects in pain management.

9) To what degree do you think it was correct to say these three analgesics work in different ways? In your answer clarify the relationship of paracetamol with the NSAIDs.

When Carter returns and notices the ibuprofen he is worried because Lucy has asthma.

10a) What are the common side effects of NSAIDs?

10b) Explain Carter's concerns regarding asthma and ibuprofen.

Lucy says she has used ibuprofen with no problems in the past and is happy to use it now.

The medical student asks about epidurals in pain relief. She knows that epidural administration involves direct introduction of the drug into the spinal cord and that this is common in some circumstances (e.g. in childbirth). She asks how this works and whether it is used in other clinical circumstances. The registrar explains to the medical student that epidural analgesia activates the system operating in the body that controls the perception of pain and that an important part of this acts in the spinal cord. In part this involves the body producing endogenous opioid peptides to help it deal with pain by their action at specific receptors on neurones on the spinal cord. Epidural opiates stimulate these spinal cord receptors.

11) Where in the spinal cord are nociceptive neurones and synapses located?

12a) What are endogenous opioid peptides called? List four examples of these.

12b) List three different types of opioid receptors.

12c) To what class of receptors do they belong? How do each of them they couple to their cellular responses when activated?

13) Summarize in a few lines how opiate analgesics work, from the level of receptors up to the perception of pain.

Lucy requests a patient controlled analgesia (PCA) when the specialist pain nurse comes to review her pain scores the next day. The nurse prescribes one after realizing that Lucy had requested more than four doses of morphine injection over 24 hours.

PCA is a method of drug delivery by which patients self-administer opioids using an infusion device that is pre-programmed. The drug is delivered either intravenously or subcutaneously when the patient presses a button if they require a dose. This avoids the need to call a nurse each time and allows for greater control. The machine is programmed to have a 'lock-out' period during which no drug can be administered, to prevent the patient from having an overdose. Patients on PCA need to be monitored for side effects and toxicity.

Lucy's PCA controls the pain brilliantly and Lucy is comfortable, except for the nausea which is a side effect of the morphine in the PCA. Antiemetics are prescribed to alleviated the nausea.

Lucy should be monitored quite closely because of the possible unwanted effects of opioids. Her blood pressure, pulse, and respiratory rates are checked regularly by the nurse and healthcare assistants looking after her.

14) What are the pharmacological actions/effects of opiates that make it necessary for patients on PCAs to be regularly monitored?

When the nurse comes to do Lucy's regular observations she realizes that Lucy's pupils are pinpoint and her breathing is laboured.

She shouts for the doctor, who comes and administers a drug called naloxone and stops the PCA.

15) What is naloxone and why was Lucy given it?

After several doses of naloxone Lucy comes round. An investigation reveals that the 'lock-out' on the PCA had not been set properly and Lucy had received three times the intended dose. The PCA is stopped and Lucy is prescribed tramadol, paracetamol, and nefopam instead.

16a) What is the mechanism of action of tramadol?

16b) What is the mechanism of action of nefopam?

Lucy is still not happy about her pain control and requests to be given co-proxamol (which contains paracetamol and an opiate called dextropropoxyphene). The pharmacist explains that co-proxamol is no longer given because of concerns over the safety of dextropropoxyphene, one of its active ingredients, which could lead to toxicity. Dextropropoxyfene has been shown in trials to be little more effective than paracetamol.

After 2 weeks Lucy is discharged home.

Two weeks later, her pain is well controlled and she returns to work.

However, a week after returning to work, Lucy finds that she has back pain that gets progressively worse. She knows this may be a consequence of the trauma associated with the traffic accident. She is reluctant to seek help because she is keen to complete her registrar training and does not want any more time off work. The 6 months she took off for stress after her divorce had set her back and she has been unable to sit her examinations to become a specialist. Carter, who has been there to support her throughout, tries but fails to convince her to seek further help.

Lucy insists she will cope and decides to use the remainder of the painkillers she was discharged with. She finds the tramadol works best. When her supply runs out, she decides to help herself to the ward supply, which she can access undisturbed whilst on call. She knows that this is wrong, but she refuses to acknowledge how dependent she has become on the tramadol.

17) What is the difference between tolerance and dependence?

---

18) Which opiate receptor is mainly implicated in dependence?

Six months later, Lucy has moved on from tramadol to diamorphine injections to alleviate her pain and 'keep her going'. Although she is worried she might be addicted she convinces herself that she will consult and get the source of her pain investigated after her exams.

Lucy's colleague notice a marked a change in her. She is now unreliable, turning up late and unkempt for work. Her consultant admonishes her and she promises to improve. However, a week later Lucy is suspended after a near-miss incident when she prescribes 500 mg of digoxin instead of 500 micrograms for a patient. Fortunately, the error was spotted by the nurse, who contacted the pharmacist. The pharmacist had been alarmed and gone up to the ward and insisted that the dose be altered by Lucy. The consultant and ward matron had been informed and Lucy, who seemed drowsy, had been sent home.

Lucy finally realized what was at stake and was easily convinced by Carter to check into a drug rehabilitation clinic.

CLINICAL CLERKING FOR LUCY IN REHABILITATION CENTRE

PC: Dependence on diamorphine leading to impaired judgement

HPC: Following car accident, pain reoccurred after resolution and became increasingly dependent on opioids

PMH: Fractured rib from road traffic accident

DH: Diamorphine (obtained illegally)

SH: Medical doctor. Divorced and lives alone. No children or dependents.

O/E, O/Q: Negative mood, nausea/vomiting, muscle aches, runny nose/watery eyes, dilated pupils, sweating, diarrhea, yawning, fever, and insomnia. Back and neck pain.

Lucy has signs of opioid withdrawal.

It is found that the pain she experiences originates from her back and neck.

Investigations:

1) X-ray : Possible spinal injury

2) Computerize tomography scan: Nil significant

3) Neurological examination: Mild spinal injury

Diagnosis: Pseudoaddiction with chronic pain caused by undiagnosed spinal injury

Is Lucy an addict? The term 'pseudoaddiction' has been introduced to cover patients with inadequately treated pain who pursue drug-seeking behaviour. Does Lucy feel she can't do without heroin because she is addicted or because she suffers pain in its absence? Pseudoaddiction allows a sort of half-way house.

Although pseudoaddictive patients become preoccupied with obtaining opiates their underlying focus is to find relief for their pain.

The good news for Lucy is that pseudoaddiction commonly resolves when patients are given adequate analgesia.

Plan:

Determine quantity of illicit drugs used

Commence equivalent regular methadone, with morphine for breakthrough pain when required

Although pain management in a drug-dependent patient is complicated, the doctor should remember that the goal is to control the patient's pain without being judgemental or letting personal values influence the decision-making process.

After calculating the amount of illicit drugs used, the doctor prescribed a dose of methadone titrated to prevent withdrawal and to provide background analgesia. He also prescribed morphine as a short-acting opioid to prevent breakthrough pain. The methadone is chosen to prevent heroin withdrawal and possibly provide additional analgesia. Lucy is assessed 1–2 hours after starting the analgesic regimen for signs of withdrawal, clinical response, and toxicity.

Following the assessment the doses of both the methadone and morphine are adjusted.

Lucy asks the doctor if they could try other non-opioid analgesia so she could be weaned off the opioids quicker.

They discuss amitriptyline, gabapentin, and pregabalin as possible options. These are analgesics used for neuropathic pain.

There is a possibility that Lucy's pain is neuropathic. They decide to transfer Lucy to the neurological ward as soon as she is over the physical withdrawal.

After investigations they diagnose spinal fracture that was missed at the earlier investigations.

They prescribe gabapentin.

19a) To what class of drug does gabapentin belong?

19b) What is its mechanism of action?

The gabapentin is very effective and Lucy can be weaned off methadone relatively quickly.

Lucy recovers and is discharged 2 months later.

With respect to her personal life, she opts to remain single and concentrate on making the best of the second chance she had been given at work.

The treatment of infections and cancer management

Despite all the advances of modern medicine, two conditions continue to be among our biggest killers: infections and cancer. Collectively they claim millions of lives each year, and yet they each start with a single cell. In the case of cancer, it is one of our own cells, and with infections, it is a microorganism. Both conditions involve cells dividing and growing, and they are examples of 'cells gone wild', in other words the growth of the cells has escaped the body's normal control mechanisms. Because of the similarity between cancers and infections, the treatments of both come under the broad term 'chemotherapy'. The ongoing challenge with chemotherapy is how to control the 'wild' cells while leaving our healthy ones intact. To understand the basis of chemotherapy we need to understand a bit about cells, in particular what makes microorganisms and cancer cells different from healthy cells so that targets for chemotherapy can be identified.

S6.1 Eukaryotes versus prokaryotes

All organisms can be divided into either eukaryotes or prokaryotes. Eukaryotes have complicated cell structures that include a nucleus where genetic material (DNA) is stored. They also contain a number of organelles (structures that have a specific function), such as mitochondria (responsible for generating the energy for the cell) and the Golgi apparatus (involved in sorting and modifying proteins). Examples of eukaryotes include animals, plants, and fungi. In contrast, prokaryotes are unicellular organisms with minimal internal structures. Their genetic material is not encapsulated, but floats freely in the cytoplasm (the inside of the cell enclosed in a membrane) and they only have simple macromolecules such as ribosomes. The main examples of these are the bacteria.

S6.2 Chemotherapy targets in microorganisms and cancer cells

To try and minimize or eliminate the toxicity of chemotherapeutic agents we have to identify elements that are unique to the 'wild' cells. Broadly speaking two areas are targets of chemotherapy: biochemical reactions and structures within the cells.

S6.2.1 Biochemical reactions

The three main biochemical reactions, classified as Class I, Class II, and Class III reactions, have been investigated as potential targets. Class I reactions involve carbon sources, such as glucose, and result in the production of precursor molecules and adenosine triphosphate (ATP), the cell's energy storage unit. The Class II reactions use ATP and the precursor molecules to produce essential 'building blocks', such as amino acids, nucleotides, and amino sugars. Examples can be seen in Figure S6.1.

These building blocks are converted by Class III reactions into macromolecules, such as proteins (from amino acids), deoxyribonucleic acid (DNA), and ribonucleic acid (RNA) (from nucleotides), and peptidoglycan and chitin (from amino sugars).

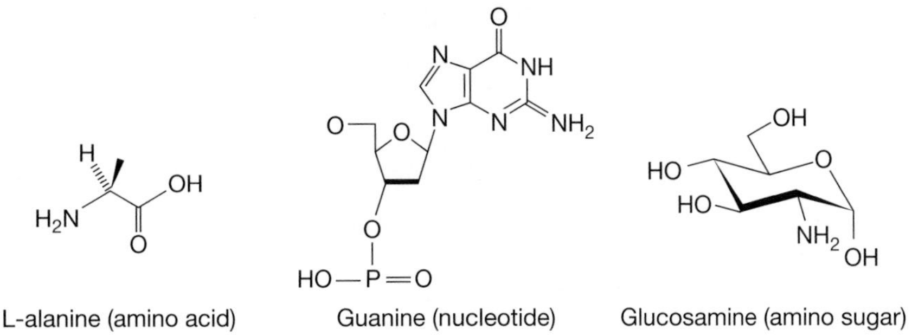

Figure S6.1 Examples of outcomes of Class II reactions.

Class I reactions are not targets of chemotherapy because many cells, including human cells, use a similar pathway, therefore there would be no selectivity. Class II reactions are used as targets as bacteria synthesise certain amino acids and vitamins (e.g. folate), but human cells do not. Examples of chemotherapy agents using Class II reactions are trimethoprim (folate antagonist—antibacterial) and fludarabine (purine antagonist—anticancer). Class III reactions are the major target of many chemotherapy agents. One example is inhibitors of peptidoglycan synthesis. As we will see in Chapter 21, peptidoglycan is a unique component of bacterial cell walls, not found in human cells, and is the target of many antibiotics. Another is the formation of ergosterol, a component of fungal cell wall not found in human cell walls, which is the mode of action of several antifungal agents.

Inhibition of protein synthesis as a chemotherapy target

An important target of several antimicrobials is inhibition of protein synthesis. Protein synthesis involves ribosomes that coordinate the 'reading' of messenger RNA (mRNA) and the subsequent building of proteins from amino acids carried on transfer RNA (tRNA). The ribosome is made up of two subunits. In humans they are the 40S and 60S. However, bacteria have 30S and 50S subunits. This difference in the ribosome make up is another target of antibacterials.

Inhibition of DNA and RNA as a chemotherapy target

The inhibition of DNA and RNA synthesis and function are important sites of action for many chemotherapy agents, therefore a more detailed explanation of the synthesis and function of DNA and RNA will help in understanding how many chemotherapy agents work.

DNA contains all the genetic information for living organisms. It comprises two long chains of polymers of nucleotides. The nucleotides consist of a base (adenine, guanine, cytosine, or thymine) and a sugar (deoxyribose). The two chains interact through cross-linking of the bases (guanine links to cytosine via a triple bond, and adenine to thymine via a double bond) (Figure S6.2).

In Figure S6.2 DNA is represented as a flat structure, but in reality it exists as a three-dimensional helix structure with the two stands twisting around each other, with a turn approximately every 10 base pairs (Figure S6.3).

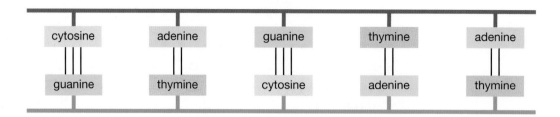

Figure S6.2 Basic structure of DNA.

In eukaryotes DNA is arranged as linear chromosomes, whereas in prokaryotes it is arranged in a circular fashion. The two main functions of DNA are to replicate to allow the cells of the organism to grow and survive, and to provide the template to produce various proteins. Both of these involve 'unwinding' the DNA and then splitting it so that it can be 'read'. To unwind the DNA an enzyme called topoisomerase is used. Once split the DNA is duplicated by the enzyme DNA polymerase. This enzyme recruits the required nucleotides and inserts them, and even 'proof reads' the insertion to make sure mistakes do not occur (if it makes a mistake, the wrong nucleotide is 'cut out' and replaced).

To produce proteins from DNA it needs to be converted to RNA (specifically mRNA). RNA differs from DNA in three ways. First, in the cell most RNA exists as a single strand. Second, where DNA has a deoxyribose unit, RNA has a ribose (a sugar) moiety. The difference is that deoxyribose is ribose with one of the hydroxyl groups replaced with hydrogen. Third, the base thymidine is replaced by uracil in RNA (i.e. the four bases are adenine, guanine, cytosine, and uracil). There are three main types of RNA: mRNA, which is used as the template for protein synthesis, tRNA, which is used to carry the amino acids that make up the protein, and ribosomal RNA (rRNA), the central component to the ribosome that translates the mRNA to produce the proteins. The first stage in producing RNA is that the DNA is again unwound and split, and then another enzyme, RNA polymerase 'reads' the DNA to produce the complementary RNA copy. There are some differences between the production of mRNA in eukaryotes and prokaryotes. Eukaryotes produce a primary transcript of the RNA, which has to undergo conversion to mature mRNA, through a number of modifications to what is called pre-mRNA, before protein synthesis is started. However, in bacteria the first transcription of the mRNA is mature and starts to produce proteins straight away.

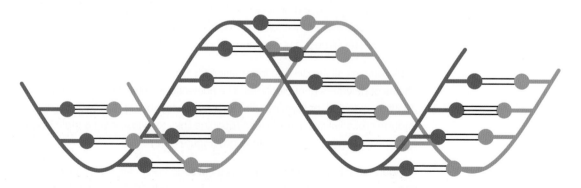

Figure S6.3 Double helix DNA.

Chemotherapy agents are used at almost any stage of this process, including:

- altering the base-pairing properties of the DNA (e.g. acriflavine—bacteria)
- inhibiting either DNA or RNA polymerase (e.g. cytarabine—cancer, aciclovir—viruses)
- inhibiting DNA gyrase (e.g. quinolones—bacteria, irinotecan—cancer)
- directly affecting DNA (e.g. bleomycin—cancer).

S6.2.2 Formed cellular structures

The other major target for chemotherapy agents is formed cellular structures, including the cell wall and organelles.

The cell wall as a target for chemotherapy

Fungi, unlike bacteria, share more similarities with human cells. However, as noted above, one unique component is the sterol ergosterol, a major component of fungal cell wall (human cells uses cholesterol). While some antifungal agents, such as imidazoles, inhibit the formation of ergosterol, others, such as the polyenes, attach to the ergosterol, forming pores that allow the contents of the fungal cell to leak out.

The polymyxin antibacterial agents, such as colistin, operate in a similar fashion and act as types of 'soaps' that disrupt the phospholipid bilayer of bacteria. Unfortunately, they are quite toxic and rarely used.

Organelles as a target for chemotherapy

Microtubules inside cells are important parts of the cytoskeleton of the cell, giving structural support. They are also an important part of cell division, forming the mitotic spindle, which separates the chromosomes during cell division (see later). They comprise polymers of tubulin dimers, a family of globular proteins. The microtubules are the target of some anticancer therapies, including taxol and the vinca alkaloids (e.g. vincristine).

S6.2.3 Cell growth

As you would imagine, targeting cancer has posed one of the greatest challenges for chemotherapy as the cells that cause cancer start as 'normal' human cells, therefore finding something that will harm the cancer cells, while leaving the healthy cells alone, is a particular problem. One of the features of cancer cells that is capitalized on is the fact that they often replicate rapidly and out of control of the body's normal constraints, therefore an understanding of normal cell growth is important.

The cell cycle

The events that occur during cell division are divided into four distinct phases. There is a fifth 'dormant' or resting phase (G_0), in which most cells that are not constantly dividing spend most of their time (Figure S6.4).

The first stage of cell division is G1, during which the cell starts to produce the various enzymes needed for DNA replication. During the S phase DNA synthesis starts and this phase ends when the chromosomes are duplicated. By the end of this phase the

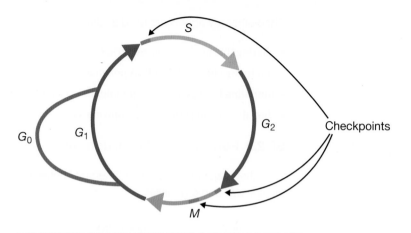

Figure S6.4 The cell cycle.

S, synthesis; G_2, gap 2; M, mitosis; G_1, gap 1; G_0, resting.

cell has effectively doubled in size. The next phase is G2, during which the microtubules are synthesised. After G2 the cell enters mitosis. During this stage nuclear division and cytoplasmic division occur. There are five stages in mitosis. In the first, called prophase, the DNA starts to condense together and centrosomes form (these are structures that coordinate the formation of the microtubules). The second phase is prometaphase, during which the nuclear membrane dissolves and the microtubules enter and attach to the genetic material. Next is the metaphase, where the chromosomes align along the midline ready to separate into the two halves of the cell. The penultimate phase is the anaphase, where the two sets of chromosomes are separated, followed by the final phase (telophase), where the two new sets of DNA condense and the nuclear envelope is formed around each. The cells then start to split, forming the two new 'daughter' cells.

Checkpoints in cell division

There are several 'checkpoints' during the cell cycle. They occur at the end of G_1 and before entering S, at the end of G_2 and before entering M, and during mitosis (M) in the metaphase, when the chromosomes are supposed to be aligned ready for separation. These checkpoints help stop cell division in response to detecting damage to the DNA to prevent the damaged DNA being duplicated and passed on to the daughter cells. They involve inhibitors of cell division that act on cyclin dependent kinases (CDK) and cyclins. The CDK and cyclin form complexes to encourage the various phases of cell division by promoting the production of the enzymes required for DNA replication. There are several inhibitors involved, but an important inhibitor at the G_1/S and G_2/M checkpoints is gene p53. Mutations to genes such as p53 are thought to be responsible for tumour formation as the mutation can allow the cell to replicate uncontrollably.

This uncontrolled replication of cancer cells is the target of most chemotherapy, as well as other tumour treatments (e.g. radiotherapy). However, this means cells that normally replicate rapidly (e.g. lining of the stomach and blood cells) are often affected by cancer chemotherapies, as we will see in Chapter 22.

Chapter 21
The treatment of infections

Everyday we share our lives with billions of organisms, including bacteria, viruses, and fungi. Most are microscopic in size and they 'live' on our skin, in our mouth, in our gut, and in every other bodily surface and orifice. Luckily, we have a range of barriers and protective mechanisms to keep these microorganisms from overwhelming us. These include obvious physical barriers such as the skin, through to our own 'army' of defenders in the form of the immune system (see Section 3). Some of these microorganisms are important for normal human functioning. For example, in Section 4 we discussed how intestinal bacteria are involved with the normal breakdown of foods such as carbohydrates. In addition, bacteria in the vagina are important for maintaining its health and preventing overgrowth by other microorganisms, particularly yeasts. These are called 'normal flora'.

However, sometimes the bacteria, fungi, and viruses can escape our defenses and result in infections. An infection can be defined as a *detrimental* colonization by an organism of a host species. This differs from the 'normal flora' by the detrimental effects caused by the presence of the organism. Infections can range from moderately irritating (e.g. infection with rhinoviruses, giving us the 'common cold') through to life threatening (e.g. septicaemia, a severe form of blood infection).

There are several stages in an infection. First, you must be exposed to the pathogen. In some cases they are present

all the time and in others you must encounter them. Second, the pathogen has to get past the host defenses, be they physical (e.g. after an injury to the skin) or immunological (e.g. because of some impairment of your immune system, such as taking immunosuppressants). Third, the organisms must multiply. Bacteria and fungi do this independently, utilizing the host nutrients and environment, while viruses use the host cells to replicate. Finally, the infection can move to other sites through the blood or lymphatic systems.

Infections can affect almost any part of the human body. However, some systems of the body are more prone to them than others. The respiratory tract is a common site for infections as Doris, our patient in Workbook 18, finds out. As noted in Chapter 11, the respiratory tract is open to the elements and relies on a number of physical (e.g. hairs in the nose and mucous) and immunological systems to protect it. Upper respiratory tract infections (those affecting the respiratory tract from the neck up) are the most common infectious presentations to GPs. These infections include the common cold and tonsillitis/pharyngitis. The common lower respiratory tract infections (those affecting the lungs and bronchi) include bronchitis and pneumonia (which Doris has).

This chapter will review the common treatments for bacterial, fungal, and viral infections.

21.1 Bacterial infections

Bacteria can be classified or described a number of ways. The first basic division is between **gram-negative** and **gram-positive** bacteria. This relates to what is called gram staining, which involves first exposing the

slide-fixed bacteria to a mixture of crystal violet and iodine, then attempting to wash the stain off with acetone, and finally counter-staining with neutral red or safranin. Gram-positive bacteria retain the first stain

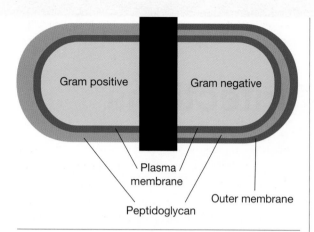

Figure 21.1 Difference between gram-positive and gram-negative bacteria.

and appear purple, while gram-negative bacteria lose the first stain and appear pink because of the counterstain. This distinction is due to differences in the makeup of the cell walls of gram-positive and gram-negative bacteria. Gram-positive bacteria have a cell wall made up mainly of **peptidoglycan**, with a small amount of proteins and polysaccharides (5–10%). Gram-negative bacteria have a more complex arrangement of layers, including a lipopolysaccharide and protein outer membrane, and a much smaller proportion of peptidoglycan (Figure 21.1).

The gram stain remains attached to the gram-positive bacteria because the crystal violet-iodide complex becomes trapped within the layers of the peptidoglycan. The peptidoglycan is a three-dimensional mesh-like structure made up of a mixture sugars (N-acetylglucosamine and N-acetylmuramic acid) and amino acids. The chains are cross-linked by enzymes called penicillin-binding proteins. The peptidoglycan mesh serves to give shape and maintain the internal pressure of the bacteria. Proteins covalently bond to the peptidoglycan structure and through this it is involved in the interaction between host cells and bacteria.

The differences in the composition of the cell walls of gram-positive and gram-negative bacteria are the target for many antibacterials. Some affect the synthesis of peptidoglycan (e.g. penicillin), while others affect protein synthesis (e.g. tetracyclines).

The other classification of bacteria is based on their shape. This includes **cocci** (round) and **bacilli** (rods). Examples of common bacteria classified this way are found in Table 21.1

The third way bacteria can be organized is into **aerobes** or **anaerobes**. Anaerobic organisms do not require oxygen to produce energy and some actually can't survive in the presence of oxygen. Aerobes require oxygen and constitute the majority of bacteria. Anaerobes produce energy through a number of mechanisms, the most common being fermentation. In contrast, aerobes often produce energy from the oxidation of fats and sugars. The difference is that aerobes can produce more energy than

Table 21.1 Some common human bacteria

	Gram positive	Example infections	Gram negative	Example infections
Cocci	*Staphylococcus aureus*	Skin/wound/blood	*Neisseria gonorrhoeae*	STI
	Staphylococcus epidermis	Skin/wound	*Neisseria meningitidis*	Meningitis
	Streptococcus pyogenes	RTI	*Moraxella catarrhalis*	RTI
	Streptococcus pneumoniae	RTI		
Bacilli	*Clostridium botulinum*	GTI	*Hemophilus influenzae*	RTI
	Clostridium difficile	GTI	*Klebsiella pneumoniae*	RTI
	Clostridium perfringens	Skin/wound	*Legionella pneumophilia*	RTI
	Clostridium tetani	Skin/wound	*Pseudomonas aeruginosa*	RTI
	Bacillus anthracis	Anthrax	*Escherichia coli*	UTI
	Bacillus cereus	GTI	*Proteus mirabilis*	UTI
	Lactobacillus species	Normal flora	*Helicobacter pylori*	GTI
	Listeria monocytogenes	CNS/blood/GTI	*Salmonella enteritidis*	GTI
	Corynebacterium diphtheriae	RTI	*Salmonella typhi*	GTI
	Propionibacterium acnes	Acne		

CNS, central nervous system; GTI, gastrointestinal tract infection; RTI, respiratory tract infection; STI, sexually transmitted infection; UTI, urinary tract infection.

the anaerobes. Examples of important anaerobes include *Actinomyces*, *Bacteroides fragilis* group and *Clostridium* spp. (including *C. tetani*, which causes tetanus, and *C. botulinum*, which causes botulism).

21.1.1 Bacterial resistance to antibiotics

While the discovery and development of antibiotics was one of the major breakthroughs in modern medicine, since then many bacteria have been progressively developing ways to resist their effects. The mechanisms of bacterial resistance can be divided into one of four types:

- enzymatic deactivation
- decreased uptake or increased efflux (removal) from the bacteria
- altered target sites
- alternative target sites ('bypass' pathways).

However, individual bacteria may exhibit more than one resistance mechanism. These resistance mechanisms can be intrinsic or acquired. The intrinsic or innate resistance is due to the biology of the bacteria. An example of this is vancomycin resistance in *Escherichia coli*. Acquired resistance can occur due to spontaneous mutations, where the 'mutant' bacteria survive and multiply (sort of 'survival of the fittest'), or by transfer of genetic material from one bacterium to another. The transfer of genetic material can involve plasmids (self-replicating circular pieces of DNA), which can transfer genes into other bacterial species. They do this by transferring genes to other plasmids or into the genome (the DNA) of the bacteria (called a transposon). The transfer via a transposon is thought to be the mechanism by which methicillin resistance was transferred in *Staphylococcus aureus*.

Although a number of causative factors have been identified, it is widely accepted that the overuse, and inappropriate use, of antibiotics has been a major contributing factor to the development of resistant bacteria.

Enzymatic deactivation

An example of this is the production of β-**lactamase** enzymes by some gram-negative and gram-positive bacteria to inactivate the β-lactams antibiotics by breaking bonds in the β-lactam ring (more later). Many β-lactamases have been identified and most affect both penicillins and cephalosporins (the two main classes of β-lactams). However, some are specific for penicillins (e.g. penicillinase produced by *Pseudomonas*), and some for cephalosporins (e.g. the AmpC enzyme produced by *Enterobacter* species).

Decreased uptake or increased removal

Some bacteria have developed ways of blocking the entry of antibiotics through the cell wall. One example is found in some resistant strains of *Pseudomonas aeruginosa*, which lack a specific **porin** (a hollow protein in the cell wall that allows antibiotics to enter the cell) and therefore are resistant to imipenem.

Another mechanism of resistance is to actively 'pump' the antibiotic out of bacteria. The 'pumps' are energy dependent and their expression is encoded into genes within the bacteria. This is thought to be one of the mechanisms of resistance to tetracyclines in the *Enterobacteriaceae* family, and the *Hemophilus* and *Moraxella* species.

Altered target sites

Bacteria may make changes to the sites of action of antibiotics once they are in the cell. One example is in the **penicillin-binding proteins**, which are responsible for peptidoglycan synthesis. Changes in this enzyme can reduce the affinity to bind cephalosporins and penicillins, resulting in resistance. Similarly, some bacteria produce proteins that protect their ribosomes, reducing their sensitivity to antibiotics that inhibit protein production through ribosomes (e.g. tetracyclines).

'Bypass' pathways

This involves production of 'false' targets for the antibiotics, thus protecting the 'real' targets. An example is the production of an alternative penicillin-binding protein. Methicillin-resistant *Staphylococcus aureus* (MRSA) produces this, and it results in the penicillin binding to the 'false' enzyme instead of the real enzyme, leaving cell wall synthesis intact.

Our patient Doris was found to have pneumonia caused by an organism resistant to vancomycin. This is a potentially dangerous situation as vancomycin is often needed when people have infections resulting from to methicillin-resistant bacteria.

21.2 Antibacterial therapy: antibiotics

There are six commonly used classes of antibacterial agents:

- β-lactams (penicillins/cephalosporins/carbapenms)
- tetracyclines
- macrolides
- quinolones
- nitroimidazoles
- aminoglycosides.

A range of less-used antibacterials, such as those used for tuberculosis, will also be discussed.

21.2.1 β-lactams

The β-lactams are some of the original antibiotics. Most were derived from fungi. However, they are synthesised today. The main subgroups of β-lactams are:

- penicillins
- cephalopsorins
- carbapenems.

Penicillins

This is the oldest of the antibiotics, being first discovered in the early 20th century by Alexander Fleming, who

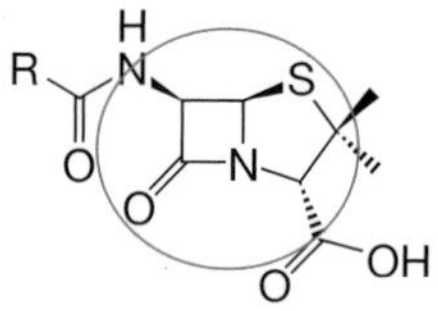

Figure 21.2 The β-lactam core of penicillins.

observed that *Penicillium* mould secreted substances that inhibited *Staphylococcus* growth. There are now several derivatives of the original penicillin, all with the same central structure, a β-lactam (Figure 21.2).

This core gives the β-lactams their activity as it is an analogue of D-alanyl-D-alanine, and binds to penicillin-binding proteins. This interrupts bacterial cell wall synthesis by stopping the cross-linking of peptidoglycan. The penicillins also cause cell lysis by inhibiting the inactivation of autolytic enzymes (which break down the cell wall). Some bacteria have faulty autolytic enzymes and these bacteria are inhibited, but not lysed, by penicillins (referred to as 'tolerant').

The pencillins can be classified by their spectrum of activity, as described in Table 21.2.

Table 21.2 Commonly used penicillins

Spectrum	Examples	Bacterial spectrum	Examples of infections they are used for
Narrow	Benzathine penicillin Benzylpenicillin (penicillin G) Phenoxymethylpenicillin (penicillin V) Procaine penicillin	Mainly gram-positive, especially *Streptococcus* sp.	Respiratory tract infections Endocarditis Meningitis
	Dicloxacillin Flucloxacillin	Mainly gram-positive, especially *Staphylococcus aureus*	Bone and joint infections Skin infections Cellulitis
Moderate	Ampicillin Amoxycillin	Mainly gram-positive and better for some gram-negative (eg *Escherichia coli*, *Haemophilus influenzae*)	Respiratory tract infections Otitis media (middle ear infection) *H. pylori* eradication
Broad	Amoxycillin + clavulanic acid	Gram-positive, including *Staphylococcus aureus* More gram-negative, including *E. coli*, *Klebsiella* sp., *Neisseria gonorrhoeae* and *H. influenzae*	Respiratory tract infections Skin/wound infections Urinary tract infections
	Piperacillin	Gram-positive and gram negative, particularly *Pseudomonas aeruginosa*	Pseudomonas infections
Extended	Piperacillin + tazobactam Ticarcillin + clavulanic acid	Broadest spectrum, including most gram-positive and gram-negative, particularly *Pseudomonas aeruginosa*	Skin infections Severe respiratory tract infections Severe sepsis

Our patient Doris was initially prescribed amoxicillin for her pneumonia. However, this is not the best choice for empiric treatment (i.e. before you know what bacteria have caused the infection) as you normally used a broad-spectrum agent to cover as many bacteria as possible.

Inactivation and resistance to penicillins The activity of penicillins can be reduced by a number of mechanisms. First, some, such as phenoxymethylpencillin, are acid labile and are broken down in the stomach, reducing their bioavailability. To overcome this, these penicillins should be taken on an empty stomach, which is 1 hour before food or 2 hours after. The second mechanism of deactivation is via β-lactamases. These enzymes hydrolyse the bonds in the β-lactam core, rendering the penicillin inactive. Some, such as dicloxacillin and flucloxacillin, are inherently more resistant to β-lactamases. However, for other penicillins the addition of clavulanic acid and tazobactam is used to improve their spectrum of activity (see Table 21.2). Both clavulanic acid and tazobactam contain a β-lactam-like core, but have little or no antibacterial activity (Figure 21.3). They are added to inhibit the β-lactamase by acting as substrates instead of the pencillin.

Other mechanisms of resistance to penicillins include altered penicillin-binding proteins that are less likely to bind penicillins. This is part of the mechanism used by methicillin (an older penicillin that is not longer used) resistant *Staphylococcus aureus* (MRSA, sometimes referred to as the 'superbug').

Administration and side effects of penicillins Most penicillins are give two to four times a day. They need to be given frequently as they need to maintain high blood levels to be effective. Most are given orally, but several of the penicillin salts (procaine, benzyl, and benzanthine), piperacillin, and ticarcillin are only given parenterally.

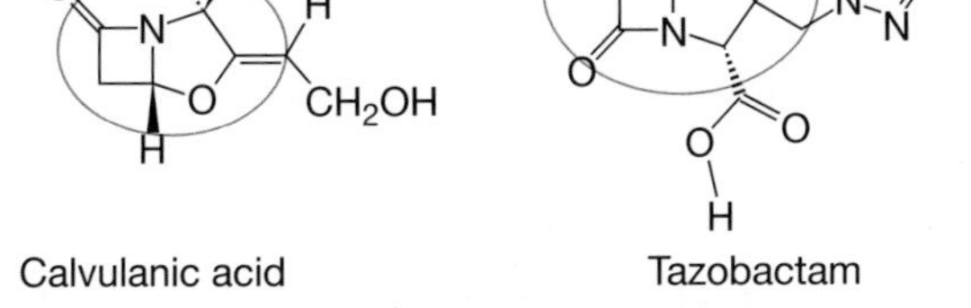

A side effect of most oral antibiotics, including the penicillins, is gastrointestinal upset, specifically mild diarrhoea. This is because antibiotics can remove the normal bacteria in the gut that are responsible for breaking down food components, including carbohydrates. Because the carbohydrates are not metabolized they cause an osmotic type of diarrhoea (see Chapter 13). If it is only mild we usually suggest the person tolerate it as it will go away once the antibiotic is stopped. However, there is a rare form of antibiotic-induced diarrhoea caused by *Clostridium difficile*. The *C. difficile* can 'overgrow' because the other bacteria in the gut that keep it under control are removed. The type of diarrhoea caused by this can be severe and is sometimes called pseudomembranous colitis. If a person experiences this, and it can occur several weeks after stopping the antibiotic, they need to seek help immediately.

Although it is possible with any antibiotic, penicillins in particular have been associated with allergic reactions, which are sometimes life threatening. However, many patients are labelled 'penicillin allergic' when in fact they are just penicillin 'intolerant' (e.g. they have had gastrointestinal upset with them). A documented severe penicillin allergy (e.g. urticaria or anaphylaxis) is a contraindication to their use, and the use of other β-lactams (e.g. cephalosporins and carbapenems) may also be contraindicated due to cross-reactivity because of the common core structure. However, patients who have Epstein–Barr virus infections (called mononucleosis or 'glandular fever') and receive ampicillin or amoxicillin can develop a diffuse, red rash (in fact it occurs in up to 90% of cases). This does not mean the person is allergic to ampicillin/amoxicillin, but it does reinforce the need to carefully assess patients with sore throats (a symptom of mononucleosis) before prescribing an antibiotic.

Penicillins are generally well tolerated and have few if any drug interactions. The drug probenecid interacts with penicillin to reduce its renal clearance (this is the main route of elimination for all penicillins). This is used therapeutically to increase the levels of penicillins to improve their effectiveness, and the combination may allow the use of oral penicillins instead of parenteral penicillins.

Cephalosporins

The cephalosporins, like penicillins, were also discovered as substances secreted by fungi (*Cephalosporium acremonium*). They have the same mechanism of action

Calvulanic acid   Tazobactam

Figure 21.3 β-lactamase inhibitors.

Table 21.3 Common cephalosporins

Generation	Examples	Bacterial spectrum	Examples of infections they are used for
First	Cefadroxil Cefradine Cefalexin (cephalexin) Cefalotin Cefazolin	Moderate spectrum Most gram-positive including *Staphylococci* and *Streptococci* Gram-negative, mainly *Klebsiella* spp. and *Escherichia coli*	Respiratory tract infections Urinary tract infections Skin and soft tissue infections Otitis media
Second	Cefaclor Cefuroxime	Mainly gram-positive and better for some gram-negative (e.g. *Neisseria gonorrhoea* and *Haemophilus influenzae*)	Respiratory tract infections Otitis media
	Cefoxitin	Also has some anaerobe activity, especially *Bacteroides fragilis*	Prophylaxis in gastrointestinal tract and gynaecological surgery
Third	Cefotaxime Ceftriaxone Cefpodoxime Cefixime	Broad spectrum Most gram-positive but not *S. aureus*. Gram-negative similar to second generation but includes *Enterobacter* spp., *Salmonella* spp., and *Serratia* spp. Better penetration into CNS.	Meningitis Respiratory tract infections Severe sepsis Skin infections
	Ceftazidime	Gram-positive and gram negative, particularly *Pseudomonas aeruginosa*	*Pseudomonas* infections (especially respiratory tract)
Fourth	Cefepime	Similar to ceftazidime but more active against gram-positive organisms	*Pseudomonas* infections (especially respiratory tract) Severe sepsis

CNS, central nervous system

as the penicillins, acting as inhibitors of cell wall synthesis by blocking penicillin-binding proteins. The cephalosporins are often grouped in terms of 'generations'. The older 'generation' has primarily gram-positive cover, while newer cephalosporins have a wide spectrum of activity, including gram-negative and gram-positive organisms (Table 21.3). Most are given two to four times a day, except **ceftriaxone**, which can be given once a day. The oral cephalosporins are mainly first-generation (**cefalexin**, **cefradine**, and **cefadroxil**) as well as **cefaclor**, **cefuroxime**, and **cefixime**; Most of the third and fourth generation are only given parenterally.

The side effect profile of cephalosporins is similar to the penicillins, and includes gastrointestinal upset and allergy. The cross-reactivity between penicillins and cephalosporins with regards allergy is about 10%, and their use is probably best avoided in penicillin-allergic patients who exhibit urticaria or anaphylaxis.

Carbapenems

The carbapenems are the third group of β-lactam antibiotics that are used, and include **imipenem**, **meropenem**, **ertapenem**, and **doripenem**. As a class

they have the widest spectrum of activity of all the β-lactams. Imipenem, doripenem, and meropenem cover gram-positive and gram-negative bacteria, including *Pseudomonas aeruginosa*, as well as providing good coverage against anaerobes, including *Bacteroides fragilis*. They do not cover MRSA or *Enterococcus faecium*, nor *Mycoplasma* or *Chlamydia*. Ertapenem has a similar spectrum, but is not as active against *P. aeruginosa* and *Enterococcus*.

Imipenem is inactivated by dehydropeptidase enzymes in the kidney. It is therefore administered with cilastin, which inhibits the dehydropeptidase enzymes. Imipenem has the shortest half-life and is given four times a day, while meropenem and doripenem are given three times a day; ertapenem has the longest half-life and is given once a day. All the carbapenems are administered parenterally. They are expensive antibiotics and tend to be reserved for complex mixed infections, such as severe septicaemia, hospital acquired pneumonia, and intra-abdominal infections.

They are well tolerated, like the other β-lactams, and have a similar spectrum of adverse effects to penicillins and cephalosporins. Neurotoxicity, such as seizures and confusion, particularly with imipenem and ertapenem, has been reported when high doses are used.

21.2.2 Tetracyclines

The tetracyclines are a group of antibiotics that were among the first antibiotics to be discovered. There are three main tetracyclines used: **tetracycline**; **doxycycline**, and **minocycline**. Other less commonly used tetracyclines include **tigecycline**, **lymecycline**, **oxytetracycline** and **demeclocycline**. They all have a common core structure (Figure 21.4).

The mode of action of tetracyclines is through blockage of protein synthesis. The synthesis of protein involves an interaction between a ribosome and messenger ribonucleic acid (mRNA). The process is detailed in Box 21.1. In bacterial cells the ribosome comprises a 50S subunit and 30S subunit. In contrast, the ribosomes of human cells have a 60S subunit and 40S subunit. This gives tetracyclines selective toxicity for bacterial cells. The tetracyclines attach to the 30S subunit and block the transcription of mRNA by inhibiting the attachment of tRNA to the A site (Box 21.1).

Resistance to tetracyclines

The two main mechanisms of resistance are by active transport out of the bacteria and modification to the ribosome, preventing the activity of tetracyclines. Some bacteria produce a membrane protein that 'pumps' tetracyclines out of the cell. The ribosomal protection can result from changes to the ribosome that stop the tetracyclines from binding, alterations to the ribosome structure so that both the tRNA and tetracycline can bind, or from dislodging of the bound tetracycline. A minor mechanism of resistance is by enzymatic deactivation, where an acetyl group is added to the tetracycline.

Uses of tetracyclines

The spectrum of activity of tetracyclines is broad, with a similar coverage of gram positive bacteria as the β-lactams, and better coverage of gram-negative

bacteria, although not as good as the extended spectrum penicillins or third/fourth generation cephalosporins. In particular, they have good activity against *Rickettsia*, *Mycoplasma*, and *Chlamydia* species, as well as some spirochetes and protozoa. The tetracyclines are used primarily for respiratory tract infections and acne. Doxycycline is also used in the prophylaxis against malaria, in the treatment of uncomplicated malaria, and to treat chlamydia. Demeclocycline is generally only used to treat the syndrome of inappropriate antidiuretic hormone (SIADH). In SIADH patients experience excessive release of antidiuretic hormone (ADH) from the pituitary, which acts on the distal convoluted tubules and collecting ducts in the kidney to cause reabsorption of water. This can result in oedema and hypertension. Demeclocycline antagonizes the effect of ADH on the kidney. Tigecycline is used for complicated skin and intra-abdominal infections (it has coverage for MRSA).

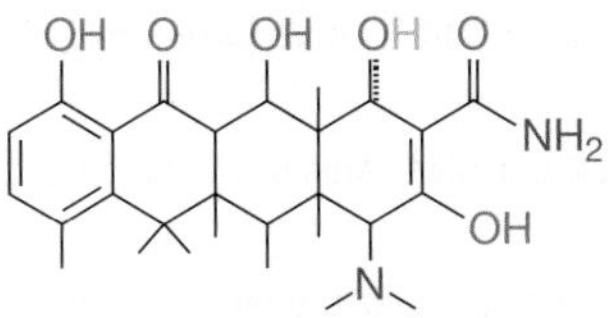

Administration and side effects of tetracyclines

The tetracyclines are usually given twice a day. However, for malaria prophylaxis, and in the treatment of acne, doxycycline is given once a day (as is minocycline for acne). The main side effect with tetracyclines is gastrointestinal upset. Both doxycycline and minocycline can be given with food to reduce this, but tetracycline should be given on an empty stomach to be absorbed. The tetracyclines chelate (bind with) large cations such as calcium, aluminium, and iron, therefore they should not be given at the same time as calcium supplements, antacids (containing magnesium and aluminium), and iron supplements. The binding to calcium also means they can be incorporated into growing bones and teeth. This leads to teeth mottling (look brown/black in patches instead of white) and reduced bone growth. The tetracyclines should therefore not be used in pregnancy or in children. Another common side effect is increasing the skins sensitivity to ultraviolet light. People taking tetracyclines need to use a good sunscreen or risk serious sunburn (this is really important when they are used for malarial prophylaxis, as malaria is usually present in warm, sunny countries around the tropics).

Figure 21.4 Tetracycline core structure.

Doris was switched to doxycycline once she could take oral medication. It is generally recommended to use oral therapy whenever possible as it is less expensive and reduces your risk of problems from the injections (e.g. inflammation of the veins or even another infection).

Box 21.1

Process of protein synthesis in bacteria

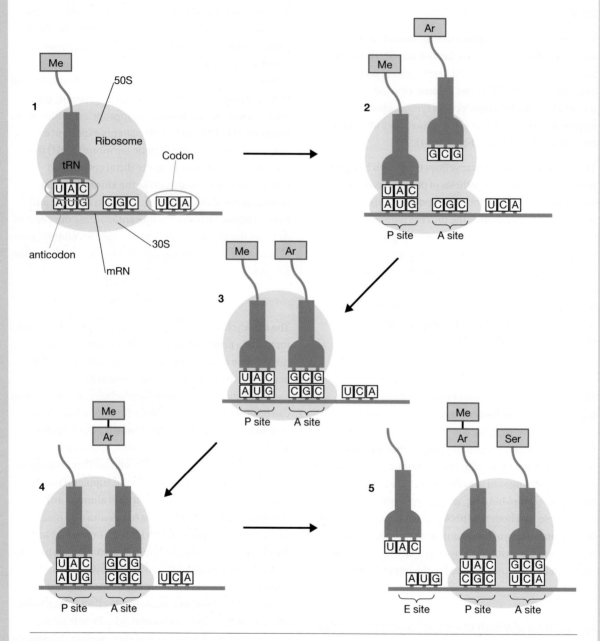

Figure a

1. mRNA is produced by RNA polymerase from DNA. It contains sequences of nucleotides, arranged in sets of three called codons. The appropriate tRNA for each of these codons has a complementary set of three nucleotides called the anticodon. The ribosome facilitates the interaction between the mRNA and tRNA. The tRNA carries an amino acid (in the example it is methionine) and is responsible for building the protein.

2. A second tRNA comes in to attach to the mRNA. It attaches to the A site of the mRNA. This is the site of action for tetracyclines, which compete with tRNA for the A site.

3. The second tRNA, carrying an amino acid (in this case argenine), attaches with the complementary base pairs (i.e. codon-anticodon interaction) This is the site of action for aminoglycosides (e.g. gentamycin), which cause abnormal codon–anticodon interactions.

21.2.3 Macrolides

The macrolides include **erythromycin** (the first discovered), **clarithromycin**, **roxithromycin**, **telithromycin**, and **azithromycin**. The structure of macrolides is complicated, with a large macrolide ring which involves a 'ring' of a large number of atoms, off which two deoxy sugars (a sugar where one OH group is replaced with a hydrogen atom) are attached. The macrolides, like the tetracyclines, act by inhibiting protein synthesis. However, they attach to the 50S subunit of the ribosome and inhibit translocation of the growing peptide chain (Box 21.1).

Resistance to macrolides

Bacteria have become resistant by two mechanisms: modification of the 50S ribosome and efflux out of the bacteria. Some bacteria develop resistance by methylation of a single adenine in the 23S rRNA (ribosomal RNA), part of the 50S subunit, which prevents binding of the macrolide. Some *Streptococcus* and *Campylobacter* produce an ATP-dependent 'pump' that removes the macrolide from the bacteria.

Uses of macrolides

The spectrum of macrolides is wider than that of the pencillins. They are particularly active against unusual (called 'atypical') respiratory organisms such as *Mycoplasma pneumonia*, *Mycobacterium avium* (important in AIDS patients), and *Legionella*. They also cover *Chlamydia*, *H. pylori*, and *Campylobacter*. The newest, telithromycin, is active against *Streptococcus pneumoniae* that is resistant to pencillins and erythromycin.

The macrolides are used primarily for respiratory tract infections, particularly when atypical agents are suspected (e.g. severe community acquired pneumonia). Erythromycin is used topically in the treatment of acne and rosacea. Clarithromycin has activity against *H. pylori,* and is used as part of triple therapy for its eradication in peptic ulcer disease (see Chapter 12). Azithromycin is useful in treating *Chlamydia* as a single dose. The macrolides are used as alternatives to penicillins, in penicillin-allergic patients, for infections such as pharangytis, tonsillitis, and impetigo (school sores).

Dosing and adverse effects of macrolides

The newer macrolides, such as azithromycin and roxithromycin, have longer half-lives and can be given once a day; erythromycin has to be given four times a day. Erythromycin and roxithromycin are best taken on an empty stomach, but if gastrointestinal upset occurs they should be taken with food. A potential problem with erythromycin and clarithromycin is that they inhibit cytochrome P450, resulting in drug interactions. The macrolides also prolong QT interval (causing delayed repolarization following depolarization, which can lead to the cardiac arrhythmia torsade de pointes) and should be used with caution with other drugs that prolong QT interval (e.g. antiarrhythmic drugs and antipsychotics such as haloperidol).

21.2.4 Other antibiotics interfering with protein synthesis

Lincosamides

Clindamycin and **lincomycin** work similarly to macrolides, binding to the 50S subunit of the ribosome. They have little or no activity against gram-negative organisms, and are active against gram-positive bacteria and anaerobes. Both are usually reserved for patients with severe gram-positive infections that are unable to receive β-lactams. Clindamycin is used topically in the treatment of acne because of its activity against *Propionibacterium acnes*. They can both cause serious gastrointestinal problems, the most serious being pseudomembranous clolitis due to overgrowth of *C. difficile*.

Chloramphenicol

Chloramphenicol is an older antibiotic that also acts through the 50S subunit. It is active against a range of gram-positive, gram-negative, and anaerobic bacteria, in particular *Bacteroides fragilis*, *Salmonella typhi*, and *Haemophilus influenzae*. It use now is largely restricted to topical use in eye and ear drops because of the potential development of aplastic anaemia when given systemically (a rare, but often fatal, blood disorder).

Fusidic acid

Fusidic acid (or sodium fusidate) is an antibiotic active primarily against gram-positive organisms such as *Staphylococcus*. It acts, similarly to macrolides, by inhibiting translocation of the tRNA with the growing peptide chain (Box 21.1). It is used for skin and soft tissue infections involving *Staphylococcus aureus* and usually in combination with rifampicin to treat MRSA. It can produce liver dysfunction and liver function should be monitored.

Linezolid

Linezolid is an oxazolidinone antibacterial that acts by inhibiting the binding of the 30S and 50S subunits together, thus preventing the initiation of protein synthesis. Like the glycopeptides and daptomycin, it is active against gram-positive organisms and is used for serious skin and soft tissue infections, and for pneumonia where organisms such as *S. aureus* that is resistant to other treatments is identified. Rare but important side effects include thrombocytopenia, anaemia, leucopenia, and pancytopenia, as well as optic neuropathy. Patients' blood counts should be carefully monitored, and they should be encouraged to report any visual disturbances.

> Doris was prescribed linezolid after her bacterial cultures were resistant to vancomycin.

Streptogramins

Quinupristin and **dalfopristin** are streptogramin antibiotics that are used together. They work synergistically to impair protein synthesis: quinupristin inhibits translocation and dalfopristin changes the structure of the 50S subunit, allowing quinupristin to bind more effectively. They are active against gram-positive organisms, in particular MRSA and vancomycin-resistant *Enterococcus faecium*. Side effects include nausea, vomiting, arthralgias, and myalgias. Liver dysfunction also can occur.

21.2.5 Quinolones

The quinolones were one of the first synthetic classes of antibiotics. The current quinolones that are used in clinical practice are all **fluoroquinolones**, which have a fluoride atom attached to the central ring (Figure 21.5) and include **ciprofloxacin, ofloxacin, levofloxacin, norfloxacin,** and **moxifloxacin**.

The major difference with the quinolones is their mode of action, as they do not interfere with cell wall synthesis (i.e. either peptidoglycan or protein), but inhibit DNA replication. As noted in the introduction, DNA exists in a helical structure that twists every 10 or so bases. These twists produce strain within the DNA structure and if the DNA is joined in a circle (as it is in a bacteria), it will contort into a new shape called a supercoil. It is a bit like what happens with the spiral cord on the handset of a telephone. If you take the handset off the cradle, stretch out the cord, and twist the handset in one direction over and over, when you try and put the handset back on the cradle the chord twists and contorts over itself. This happens with the DNA and it is why we can pack so much DNA into a cell. For example, if you stretch out a single molecule of human DNA it would extend for over 2 m. Yet it is housed in a cell with a nucleus of only a few micrometers across. However, while it needs to be packed to be able to be stored inside the cell, the cell must also be able to 'unwind' it again to be able to use the DNA. To do this the supercoil needs to be 'relaxed' and this is done by a type II topoisomerase (DNA gyrase

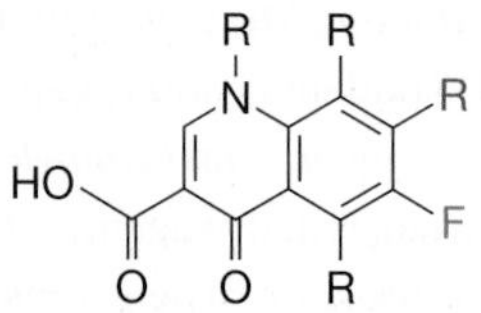

Figure 21.5 Central structure of fluoroquinolones.

and topoisomerase IV). Fluoroquinolones act by binding reversibly to DNA gyrase and topoisomerase IV, stopping DNA transcription and replication.

Resistance to quinolones

Quinolone resistance can develop quite quickly by one of two main mechanisms. First, is an alteration in GryA (one of the subunits of DNA gyrase) or ParC (a subunit of topoisomerase IV). This prevents the quinolone from binding to the DNA complex. The second mechanism is through reduced concentration of quinolones in the bacteria by blocking uptake or increased efflux. Some resistant bacteria have a decreased expression of porins, while others have increased expression of efflux pumps, which actively remove quinolones from the bacteria.

The rapid development of resistance has been put down, in part, to the excessive use of these antibiotics worldwide. Their broad spectrum of action (see later) has made them attractive as first-line antibiotics and currently they are the most widely prescribed antibiotics. To make matters worse, there has been excessive use in animals as a growth-enhancer. Together, this has dramatically reduced the effectiveness of this very valuable group of antibiotics.

Use of quinolones

Older quinolones, such as nalidixic acid, are used largely for urinary tract infections. The newer fluoroquinolones, which have the addition of the fluoride moiety, have a greater spectrum of bacterial coverage and better bioavailability. They generally have good activity against gram-negative bacteria, in particular *Haemophilus influenzae* (not norfloxacin) and *Pseudomonas aeruginosa*. They are active against some gram-positive bacteria, *Legionella*, and some mycobacteria. Ciprofloxacin and norfloxacin have the most limited spectrum for gram-positive bacteria and no coverage of anaerobes. Moxifloxacin has the widest coverage, including many gram-positive bacteria and anaerobes, but is not as active as ciprofloxacin against *Pseudomonas*. Ofloxacin, levofloxacin, moxifloxacin, and ciprofloxacin are used mainly for serious respiratory tract infections, particularly where atypical organisms such as *Pseudomonas* are suspected and where there is resistance to cheaper alternatives. They are also used for some skin and soft-tissue infections. Norfloxacin is used mainly for complicated urinary tract infections and for some gastrointestinal infections such as travellers' diarrhoea.

Given the rapid development of resistance and their cost, their use should be reserved to try and prolong their clinical utility.

Administration and side effects of quinolones

The fluoroquinolones can usually be given once or twice a day; moxifloxacin is only used once a day. Like all antibiotics they can cause antibiotic-induced diarrhoea due to *Clostridium difficile* overgrowth, and like tetracyclines they increase the sensitivity of the skin to ultraviolet light. Their use has been associated with damage to growing cartilage in animals, although human studies are lacking. However, they should only be used with caution in children. They have been linked with tendonitis and patients should be advised to stop the medication and stop exercising (there have been reports of tendon rupture, particularly in athletes) if they experience tendon pain or inflammation. The fluoroquinolones inhibit CYP3A4 (ciprofloxacin and norfloxacin also inhibit CYP1A2) and therefore they have a number of potential drug interactions (e.g. warfarin).

21.2.6 Nitroimidazoles

This is a small class of antibiotics comprising **metronidazole** and **tinidazole**. Structurally they are related to the imidazole group of antifungal agents (see section 21.3), but they are not used as antifungal agents (Figure 21.6).

Although they are taken up by both aerobic and anaerobic bacteria, their action is targeted in anaerobes. Once inside the bacteria the nitro group is reduced by ferredoxin, and the products of this process interfere with DNA synthesis. The selectivity for anaerobes appears to come from the need for an anaerobic (oxygen-free) environment for this reduction to occur.

Resistance to nitroimidazoles

There is increasing evidence of resistance to metronidazole in a number of important gastrointestinal organisms, including *H. pylori*. However, the exact mechanism is still

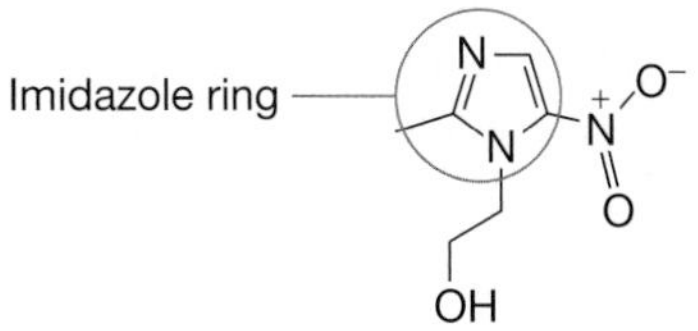

Figure 21.6 Metronidazole.

to be fully elucidated. One potential resistance pathway appears to be due to mutations in the *rdxA* gene, which results in a modification to nitroreductase. The prevalence of resistance is particularly high in people from developing countries, where metronidazole is used extensively to treat gastrointestinal infections.

Use of nitroimidazoles

Their activity against gram-negative anaerobes makes nitroimidazoles useful in the treatment of some gastrointestinal infections, including *H. pylori*. Metronidazole is the drug of choice for *C. difficile* infections. They are used for protazoal diseases, including bacterial vaginitis (caused by *Gardnerella vaginalis*) and giardiasis (caused by *Giardia lamblia*), and as prophylaxis prior to colorectal and abdominal surgery (to protect against gut anaerobes such as *Bacteroides* spp.). Metronidazole is also used topically to treat rosacea (sometimes called 'adult acne' as it has a similar appearance), although its mechanism of action for this condition is unclear.

> Our patient Doris was prescribed metronidazole after she developed aspiration pneumonia, which involves the gut contents, including bacteria from the gut, being inhaled into the lung. Unfortunately, later she developed *C. difficile* overgrowth despite being on metronidazole, so had to be prescribed a second-line agent (vancomycin).

Administration and side effects of nitroimidazoles

Metronidazole is given two to three times a day, while tinidazole is often given a single dose because of its long half-life (11–14 hours). Metronidazole can be given intravenously. However, it is well absorbed rectally, and this may be preferable to the parenteral route.

The main side effects are gastrointestinal, including gastrointestinal upset and causing a metallic taste. They can also cause central nervous system effects,, including dizziness and headaches. Metronidazole can rarely cause a disulfiram-like reaction with alcohol (disulfiram is a drug used to treat alcohol abuse by interfering with the breakdown of alcohol and causing a severe reaction, including nausea, vomiting, flushing, and tachycardia). Patients taking metronidazole should therefore not drink alcohol (although it is a potential with tinidazole, it has only been reported with metronidazole). Metronidazole and tinidazole are metabolized by the cytochrome P450 enzyme system, and metronidazole may increase the

levels of some drugs, including warfarin. Overall, tinidazole is better tolerated and has fewer reported interactions.

21.2.7 Aminoglycosides

The aminoglycosides are an older group of antibiotics derived from two bacterial species, *Streptomyces* (aminoglycosides that end in -mycin, such as streptomycin) and *Micromonospora* (aminoglycosides that end in -micin, such as gentamicin). The commonly used aminoglycosides are **amikacin**, **gentamicin**, **tobramycin**, **neomycin**, and **streptomycin**. They work by a couple of different mechanisms. First, they bind to the 30S subunit of the ribosome and interfere with protein synthesis by affecting the interaction between tRNA and mRNA. Second, they cause transient holes in the cell membrane of bacteria by displacing Mg^{++} and Ca^{++} in the cell membrane that links polysaccharides and lipopolysaccharides. It is the latter mechanism that is thought to confer the bactericidal effects of aminoglycosides, compared to tetracyclines, which also inhibit protein synthesis via the 30S subunit but are not bactericidal. They are mainly active against gram-negative organisms and have little activity against anaerobes because their uptake into bacteria is an active, energy-dependent system, and anaerobes have less energy to take up the aminoglycosides.

Resistance to aminoglycosides

Aminoglycoside resistance occurs through one of three mechanisms. The first is through inhibition of the uptake into bacterial cells. This is thought to be chromosomally mediated and produces moderate resistance to all aminoglycosides. The second mechanism is through alteration to the binding site on the 30S subunit. This mainly affects streptomycin, as most of the other aminoglycosides attach to multiple sites on the 30S subunit. The third mode of resistance, and the most common, is due to enzymatic modification of the aminoglycosides inside the bacteria. There are three groups of enzymes involved:

- N-acetyltransferases—cause acetylation of an amino group
- O-adenyltransferases—cause adenylation of hydroxyl group
- O-phosphotransferases—cause phosphorylation of a hydroxyl group.

The genes for these are found on plasmids and transposons, and they produce the most significant resistance to aminoglycosides. However, there are differences across the aminoglycosides in their susceptibility to enzymatic modification, with amikacin being the least likely to be inactivated by enzymes.

Uses of aminoglycosides

Because of their potential toxicity (see later) the aminoglycosides are reserved for serious gram-negative infections. They are used for respiratory tract infections (e.g. serious pneumonia), meningitis, renal infections, endocarditis, and sepsis. Tobramycin has slightly better coverage against *Pseudomonas aeruginosa*, but not against other gram-negative bacteria. Neomycin is used topically in ointments, although it can cause sensitization, and orally to sterilize the gut. Generally, gentamicin is the aminoglycoside of choice because it is usually effective and inexpensive; amikacin should be reserved for patients with organisms resistant to gentamicin because of its cost.

Administration and side effects of aminoglycosides

None of the aminoglycosides are absorbed orally, therefore they must be given parenterally for a systemic effect (note: neomycin is given orally but it acts locally in the gut, and is not absorbed). They are usually given by intravenous infusion once a day. Because they are renally cleared, largely unchanged, their dosage must be adjusted in patients who have reduced kidney function. Initial doses are chosen based on lean body weight and creatinine clearance (a measure of renal function). In patients with impaired renal function subsequent doses can be adjusted in one of two ways. First, the dose given every 24 hours can be reduced. Second, the interval between doses can be extended, while maintaining the same dose. Either method can be calculated using formulas, nomograms, or, most commonly today, using computer programs.

The aminoglycosides have a range of adverse events, the most serious being ototoxicity and nephrotoxicity. All aminoglycosides are toxic to the cells of the ears, but they differ in their effects on hearing (cochlear toxicity) versus balance (vestibular toxicity). Gentamicin has a greater effect on the vestibular apparatus and tends to cause issues with balance rather than hearing loss. Amikacin has fewer vestibular effects and is more likely to cause deafness. The ototoxicity and nephrotoxicity are dose related and potentially worsened by other ototoxic (e.g. loop diuretics) or nephrotoxic (e.g. non-steroidal anti-inflammatories and angiotensin-converting enzyme inhibitors) drugs, therefore careful monitoring of levels and the use of short courses (less than 7 days) is recommended. Both nephrotoxicity and ototoxicity are usually reversible, although permanent damage to the ear has been documented. Patients should be encouraged to report signs of dizziness, vertigo, and 'ringing in the ear'.

21.2.8 Other antibiotics that interfere with DNA synthesis

Two antibiotics, **trimethoprim** and **sulfamethoxazole** (a **sulphonamide**), interfere with the production of thymidine triphosphate, one of the four nucleosides used in the synthesis of DNA, by inhibiting folate production in the bacteria. Trimethoprim inhibits dihydrofolate reductase, while sulphonamides act as an analogue of para-aminobenzoic acid and compete for dihydropteroate synthetase (Figure 21.7).

Although human cells also use folic acid to synthesize DNA, unlike bacteria, we can get our folic acid from our diet and do not need to synthesize it. A combination product with both sulfamethoxazole and trimethoprim (called co-trimoxazole) was used commonly for respiratory tract infections, but it has been largely phased out because of adverse reactions to the sulphonamide. Trimethoprim alone is now one of the antibiotics of choice for urinary tract infections, as well as prostatitis and epididymo-orchitis. Co-trimoxazole is used largely now as a treatment for *Pneumocystis jiroveci (carinii)* pneumonia (PCP), an opportunistic respiratory tract infection in patients with HIV.

21.2.9 Antibiotics against *Mycobacteria*

Mycobacteria are a group of aerobic bacteria that can cause serious respiratory tract infections. They have a distinct, hydrophobic cell wall containing mycolic acid or mycolate, giving it a waxy consistency (*myco* is Latin for wax). Because the cell wall is not typically gram-positive or gram-negative, *Mycobacteria* can be very difficult organisms to treat. The two main respiratory diseases they cause are tuberculosis (TB, mainly caused by *Mycobacterium tuberculosis*) and a similar condition called mycobacterium avium complex (MAC, caused by

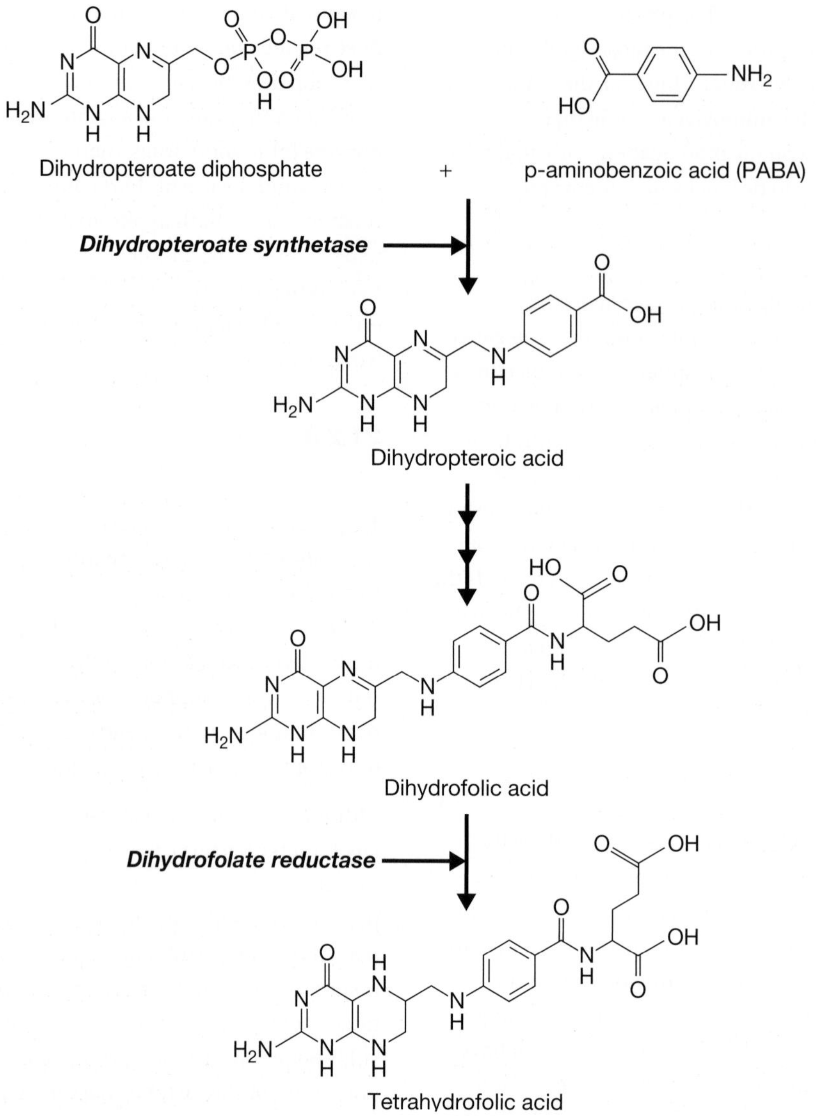

Figure 21.7 Folate synthesis.

various *Mycobacterium avium* subspecies). The latter is another opportunistic infection in patients with HIV.

Tuberculosis is one of the most prevalent infections in the world, with about a third of the population infected at any one time. It is spread by droplets through coughing or sneezing, but the majority of people exposed will not develop clinical disease and can remain as asymptomatic carriers. Given the number of people affected, and the nearly two million deaths each year, TB is one of the world's most important infections.

Several of the antibiotics discussed above are used in the treatment of TB and MAC, including macrolides (section

21.2.3) and streptomycin (section 21.2.7). Other antibiotics include:

- rifamycins
- dapsone
- ethambutol
- isoniazid
- pyrazinamide
- clofazimine
- capreomycin.

Because of rapid resistance, multi-drug therapy is usually used.

Rifamycins

The rifamycins used clinically are **rifampicin** and **rifabutin**. They are both complex structures and they act by inhibiting the synthesis of mRNA from DNA by binding to DNA-dependent RNA polymerase. They only affect prokaryotic cells (i.e. cells without a nucleus, such as bacteria) and their lipid solubility makes them useful in treating disseminated TB that can pass into the brain. The main side effects are gastrointestinal upset and discolouration of bodily fluids (e.g. urine turns orange/red). Both are inducers of cytochrome P450 and can decrease the concentration and effectiveness of many drugs, although rifabutin is a weaker inducer than rifampicin.

Dapsone

Dapsone, like sulphonamides, acts as inhibitor of folate synthesis by acting as an analogue of p-aminobenzoic acid. It is used mainly for the treatment and prevention of PCP infections, and for treating leprosy (caused by *Mycobacterium leprae* and *Mycobacterium lepromatosis*). The main side effect is dose-related asymptomatic haemolytic anaemia. It can rarely cause hepatic dysfunction and what is called 'dapsone syndrome', which involves a rash, jaundice, eosinophilia, and fever, and is usually reversible on stopping therapy.

Ethambutol

Ethambutol is another complex molecule used to treat TB and MAC. It acts by inhibiting arabinosyl transferases, which are involved in arabinogalactan synthesis in mycobacterium. The arabinogalactan forms a complex with mycolic acid and peptidoglycan in the cell wall. Thus ethambutol inhibits cell wall development and is bacteriostatic. The main side effect is optic neuritis, which can present as decreased visual acuity or colour blindness, and is usually reversible on stopping therapy.

Isoniazid

Isoniazid is a pro-drug that is activated by catalase-peroxidase enzyme KatG in the mycobacterium. Once activated it forms a complex with nicotinamide adenine dinucleotide, and this complex blocks the synthesis of mycolic acid. Side effects include peripheral neuritis, and it is recommended that patients be prescribed pyridoxine 25 mg with each dose to reduce the risk. Other rare effects include hepatitis and optic neuritis.

Pyrazinamide

Like isoniazid, **pyrazinamide** is also a pro-drug that is converted by pyrazinamidase in the mycobacteria to pyrazinoic acid. This is active only in an acid pH, thus the activity of pyrazinamide declines as the pH rises (i.e. once inflammation subsides). Although the exact effect of pyrazioic acid on the cells is uncertain, one proposed mechanism is its action as a weak acid and affecting the cell wall transport functions by 'de-energizing' the cell wall. The common side effects are arthralgia and hyperuricaemia. It can also rarely cause liver dysfunction.

Clofazimine

Clofazimine is a fat-soluble antibiotic used to treat leprosy and MAC belonging to the class called riminophenazines. Its exact mechanism of action is still to be elucidated, but one proposed mechanism is interruption to DNA replication by binding to guanine bases on DNA. The main side effect is deposition in the skin, causing a pink to brownish/black appearance, which can worsen on sun exposure. Patients can be assured that this will return to normal once the drug is stopped.

Capreomycin

Capreopmycin is an aminoglycoside-like antibiotic. Like aminoglycosides, it appears to work by inhibiting protein synthesis by binding to the ribosome, possibly both the 50S and 30S subunits. It also shares many of the adverse effects of aminoglycosides, including ototoxicity and nephrotoxicity. It is generally reserved for patients who have failed or cannot take other first-line treatments.

21.2.10 Other antibiotics

Glycopeptides

Vancomycin and **teicoplanin** are glycopeptide antibiotics, with teicoplanin having a longer duration of action, allowing once daily administration. They both inhibit cell wall synthesis in gram-positive bacteria by inhibiting the incorporation of N-acetylmuramic acid and N-acetylglucosamine peptide into peptidoglycan. They are active only against gram-positive bacteria and are used in the treatment of MRSA and other severe infections in patients where β-lactams are contraindicated. Vancomycin is also used to treat *C. difficile* infections in patients who are intolerant of, or where resistance exists to, other agents such as metronidazole. It is given orally for *C. difficile* because it is not absorbed and acts locally in the gut on the bacteria. The lack of oral absorption (<1%) means there are no issues with systemic toxicity. The well-known side effect of intravenous vancomycin is 'red man' syndrome, which is an allergic reaction where patients exhibit pruritus and an erythematous (red) rash covering the face, neck, and upper torso, which can be accompanied by dyspnoea and hypotension. The reaction can be reduced by slow (over 60 minutes) infusion and pre-treatment with antihistamines.

Lipopeptides

Daptomycin is a new lipopeptide antibiotic derived from *Streptomyces roseosporus* found in soil. It has a unique mechanism of action that causes rapid depolarization of the cell membrane through potassium efflux. This disrupts DNA, RNA, and protein synthesis. It is active against gram-positive organisms, including MRSA, and is reserved for complicated skin and soft tissue infections. Side effects include nausea and diarrhoea, and, rarely, myopathies. Patients should have their creatine kinase monitored and be asked to report any muscle pain or weakness.

Polymyxins

Colistin and **Polymyxin B** are polymyxin antibiotics. They act by biding to lipopolysaccharides in the outer membrane of gram-negative bacteria and cause disruption to the cell membrane in a similar fashion to detergents (i.e. they have both a hydrophilic and hydrophobic component). They are active against *Pseudomonas aeruginosa*, *Enterobacteriaceae*, and *Klebsiella pneumoniae*. However, their renal and neurotoxicity have limited their use. Colistin is used by mouth for gut sterilization, and by inhalation for the treatment of *P. aeruginosa* in cystic fibrosis. Colistin is used parenterally for the treatment of multi-drug resistant gram-negative infections where other agents cannot be used.

Nitrofurantoin

Nitrofurantoin is a bacteriostatic antibiotic with activity against gram-positive organisms, but limited or no activity against gram-negative bacteria or anaerobes. It is taken into bacteria, where it is converted by nitrofuran reductase, a flavoprotein, to unstable intermediates that cause damage to DNA, ribosomes, and other macromolecules. Because of its multiple sites of action, resistance to nitrofurantoin is relatively low. It is used primarily for complicated urinary tract infections, but is second or third line because of its toxicity, which includes gastrointestinal upset, allergic reactions, hepatotoxicity, pulmonary toxicity, and peripheral neuropathy.

21.2.11 Bactericidal versus bacteriostatic activity

It has been noted that some antibiotics have bactericidal (killing bacteria) activity, while others are bacteriostatic (stopping the growth of bacteria). Examples of bactericidal antibiotics include the aminoglycocides, β-lactams, fluoroquinolones, cotrimoxazole, and nitrofurantoin. Agents such as macrolides, tetracyclines, and lincosamides are usually considered bacteriostatic. However, this classification is not clearly delineated. Some antibiotics possess bacteriostatic properties against some bacteria, while they are bactericidal against others. An example of this is penicillin, which is bacteriostatic against enterococci, but bactericidal against pneumococci. Others are bacteriostatic at some doses, while bactericidal at others. While intuitively it would seem that it is more desirable to kill the bacteria, rather than just inhibit its growth, the clinical significance of the difference in many infections is unclear. In the majority of situations, provided you can stop the bacteria from growing, you can allow the bodies normal defence system to get rid of it. However, for some serious infections, such as endocarditis, meningitis, and infections in patients with impaired immune systems, bactericidal antibiotics are the preferred treatment. Bactericidal antibiotics may also confer some advantage in that there is often less resistance if you can kill the bacteria, rather than just slow its growth.

21.2.12 Post-antibiotic effects

For several decades it has been observed that the effects of some antibiotics can continue well after the levels of the antibiotic are undetectable. This has been referred to as the post-antibiotic effect (PAE). Antibiotics reported to have significant PAE include the aminoglycosides and quinolones. By contrast, β-lactams and vancomycin have little or no PAE for many organisms. The difference is, in part, due to their mechanism of action, with drugs that affect DNA and protein synthesis more likely to demonstrate PAE, compared to those that only affect cell wall synthesis. However, the PAE can also differ with the same antibiotic in different bacteria. For example, with aminoglycosides, they have a short PAE (½–2½ hours) for methicillin-sensitive *S. aureus*, but a longer PAE (up to 3½ hours or more) for *P. aeruginosa,* and *E. coli.* The main consequence of PAE is probably in designing treatment regimens. The consistent PAE with aminoglycosides has allowed us to move away from trying to keep the levels above the minimum inhibitory concentration by giving doses several times a day, to now giving the aminoglycosides once a day, which allows levels to drop very low between dosing, thus minimizing toxicity.

21.3 Fungal infections

Fungi are more complex organisms than bacteria. They are one of the five 'kingdoms' of life forms (others are plants, animals, protista, and monera—**prokaryotes**), and probably resemble animal cells more than the other cellular forms. Unlike bacteria (prokaryotic), fungi contain a nucleus (eukaryotic) and represent the latter stages in evolution. Apart from a nucleus, **eukaryotes** often contain other intracellular structures, including mitochondria, Golgi bodies, and vacuoles.

21.3.1 Fungal cell walls

Unlike bacterial cell walls, which are composed primarily of lipopolysaccharides and peptidoglycan, fungal walls are made up of four layers: phospholipid plasma membrane comprising mainly ergosterol, chitin, glucans, and mannoproteins (Figure 21.8).

Chitin is a polysaccharide made of N-acetylglucosamine (derived from glucose). Apart from fungi, it is found in the exoskeleton of insects and crustaceans. β-**glucans** comprise polysaccharides of D-glucose and are found in fungi and some bacteria. The outer layer comprises **mannoproteins**, which are proteins containing a large number of manose groups (an isomer of glucose).

21.3.2 Classification of fungi

Fungi can be classified in a number of ways, for example based on their shape or appearance. Yeasts tend to be unicellular and spherical in shape, while moulds are often filamentous, growing in branches made up of hyphae, which form a mycelium (Figure 21.9). Some organisms are dimorphic, existing as yeasts or moulds depending on the temperature.

Clinically we often classify fungal infections as superficial, cutaneous, subcutaneous, or systemic (or deep). The latter is also divided into primary, which can establish infections in a normal host, and opportunistic organisms, which occur in hosts with an impaired immune system. Examples of some of the human mycoses and their causative organisms are given in Table 21.4.

21.3.3 Tinea infections

Tinea is the most common fungal infection to affect humans, with up to 70% of the population reported to suffer from tinea pedis (athlete's foot) at some time in their life. The main causative organisms are dermatophytes, which are organisms that obtain their nutrients from the keratin in our skin. The fungi involved include *Epidermophyton*, *Trichophyton*, and

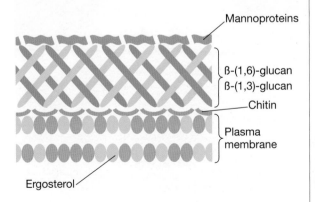

Figure 21.8 Composition of fungal cell walls.

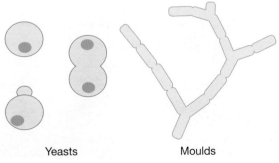

Figure 21.9 Yeasts versus moulds.

Table 21.4 Human mycoses classified by depth of infection

Example infection	Causative organisms	Prevalence
Superficial mycoses		
Black piedra	*Piedraia hortae*	Rare
White piedra	*Trichosporon beigelii*	Common
Pityriasis (Tinea) versicolor	*Malassezia furfur*	Common
Seborrheic dermatitis	*Malassezia furfur*	Common
Dandruff	*Malassezia furfur*	Common
Cutaneous mycoses		
Tinea (including ring worm)	*Epidermophyton*, *Microsporum*, and *Trichophyton* spp.	Common
Cutaneous candidiasis	*Candidia albicans* and other *Candida* spp.	Common
Subcutanous mycoses		
Sporotrichosis	*Sporothrix schenckii*	Rare
Chromoblastomycosis	*Fonsecaea*, *Phialophora*, *Cladosporium* spp.	Rare
Systemic mycoses – primary		
Histoplasmosis	*Histoplasma capsulatum*	Rare
Coccidioidomycosis	*Coccidioides immitis*	Rare
Systemic mycoses – opportunistic		
Candidiasis	*Candida albicans* and other *Candida* spp.	Common
Cryptococcosis	*Cryptococcus neoformans*	Rare/common
Aspergillosis	*Aspergillus fumigatus*	Rare

Microsporum species. They exist all the time on our skin, but only become problematic when there is damage to skin allowing them to infiltrate the keratin layer. They facilitate this by producing keratinises and proteinases that help them penetrate the outer skin layers. Once established they can cause peeling of the superficial layers of the skin (tinea pedis) or a scaly plaque with a raised, vesicular-like skin eruption at the edges (tinea corporis – ringworm) (Figure 21.10). Tinea pedis often causes intense itching.

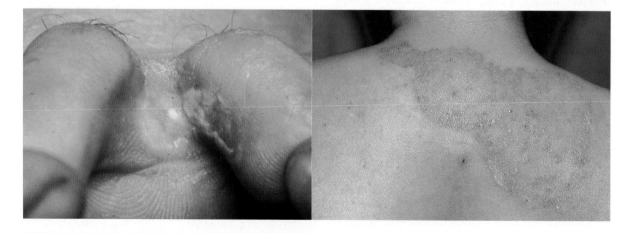

Figure 21.10 Two common types of tinea.

Table 21.5 Main types of human tinea infections

Location	Type of tinea	Common name/ alternative name
Foot	Tinea pedis	Athlete's foot
Body	Tinea corporis	Ringworm
Fingernails and toenails	Tinea unguium	Onychomycosis
Groin	Tinea cruris	Jock itch/crotch itch/ dhobi itch/scrot rot
Face	Tinea faciei	N/A
Beard line (men)	Tinea barbae	Barbers itch
Scalp	Tinea capitis	Scalp ringworm
Hand	Tinea manuum	N/A

N/A, not applicable.

Tinea can appear just about anywhere on the body and the different types of tinea are classified according to their location (Table 21.5).

Rarely, tinea can be caused by *Candida* spp., particularly if a person is immunosuppressed (see section 21.3.4).

21.3.4 Candida infections

Candida, in particular *Candida albicans*, is another common source of fungal infection in humans. The two main sites are in the oropharyngeal region (mouth, tongue, and throat—oral thrush) and in women the vagina (vaginal thrush). This is another organism that is usually present all the time, but is kept in check by our immune system and, in the case of the vagina, by the presence of normal bacteria that keep it under control. Just like tinea, candidal infections require some alteration to the normal system to gain a foothold. In the case of oropharyngeal infections, this can occur with the use of inhaled corticosteroids, which suppress the normal human immune system in and around the mouth. Vaginal candidiasis is sometimes caused by broad-spectrum antibiotics, which remove the bacteria that normally suppress the *Candida* in the vagina. Both types can also be caused by other things that suppress our normal immune response, in particular poorly controlled or undiagnosed diabetes mellitus.

21.3.5 Tinea versicolour

Although less common than *Candida* and dermatophyte infections, tinea versicolour affects more than 1% of the population, with a higher incidence in warmer, humid environments (up to 50% prevalence). It is a benign superficial infection of the skin caused by the yeast *Malassezia furfur* (formally called *Pityrosporum ovale*), the organism associated with seborrheic dermatitis and dandruff. It produces patches on the skin that change colour. In dark-skinned people it tends to cause paler spots (hypopigmentation), while in fair-skinned people it causes darker spots (hyperpigmentation). The yeast is thought to live off lipids on the skin, and so areas high in lipid production, such as the back and chest, are common sites for the lesions.

21.4 Treatment of fungal infections

Just like many bacterial infections, treating fungal infections is largely aimed at targeting cell wall synthesis. As fungal cells closely resemble human cells, it has been important to exploit the differences in the cell wall synthesis to avoid toxicity. In this case, the main difference is in the use ergosterol by fungi in cell wall synthesis, compared to cholesterol by human cells. The main targets of pharmacological agents in inhibiting ergosterol synthesis are outlined in Box 21.2.

The main antifungal agents used are:

- imidazoles and triazoles (referred to collectively as the 'azoles')
- terbinafine
- polyenes
- amorolfine
- griseofulvin.

Some lesser-used agents will also be discussed, including those targeted at dandruff and seborrheic dermatitis.

21.4.1 The 'azole' antifungals

This group includes the largest number of antifungal agents. The imidazoles include **miconazole, ketoconazole, clotrimazole, econazole, butoconazole**, and **bifonazole**. The triazoles are **fluconazole, itraconazole, voriconazole,**

Box 21.2
Synthesis of ergosterol

Figure b

1. Squalene is synthesised from isopentenyl pyrophosphate (IPP) and dimethylallyl pyrophosphate (DMAPP). It is converted to squalene epoxide by squalene epoxidase. This is the site of action for terbinafine.

2. Squalene epoxide is converted to lanosterol by lanosterol synthetase.

3. Lanosterol is converted to 14-demethyl lanosterol by C14-demethylase, a cytochrome P450 enzyme. This is the site of action for the azole antifungals (e.g. clotrimazole).

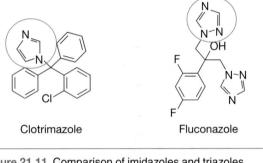

Clotrimazole

Fluconazole

Figure 21.11 Comparison of imidazoles and triazoles.

and **posaconazole**. Both groups share similar structures (Figure 21.11), but the triazoles have the advantage of all being able to be given orally for systemic treatment (although ketoconazole can also be given orally).

All 'azoles' work by inhibiting C14 demethylase, which is involved in the synthesis of ergosterol (Box 21.2). The topical imidazoles (clotrimazole, econazole, ketoconazole, butoconazole, bifonazole, and miconazole) are active against dermatophytes and *Candida* spp. The use of the different topical imidazoles and their formulations is outlined in Table 21.6.

Table 21.6 Imidazole antifungal agents

Imidazole	Formulation	Clinical use
Clotrimazole	Cream	Tinea (including versicolour) Candida nappy rash Vulvovaginal candidiasis
	Pessary	Vuvlovaginal candidiasis
	Lotion	Tinea
Miconazole	Cream	Tinea (including versicolour) Candida nappy rash Vulvovaginal candidiasis
	Lotion	Tinea
	Tincture	Onychomycosis
	Powder	Tinea pedis
	Oral gel	Oropharyngeal candida (thrush)
	Shampoo	Seborrheic dermatitis/dandruff
Econazole	Cream	Tinea (including versicolour)
	Foaming solution	Tinea versicolour
Bifonazole	Cream	Tinea (including versicolour)
Ketoconazole	Cream	Tinea (including versicolour)
	Shampoo	Seborrheic dermatitis/dandruff
Butoconazole	Cream	Vulvovaginal candidiasis

Apart from being available in different formulations, the imidazoles differ in the frequency they are used to treat tinea. Clotrimazole, econazole, and miconazole are all used two or three times a day, whereas ketoconazole and bifonazole are used only once a day.

The systemic 'azoles' (ketoconazole, fluconazole, itraconazole, posaconazole, and voriconazole) are used for a variety of systemic and topical fungal infections. Fluconazole is used to treat vulvovaginal candidiasis, but is generally reserved for patients who have failed or are intolerant to topical imidazoles. It is also used for a number of systemic infections, including *Cryptococcosis*, *Coccidioidomycosis*, and *Histoplasmosis*, as well as some *Candida* infections (except *C. krusei* and *C. glabrate*). Ketoconazole and itraconazole are used for dermatophyte, tinea versicolour, and *Candida* infections in patients who are intolerant to, or failed on, topical treatment or in difficult-to-treat areas. Both posaconazole and voriconazole are generally reserved for patients with severe systemic fungal infections in those who failed or cannot tolerate the other systemic antifungals; voriconazole may be the drug of choice for treatment of life-threatening aspergillosis.

The main side effects of oral azoles are gastrointestinal. Some less common but serious adverse effects include heart failure (itraconazole), thrombocytopenia (voriconazole), and hepatotoxicity (ketoconazole). The systemic azoles have a number of potential drug interactions. First, both itraconazole and ketoconazole are better absorbed in an acidic environment and therefore their absorption can be reduced in patients on proton pump inhibitors or even histamine-2 receptor antagonists. The systemic azoles inhibit several cytochrome P450 enzymes, particularly CYP3A4. Thus, they interact with a number of medicines, and these should be checked before starting therapy. Single does fluconazole, which is used to treat simple vulvovaginal candidiasis, is generally unlikely to cause significant interactions, except possibly with warfarin, when international normalized ratios should be monitored. Fluconazole and voriconazole can prolong the QT interval and may interact with other drugs that prolong the QT interval (e.g. some antiarrhythmics and some macrolide antibiotics) to produce torsades de points (a potentially serious cardiac arrhythmia).

21.4.2 Terbinafine

Terbinafine is an allylamine. It works by inhibiting squalene epoxidase and stops conversion of squalene to squalene epoxide, an early step in ergosterol synthesis (Box 21.2). It is active against a broad range of dermatophytes and *C. albicans*. Terbinafine is available in topical (creams, gels, and a special 'film-forming solution') and oral preparations. The topical preparations are used to treat tinea, and compared to azoles are effective after only 7 days of treatment, compared to 2–4 weeks with most azoles (the 'film-forming solution' preparation only has to be applied once). The oral tablets are used for difficult-to-treat infections such as onychomycosis (tinea unguium) or where topical therapy has failed or is not tolerated.

Like the azoles, gastrointestinal side effects are common, including taste disturbance. Rare side effects include hepatitis and hepatic failure. Terbinafine is an inhibitor of CYP2D6. However, it has fewer important interactions compared to azoles. It may increase the levels of some tricyclic antidepressants, including imipramine and nortriptyline, and the serotonin–noradrenaline reuptake inhibitor venlafaxine.

21.4.3 Polyenes

This is one of the oldest class of antifungals and includes **amphotericin B** and **nystatin**. Both are large, complex structures that consist of a ring of molecules, including many carbon–carbon double bonds (hence polyene), and multiple hydroxide groups. The polyene molecule attaches to ergosterol and forms 'pores' in the cell membrane that allow the contents of the cell to leak out (Figure 21.12).

Amphotericin remains the antifungal of choice for many serious systemic fungal infections, with activity against most fungi except dermatophytes, and only some of the newer azoles (e.g. posaconazole and voriconazole) have a

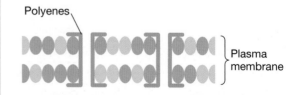

Figure 21.12 Action of polyene antifungals.

wider spectrum. Furthermore, resistance to amphotericin is rare. Amphotericin is also used for the treatment of oral thrush. It is given intravenously for systemic infections and by lozenge for oral thrush. The intravenous preparation can be quite toxic, causing phlebitis (inflammation of the blood vessels), infusion reactions (e.g. fever, chills, and hypotension), and nephrotoxicity. To reduce some of these side effects the newer intravenous preparations combine amphotericin with lipids either as a lipid complex or as liposomes. However, these are significantly more expensive than regular intravenous amphotericin preparations.

> Doris was initially treated with nystatin when she develops oral thrush, a not uncommon side effect of broad-spectrum antibiotics. Unfortunately, it failed to treat the infection and she needed an oral azole.

21.4.4 Amorolfine

Amorolfine is an antifungal agent that targets two parts of the synthesis of ergosterol, D14-reductase, and D-7,8-isomerase (Box 21.2). It is active against a broad range of dermatophytes and *Candida* spp. It is used only for treating onychomycosis and is applied as a nail lacquer. However, it is mainly useful for superficial, distal nail infections, with oral therapy better for proximal or nail-bed involvement. It is generally well tolerated, with local reactions to the nail lacquer being the main side effects.

21.4.5 Griseofulvin

Griseofulvin is an oral antifungal used to treat cutaneous mycoses. It acts by binding to tubulin and therefore blocks microtubule formation within the fungi, which interferes with cell division. This effect on the mitotic spindle has seen griseofulvin investigated as a potential treatment for cancer. Griseofulvin is only active against dermatophytes and is used to treat tinea infections where other treatments have failed; it is the preferred treatment of tinea capitis.

Griseofulvin is generally well tolerated, but can cause gastrointestinal upset and increase the skin's sensitivity to the sun. It interacts with a number of drugs and can cause reduced effectiveness of the oral contraceptive pill and warfarin. Griseofulvin should be taken with food or milk to increase its absorption.

21.4.6 Other antifungals used to treat dermatological mycoses

Ranges of antifungal agents, most available without a prescription, have been used to treat topical mycoses such as tinea pedis, tinea corporis, and tinea versicolour. These include:

- tolnaftate
- compound benzoic acid ointment (Whitfield's ointment)
- undecenoates
- zinc pyridinethione
- selenium sulfide
- piroctone olamine
- ciclopirox olamine.

However, several of these have been superseded by the 'azoles' and other newer antifungals.

Tolnaftate

Tolnaftate is one of the oldest antifungal agents. Despite this, its exact mechanism of action is unclear, but it has been postulated that it may block squalene epoxidase (similar to terbinafine) and therefore interfere with ergosterol synthesis. It is only active against dermatophytes and is mainly used for tinea pedis.

Compound benzoic acid ointment

Compound benzoic acid ointment (Whitfield's ointment) is a combination of benzoic acid and salicylic acid in a greasy base. It is the benzoic acid that is thought to have antifungal activity, and it enters the fungal cell, lowers the internal pH of the fungi, and interferes with fungal cell growth. It is used primarily for tinea infections, such as tinea corporis, but it is cosmetically less acceptable than the newer antifungals because of the greasy nature of the base.

Undecenoates

The undecenoates include **zinc undecenoate** and **undecenoic acid**. Undecenoic acid, also called undecylenic acid, is an organic fatty acid derived from castor oil. The exact mechanism of its antifungal action is still unclear, but may include disruption of the pH of the fungal cell and inhibition of the conversion of yeasts into the hyphal form. It is used for tinea pedis and onychomycosis.

Zinc pyridinethione and selenium sulfide

Both **zinc pyridinethione** (also called **pyrithione zinc**) and **selenium sulfide** have been used as antidandruff shampoos for decades. Their mechanism of action is uncertain, but they appear to be effective against *Malassezia furfur*, and are used to treat seborrheic dermatitis (dandruff) and tinea versicolour. An added benefit in seborrheic dermatitis is that they have antimitotic activity, reducing epithelial cell growth.

Piroctone olamine and ciclopirox olamine

Piroctone olamine and **ciclopirox olamine** are two of the newer antidandruff treatments. They are both active against *M. furfur* and used mainly for seborrhoeic dermatitis. Their pharmacology is not well understood. However, it has been postulated that ciclopirox interferes with cell division and DNA repair in fungi.

21.5 Viral infections

Viruses are the smallest of the infective organisms. They are also arguably the simplest in their structure. Despite this they can result in significant morbidity, and in some cases, such as HIV, high mortality. The basic structure of a virus contains two or three parts. At the core is a piece of DNA or RNA. Surrounding this is a protein coat that protects the DNA/RNA (capsid), and in some cases this is then covered in a lipoprotein outer layer to protect the virus when it is outside the host cell (more later).

21.5.1 Classification of viruses

Broadly speaking viruses are classified by their genetic material (DNA vs RNA), the number of strands of genetic material (single strand vs double strand), and the 'sense' of the genetic material (positive, negative, and both—ambisence). The sense relates to whether it is a positive or negative copy of the genetic material. For example, positive-sense viral RNA is the same as viral mRNA and can be translated easily by the host cell, whereas negative-sense viral RNA is a complementary copy of mRNA and therefore must be converted to positive-sense RNA by an RNA polymerase before

translation. Some examples of human viruses classified this way can be found in Table 21.7.

21.5.2 Life cycle of the virus

Viruses are the ultimate parasites. Unlike bacteria and fungi they are unable to replicate by themselves and use the host (human) cells to copy their genetic material. This is partly what makes treating them so difficult, as stopping viral reproduction can lead to healthy cells being prevented from replicating.

There are five key phases in the life cycle of a virus:

- exposure to the virus
- entry into the cells
- replication of the virus
- shedding of the virus
- laying dormant (latency).

Exposure to the virus

Just like bacteria and fungi, you must be exposed to a virus to be infected. Intact skin is a good barrier to viruses.

Table 21.7 Examples of human viral conditions

Type of virus	Example viruses	Example clinical conditions
dsDNA	Adenoviruses, herpes virus	Common cold (adenovirus), cold sores (herpes simplex I)
ssDNA	Parvovirus	Erythema infectiosum—fifth disease (parvovirus B19)
dsRNA	Reoviruses	Gastroenteritis (rotavirus)
(+)ssRNA	Picornavirus	Polio (poliovirus), common cold (rhinovirus)
(−)ssRNA	Rhabdoviruses, orthomyxoviruses	Rabies (rabies virus), influenza (influenza A)
ssRNA-RT	Retroviruses	HIV (human immunodeficiency virus 1)
dsDNA-RT	Hepadnaviruses	Hepatitis B (hepatitis B virus)

ds, double strand; ss, single strand; (+), positive sense; (−), negative sense; RT, uses reverse transcriptase

However, a cut or direct inoculation, such as from a mosquito or sharing infected needles, is how viruses such as HIV and hepatitis can enter the body. Many others enter through the mucosa (e.g. the rhinoviruses that cause the common cold), as it poses less of a barrier compared to the skin.

Entry into the cells

Once inside the body the virus has to enter the cell to replicate. To do this the virus uses receptors on its outer surface to attach to complementary receptors on the host cell. This then allows the surface proteins of the virus and the host cell to interact. Once attached to the outer surface the virus enters through one of a number of different mechanisms depending on the virus. One method is by membrane fusion, in which the membrane of the virus fuses with the membrane of the cell and then releases the contents into the cell (Figure 21.13). This is the method used by influenza A virus and HIV. The other popular method of entering the cell is via endocytosis. This involves getting the cell to engulf the virus within a pocket of the cell membrane (vacuole) (Figure 21.14). This is also called phagocytosis and is used by some immune cells to remove foreign particles. Examples of viruses that do this include coxsackie virus (causes hand, foot, and mouth disease), hepatitis C, and poliovirus.

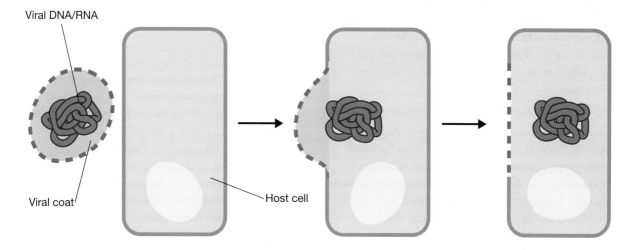

Figure 21.13 Viral entry by membrane fusion.

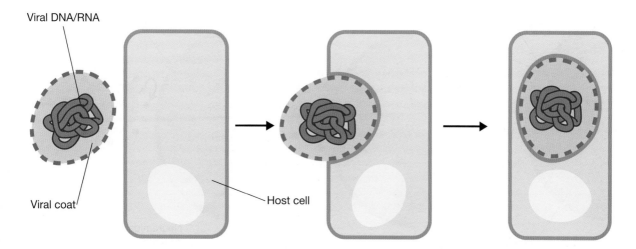

Figure 21.14 Viral entry by endocytosis.

Viral replication

The method of viral replication is dependent on the type of genetic material in the virus. The DNA viruses (double-strand DNA and single-strand DNA) generally must enter the host's nucleus to replicate. They then use the host cells polymerase to duplicate the viral genetic material, therefore these viruses are often dependent on the stage of the cell cycle to reproduce and require the host cell to be undergoing replication so that the polymerases are active.

The RNA viruses can usually replicate in the cytoplasm of the cell. Single-stranded RNA viruses with a positive sense (e.g. picornaviruses) can directly access cytoplasmic enzymes such as RNA polymerase to replicate. The negative-sense single-strand RNA viruses (e.g. rabies virus) must first be transcribed by viral polymerase into a positive form, and this is used as a template to generate proteins and another 'negative' copy of the RNA.

The single-stranded RNA viruses that use a viral reverse transcriptase, such as HIV, undergo several steps to replicate. Given the importance of HIV it has been well investigated. The details of the replication of HIV are outlined Box 21.3. Briefly, the virus attaches to the outside of a CD4+ T-cell and enters the cell by fusing with the membrane (see Figure 21.13). Once inside the single-strand of RNA is converted to DNA by reverse transcriptase. This is then spliced into the host DNA and copied to produce a pro-virus in the nucleus. From this mRNA is produced and translated to produce proteins, and new viral RNA is produced.

Viral shedding

The fourth phase in the viral life cycle is viral shedding, where the virus leaves the host cell and can then infect other cells. Three main mechanisms are used. First, cells can use the host cell's own membrane to form its envelope. This is called budding and is used by herpes simplex and smallpox viruses. The second method is to cause the host cell to die (apoptosis), releasing the virus or, more commonly, having the virus taken up by macrophages that come to remove the dead cells and transported to another site. The third is by exocytosis, which is a reverse of the way some viruses enter cells (see Figure 21.14).

Viral latency

Some viruses can 'hide' inside a host cell, lying dormant until something happens to start the replication cycle again. Examples include the herpes simplex (causing cold sores) and varicella (causing shingles) viruses. The triggers are often unknown, but stress or modifications to the immune system can reactivate the virus. Apart from meaning that for some viruses once infected you are always at risk of another viral infection, other viruses, such as some human papillomaviruses (a virus associated with skin and other types of warts), have been associated with causing uncontrolled cell division down the track, leading to cancer (e.g. cervical cancer).

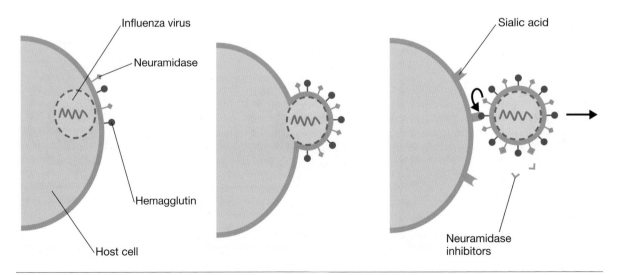

Figure 21.15 Action of neuramidase inhibitors.

Box 21.3
HIV replication

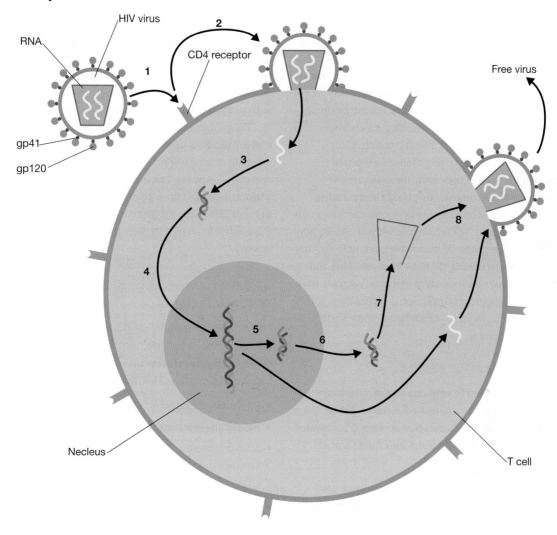

Figure c

1. The HIV has glycoproteins on its outer surface that interact with the CD4 receptors on CD4+ T-cells. The interaction is stabilized by an interaction between the glycoproteins and another receptor, CXCR4 or CCR5 cytokine receptor, which is co-located with the CD4 receptor.

2. The virus then enters the cell by fusing with the outer membrane of the T-cells, depositing the single-stranded positive-sense RNA into the T-cell along with viral reverse transcriptase, integrase, and protease. This is the site of action for fusion inhibitors (e.g. enfurvtide and maroviroc).

3. The viral RNA is converted to double-stranded DNA by viral reverse transcriptase. This is the site of action for the reverse transcriptase inhibitors (e.g. zidovudine and nevirapine).

4. The double-stranded DNA enters the nucleus and is incorporated into the host DNA via viral integrase. This is the site of action for integrase inhibitors (e.g. raltegravir).

5. The integrated DNA is transcribed and from this mRNA is produced. New viral RNA is also produced.

6. The mRNA leaves the nucleus and interacts with the host ribosomes and creates polypeptides.

7. The polypeptides are cleaved by viral protease into the viral coat as well as new viral reverse transcriptase, integrase, and protease. This is the site of action of protease inhibitors (e.g. saquinavir and ritonavir).

8. The new virus is assembled and released by the cell.

21.6 Treatment of viral infections

Unlike fungal and bacterial infections, where a lot of emphasis has been placed on pharmacological treatment, for vial infections prevention is often the preferred course. This is largely driven, as we will see, by the difficulty in treating viruses. Prevention for some viruses, particularly the common cold and HIV, is about limiting or stopping contact with the virus in the first place. For the common cold this means good hygiene (washing hands frequently) and covering your nose and mouth if you cough or sneeze. For HIV it means using barrier methods of contraception, such as condoms. The reason these measures are so important is that unlike several other viruses, we have not been able to develop a vaccine yet for these two conditions. While vaccines will not usually stop the virus entering the body, they are important in limiting their effects by preventing the virus from attaching and infecting the host cells it needs to replicate. Vaccines have been developed for several pathogens, including polio, smallpox, rubella, measles, varicella, hepatitis A and B, and influenza viruses.

21.6.1 Vaccines for viruses

There are several types of viral vaccines, but the main types are killed and live-attenuated vaccines. Killed vaccines contain whole viruses that have been inactivated by chemicals or heat. Examples include influenza and hepatitis A.

Live-attenuated vaccines contain living viruses that have been modified to stop them from spreading too quickly. This means that they produce a more long-lasting immune response and may not need boosters (unlike killed vaccines, which often need boosters annually or every few years). The disadvantages of live-attenuated vaccines are that because they are alive they can cause infection in people who are immunocompromised (e.g. HIV). Examples include rubella and measles.

A third type of viral vaccine uses a protein subunit from the viral coat. An example of this is the human papillomavirus vaccine (HPV).

The vaccines work by priming the immune system so that when the body encounters the features of the viral coat down the track ('memory') it can mount a quick response, leading to destruction and removal of the virus. This works fine if the virus is stable and exists in a few basic forms. The problem comes with things like the common cold, where there are over 100 different variants. Hence, there is no vaccine yet for the common cold. In the case of influenza there are a number of different subtypes that have been identified. They are all labelled with HxNx, where x is a number. For example H1N1 was associated with swine flu, while H5N1 caused what was called avian flu. The subtypes that are around change from year to year and the vaccines used against influenza are based on an estimate of what will predominate in the next influenza season (i.e. winter). This is usually done by looking at the major subtypes in the winter of the opposite hemisphere the year before (i.e. for the northern hemisphere what was the predominant type in the southern hemisphere winter).

21.6.2 Pharmacological treatment of viral infections

The different treatments are grouped largely around specific types of viral infections. The ones we will concentrate on are influenza, herpes and cytomegalovirus, and HIV. The groups are as follows:

- inhibitors of viral coat disassembly (influenza)
- neuramidase inhibitors (influenza)
- DNA polymerase inhibitors (herpes and cytomegalovirus)
- viral entry inhibitors (HIV)
- reverse transcriptase inhibitors (HIV)
- integrase inhibitors (HIV)
- protease inhibitors (HIV).

Inhibitors of viral coat disassembly

The main drug in this group is **amantadine**, which is also used for Parkinson's disease. When influenza viruses enter a cell the M2 protein in the viral coat allows hydrogen ions to enter the virus, acidifying the virus, which allows the viral coat to dissociate and deposit the viral contents for replication. Amantadine works by inhibiting M2 in the viral coat. It is associated with a number of side effects, including central nervous system effects such as hallucinations and confusion. This, combined with a lack of significant efficacy, has seen it largely replaced by vaccination in the prevention, and by neuramidase inhibitors in the treatment, of influenza.

Neuraminidase inhibitors

The neuraminidase inhibitors stop the release of the influenza virus from the cell. Once the influenza virus has replicated and re-assembled it leaves the cell by exocytosis, budding from the cell using part of the cell membrane to form a new viral coat. On the surface of this coat is hemagglutinin, which binds with sialic acid on the host cell, and neuraminidase. To be released, the neuraminidase on the viral coat breaks the bond, allowing the virus to float free (Figure 21.15). The neuraminidase inhibitors **oseltamivir** and **zanamavir** stop the virus from separating from the host cell.

Oseltamivir is given orally, while zanamivir is inhaled. Both should be started as soon as possible to be effective, and they are not recommended to be introduced more than 48 hours after symptoms started. On average they reduce the duration of the symptoms by 1.5–2 days. Both are generally well tolerated with gastrointestinal side effects the most prominent for oseltamivir.

DNA polymerase inhibitors

This group includes the guanine analogues (**aciclovir**, **famciclovir**, **ganciclovir**, **penciclovir**, **valaciclovir**, and **valganciclovir**) and nucleoside analogues (e.g. **idoxuridine**, **ribavirin**, **cidofovir**, and **foscarnet**).

Guanine analogues

These are used primarily for herpes simplex and varicella (aciclovir, famciclovir, and valaciclovir), and treatment or prevention of cytomegalovirus (CMV) infections (ganciclovir and valganciclovir). Herpes simplex causes cold sores and, while not life threatening in most people, it can be quite unpleasant and embarrassing (Figure 21.16). Varicella zoster virus (also called herpes zoster or just zoster) causes chickenpox in children (usually) and shingles in adults. While shingles is also not life threatening, it can cause persistent neuropathic pain, which can be very difficult to treat (Figure 21.16). CMV is a potentially severe infection in patients who are immunocompromised (e.g. HIV) and it can cause lung, gastrointestinal, and retinal infections.

> Poor Doris develops shingles after all the infections she has had. It is likely her immune system was not at is best. Viruses like varicella lie dormant in nerves and then being 'run down' can spark it off.

Guanine analogues, as the name suggest, share structural similarity to the nucleobase guanine. Guanine is first converted to guanosine monophosphate (GMP) by thymidine kinase, this is subsequently further phosphorolated to guanosine triphosphate (GTP), which is then used in DNA synthesis (Figure 21.17). The guanine analogues replace guanine in the production of GMP and therefore inhibit DNA synthesis. Their selectivity comes from being preferentially converted by viral thymidine kinase, thus having little effect on the host cell.

Famciclovir, aciclovir, valaciclovir, and valganciclovir are administered orally, while gangciclovir is only given intravenously. Aciclovir is also available intravenously and in a topical preparation for herpes simplex. Penciclovir is only used topically. Valgangciclovir and valaciclovir are pro-drugs converted to ganciclovir and

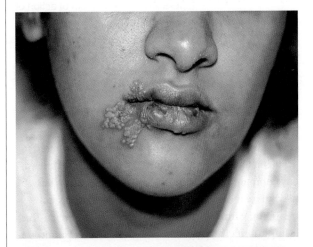

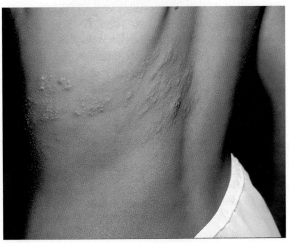

Figure 21.16 Examples of cold sores and shingles.

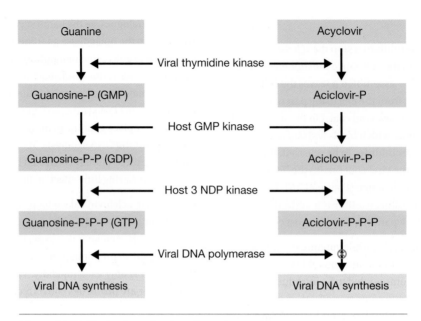

Figure 21.17 Mechanism of action of guanine analogues.

GMP, guanine monophosphate; GDP, guanine diphosphate; GTP, guanine triphosphate; NDP, nucleoside diphosphate kinase.

aciclovir, respectively, in the liver, while famciclovir is the pro-drug of penciclovir. Both famciclovir and valaciclovir have better oral bioavailability compared to aciclovir, and less frequent dosing (two or three times a day compared to five times a day for aciclovir). When used to treat varicella zoster the patient should start treatment within 72 hours to have maximum effect. This is important given the risk of long-term neuropathic pain with untreated zoster. When used for herpes simplex, topical treatment needs to start at what is called the prodrome (when the skin is tingling or itching, but the blisters have not appeared yet). This is because this is time when the virus is replicating. Once the blisters appear the virus has stopped reproducing and applying aciclovir will do very little. Because of their selectivity the guanine analogues are generally well tolerated.

Nucleoside analogues **Idoxuridine** is an analogue of deoxyuridine. It closely resembles thymidine and is incorporated in place of it during DNA synthesis. However, the presence of an iodine atom stops the base pairing, thus inhibiting DNA synthesis. However, unlike the guanine analogues, it is not as selective and is also incorporated into human DNA. It is used topically for the treatment of cold sores, sometimes combined with

lignocaine. It is much less effective than aciclovir and has a limited role in herpes simplex virus (HSV) infection.

Ribavirin **Ribavirin** is a nucleoside analogue that is active against a range of RNA and DNA viruses. It is used primarily in the treatment of respiratory syncytial virus (RSV; a very severe respiratory pathogen) infections, and in combination with interferon-α in the treatment of hepatitis C. Ribavirin is transported into cells, where it is phosphorylated to mono-, di-, and tri-phosphate versions. The mono-phosphate version inhibits inosine monophosphate dehydrogenase, leading to a reduced production of GTP, an essential part of viral RNA synthesis. The triphosphate form is thought to inhibit RNA polymerase as well as causing mutations in the synthesized RNA.

Ribavirin is given by inhalation for RSV and subcutaneously with interferon for hepatitis C. When given parenterally with interferon it can cause a number of serious reactions, including blood dyscrasias, injection site reactions, and flu-like symptoms. These may be due to the interferon as the incidence is higher in patients who are interferon-naive. Because it may affect human DNA synthesis, and is a potential teratogen, caution needs to be taken when administering this drug.

Cidofovir Cidofovir is a nucleotide phosphonate derivative used in the treatment of CMV, but also has activity against human papillomavirus and herpes simplex virus. It is phosphorylated to the active diphosphorylated form by cellular monophosphate kinase and pyruvate kinase, and does not require viral enzymes. The diphosphate cidofovir acts as inhibitor of CMV DNA polymerase or as alternative substrate for DNA polymerase, and it inhibits CMV polymerase at one hundredth of the concentration that it inhibits human DNA polymerase. Cidofovir has greater toxicity than the guanine analogues, including renal dysfunction and neutropenia, and is potentially carcinogenic, therefore it is usually used second line when other agents, such as valgangciclovir and gangciclovir, are unable to be used.

Foscarnet Foscarnet is a relatively simple molecule with the formula $HO_2CPO_3H_2$. It is an analogue of **pyrophosphate**, and interferes with exchange of pyrophosphate from deoxynucleoside triphosphate during viral replication by binding to a site on DNA polymerase. It interferes with viral DNA polymerase at levels that are much lower than would affect human DNA polymerase. Also, because it does not require viral or cellular enzyme to covert it to its active form, it can work in situations where resistance has occurred (e.g. due to loss of thymidine kinase activity with some guanine analogues). Like cidofovir it is fairly toxic, causing renal dysfunction and electrolyte disturbances, and should also be reserved as second- or third-line treatment of CMV or herpes simplex infections in patients with HIV.

Viral entry inhibitors

The first stage in HIV infection is entry of the viral particle into the host T-cell. This starts by having the gp120 on the surface of the HIV interacting with CD4 receptor on the T-cell. This causes a conformational change in the gp120 that exposes another glycoprotein, gp41, and causes the gp120 to bind to a co-receptor located near the CD4 receptor (either CCR5 or CXCR4). The exposed gp41 then penetrates the T-cell membrane and promotes the fusion of the viral and T-cell membranes.

Maraviroc is a slowly reversible inhibitor of the CCR5 receptor. Early in HIV infection the predominant co-receptor appears to be the CCR5 receptor, whereas in later stages of the infection the CXCR4 co-receptor dominates. This can be established using a Trofile assay. Maraviroc is given orally twice a day and is generally well tolerated, with the most common side effects being gastrointestinal. It is metabolized by the cytochrome P450 CYP3A4 isosyme and therefore can interact with inducers (e.g. rifampicin, used for tuberculosis in patients with HIV) or inhibitors (e.g. ketoconazole, used for fungal infections in patients with HIV) of this isozyme.

Enfuvirtide (also called T-20) binds to gp41 and prevents the formation of an entry pore for the virus. It is not stable orally so is given by subcutaneous injection twice a day. The main adverse effects are injection site reactions, which are greatest in the first week of therapy. Occasionally patients can be allergic and they should report signs of allergy. Enfuvirtide is not metabolized by CYP450, therefore it is not subject to the interactions seen with maraviroc.

Reverse transcriptase inhibitors

The reverse transcriptase inhibitors (RTIs) were the among first treatments developed for HIV. They are divided into three broad categories:

- nucleoside analogue reverse transcriptase inhibitors
- nucleotide analogue reverse transcriptase inhibitors
- non-nucleoside reverse transcriptase inhibitors.

Reverse transcriptase is required by HIV to generate a double-stranded DNA sequence that can be then incorporated into host DNA (see Box 21.3).

Nucleoside analogue RTIs The first nucleoside analogue RTI (NARTI), and in fact the first drug marketed for HIV in the late 1980s, was zidovudine. Since then several others have been developed, including abacavir, didanosine, emtricitabine, lamivudine, and stavudine. All NARTIs require activation by phosphorylation. However, the pathways of this activation are dependent on which nucleoside they resemble (Figures 21.18 and 21.19). An understanding of these pathways is important as it explains some of the drug interactions and therefore logical combinations, with these agents. For example, it is not logical to give both zidovudine and stavudine together as they both compete for the same phosphorylation pathway. Once phosphorylated to the triphosphate form the NARTIs attach to reverse transcriptases and are incorporated into the DNA. However, because they lack a hydroxyl group at the 3'

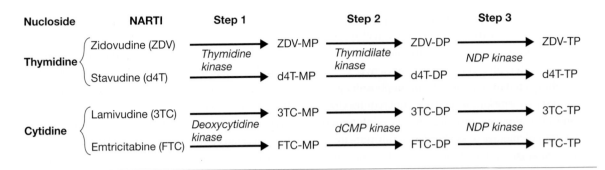

Figure 21.18 Conversion of pyrimadine analogues.

dCMP, deoxycytidine monophosphate; DP, diphosphate; MP, monophosphate; NDP, nucleoside diphosphate; TP, triphosphate.

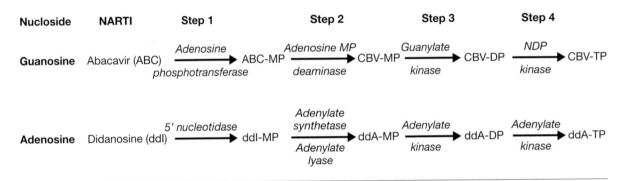

Figure 21.19 Conversion of purine analogues.

CBV, carbovir; ddA, dideoxyadenosine; DP, diphosphate; MP, monophosphate; NDP, nucleoside diphosphate; TP, triphosphate.

position on the sugar moiety, DNA synthesis is terminated.

The NARTIs are generally given once or twice a day. Simplifying the regimen is important as compliance with therapy is paramount. The side effects include gastrointestinal upset and anorexia, as well as potentially severe hepatic damage, including lactic acidosis. Other side effects include lipodystrophy (loss of fat from the periphery and deposition intra-abdominally), hyperglycaemia, and hyperlipidemia.

The NARTIs are not metabolized by CYP450 and most are cleared by the kidneys. The main interactions seem to come from combinations of NARTIs, and the following should be avoided:

- stavudine with didanosine or zidovudine
- lamivudine with emtricitabine.

Nucleotide analogue RTIs A rate-limiting effect in activating NARTIs such as zidovudine is phosphorylation by thymidine kinease. Nucleotide analogue RTIs

(NtARTIs), such as **tenofovir**, do not require this first step as they already contain the first phosphate group. Tenofovir is administered orally as the pro-drug tenofovir disoproxil fumarate, which is converted by diester hydrolysis to its active form. The tefnofovir is then converted to a monophosphate and then diphosphate form by adenosine monophosphate kinase and nucleoside diphosphate kinase. Once in the diphosphate form it acts like the NARTI didanosine as an analogue of the purine adenosine. The combination of didanosine with tenofovir should be avoided because it is associated with treatment failure and increased toxicity of didanosine. Tenofovir is given once a day and has a similar range of side effects as the NARTIs. It is primarily excreted unchanged in the urine.

Non-nucleoside reverse transcriptase inhibitors This class includes **delavirdine, efavirenz, etraverine,** and **nevirapine.** The non-nucleoside reverse transcriptase inhibitors (NNRTIs) are chemically diverse and, unlike the NARTIs, they bear no resemblance to the normal DNA building blocks.

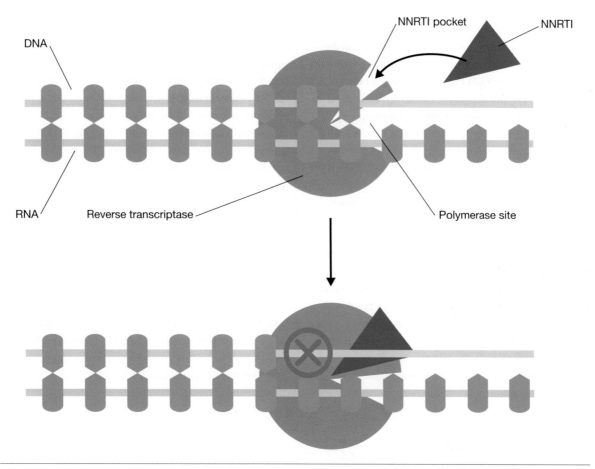

Figure 21.20 Mechanism of action of non-nucleoside reverse transcriptase inhibitors.

NNRTI, non nucleoside reverse transcriptase inhibitor. Adapted from Clavel F, Hance AJ. HIV drug resistance. *N Engl J Med* 2004; 350(10): 1023–1035.

The NNRTIs attach to a hydrophobic binding site (called the NNRTI 'pocket') near the polymerase activity site on RTI. Once bound they cause a conformational change in the enzyme that stops its activity (Figure 21.20).

Efavirenz and nevirapine are given orally once a day, etravirine is given twice a day, and delaverdine is given three times a day. The NNRTIs are metabolized by the cytochrome P450 system and therefore have numerous potential drug interactions. They share a similar range of side effects as the NARTIs, with rash a particular problem, and hepatic dysfunction with nevirapine.

Integrase inhibitors

Once the viral RNA has been converted to DNA by reverse transcriptase, it is then incorporated into the host DNA for replication by the enzyme integrase (Box 21.3). **Raltegravir** is the first commercially available integrase inhibitor. Integrase works by first forming a bond with the viral DNA, producing a stable pre-integration complex. The pre-integration complex then moves from the cytoplasm to the nucleus, where the viral DNA is transferred to host DNA. To do this integrase first cuts two nucleotides from the 3' end of the viral DNA and then inserts these into the host DNA in a process called strand transfer. Raltegravir blocks strand transfer by binding to divalent metals within the active site of the HIV integrase. The unintegrated complex is then deactivated by normal cellular DNA repair mechanisms. Raltegravir is metabolized by glucuronidation and not by CYP450. There is a reported in interaction between it and rifampicin, with levels decreased during rifampicin therapy. Proton pump inhibitors increase raltegravir solubility and can increase its toxicity. Raltegravir is given orally twice a day and is generally well tolerated.

Protease inhibitors

Proteases are carried by the HIV virus and are used in the final stages of replication to enable assembly of the particles of the viral core (Box 21.3). Proteases cleave the polyproteins, formed from the mRNA produced from the viral DNA, at the appropriate places. Protease inhibitors (PIs) suppress cleavage of Gag and Gag-pol protein precursors, which inhibits maturation of the budding HIV viruses. The first generation PIs are ritonavir, saquinavir, and indinavir. The second generation are atazanavir, darunavir, fosamprenavir, lopinavir, and tipranavir. All protease inhibitors are metabolized by cytochrome P450 (usually CYP3A4), with ritonavir also metabolized by CYP2D6. They are inhibitors if this system and therefore have numerous potential drug interactions. Ritonivir is the most potent inhibitor of the class and it is used almost exclusively now at low doses to boost the levels of other PIs as it is poorly tolerated at antiretroviral doses. The PIs are given orally once or twice a day. The adverse events are similar to the NARTIs. Gastrointestinal side effects are common, with ritonavir and saquinavir more likely to cause abdominal pain. Hepatotoxicity is also more common with ritonavir.

Combination therapy and resistance with HIV treatment

Unfortunately, resistance to antivirals in HIV can occur quite rapidly. The HIV replicates rapidly, with untreated patients having between 10^7 and 10^8 infected cells in their lymphatic system. Mutations that give a virus an selective advantage will therefore quickly allow them to increase in number by simple Darwinian selection (i.e. survival of the fittest). Thymidine analogue mutations promote removal of the NARTIs from the DNA, leading to resistance to NARTIs and NtARTIs. Mutations also reduce the binding affinity for NNARTIs and PIs. There are also alterations to the HR1 domain of the gp41 that causes resistance to enfuvirtide.

In an attempt to minimize resistance, combination therapy is now recommended for all patients. Guidelines vary widely, but regimens consisting of two NARTIs, an NARTI and tenofovir, or one NARTI with either a NNRTI or a PI have been suggested. The integrase and viral entry inhibitors are usually reserved for patients who fail treatment with NARTI/NtARTIs and/or PIs.

SUMMARY OF DRUGS USED FOR INFECTIONS

Therapeutic class	Drug	Mechanism of action	Common clinical uses	Comments	Examples of adverse drug reactions
β-lactams	Penicillins: benzylpenicillin (penicillin G) phenoxymethylpenicillin (penicillin V) flucloxacillin amoxycillin amoxycillin + clavulanic acid piperacillin piperacillin + tazobactam ticarcillin + clavulanic acid	Blocks the synthesis of cell-wall mucopeptide, thereby exerting a bactericidal effect against actively replicating bacteria	Infection See Table 21.2 for details	Most given three to four times daily to maintain plasma concentration See Table 21.2 for details of spectrum	Gastrointestinal Anaphylaxis (10% cross-sensitivity between penicillin and cephalosporines)
	Cephalopsorins: First generation cefadroxil cefradine cefalexin (cephalexin) cefalotin cefazolin Second generation cefaclor cefuroxime cefoxitin Third generation cefotaxime ceftriaxone cefpodoxime cefixime ceftazidime Fourth generation cefepime		Infection See Table 21.3 for details	Most given three to four times daily to maintain plasma concentration First generation mainly oral and other generations mainly intravenous administration See Table 21.3 for details	
	Carbapenems: imipenem meropenem ertapenem doripenem	Inhibit bacterial cell wall synthesis following attachment to penicillin binding proteins	Septicaemia, hospital-acquired pneumonia Intra-abdominal infections (Reserved for complex mixed infections; widest spectrum of activity of all the β-lactams)	Parenteral administration Imipenem administered with cilastin, a dehydropeptidase inhibitor Imipenem has the shortest half-life and is given QDS Meropenem and doripenem given TDS Ertapenem given once a day	Gastrointestinal Neurotoxicity

Therapeutic class	Drug	Mechanism of action	Common clinical uses	Comments	Examples of adverse drug reactions
Tetracycline	Tetracycline, Doxycycline, Minocycline, Tigecycline, Lymecycline, Oxytetracycline, Demeclocycline	Attach to the 30S subunit and block the transcription of mRNA by inhibiting the attachment of tRNA to the A site (Box 21.1)	Respiratory tract infections, Acne, Malaria, SIADH (demeclocycline)	Administer once or twice daily. Good activity against *Rickettsia*, *Mycoplasma*, *Chlamydia*, spirochetes, and protozoa. Not to be taken in pregnancy	Gastrointestinal upset, Teeth mottling, Photosensitivity
Macrolides	Erythromycin, Clarithromycin, Roxithromycin, Telithromycin, Azithromycin	Attach to the 50S subunit of the ribosome and inhibit translocation of the growing peptide chain	Respiratory tract infections, *Chlamydia*, H. pylori, and *Campylobacter*	Older ones given four times daily, newer ones once daily. Activity against *Mycoplasma pneumonia*, *Mycobacterium avium* *Legionella*. Telithromycin, active against penicillin-resistant *Streptococcus pneumoniae* Inhibit CYP450, resulting in drug interactions	Prolong QT interval
Other antibiotics interfering with protein synthesis	Lincosamides: clindamycin lincomycin	Attach to the 50S subunit of the ribosome and inhibit translocation of the growing peptide chain	Infections (usually reserved for severe gram-positive infections, second-line to β-lactams) Acne (*Clindamycin*)	Active against gram-positive bacteria and anaerobes Active against *Propionibacterium* acnes	Gastrointestinal (most serious is pseudomembranous clolitis caused by overgrowth of *C. difficile*)
	Chloramphenicol		Infections (gram-positive, gram-negative, and anaerobic bacteria)	Active against *Bacteroides fragilis*, *Salmonella typhi*, and *Haemophilus influenzae* Largely restricted to topical use in eye and ear drops because of adverse drug reactions	Aplastic anaemia (systemic application)
	Fusidic acid (or sodium fusidate)	Inhibits the translocation of the tRNA with the growing peptide chain	Gram-positive infections MRSA (in combination with rifampicin)	Active against *Staphylococcus* in skin and soft tissue	Liver dysfunction
	Linezolid	Inhibits the binding of the 30S and 50S subunits together, preventing initiation of protein synthesis	Gram-positive organisms MRSA pneumonia	Serious skin and soft tissue infection	Thrombocytopenia, Anaemia
	Streptogramins: quinupristin dalfopristin	Work synergistically to impair protein synthesis: quinupristin inhibits translocation and dalfopristin changes the structure of the 50S subunit, allowing quinupristin to bind more effectively	MRSA VRE	Active against gram-positive organisms	Nausea, Vomiting, Arthralgias, Myalgias, Liver dysfunction

Therapeutic class	Drug	Mechanism of action	Common clinical uses	Comments	Examples of adverse drug reactions
Quinolones	Fluoroquinolones: ciprofloxacin ofloxacin levofloxacin norfloxacin moxifloxacin	Bind reversibly to DNA gyrase and topoisomerase IV, stopping DNA transcription and replication	Urinary tract infections Respiratory infections Soft tissue infections	Taken once to twice daily activity against gram-negative bacteria (*Haemophilus influenzae* (not norfloxacin), *Pseudomonas aeruginosa*) and some gram-positive bacteria (Legionella and some mycobacteria) Inhibit CYP3A4, leading to interactions	Tendonitis Pseudomembranous colitis caused by overgrowth of *C. difficile* Photosensitivity
Nitroimidazoles	Metronidazole Tinidazole	Once inside the bacteria the nitro group is reduced by ferredoxin, and the products of this process interfere with DNA synthesis	*H. pylori* *Clostridium difficile* Bacterial vaginitis Giardiasis Rosacea (topical)	Surgical prophylaxis to protect against gut anaerobes, e.g. *Bacteroides* spp.) Interacts with alcohol, causing a disulfiram-like reaction Metabolized by cytochrome P450, causing interaction	Gastrointestinal effects Metallic taste Dizziness Headaches (Tinidazole better tolerated and has fewer reported interactions)
Aminoglycosides	Amikacin Gentamicin Tobramycin Neomycin Streptomycin	1) Bind to the 30S subunit of the ribosome and interferes with protein synthesis by affecting the interaction between tRNA and mRNA 2) Cause transient holes in the cell membrane of bacteria by displacing Mg^{++} and Ca^{++} in the cell membrane that links polysaccharides and lipopolysaccharides, leading to bactericidal effects	Respiratory tract infections Meningitis Renal infections Endocarditis Sepsis	Serious gram-negative infections Tobramycin has slightly better coverage against *Pseudomonas aeruginosa*, but not for other gram-negative bacteria	Ototoxicity Nephrptoxicity
Other antibiotics that interfere with DNA synthesis	Trimethoprim Sulfamethoxazole (a sulphonamide)	Interfere with the production of thymidine triphosphate, one of the four nucleosides used in the synthesis of DNA, by inhibiting folate production in the bacteria Trimethoprim inhibits dihydrofolate reductase, while sulphonamides act as an analogue of para-aminobenzoic acid competing for dihydropteroate synthetase	UTI Treatment and prevention of (*Pneumocystis jiroveci, P. carinii*) pneumonitis, toxoplasmosis, nocardiosis (combination of both)	Drug containing combination of trimethoprim and sulfamethoxazole usually reserved for opportunistic infections of HIV	Steven Johnson's (co-trimoxazole)
Antibiotics against *Mycobacteria*	Rifamycins: rifampicin rifabutin	Inhibit the synthesis of mRNA from DNA by binding to DNA-dependent RNA polymerase	TB (useful in treating disseminated TB, which can pass into the brain)	Only affect prokaryotic cells (i.e. cells without a nucleus such as bacteria) Induces CYP450 leading to interactions	Gastrointestinal Discolouration of bodily fluids
	Dapsone	By acting as an analogue of para-aminobenzoic acid, they inhibit folate synthesis The main side effect is dose-related asymptomatic haemolytic anaemia	PCP infections Leprosy	Activity against *Mycobacterium leprae* and *Mycobacterium lepromatosis*)	Hepatic dysfunction 'dapsone syndrome' (involves a rash, jaundice, eosinophilia, and fever)

Therapeutic class	Drug	Mechanism of action	Common clinical uses	Comments	Examples of adverse drug reactions
	Ethambutol	Inhibits arabinosyl transferases, which is involved in arabinogalactan synthesis in mycobacterium. The arabinogalactan forms a complex with mycolic acid and peptidoglycan in the cell wall. Ethambutol thus inhibits cell wall development	TB MAC		Optic neuritis
	Isoniazid	Activated to form a complex that blocks the synthesis of mycolic acid	TB	Pyridoxine co-prescription recommended to reduce risk of peripheral neuritis	Peripheral neuritis Hepatitis Optic neuritis
	Pyrazinamide	A pro-drug that is converted to pyrazinoic acid, which acts as a weak acid affecting the cell wall transport functions by 'de-energising' the cell wall		Active only in an acid pH, thus the activity of pyrazinamide declines as the pH rises (i.e. once inflammation subsides)	Arthralgia Hyperuricaemia Liver dysfunction
	Clofazimine	Thought to interrupt DNA replication by binding to guanine bases on DNA	Leprosy MAC	Belongs to a class called riminophenazines	Skin deposition, causing pink to brownish/black appearance
	Capreomycin	Appears to work by inhibiting protein synthesis by binding to the ribosome, possibly both the 50S and 30S subunits		Generally reserved as second- or third-line option	Ototoxicity Nephrotoxicity
Other antibiotics	Glycopeptides: vancomycin teicoplanin	Both inhibit cell wall synthesis in gram-positive bacteria by inhibiting the incorporation of N-acetylmuramic acid and N-acetylglucosamine peptide into peptidoglycan	MRSA (serious infections when β-lactams contraindicated) Clostridium difficile (oral vancomycin for local effect)	Both active only against gram-positive bacteria. Teicoplanin administered once daily. Oral vancomycin molecules too large for absorption	Red man syndrome (vancomycin)
	Lipopeptides: daptomycin	Causes rapid depolarization of the cell membrane through potassium efflux, disrupting DNA, RNA, and protein synthesis	MRSA Complicated skin and soft tissue infections	Creatine kinase should be monitored. Any muscle pain should be reported	Nausea Diarrhoea Myopathy
	Polymyxins: colistin polymyxin B	Bind to lipopolysaccharides in the outer membrane of gram-negative bacteria, causing disruption to the cell membrane similar to detergent effect (i.e. they have both a hydrophilic and hydrophobic component)	Gut sterilization P. aeruginosa in cystic fibrosis. (Colistin) Multi-drug resistant gram-negative infections	Effective against Pseudomonas aeruginosa, Enterobacteriaceae, and Klebsiella pneumoniae. Colistin nebulised for cystic fibrosis	Renal toxicity Neurotoxicity
	Nitrofurantoin	Within bacteria, it is converted by nitrofuran reductase, a flavoprotein, to unstable intermediates that cause damage to DNA, ribosomes, and other macromolecules	Urinary tract infections second-and thrid-line)	Activity against gram-positive organisms and anaerobes. Resistance to nitrofurantoin is relatively low because of many sites of action	Gastrointestinal upset Allergic reactions Hepatotoxicity

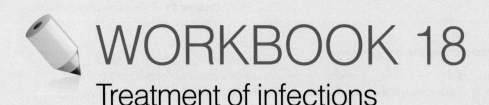

WORKBOOK 18
Treatment of infections

Doris Kaiser: a simplified case history

Monique is glad she stopped by to visit her mum–in-law, Doris, at her nursing home. As soon as she saw her Monique knew Doris was very unwell. After talking to Doris, Monique is very concerned and insists that a doctor be called to asses her. One hour later the doctor finally comes to see her.

What Doris had described to her over the phone as a dry cough had worsened over the last 2 days and last night the cough had produced bloodstained sputum. Doris also admitted that she felt a sharp pain when she coughed. She felt warm to Monique's touch and sounds as if she is struggling to catch her breath. She admits to feeling feverish and under the weather.

The doctor asks Doris a couple of questions and listens to Doris's chest

A table of clinical clerking abbreviations is given on page xi.

GP NOTES FOR CONSULTATION WITH DORIS

Age: 66 years

PC: Painful and productive cough, shortness of breath and fever

HPC: A 4-day history of cough. Initially dry but 3 days later produced blood-stained sputum. Also became feverish on day 3. Increasing shortness of breath and sharp pain on coughing. Feels generally weak and unwell.

> *Her symptoms could be indicative of any one of the following diseases:*
>
> * *congestive heart failure*
> * *pulmonary embolism*
> * *acute bronchitis*
> * *pneumonia.*

PMH: Stroke 2 years ago with residual paralysis

Doris is recovering from a severe stroke which she suffered 2 years ago. The stroke left her paralysed on one side, although she is much improved and can now eat solid food and is mobile with help.

How is the stroke linked to her symptoms?

- *Foreign substances are normally prevented from moving into the lower respiratory tract of healthy individuals through the action of nasal hair, ciliated mucosal cells, mucus, saliva enzymes, and swallowing.*

- *Neurological diseases such as strokes could hinder this and facilitate aspiration of respiratory tract secretions into the lungs.*

- *These diseases also inhibit a patient's gag reflex, making it difficult for them to cough out the respiratory aspirates.*

- *As a consequence foreign matter can make its way into the lower airways and could ultimately cause infections, such as pneumonia.*

DH:

Aspirin

Dipyridamole

SH: Rehabilitating from stroke in nursing home. Married and has two children, both grown up.

O/E:

Auscultation (listening to breath with stethoscope): Abnormal sounds

Mini mental test score: 7

Respiratory rate: 32

Pulse rate: 104 beats per minute

Blood pressure: 85/55 mm Hg

Oximetry: O_2 saturation = 91%

The initial diagnosis of pneumonia is made through a combination of:

1 Assessing symptoms and patient's medical history

- *Cough, fever, malaise: symptoms of pneumonia and other respiratory tract infections*

- *Sharp pain: symptom of pneumonia and pulmonary embolism*

- *Stroke history: predisposes to pneumonia*

- *Lives in home: increased colonization of oropharynx with pathogens*

- *Age: older patients have higher risks*

2 Examining the patient for signs such as

- *breath sounds: abnormal sounds indicate reduced air entry*

- *respiratory rate: increased respiratory rate signifies increased risk*

- *pulse: increased pulse indicates increased risk*

- *mental test score: tests confusion status, less than 8 signifies higher risk*

- *blood pressure: low blood pressure signifies higher risk*

After initial diagnosis using physical examination and history, the patient's risk of mortality is assessed. A number of methods used have been used:

Fine and colleagues method

Also called the Pneumonia Severity Index (PSI). Takes into consideration age, gender, laboratory data and co-morbidities to categorize patients using point allocation. The total scores are tallied and used to categorize the patient. Patients in categories I and II should be treated in the community whilst those in categories III and V should be admitted to hospital.

2 CRB-65 method

This method allocates one point each if:

- *patient is confused (using mental test scoring: asking the patient simple questions like date, name, and place)*
- *respiratory rate 30 per minute or more*
- *blood pressure low: systolic <90 mm Hg or diastolic <60 mm Hg*
- *age 65 years or over.*

Patients with a score of 1 or 2 should be considered for hospitalization and those with a score of 3 or 4 require urgent hospitalization.

There a couple of modified version of these methods. The CORB (confusion, oxygen, respiratory rate, blood pressure) score does not use age, but includes oxygen (a PaO$_2$* of <60 mm or O$_2$ of ≤90% adds 1 point). CURB (confusion, urea, respiratory rate, blood pressure) substitutes urea for age (a urea of ≥ 7.0 mmol/L adds 1 point).

*PaO$_2$= partial pressure of oxygen, which is a measure of how much, oxygen is in the blood.

Doris' has a CRB-65 of 4. She has a high risk of death and should be hospitalized urgently! The impression is that she has got pneumonia but without radiographic evidence using X-ray, pulmonary embolism (a blood clot in her lungs) cannot be ruled out.

Initial differential diagnosis:

Severe community acquired pneumonia

Pulmonary embolism

Plan:

Admit to hospital

HOSPITAL ADMISSION CLERKING AND REGISTRAR WARD ROUND RECORDS FOR DORIS

Biochemistry:

1) White cell count = 16 x 10^9 (reference 4–11 x 10^9)

2) Urea = 10 mmol/L (reference <7 mmol/L)

3) Others within range

Elevated white cell count signifies bacterial infection.

Elevated urea level signifies higher risk.

4) Arterial blood gases: pH = 7.47 (reference 7.38–7.45)

PO_2 = 75 mm Hg (reference 80–100 mm Hg)

> *Doris' oxygen saturation is low and signifies hypoxemia, indicating that she needs to be given oxygen.*

5) Gram stains: Mixed negative and positive

> *The gram stain refers to whether the sputum culture stains or not when mixed with a combination of dyes and viewed under a microscope. The implication of this is more complex than just a colour; gram-positive and -negative bacteria have many other differences that significantly influence the choice of antimicrobial agents as well as prognosis.*

Severity assessment: CRB-65 = 4

Diagnosis: Severe community acquired pneumonia

Plan:

1) Chest X-ray

2) Send sputum samples to microbiology for culture and sensitivity

3) Send blood samples to microbiology for culture and sensitivity

4) Urine antigen tests for *Legionella* and *Pneumococcus*

5) Commence empiric treatment with intravenous amoxycillin

6) Admit to intensive care unit

7) Contact microbiology for advice

PART 1

The registrar explains to Monique that Doris has to be admitted to intensive care for respiratory support because of her symptoms. He explains that samples have been sent to identify the exact bacteria. In the interim they have decided to use the antibiotic recommended for severe community acquired pneumonia.

1) List three infectious organisms that are targets of antimicrobial agents.

2a) Explain the term 'selective toxicity', which is used to describe the rationale for antimicrobial drugs.

2b) What are the differences between prokaryotes and eukaryotes?

3a) Explain the procedure used to identify pathogens as either gram-positive or gram-negative.

3b) How do gram-positive and gram-negative bacteria differ from each other?

Explain in detail the significance of these differences.

4a) Describe the three classes of biochemical reactions that lead to bacterial cell wall formation.

4b) Which of these three classes are targeted by the cefuroxime used for Doris?

5a) What class does amoxycillin belong to?

5b) Describe the mechanism of action of this class to which amoxycillin belongs.

6) Amoxycillin is also available in combination with clavulanate. What is the role of clavulanate?

The registrar comes by and stops the amoxycillin. His consultant has recommended the following treatment:

- a second- or third-generation cephalosporin combined with a macrolide

or

- a quinolone combined with benzylpenicillin.

7a) What is the mechanism of action of cephalosporins?

7b) Explain how the different classes of cephalosporins differ.

8a) Explain the difference between bacteriostatic and bactericidal.

8b) List one example each of bacteriostatic and bactericidal antimicrobial agents.

9) What is the mechanism of action of macrolides?

10a) Describe the mechanism of action of quinolones.

10b) Which pathogens are generally targeted by quinolones?

10c) Describe one mechanism of resistance to quinolones. Why is resistance such a problem with this class of antibiotic?

PART 2

The consultant arrives and he has been contacted by the infectious disease department. Based on local sensitivity patterns, they have recommended the combination gentamicin and ciprofloxacin.

11a) To what class does gentamicin belong? Describe the mechanism of action of gentamicin.

11b) What pathogens are targeted by gentamicin?

11c) Describe the pharmacokinetic of gentamicin. What are the implications for dosing?

Two days later microbiology ring with the culture and sensitivity results, and recommend that the gentamicin be replaced with linezolid. The microbiologist reports that vancomycin-resistant *Staphylococcus aureus* and *M. pneumonia* were isolated. He tells the consultant that the next options are either quinupristin plus dalfopristin, daptomycin or co-trimoxazole.

12) What is the mechanism of action of vancomycin?

13a) Describe the action of linezolid.

13b) What are the adverse drug reactions of linezolid which necessitate extra blood monitoring for patients?

14) Describe the mechanism of action of daptomycin.

15a) What two drugs make up co-trimoxazole?

15b) Explain the mechanism of action of each component in co-trimoxazole.

Three days later Doris has improved significantly and has been discharged to the ward from intensive care. The ciprofloxacin is changed to doxycycline, which was not prescribed on intensive care because it can only be given orally.

16a) What is the mechanism of action of tetracyclines?

16b) Why are tetracyclines contraindicated in children?

16c) Identify three things that interact with tetracyclines and the mechanism of their interaction.

On day 4, Doris complains of pain and has started coughing and wheezing again. The shortness of breath and increased respiratory rate are back.

X-ray is performed and blood tests are done. All of these, together with her history of nasogastric feeding on intensive care, suggest aspiration pneumonia.

Metronidazole, in combination with penicillin, is prescribed to treat this. Clindamycin is also indicated for aspiration pneumonia but rarely used.

17a) What is the mechanism of action of metronidazole?

17b) What can happen if alcohol is consumed by a patient on metronidazole?

17c) What is the other antibiotic in the same class as metronidazole and how does it differ from metronidazole?

Doris improves over the next 5 days but develops diarrhoea on the 6th day. She also has oral thrush for which she is prescribed nystatin suspension 1 ml four times a day.

Her diarrhoea is confirmed as *Clostridium difficile* toxin (CDT) associated. She is prescribed oral vancomycin because she developed the diarrhoea whilst taking metronidazole, the first line agent for CDT. She has also developed a Urinary tract infection and trimethoprim is prescribed for that.

18) Explain how *Clostridium difficile* overgrowth develops.

19) Explain why vancomycin is used orally as opposed to intravenously to treat CDT.

Doris develops oral trush and is prescribed an antifungal called nystatin. The oral trush is an infection caused by candida albicans which proliferates after the use of bacteria that affect the normal oral flora. The nystatin does not seem to work for the fungal mouth infection, so fluconazole is prescribed instead.

20a) How does the mechanism of action of nystatin differ to that of fluconazole?

20b) What drug interactions do you have to be careful of with fluconazole?

Doris recovers after 2 weeks and can be discharged.

Three months later she develops a painful rash around her back. She sees her GP, who diagnoses her with shingles. He explains that it probably has occurred because she has been so run down with all the illnesses that she has had of late. He gives her a prescription for famciclovir and tells her she must go and get the tablets today and start taking them.

21a) What is the virus that causes shingles?

21b) How do viruses replicate and how does this differ from bacteria and fungi?

22a) What is the mechanism of action of famciclovir?

22b) Why was it important that Doris start her famciclovir that day?

Doris' GP suggests that she gets a vaccination against influenza.

23a) What type of vaccination is influenza and how is it produced?

23b) How does rubella vaccine differ from influenza vaccine?

Doris recovers from her shingles, but the rash takes several weeks to go away. She hopes she never has to take another antimicrobial again!

Chapter 22
Cancer chemotherapy

To be told you have cancer is probably one of the most dreaded diagnoses a person can hear. It is estimated that over 12 million people worldwide are diagnosed and over 7 million die each year from cancer. However, while the prognosis of some cancers is poor (e.g. lung cancer), others respond well to treatment (e.g. basal cell carcinomas). A person's prospects are dependent on a number of factors, including the site of the cancer, how advanced the cancer is (including if it has spread or not), and how abnormal the cells are (called the 'grade'). Other aspects that affect your prognosis include your age and general health (measured by 'performance status').

In this chapter we will review the causes of cancer and the common chemotherapy agents used to treat various cancers. As we will see, treating cancer poses a range of problems, mostly because it involves using drugs that are toxic to growing cells. This leads to a range of problems, as the patient in our workbook, Ngozi, found when she lost her hair and suffered severe gastrointestinal side effects (both effects involve cells that are naturally rapidly dividing).

22.1 Causes of cancer

The exact cause of most cancers is still unknown. However, it is generally thought that the underlying causes relate to mutations or damage to mechanisms that normally prevent 'errors' from being passed on from cell to cell. As noted in the introduction, there are several 'check points' in the cell cycle that prevent a cell from starting to replicate if there is damage to the DNA. In addition, the process of DNA replication itself includes 'proof reading', which ensures that DNA is assembled correctly and incorrect portions are 'chopped out'. A third protective mechanism is apoptosis, or programmed cell death. Apoptosis is initiated in response to cellular damage or stress. Several cellular signals control apoptosis. Some come from the mitochondria, the cell's 'powerhouse', and include the second mitochondria-derived activator of caspases and cytochrome c, which forms a complex that activates capsases. The capsases stop the action of enzymes that normally inhibit apoptosis. The other source of signalling for apoptosis comes from cytokines outside the cell from the tumour necrosis factor (TNF) family.

These send cellular signals that cause activation of capsases. The net result is the cell shrinks, the nucleus condenses, and then the cell breaks down. It is finally removed by phagocytic cells such as macrophages.

Proto-oncogene is the name given to 'normal' genes that produce the proteins related to apoptosis, which mutates or up-regulates and turns a healthy cell into a cancer cell. When this occurs it is called an oncogene. Several mechanisms are related to the conversion of a proto-oncogene, including:

- changes in the protein structure that result in increased activity or loss of regulation of the gene
- increased levels of proteins due to reduced breakdown or increased production due to duplication of genes
- chromosomal abnormality resulting in translocation of one part of a gene to another.

Oncogenes have been classified by the effects they have (Table 22.1).

Table 22.1 Examples of oncogenes

Classification	Example	Function
Stimulators of cell division	Abl	Tyrosine kinase involved in cell differentiation and division
	c-Jun	Combines with c-Fos for early response transcription factor
	c-Myc	DNA-binding protein that acts as a transcription factor
	Ras	GTPase involved with growth factors to increase cell division
Inhibitors of cell division	NF1	Gene that suppresses the Ras signalling pathway
	p53	Gene that arrests cell division and allows DNA repair
Regulators of apoptosis	Bax	Stimulates mitochondria to release pro-apoptotic signals
	Bcl-2	Inhibits release of pro-apoptotic signals from mitochondria

Adapted from: Doan, T., Melvold, R., Viselli, S., Waltenbaugh, C., eds. *Immunology*. Baltimore, Lippincott Williams & Wilkins 2008.

Agents that cause cancer are referred to as carcinogens, and agents that cause mutations are called mutagens. While the two terms have a lot in common, they are not synonymous. Many mutagens do cause cancer, and examples of chemical mutagens include the elements of tobacco smoke (lung cancer) and asbestos (mesothelioma). The best example of radiation as a mutagen is ultraviolet light, which can lead to skin cancer. However, alcohol is a chemical carcinogen, but not a mutagen. Alcohol is thought to promote cancer by encouraging cell division, giving less time for damage to the DNA to be repaired and increasing the risk of duplication of defective cells. Viruses and bacteria have both been associated with causing cancer. There are more cancers associated with viruses (e.g. cervical cancer from human papillomavirus, liver cancer from hepatitis B or C) than bacteria (e.g. gastric cancer caused by *H. pylori*). This is probably not surprising given that viruses use the host cell's own enzymes, including sometimes the host DNA, to replicate. Other causes of cancer include hormones, which cause increased cell replication (e.g. oestrogens), immune deficiency (e.g. patients with HIV are at increased risk of Kaposi's sarcoma and non-Hodgkin's lymphoma), and inherited tendencies to develop cancer (e.g. inherited mutations in genes that are associated with breast cancer).

22.2 Classification of cancers

Cancers can be classified in a number of ways, including the site of the cancer, the type of tissue (histology), the abnormality of the cells (grading), and the extent of the disease (staging). The international standard for the classification is the International Classification of Diseases for Oncology, Third Edition (ICD-O-3). Cancers can be organized into six categories based on the type of tissue or system affected. Examples are outlined in Table 22.2.

Our patient in the workbook for this chapter, Ngozi, had a carcinoma involving the milk ducts of the breast.

Grading of cancers is based on biopsies and reflects how 'normal' or differentiated ('mature') the cells look. There are four grades:

Grade 1   Well-differentiated (low grade)

Grade 2   Moderately differentiated (intermediate grade)

Grade 3   Poorly differentiated (high grade)

Grade 4   Undifferentiated (high grade)

There are two main ways cancers are 'staged'. One is called the 'TNM' system, which is based on the extent of the tumour (T), the spread to the lymph nodes (N), and the presence of metastasis (M). Numbers are then added to show the levels of each. For example, for the extent of the tumour (T), T0 means no sign of tumour, Tis means the tumour is in situ (i.e. only on the surface and no spread to surrounding tissue), and T1 to T4 are increasing in size and involvement of tissue. If someone has breast cancer that is grade T3 N2 M0 it means it is a large tumour that

Table 22.2 Cancers classified by tissue/system affected

Type of cancer	Body system/tissue affected	Example
Carcinoma	Epithelial tissue or lining of the body Two types: from organs or glands (adenocarcinoma) squamous tissue (squamous cell carcinomas)	Renal cell carcinoma (kidney) Basal cell carcinoma (skin)
Sarcoma	Supportive and connective tissue such as bones, tendons, cartilage, muscle, and fat	Rhabdomyosarcoma (striated muscle)
Myeloma	Plasma cells of the bone marrow	Multiple myeloma
Leukaemia	Haemopoietic (blood) cells	Acute myelogenous leukaemia Acute lymphoblastic leukemia Chronic lymphocytic leukemia Chronic myelogenous leukemia
Lymphoma	Glands or nodes of the lymphatic system	Non-Hodgkin's lymphoma
Mixed	More than one type of tissue/system	Adenosquamous carcinoma

has spread to nearby lymph nodes, but not to other parts of the body.

The staging of Ngozi's tumour was very similar to the above example, but slightly smaller (T2) and less spread (N1). Fortunately, she also had no metastases (M0).

The second ways cancers are staged is a numerical system:

Stage 0   Cancer in situ

Stage I   Cancer limited to the tissue of origin, evidence of tumour growth

Stage II   Limited local spread of cancerous cells

Stage III   Extensive local and regional spread

Stage IV   Distant metastasis

As noted above, staging and grading can help with prognosis (higher grades/stages usually indicate poorer prognosis) and with the choice of treatment.

The other broad categories applied to cancers are 'benign' and 'malignant'. The difference is benign tumours do not invade surrounding tissue and cannot metastasize. They are usually reasonably well differentiated and often slow growing. This contrasts to malignancies, which have rapid growth rates, invasion of surrounding areas, and can metastasize.

22.3 Pharmacological treatment of cancer

The main feature of cancer cells that is targeted by chemotherapy is their rapid reproduction. Thus, treatments are aimed at different parts of cell replication, including the signals that promote cell replication, DNA synthesis, DNA replication, RNA production, and protein and enzyme synthesis from RNA.

An important related feature of some solid tumours is the ability to induce angiogenesis. The term 'angiogenesis' refers to the growth of new blood vessels from existing ones. It is not unique to cancers and occurs during wound healing. Angiogenesis results from the new, growing cells needing oxygen and nutrients to continue to expand. Cancer cells promote this by

releasing growth factors, including vascular endothelial growth factor A (VEGF-A) and basic fibroblast growth factor (bFGF). VEGF-A is the main growth factor associated with angiogenesis. It causes increased migration and mitosis of endothelial cells, creation of the vessel lumen, and vasodilatation by releasing nitric oxide, by attaching to tyrosine kinase receptors (the VEGF 1 or 2 receptors). bFGF also increases endothelial cell production and helps arrange the endothelial cells into tube-like structures. It is more potent than VEGF in inducing angiogenesis. As we will see later, angiogenesis has become one of the new targets of anticancer treatments.

There are many ways to classify anticancer drugs. Traditionally this has been based on the mode of action, and the four broad categories have been cytotoxic drugs (e.g. alkylating agents, mitosis inhibitors, etc.), hormonal therapies (e.g. steroids and anti-hormonal treatments), immunotherapy (e.g. interferon), and 'other' or 'miscellaneous'. The rapid development of new and novel treatments has meant that the latter category ('other') has grown in size. In this chapter we will consider the drugs divided into their therapeutic targets. While this means some 'classes' of therapies may appear in more than one category (e.g. monoclonal antibodies, which all act by similar mechanism, are used as inhibitors of tumour cells and directed against vascular endothelium where they affect angiogenesis), the grouping is useful as a way of understanding the combination drug regimens that are used in cancer chemotherapy. The classification based on therapeutic targets is outlined in Table 22.3.

Another term applied to chemotherapy is neoadjuvant and adjuvant chemotherapy. A neoadjuvant chemotherapy is given to patients prior to surgery or radiation, with the aim of reducing the size of the tumour mass. Examples where this is used are breast, colorectal, and lung cancer. Adjuvant chemotherapy refers to giving chemotherapy *after* surgery or radiotherapy and aims to improve survival.

22.3.1 Chemotherapy targeted at the tumour DNA

This is the largest, and oldest, collection of anticancer treatments. This group can be further subdivided into those that cause breakage of DNA, those that inhibit the synthesis of DNA, and those that modify specific genes. Some examples are outlined in Table 22.4.

Side effects common to chemotherapy targeted at tumour DNA

Most of the drugs that affect tumour DNA are cytotoxic (exceptions are those that modify genes) and share a number of common side effects. The systems affected are those where cells are rapidly duplicating, including the bone marrow, gastrointestinal tract, hair, and reproductive system.

Bone marrow suppression Bone marrow suppression can result in anaemia (low red blood cells), thrombocytopenia (low platelets), and neutropenia (low white cells), leading to tiredness, shortness of breath, increased bleeding, bruising, immunosuppression, and infections. Of particular concern has been neutropenia, which increases the risk of infection. This is often controlled using colony-stimulating factors, specifically granulocyte colony stimulating factors (G-CSF) that encourage the production and differentiation of neutrophils from stem cells (primitive cells that can evolve into a number of different blood cells). The anaemia is sometimes treated with erythropoietin, which attaches to erythropoietin receptors on erythroid progenitor cells, resulting in increased reticulocytes (immature red blood cells).

Gastrointestinal effects The major side effect reported is nausea and vomiting. A number of mechanisms have been proposed for

Table 22.3 Classification of anticancer treatments

Broad target	Sub-target	Examples
Tumour	DNA	Alkylating agents, topoisomerase inhibitors, antimetabolites, antihormones
	RNA	Platinum compounds, cytarabine
	Proteins	Vinca alkaloids, trastuzumab
Endothelium/extracellular matrix	DNA	Combretastatin[a]
	Proteins	Thalidomide, bevacizumab
	Metalloproteinases	Prinomastat[a]
Immune system	Lymphocytes and macrophages	Interferons

[a.] Investigational

Adapted from Espinosa E, Zamora P, Feliu J, González Barón M. Classification of anticancer drugs—a new system based on therapeutic targets. *Cancer Treatment Reviews* 2003; 29: 515–23.

Table 22.4 Chemotherapy agents targeted at the DNA

Target	Group	Examples
DNA breakage	Alkylating agents	Nitrogen mustards, nitrosoureas, alkyl sulphonates, aziridines
	Non-classical alkylating agents	Dacarbazine, temozoloamide, procarbazine
	Cytotoxic antibiotics	Bleomycin, mitomycin
	Platinum compounds	Cisplatin, carboplatin
Inhibit DNA synthesis	Anthracyclines	Doxorubicin, idarubicin
	Podophyllotoxins	Etoposide
	Topoisomerase inhibitors	Topotecan, irinotecan
	Antimetabolites	Folate antagonists, pyrimidine analogues, purine analogues
Modify genes	Antihormones	Anti oestrogens, anti androgens, aromatase inhibitors, LH-RH antagonists
	Retinoids	Bexarotene
	Interferons	Interferon alpha

LH-RH, luteinizing hormone-releasing hormone.

chemotherapy-induced nausea and vomiting, but the most accepted is that chemotherapy results in release of serotonin (5-hydroxy tryptamine, 5-HT) from the entrochromaffin cells found in the mucosa of the upper part of the small intestine. This stimulates 5-HT_3 receptors on vagal afferent nerve fibres, which sends a signal through the nucleus tractus solitarius (a region of the brain stem) and onto the vomiting centre. The most common treatment of chemotherapy induced nausea and vomiting involves the 5-HT_3 antagonists such as ondansetron (see Chapter 12). Chemotherapy agents differ in their propensity to cause nausea and vomiting, with the highest risk being treatments involving platinum compounds and the lowest risk agents such as the vinca alkaloids (see later).

Mucositis (inflammation of the mucosa that can lead to ulceration and pain), particularly of the mouth, is another gastrointestinal side effect seen with cytotoxic drugs. It is best managed with good oral hygiene and can be alleviated by sucking on ice chips.

Diarrhoea is also associated with some chemotherapy. It can lead to dehydration and is treated with loperamide (see Chapter 13) or, in severe cases, with octreotide (a drug that mimics somatostatin, which inhibits gastric secretions and motility).

Alopecia Partial or complete loss of hair (alopecia) is common with many cytotoxic agents. It is usually reversible, but once stopped the hair that returns can be of a different colour or texture. The scalp is usually the worst affected, but there can be loss of eyebrows and beards.

Infertility An important and quite distressing side effect of cytotoxic agents is infertility. It can affect both males and females, and sometimes is not reversible on stopping therapy. Patients of childbearing age need to be carefully counselled before treatment and possible options such as freezing sperm or ovum may be investigated.

Ngozi suffered several of these side effects, but in particular the nausea/vomiting and hair loss. She also suffered mucositis and infections from the bone marrow depression. These side effects, in combination with the fear of having cancer, can lead to psychological problems, particularly depression, which Ngozi suffered from.

Alkylating agents

The alkylating agents work by forming covalent bonds across the strands of DNA. They do this by forming an unstable molecule called a carbonium ion, a carbon atom with a net positive charge. This carbonium ion then binds to the 7-nitrogen on the guanine molecule in DNA. The alkylating agents used as chemotherapy are referred to as dialkylating or bifunctional. This means they can form this carbonium ion on two ends of the molecule and therefore bind to two guanine molecules in the DNA, producing the cross-linking (Figure 22.1).

The alkylating agents can impact on any part of the cell cycle, but their main effect is in the synthesis (S) phase. Cells that are in the resting phase (G_0) have sufficient time to 'repair' the damage that alkylating agents may do. This repair involves excision of the cross-linked nucleotides and new ones being inserted. Thus, alkylating agents have some specificity for cancer cells as they target cells that are proliferating.

The alkylating agents share common side effects. They all suppress bone marrow, leading to immunosuppression. This has been exploited with some agents having been employed as immunosuppressants in patients undergoing organ transplant. The risk of gastrointestinal side effects, especially nausea and vomiting, tends to be moderate to high, and they are more likely than other cytotoxic drugs to cause infertility.

Nitrogen mustards These agents are similar in structure to mustard gas, a toxic chemical used in warfare that was developed at the beginning of last century. One of the original nitrogen mustards was **mustine**. However, this is no longer used. The nitrogen mustards have two chlorethyl groups and a general formula of Cl-CH_2CH_2-R-CH_2CH_2-Cl. The chloride atoms are called the 'leaving group' and in alkaline or neutral pH the Cl is removed and the side chain (CH_2CH_2) undergoes cyclization to form an immonium ion (a three-member ring with a positive charge). This structure is very unstable and opens to form the carbonium ion, which then reacts with the nitrogen on guanine. The 'R' group varies from a simple molecule (CH_3N) in **mechlorethamine**

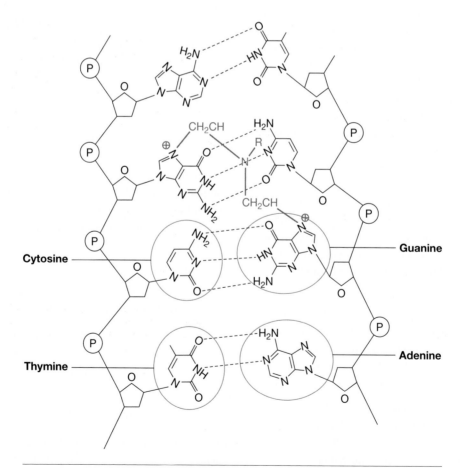

Figure 22.1 Cross-linking of DNA helix by a nitrogen mustard alkylating agent.

(mustine), through to a complex, cyclic structure seen in **cyclophosphamide** and **ifosfamide**.

Cyclophosphamide is one of the most commonly used nitrogen mustards. It is a pro drug and must be converted by hepatic cytochrome P450 enzymes (CYP2B6 and CYP3A4) to 4-hydroxy-cyclophosphamide. This exists in equilibrium with its tautomer aldophosphamide, which is partly converted into the cytotoxic agent phosphoramide mustard and acrolein (Figure 22.2). The metabolism by cytochrome P450 means there are a number of potential drug interactions with inhibitors and inducers of this system.

Cyclophosphamide has less toxicity in the bone marrow, liver, and gastrointestinal tract because in these areas the cells have abundant supplies of aldehyde dehydrogenase and therefore convert most of the aldophosphamide to carboxyphosphamide. However, bone marrow suppression is possible. A major, but rare, toxicity of cyclophosphamide is haemorrhagic cystitis (a severe inflammation of the bladder wall), which is caused by accumulation of acrolein in the urine. It can be limited by making sure that the patient drinks plenty of water and goes to the toilet frequently, emptying their bladder completely when they go. Because haemorrhagic cystitis can be life threatening, the drug mesna, which has sulphhydryl groups that interact with the acrolein and neutralizes it (Figure 22.2), can be given by intravenous infusion. Cyclophosphamide is given orally and intravenously, and is used for a variety of solid tumours and as an immunosuppressant.

Ifosfamide has a similar structure to cyclophosphamide and is also converted in the liver to its active form, which is eventually converted to isophosphoramide mustard. Like cyclophosphamide, it also produces acrolein and mesna is routinely used with it. Because it is converted to the 4-hydroxy form at a slower rate than cyclophosphamide, it has a different spectrum of adverse effects and appears to be less toxic than cyclophosphamide to the bone marrow. It is only given intravenously and is used for a variety of tumours, including sarcomas, lymphomas, and ovarian, cervical, testicular, breast, and lung cancer.

Chlorambucil and **melphalan** have simple structures compared to ifosfamide and cyclophosphamide, and do not require conversion in the liver to be active. They were developed as derivatives of the original nitrogen mustard, mustine, with an aromatic ring placed next to the nitrogen. This reduced the reactivity of the molecule, making them less toxic and allowing them to be given orally. Chlorambucil is rapidly almost completely absorbed orally, whereas melphalan's absorption is more variable. The main side effect with chlorambucil is the potential to cause Steven–Johnson syndrome (a severe and potentially life-threatening skin reaction), whereas pneumonitis and pulmonary fibrosis are possible with melphalan. Chlorambucil can be used for chronic lymphocytic leukaemia, non-Hodgkin's lymphoma, and Hodgkin's disease. Melphalan is indicated for multiple myeloma, advanced ovarian adenocarcinoma, advanced

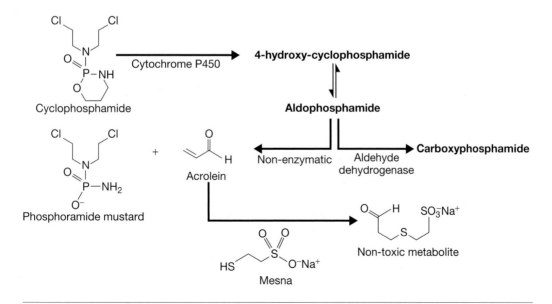

Figure 22.2 Conversion of cyclophosphamide to the active nitrogen mustard.

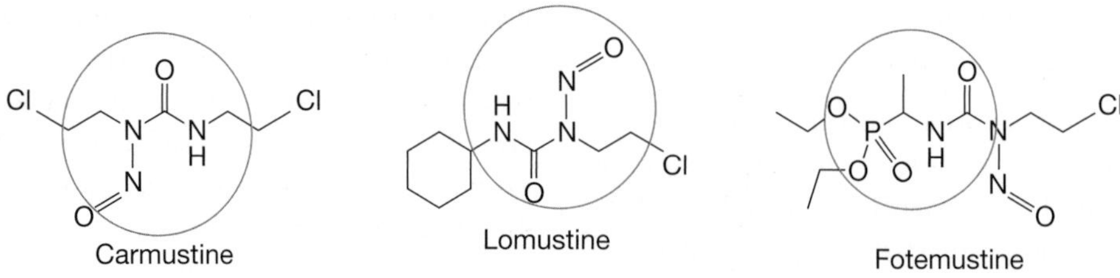

Figure 22.3 Structure of nitrosoureas.

breast cancer, childhood neuroblastoma, polycythaemia vera, and malignant melanoma. However, both have been largely replaced by more effective treatments for several of these tumours.

Estramustine is a combination of estradiol and mustine. It has the actions of both an alkylating agent and a hormonal agent, and will be discussed under hormonal drugs.

Nitrosoureas The nitrosoureas get their name because they contain a nitroso group (R-NO) and urea ((NH_2)$_2$CO). The common central nitrosourea structure is outlined in Figure 22.3.

The mechanism of action of nitrosoureas is not as well established as that of the nitrogen mustards. They share the ability to form carbonium ions and thus cross-link DNA, as nitrogen mustards do. The cross-linking occurs in all nitrosoureas, despite the fact that **lomustine** and **fotemustine** only have one chlorethyl moiety (CH_2CH_2-Cl). They do this by a different mechanism to the nitrogen mustards. The first step is similar, with the molecule rapidly binding to the 7-nitrogen on guanine. The next cross-link, however, occurs more slowly and happens at the 6-oxygen on another guanine. In addition to DNA cross-linking, the nitrosoureas also form isocyanates (O=C=N-R), which can carbamoylate proteins, predominantly lysine. However, this is not a major part of their cytotoxicity.

Carmustine (also called BCNU) is rapidly metabolized by the liver and is given intravenously. It is also available as implants for local effect in the brain. Fotemustine, while not as rapidly metabolized as carmustine, it is also given intravenously, whereas lomustine (also called CCNU) is given orally. A common feature of the nitrosoureas is their high lipid solubility. This means that they pass through the blood–brain barrier, a unique feature that has seen them used for brain and cerebrospinal tumours. Carmustine and lomustine are used for non-Hodgkin's

lymphoma, Hodgkin's disease, and brain tumours. Fotemustine is used primarily for malignant melanoma. Nausea and vomiting are common side effects of the nitrosoureas, and they are also associated with delayed bone marrow suppression (4–6 weeks after treatment). Carmustine has been associated with pulmonary fibrosis and causes injection site pain.

Alkyl sulphonates **Busulfan** and **treosulfan** are in this group. They have no structural relationship to the nitrogen mustards and nitrosoureas, as they lack any chlorethyl moiety (Figure 22.4.). However, they still react with guanine in DNA. Busulfan does this by what is called an S_N2 reaction. The S_N2 reaction, also called bimolecular nucleophilic substitution, involves an interaction between a nucleophile (a molecule that donates electrons) and an electrophile (a molecule that attracts electrons). In this case, the nucleophile is the 7-nitrogen on guanine, and the electrophile is the carbon next to the mesylate group on either end of busulfan (Figure 22.4).

Treosulfan has a similar structure to busulfan, but differs in having two hydroxyl groups (Figure 22.5). This changes its mechanisim of action and it has to be activated by being converted to epoxides in the body (e.g. L-diepoxybutane). It is the epoxides that then form the cross-links with DNA.

Busulfan is well absorbed orally and is metabolized to methanesulfonic acid, and other inactive metabolites,

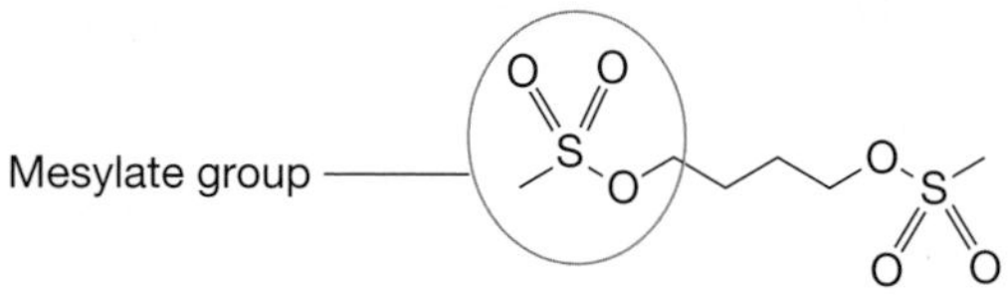

Figure 22.4 Busulfan structure.

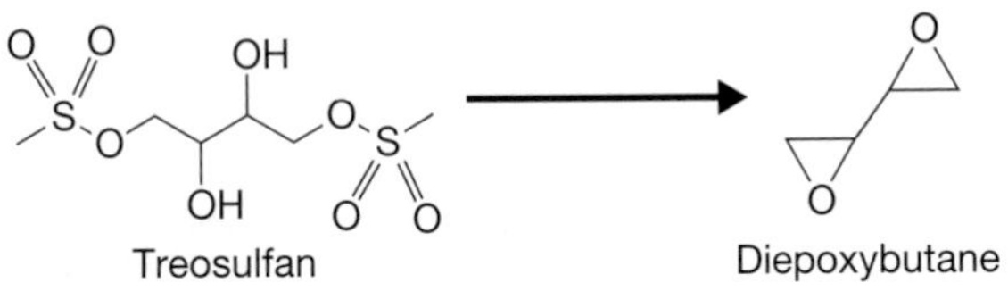

Figure 22.5 Conversion of treosulfan to its active metabolite.

with a half-life of about 2.5 hours. Treosulfan can also be given orally and has a half-life of about 2 hours. Bone marrow suppression is the main side effect of concern. Pulmonary fibrosis and skin hyperpigmentation are also possible adverse effects. Busulfan is used for myeloid leukemia (intravenously and orally), and myelofibrosis and polycythemia vera (orally). It is also used as conditioning treatment prior to stem-cell (haematopoietic) transplantation. Treosulfan is used for ovarian cancer.

Aziridines The core structure of this class is an aziridine group, a three-member heterocycle with an amine group (NH) and two methylene groups (CH$_2$). **ThioTEPA** (N,N',N'-triethylenethiophosphoramide) is the main member of this class currently used. Although mitomycin also contains an aziridine group, it is considered under the class of cytotoxic antibiotics (see later). ThioTEPA has a similar mechanism of action to the nitrogen mustards, but is more active at acid pH. It does not form an immonium ion, rather its reactivity

comes from the existing three-member aziridine rings in its structure. It is rarely used systemically and is used locally, by instillation, in treating bladder cancers. It has also been used for breast and ovarian cancer. Bone marrow suppression is the major side effect, which can occur after bladder instillation.

Non-classical alkylating agents

This group includes the tetrazines (**dacarbazine** and **temozolomide**) and **procarbazine**.

Tetrazines Dacarbazine (also called DTIC) was the first agent in this class. It is inactive and requires conversion in the liver by cytochrome P450 (CYP1A2) to methyltriazenyl-imidazole-carboxamide (MTIC). This non-enzymatically breaks down into 5-aminoimidazole-4-carboxamide and methyldiazonium ion. The latter interacts with DNA to methylate the 6-oxygen and 7-nitrogen on guanine. However, it does not cross-link as the nitrogen mustards do (Figure 22.6).

Temozolamide has a similar structure to dacarbazine and is also converted to 5-aminoimidazole-4-carboxamide (AIC) and the methyldiazonium ion. However, unlike dacarbazine, it does not require hepatic conversion to the intermediate MTIC, rather it converts to MTIC in the presence of water at physiological pH.

Dacarbazine is given intravenously, while temozolamide is given orally. Temozolamide has good penetration into the central nervous system and is used for brain tumours

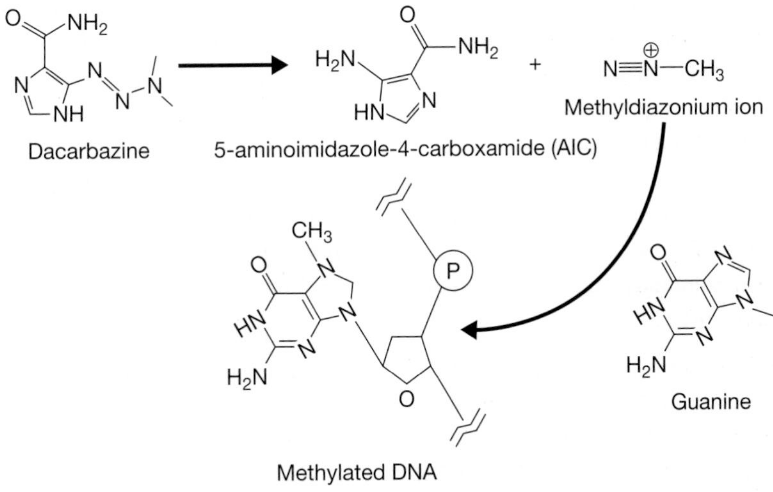

Figure 22.6 Mechanism of action of dacarbazine.

(e.g. glioma). Dacarbazine is used for soft tissue sarcomas, malignant melanoma, and Hodgkin's disease. The most prominent side effects are bone marrow suppression, and nausea and vomiting. Both dacarbazine and temozoloamide are metabolized in the liver and their elimination half-lives are 5 and 2 hours, respectively.

Procarbazine Procarbazine also works by methylation of DNA. It is structurally unrelated to dacarbazine and temozolamide, and is first converted to azoprocarbazine either non-enzymatically or by cytochrome P450. The azoprocarbazine is the active moiety that breaks down to isopropylformyl benzamide and the methyldiazonium ion (see Figure 22.6). Like temozalamide it is used for some brain cancers, and is also used for non-Hodgkin's lymphoma and Hodgkin's disease. It is given orally, and has a similar spectrum of side effects as the tetrazines. It is a weak monoamine oxidase inhibitor (see Chapter 19), but dietary changes are usually not required. Procarbazine can also cause a disulfuram-like reaction, similar to metronidazole, when alcohol is consumed (see metronidazole in Chapter 21). It is eliminated by the kidneys as N-isopropyl-terphthalamic acid.

Cytotoxic antibiotics

This group includes the anthracyclines (e.g. doxorubicin) and another group also derived from the *Streptomyces* bacterial species (e.g. bleomycin). Actinomycin, also derived from *Streptomyces*, works primarily by inhibiting RNA polymerase and will be described later under drugs targetting RNA.

Anthracyclines This group includes **doxorubicin**, **idarubicin**, **daunorubicin**, **epirubicin**, and the derivative **mitoxantrone**. Daunorubicin was the first of this class to be discovered and it came from bacteria, *Streptomyces peucetius*. This was closely followed by doxorubicin (also called hydroxydaunorubicin), which has become the most widely used of this class. The anthracyclines share a common central structure based on anthraquinone (Figure 22.7).

There have been several proposed mechanisms of action for the anthracyclines. First, the planar ring structure intercalates between DNA strands, causing structural distortion of the DNA and stopping both DNA and RNA synthesis. Second, the anthracyclines inhibit topoisomerase, the enzyme required for DNA replication. Topoisomerase exists in three main forms:

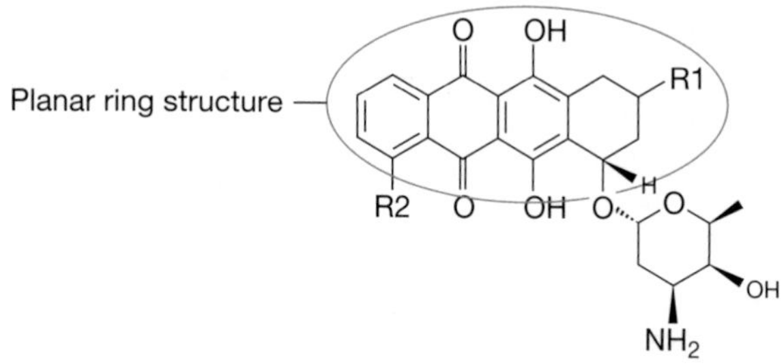

Figure 22.7 Common central structure of anthracyclines.

type I, type II and type III. Type I and type III topoisomerase cause a single-strand break in DNA, whereas type II produces a double-strand break. Anthracyclines are thought to bind to type II, specifically the subfamily type IIα. The topoisomerase IIα cuts both strands of DNA, allows a second double-strand to pass through, and then rejoins the DNA strands (Box 22.1). This process is essential to disentangle the two daughter strands of DNA during cell replication. To do this the topoisomerase forms a complex with the cut ends of the DNA. Anthracyclines are thought to stabilize this complex, thus arresting its action. A third mechanism relates to iron-dependent oxidation, which leads to the production of free radicals that further damage the DNA.

Apart from the other side effects of cytotoxic drugs, the anthracyclines are associated with cardiac toxicity, and liposomal formulations of doxorubicin have been developed to try to reduce this adverse effect. Patients on these drugs need to have their cardiac function monitored, including ECG and left ventricular ejection fraction. The anthracyclines can result in necrosis if extravasated (injected into the tissues instead of the veins). However, the risk is minimal with mitoxantrone. Idarubicin is the only one of this class that can be given orally. The anthracyclines are largely bound to tissue in the body and eliminated by hepatic metabolism.

Doxorubicin is used for a wide range of malignancies, including breast, bladder, and lung cancer, lymphomas, sarcoma, leukaemia, and multiple myeloma. Epirubicin is used for breast cancer, while idarubicin is used for various types of leukemia. Mitoxantrone is used for non-Hodgkin's lymphoma, acute myeloid leukaemia, and breast and prostate cancer.

Box 22.1

Action of topoisomerase II

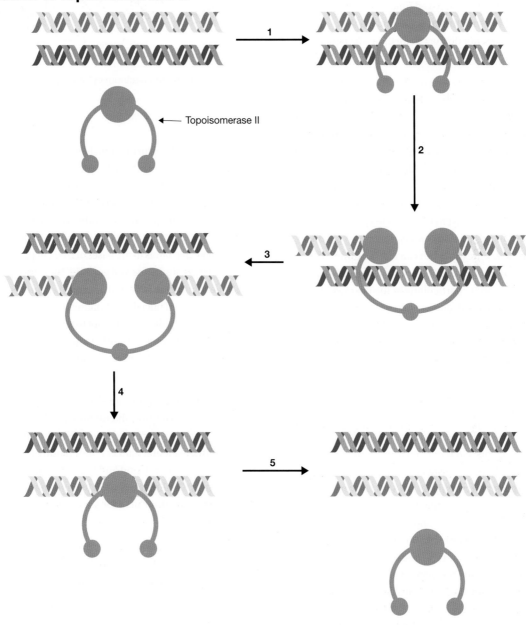

Figure a

1. Topoisomerase II (topo II) binds with one of the DNA double helixes and causes a double-strand break.

2. The cut ends of the DNA complex with the topo II and the topo II then splits the DNA apart. **This is the site of action of the anthracyclines (e.g. doxorubicin) and the podophyllotoxins (e.g. etoposide).**

3. The second DNA double helix passes through the split in the first DNA.

4. The topo II closes the gap and binds the ends of the first DNA double helix back together.

5. The topo II then dissociates, leaving the second DNA double helix now on the other side of the first DNA double helix.

Adapted from: McLeod HL. Epipodophyllotoxins In: Schellens JHM, McLeod HL, Newell DR. *Cancer clinical pharmacology.* Oxford: Oxford University Press, 2005.

Other *Streptomyces*-derived antibiotics This group includes **mitomycin** and **bleomycin**. Although these are natural products also derived from *Streptomyces* species, they have little structural resemblance to the anthracyclines, nor do they share their mechanism of action.

Bleomycin is actually part of a family of peptides called the bleomycins, with the predominant peptide being bleomycin A_2. Bleomycin binds metal ions, in particular copper and iron. When it complexes with iron (Fe^{++}) in the presence of oxygen it forms a very reactive bleomycin-iron-hydroperoxide, which then leads to oxidation and breaking of DNA strands. It can produce both single-strand and double-strand breaks, in the ratio of about 10:1. Bleomycin is cell-cycle specific, affecting G_2 and M phases predominantly. It tends to produce little myelosuppression, but can cause pulmonary fibrosis in approximately 10% of patients and changes in skin pigmentation, particularly in the flexures. It has also been associated with allergic reactions in about 1% of lymphoma patients. Bleomycin is given parenterally for the treatment of a range of solid tumours, including carcinoma of the testes, non-Hodgkin's lymphoma, and squamous cell carcinomas. Bleomycin is eliminated by the kidneys and dosage adjustments are required in renal failure.

Mitomycin is structurally similar to the aziridine alkylating agents and is derived from *Streptomyces lavendulae*. Its mechanism of action is the same as the alkylating agents (cross-links DNA). It is given intravenously in the treatment of gastrointestinal tumours (e.g. stomach, pancreatic, and colon) and instilled for the treatment of bladder cancer. Bone marrow suppression is the main side effect and can be delayed for several weeks after treatment. Rare reactions include pulmonary toxicity and haemolytic uraemic syndrome (characterized by low platelets and renal failure). Mitomycin is cleared by the liver and has a short half-life (around 1 hour).

Platinum compounds

Cisplatin, the first of this group, was discovered in the late 1800s and was subsequently found to inhibit *E. coli* replication. Because of its toxicity, a number of analogues have been developed, including **carboplatin** and **oxaliplatin**. As their name suggests, they all share the same core of a platinum molecule, a transition metal (Figure 22.8).

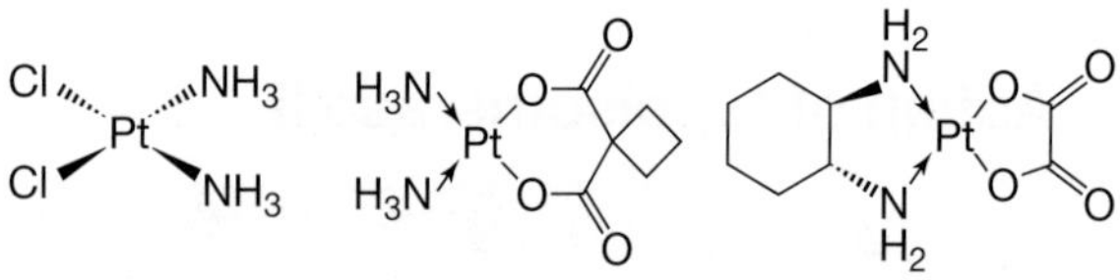

Cisplatin   Carboplatin   Oxaliplatin

Figure 22.8 Common platinum cytotoxics.

Their overall mechanism of action is analogous with the nitrogen mustards and other alkylating agents. The first step involves aquation of the molecules, during which water replaces a ligand. In the case of cisplatin, the leaving group is chloride, for carboplatin it is dicarboxycyclobutane, and for oxaliplatin it is oxalate. This results in a reactive intermediate that binds to the bases of DNA, in particular the 7-nitrogens of adenine and guanine. The cross-linking causes bending of the DNA and denaturing (a process by which proteins and nucleic acids loose their structure) of the DNA strand. While cells attempt to repair this damage, if sufficient it can prompt apoptosis. Other mechanisms that may be involved include effects on the immune system that increase monocyte function.

The platinum compounds are all given intravenously and used for a variety of solid tumours, including ovarian and head and neck cancer (cisplatin and carboplatin), testicular cancer (carboplatin), bladder cancer (cisplatin), and lung and brain tumours (carboplatin). Oxaliplatin is used in combination with fluorouracil and folinic acid for advanced colorectal cancer.

As noted above, cisplatin has the greatest toxicity of the platinum compounds. It is more likely to cause vomiting, renal toxicity, and neuropathy compared to carboplatin, and the latter may not be reversible. Carboplatin has more effect on bone marrow and platelets. Oxaliplatin is also associated with neurotoxicity. The nephrotoxicity with cisplatin means it cannot be used in patients with impaired renal function (creatinine clearance <40 mL/min), while dosage adjustment is usually not required with oxaliplatin unless there is severe renal impairment (e.g. creatinine clearance <20 mL/min). Cisplatin and oxaliplatin are extensively bound to protein in the body, unlike carboplatin. All of the platinum compounds undergo extensive renal elimination.

Podophyllotoxins

Podophyllotoxin, a non-alkaloid toxin found in the American mayapple and used to treat warts, is the precursor for the cytotoxic agents **etoposide** (also called VP-16) and **teniposide** (also called VM-26). This group is also called the epipodophyllotoxins. They work by the same mechanism as the anthracycline chemotherapy agents and bind to topoisomerase II (Box 22.1). However, unlike the anthracyclines, they do not intercalate DNA. Teniposide is almost identical to etoposide, but about 10 times as potent. Etoposide is given orally and intravenously, while teniposide is only given intravenously. They are used for a variety of tumours, but teniposide is used mainly for paediatric malignancies (e.g. acute lymphoblastic leukaemia and neuroblastoma). Etoposide is used for lung cancers, lymphomas and testicular cancer (phosphate salt). Teniposide is primarily metabolized in the liver, whereas etoposide is both renally cleared unchanged and metabolized, with half-lives of 5 hours and 4–11 hours, respectively. The main side effect of both is bone marrow suppression, mainly affecting leukocytes. Occasionally patients can suffer allergic reactions from the intravenous formulations, although the actual cause (i.e. drug versus the vehicle) is uncertain and the incidence is less with the water-soluble phosphate salt.

Topoisomerase I inhibitors

As previously discussed, there are three types of topoisomerase (types I, II, and III) in mammalian cells, although type I and II predominate. Topoisomerase I is sub divided into type IA and type IB. The role of topoisomerase I is in relaxation and coiling of the DNA. It does this by making a break in one strand of the DNA helix, compared to both strands with type II (see Box 22.1). The enzyme then 'holds on' strongly to one cut end and allows the other to rotate, then re-attaches the strand together. Another difference is that the type I enzyme does not require energy to undertake its activity, whereas type II requires ATP.

Camptothecin, derived from the bark of *Camptotheca acuminata* (commonly known as the 'happy tree'), was one of the original topoisomerase I inhibitors. However, because of its low solubility and poor adverse effect profile, derivatives such as **irinotecan** and **topotecan** have been developed. The topoisomerase inhibitors stop DNA synthesis by binding to and stabilizing the DNA/ topoisomerase complex, and therefore are specific for the S phase of cell replication.

Irinotecan is a pro-drug that is converted by hydrolysis to SN-38, the active moiety. The SN-38 is subsequently metabolized by hepatic uridine diphosphate-glucuronyltransferase (UGT) to an inactive glucuronide, and the half-life is about 11 hours. Patients who have Gilbert's syndrome, a deficiency in the glucuronuyltransferase, are unable to metabolize irinotecan and can suffer severe side effects. Irinotecan is used with other cytotoxics in the treatment of colorectal cancer and is given intravenously. Apart from the usual side effects of chemotherapy it is particularly associated with causing diarrhoea. This can be in part due to the cholinergic effects of irinotecan. The acute cholinergic effects include diarrhoea, cramping, rhinitis, and sweating, while the chronic effects are predominantly diarrhoea. Patients who develop the acute cholinergic effects can be treated with atropine, while those who develop chronic diarrhoea are usually treated with loperamide (see Chapter 13). The cholinergic effects can also worsen or precipitate asthma. Irinotecan can cause bone marrow suppression, especially neutropenia.

Topotecan is a more recent development and has a better gastrointestinal side effect profile than irinotecan. Unlike irinotecan it does not require conversion for activity. It is partly excreted unchanged in the urine and partly metabolized by hydrolysis to a less active metabolite. It is also administered intravenously and is used in combination with other agents in the treatment of ovarian, cervical, and small-cell lung cancer. The main side effect of concern is myelosuppression, including anaemia, leukopenia, and thrombocytopenia.

Antimetabolites

This group is also one of the oldest classes of drug. Antimetabolites work by acting as 'false' versions of DNA and RNA building blocks or by stopping the synthesis of DNA/RNA precursors. This class can be further subdivided in folate antagonists, purine analogues, and pyrimidine analogues.

Methotrexate is the best-known example of the folate antagonists. It works by inhibiting dihydrofolate reductase (DFR), the enzyme responsible for conversion of dihydrofolate to tetrahydrofolate (Figure 22.9). Tetrahydrofolate is essential in the production of purine bases and thymidine, both of which are required for DNA, RNA, and protein synthesis.

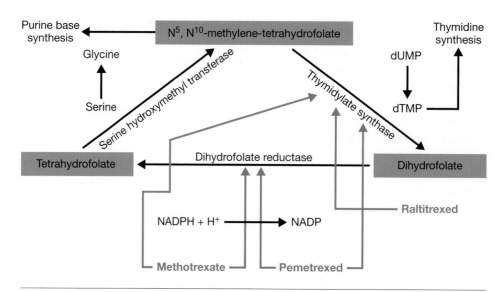

Figure 22.9 Synthesis of tetrahydrofolate and the targets of folate antagonists. dUMP, 2'-deoxyuridylate monophosphate; dTMP, 2'-deoxythymidylate monophophosphate; NADPH, nicotinamide adenine dinucleotide phosphate. Adapted from: Zaboikin M, Srinivasakumar N, Schuening F. Gene therapy with drug resistance genes. *Cancer Gene Therapy* 2005; 13: 335–45.

The folate antagonists all share a structural similarity with folic acid, but a key alteration is the substitution of a hydroxyl group with an amino group, which changes them from substrates to tight-binding inhibitors of the essential enzymes. Because of their effect on DNA synthesis, they target the S phase of cell replication and, like many other cytotoxic agents, are more selective for rapidly dividing cells.

Methotrexate is taken up into cells and converted, as folic acid is, to a polyglutamate. This then binds to the DFR, and has 1000 times the affinity that folic acid has for DFR. The methotrexate polyglutamate also has some effect on thymidylate synthetase (TS), which is important in producing the precursor for thymidine. The net effect is depletion of tetrahydrofolate, leading to impairment of DNA and RNA synthesis through the effects on the production of 2'deoxythymidylate monophosphate (dTMP). Methotrexate is given both orally and parenterally in the treatment of a range of solid tumours, leukaemia, and lymphoma. It is also used in much lower doses in the treatment of psoriasis (see Chapter 8) and rheumatoid arthritis (see Chapter 9). At the doses used in chemotherapy it can cause serious bone marrow suppression and pulmonary toxicity. If very high doses are used then folinic acid is used as a 'rescue'. Folinic acid is the 5-formyl derivative of tetrahydrofolic acid. It does not require DFR to convert it to tetrahydrofolic acid and

therefore allows cells to continue DNA/RNA synthesis when DFR inhibitors are used. Other side effects include nausea and vomiting, and mucositis. Methotrexate is cleared by the kidneys and should not be used if there is severe renal failure. It can also cause liver toxicity and liver enzymes should be monitored.

Pemetrexed is a folate antagonist that, like methotrexate, is transported into cells and converted to a polyglutamate. Its primary site of action is on TS, but it also has some inhibitory effect on DFR and 5-phosphoribosylglycinamide formyltransferase, which is involved in the formation of purines from 10-formyltetrahydrofolate, a derivative of tetrahydrofolate. Pemetrexed's main role is in the treatment of mesothelioma, a lung cancer caused by exposure to asbestos with a poor prognosis, as well as small-cell lung cancer. Like methotrexate it can cause bone marrow suppression, nausea and vomiting, and mucositis, but does not have the pulmonary toxicity of methotrexate. Patients are given folic acid (not folinic acid) to reduce the toxicity. Pemetrexed is renally cleared, with a half-life of 2–4 hours. Dosage adjustment is required in renal failure.

Raltitrexed is also structurally related to folic acid and, like the other folate antagonists, must be polyglutamated to become active. It acts primarily by inhibiting TS, with little effect on DFR. It has a better side effect profile than methotrexate and it is used for palliation of colorectal cancer. The main side effects are gastrointestinal and myelosuppression. Raltitrexed is cleared by the kidney and the dose must be reduced in patients with renal impairment.

Purine analogues Purines, adenine, and guanine make up half the nucleotides of DNA and RNA. The purine analogues mimic the structure if purines and act as 'false' substrates in DNA and RNA synthesis. **6-Mercaptopurine** (6-MP) and **tioguanine** (thioguanine) are analogues of guanine, and **fludarabine** and **cladribine** are adenine analogues.

6-Mercaptopurine has been used for over 50 years. It is the active metabolite of azathioprine, and like azathioprine it is also used as an immunosuppressant in inflammatory diseases such as inflammatory bowel disease. It undergoes a number of different metabolic transformations in cells (Figure 22.11).

The 6-MTITP produced from 6-MP, and its diphosphate and monophosphate precursors, collectively inhibit purine synthesis. The 6-TGTP is incorporated as a 'false' nucleotide into DNA in place of guanine and causes strand breaks. As outlined in Figure 22.10, the other guanine analogue, tioguanine, undergoes simple metabolism to thioguanine monophosphate, and this is subsequently converted to 6-TGTP and integrated into DNA.

Both 6-MP and tioguanine are broken down by xanthine oxidase. This is the enzyme inhibited by allopurinol, a drug used for gout, and the combination of 6-MP and allopurinol should be avoided or the dose of 6-MP reduced to one quarter (the interaction does not appear to be a problem with tioguanine as it is largely eliminated by hepatic metabolism). Mercaptopurine and tioguanine are given orally, and they are used in the treatment of acute and chronic leukemias. Both share the same side effects of bone marrow and mucositis, and they can cause liver dysfunction.

Fludarabine is rapidly de-phosphorylated in the plasma to arabinofuranosyl-fluoroadenine (F-ara-A). This is taken up into cells where it is phosphorylated into its active form fludarabine triphosphate (F-ara-ATP), which blocks DNA and RNA polymerase, DNA ligase, and DNA primase. The monophospate form (F-ara-AMP) is also incorporated, in place of adenine, into DNA and causes DNA chain termination during replication.

Cladribine has a similar structure to fludarabine, except the fluoride moiety is replaced with chloride and it lacks the phosphate group. It is taken up into cells and, like fludarabine, is then phosphorylated in to its active form (cladribine triphosphate), which has similar effects to fludarabine triphosphate. The cladribine triphosphate also stimulates capsases, which triggers apoptosis.

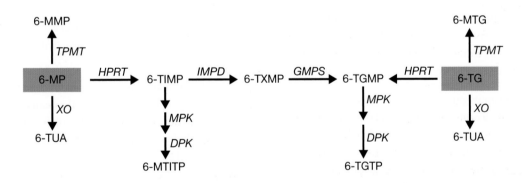

Figure 22.10 Metabolism and transformation of 6-mercaptopurine and thioguanine. 6-MP, 6-mercaptopurine; 6-MMP, 6-methylmercaptopurine; 6-TUA, 6-thiouric acid; 6-MTIMP, 6-methylthioinosine monophosphate; 6-MTITP, 6-methylthioinosine triphosphate; 6-TIMP, 6-thioinosine monophosphate; 6-TXMP, 6-thioxanthosine monophosphate; 6-TGMP, 6-thioguanine monophosphate; 6-TGTP, 6-thioguanine triphosphate; 6-TG, 6-thioguanine; 6-MTG, 6-methylthioguanine; *XO*, xanthine oxidase; *TPMT*, thiopurine S-methyl transferase; *HPRT*, hypoxanthine phosphoribosyl transferase; *IMPD*, inosine monophosphate dehydrogenase; *GMPS*, guanosine monophosphate synthetase; *MPK*, monophosphate kinase; *DPK*, diphosphate kinase. Adapted from: Derijks LJJ, Gilissen LPL, Hooymans PM, Hommes DW. Thiopurines in inflammatory bowel disease. *Alimentary Pharmacology & Therapeutics* 2006; 24: 715–29.

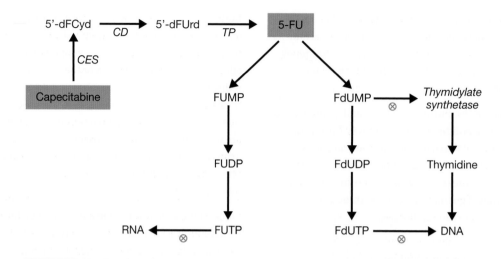

Figure 22.11 Activity of fluorouracil and capecitabine. 5'-dFCyd, 5'dexoy-5'fluorocytidine; 5'-dFUrd, 5'-deoxy-5'-fluorouridine; *CES*, carboxylesterase (liver); *CD*, cytidine deaminase; *TP*, thymidine phosphorylase; 5-FU, 5-fluourouracil; FUMP, fluorouracil monophosphate; FUDP, fluorouracil diphosphate; FUTP, fluorouracil diphosphate; FdUMP, fluorodeoxyuridylate monophosphate; FdUDP, fluorodeoxyuridylate diphosphate; FdUTP, fluorodeoxyuridylate triphosphate.

Fludarabine is given orally and intravenously, and cladribine intravenously, in the treatment of chronic lymphocytic leukaemia. Cladribine is also used for hairy cell leukaemia. Bone marrow suppression is the most important side effect with both drugs. This can last for several weeks and immunosuppression can last for several months because of effects on CD4 T-cells. Both are also associated with neurotoxicity at high doses and cladribine can cause fever (in the absence of infection) in patients with hairy cell leukaemia. Fludarabine is excreted by the kidneys as the de-phosphorylated form and approximately 50% of cladribine is renally excreted.

Pyrimidine analogues Pyrimidines make up the other half of the nucleoside bases found in DNA and RNA. In DNA they are thymine and cytosine, while RNA uses uracil and cytosine. The pyrimidine analogues are divided into those that are related to uracil (e.g. **5-fluorouracil** and **capecitabine**), and those that mimic cytosine (e.g. **cytarabine** and **gemcitabine**).

5-Fluorouracil (5-FU) is one of the oldest agents in this class. It is active within the cells through one of two metabolic pathways (Figure 22.11). In one pathway, it is converted to a fluorouracil triphosphate, which is then incorporated in to RNA in place of uracil. In the other, it is converted to fluorodeoxyuridylate monophosphate (FdUMP). The fluoride ion makes it a potent inhibitor of

thymidylate synthetase, which is important in the production of thymidine (see Figure 22.11). The FdUMP is also further phosphorylated into a triphosphate, which can be incorporated into DNA, causing instability in the DNA.

Capecitabine is a pro-drug of 5-FU. It is active orally, unlike 5-FU, and is converted through three steps to 5-FU (Figure 22.11). The final step, involving thymidine phosphorylase, is more active in cancer cells and therefore gives capecitabine some selectivity for malignancies.

Both 5-FU and capecitabine are used for solid tumours, including colon and breast cancer. They cause myelosuppression, diarrhoea, and cardiac toxicity. 5-FU is metabolized largely by intracellular catabolism (see Figure 22.11), while capecitabine is metabolized in the liver.

Cytarabine (also called Ara C or cytosine arabinoside) is an analogue of deoxycytidine and affects DNA in a number of ways. First, it is phosphorylated to a triphosphate (Ara CTP), which is an inhibitor of DNA polymerase that is required for DNA replication and repair. However, more important for its cytotoxic activity is the incorporation of cytarabine into DNA, which tumour cells can only remove slowly. It is given intravenously for the treatment of a range of leukaemias and non-Hodgkin's lymphoma. Cytarabine is metabolized hepatically to the inactive uracil arabinoside, which is subsequently excreted by the kidneys. The main dose-limiting side effect is bone marrow suppression. High doses can cause central nervous system and gastrointestinal toxicity.

Gemcitabine resembles deoxycytidine and cytarabine, with two molecules on the deoxyribose sugar replaced with fluoride molecules. Like cytarabine it is converted to a triphosphorylate and competes with deoxycytidine triphosphate (dCTP) to inhibit DNA synthetase. It also inhibits ribonucleoside reductase, depleting deoxyribonucleotides needed for DNA synthesis. Gemcitabine triphosphate, like cytarabine, is incorporated into DNA, causes DNA strand termination, and is resistant to being repaired by the usual cellular mechanisms. It is used for the treatment of small-cell lung cancer, and bladder, breast, and ovarian cancer. Compared to many other cytotoxics it has a much better side effect profile, causing much milder and transient bone marrow suppression. Common side effects are nausea, diarrhoea, and flu-like symptoms. Most of the gemcitabine is excreted in the urine and doses need to be reduced in renal failure.

Hormone and anti-hormonal therapy

Hormones play an important role in cellular functions by acting on receptors to produce the up- and down-regulation of genes. Tissues and organs related to sexual function (e.g. prostate, testes, and breast) are particularly sensitive to the action of sex hormones (e.g. androgens, oestrogens, and progestogens), which can enhance or inhibit their growth. This has therefore become a target of treatment for cancers of these tissues. However, it should be noted that many hormonal therapies only slow the growth rather than 'kill' the cancer cells, and therefore are used for palliation (i.e. does not cure but reduces the symptoms and/or prolongs survival).

There are several approaches to hormonal anticancer treatment. First, hormones that inhibit growth of tissues can be used. An example of this is the use of oestrogens in the treatment of prostatic tumours. Increasing oestrogen levels produces a negative feed back on the anterior pituitary, leading to a decrease in luteinizing hormone release, resulting in a decrease in testosterone levels. They may also increase sex hormone binding globulin, further reducing androgen levels, and may have a direct effect on the tumour cells. Both **diethylstilboestrol** and

ethinylestradiol are used. However, they are poorly tolerated and not used as first-line treatment. A more recent advance has combined oestrogens with an alkalyating agent in the treatment of prostate cancer. **Estramustine** contains a molecule of estrogen (oestradiol) and a molecule of nitrogen mustard (mechlorethamine, also called mustine). It is given orally for advanced prostate cancer and has the side effects of both alkylating agents and oestrogens (i.e. gynaecomastia and cardiovascular disorders, see Chapter 15).

A second approach is to block the effect of the hormone on the tissue. Agents that act in this way are referred to as hormone antagonists (or anti-hormonal therapy). Anti-oestrogens are used in hormone-dependent breast cancer and anti-androgens in prostate cancer. A third approach is to reduce the production of hormones.

Anti-oestrogens Tamoxifen is probably the best-known oestrogen receptor antagonist (also called selective estrogen receptor modulators, SERMs). There are two forms of the oestrogen receptor, ERα and ERβ. Both are nuclear receptors, similar to many other steroid receptors, and it is ERα that is involved in breast cancer. Oestrogen receptors are found in the cytoplasm and when activated migrate to the nucleus, where they influence DNA, mRNA, and finally protein production. Some receptors are also found on the cell surface membrane and can complex with tyrosine kinases (e.g. epidermal growth factor receptor, HER2), and can influence mitosis through the mitogen-activated protein kinase pathway. Tamoxifen is a triphenylethylene derivative that has little structural similarity to oestrogen. It is administered orally and extensively metabolized in the liver by cytochrome P450 into active metabolites, one of which (endoxifen) is 100 times more potent as an inhibitor of oestrogen receptors (Figure 22.12).

Not all breast cancers express oestrogen receptors and tamoxifen should only be used in receptor-positive patients. The side effects of tamoxifen are related to its anti-oestrogenic activity and include hot flushes, fluid retention, and menstrual irregularities. While tamoxifen is an antagonist in breast tissue, it has oestrogenic effects on the endometrium and is associated with a small increased risk of endometrial cancer.

Toremifene is another SERM, with an identical structure to tamoxifen except for an additional single chloride molecule. It is also given orally and metabolized in the liver, with some active metabolite. Its effectiveness and

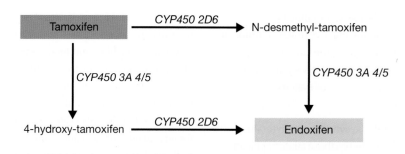

Figure 22.12 Metabolism of tamoxifen. Adapted from: Jin Y, Zeruesenay D, Stearns V, *et al.*: CYP2D6 genotype, antidepressant use, and tamoxifen metabolism during adjuvant breast cancer treatment. *Journal of the National Cancer Institute* 2005; 97: 30–9.

safety profile are almost identical to tamoxifen, except there is limited evidence that it may have less effect on the endometrium. However, further clinical experience is required to evaluate this.

Fulvestrant is chemically unrelated to the other oestrogen receptor antagonists. Unlike tamoxifen and toremifene it occupies the receptor and produces a conformational change that causes down-regulation of the oestrogen receptors (hence it is in a class called selective estrogen receptor down-regulators, SERDs) and reduced binding of receptor complex to oestrogen response elements in the cell. The result is that it has no oestrogenic effects on the endometrium and bones. However, it still has the anti-oestrogenic side effects of tamoxifen (e.g. hot flushes). It is given by subcutaneous injection.

Anti-androgens These are broadly divided into steroidal (e.g. **cyproterone acetate**) and non-steroidal (e.g. **flutamide**). Cyproterone acetate is chemically related to17-hydroxyprogesterone and inhibits androgen receptors. The androgen receptor, like the oestrogen receptor, is a nuclear receptor that regulates genes, resulting increased transcription of mRNA and subsequent production of selected proteins. Among these is the production of IGF-1, a potent promoter of cell growth. The exact mechanism by which cyproterone blocks androgen receptors is not well understood and competition for binding of the receptor only partly explains its effect. Apart from blocking androgen receptors, cyproterone also inhibits oestrogen, progestin, mineralocorticoid, and glucocorticoid receptors. This helps with its chemotherapeutic effects (e.g. causing decreased production of testosterone), but also leads to some of its adverse effects, which include decreased

libido, oedema, hot flushes, mood changes, and insomnia. It can also rarely cause hepatotoxicity. It is given orally and is metabolized by the CYP3A4 to an active metabolite.

Flutamide is the oldest of the non-steroidal anti-androgens, and has now been largely replaced by others, including **bicalutamide** and **nilutamide** because of better side effect profiles. As the name suggests, non-steroidal anti-androgens have no structural similarity to the androgens. Flutamide is a pro-drug, which is α-hydroxylated into its active form of hydroxyflutamide. This is a competitive inhibitor of the androgen receptor and, unlike cyproterone, it has no effect on androgen production and may actually be associated with an increase in testosterone levels. This may cause one of its side effects, fluid retention, which can exacerbate heart failure. Other side effects include nausea and diarrhoea, gynecomastia (sometimes with reversible galactorrhea), and hot flushes. Although rare, it is also associated with serious liver dysfunction. Bicalutamide and nilutamide are structurally related to flutamide and equally efficacious. Both are active without conversion, with only the *R*-isomer of bicalutamide being active. They are less likely to cause diarrhoea compared to flutamide and are both given orally once a day (compared to three times a day for flutamide). Nilutamide is associated with serious pneumonitis, which is reversible.

Agents that reduce the production of sex hormones The third approach to the hormonal therapy of cancers is to stop or reduce the production of the hormones, rather than blocking their effects. An important pathway in the production of oestrogen is the conversion of testosterone to oestradiol, and androstenedione to oestrone, by aromatase (see Chapter 15, Figure 15.3). Aromatase is part of the cytochrome P450 superfamily of enzymes and is found in brain, skin, gonads, and adipose tissue. The latter is an important source of the production of oestrogens in post-menopausal women. Aromatase produces a series of hydroxylations of testosterone to produce oestradiol. The original aromatase inhibitor was **aminoglutethimide**, a drug discovered accidentally while developing new anticonvulsants. However, it had a poor side effect profile because it was not selective for aromatase and inhibited the production of all cholesterol-derived sex hormones. This resulted in the development of the new aromatase-selective inhibitors, which is one of the most recent advances in the treatment of breast cancer. **Anastrozole** was the first of this group to be discovered. It is a non-steroidal (i.e. it bears no resemblance to oestrogens) reversible inhibitor of aromatase (Figure 22.13). Anastrozole's structure includes a triazole ring that binds to the iron in the heme moity of the enzyme (this is similar to the mechanism by which triazole antifungals inhibit cytochrome P450 in the liver). It reduces conversion of testosterone/androstenedione by over 95%. It is given orally and metabolized in the liver by N-dealkylation, hydroxylation, and glucuronidation to inactive triazole, hydroxy-anastrozole, and anastrozole glucuronide. Side effects include those expected of depleted oestrogen levels, including hot flushes, vaginal dryness, thinning hair, and reduced bone mineral density, as well as headache, arthralgias, and peripheral oedema. Despite its mechanism of action, it does not appear to significantly inhibit the metabolism of other drugs by cytochrome P450 in the liver. **Letrozole** is the other non-steroidal reversible antagonist, and it has a triazole ring like anastrozole. It has similar efficacy and side effects to anastrozole and is given orally. Letrozole is metabolized by cytochrome P450 in the liver to an inactive carbinol metabolite, but also lacks significant interactions.

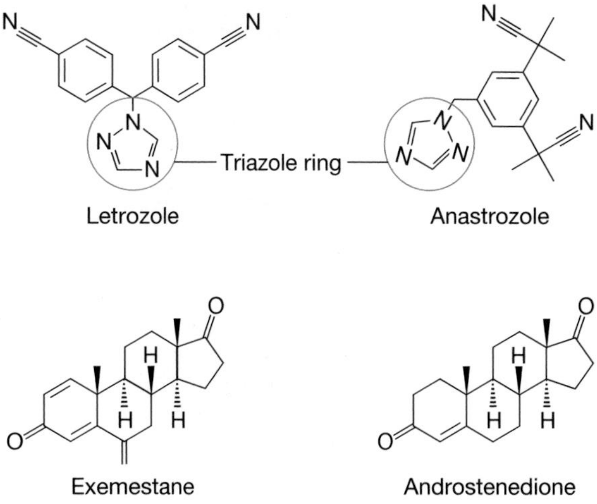

Exemestane is an aromatase inhibitor but, unlike anastrozole and letrazole, is structurally related to androstenedione (a precursor to testosterone) and is an irreversible inhibitor (Figure 22.13). It acts as a substrate for aromatase and is converted to an intermediate that binds covalently to the enzyme. This complex then leads to degradation of the enzyme and therefore is sometimes referred to as a 'suicide substrate'. It is given orally in the treatment of breast cancer in post-menopausal women. It has a similar side effect profile to the non-steroidal agents

Figure 22.13 Structures of the key aromatase inhibitors and androstenedione.

and is metabolized in the liver to inactive metabolites, predominantly 17-hydroxyexemestane.

A range of drugs are also used to inhibit the production of male sex hormones, in particular testosterone. The release of testosterone is modulated through the luteinizing hormone (LH) and follicle-stimulating hormone (FSH) from the pituitary, which are in turn regulated by gonadotropin-releasing hormone (GnRH, also called luteinizing hormone-releasing hormone) from the hypothalamus (Figure 22.14). GnRH is a neuropeptide released from the hypothalamus into the hypophysial portal blood vessels, which feed directly to the pituitary. When it reaches the pituitary it interacts with a GnRH receptor, which is a G-protein coupled receptor on gonadotrope cells. This stimulates the gonadotope cells to synthesize and release FSH and LH. While it may seem somewhat counterintuitive, we use GnRH analogues (not antagonists) to reduce testosterone levels in prostate cancer. The reason is that when given intermittently GnRH leads to an increase in testosterone production. However, if the GnRH receptors are continuously stimulated it causes the receptors to internalize, and there is a down-regulation of the action of GnRH activity. Thus, when GnRH analogues are used continuously you get an initial increase in testosterone production (called a 'flare') and then 10 days or so later production is suppressed due to a chemical-induced hypogonadism (i.e. a lack of function in the testes). To combat the flare, androgen antagonists (e.g. biclutamide, see above) are often given

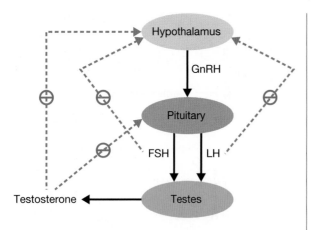

Figure 22.14 Normal control and release of testosterone. GnRH, gonadotropin-releasing hormone; FSH, follicle stimulating hormone; LH, leuteinizing hormone; - - ⊖ - - - indicates negative feedback inhibiting release of hormones.

with GnRH initially. The GnRH agonists used in cancer chemotherapy include **goserelin**, **leuprorelin**, **triptortelin**, and **buserelin**. Goserelin is also used in oestrogen-positive breast cancer to have the same effects on oestrogen production.

> Our patient, Ngozi, received goserelin because her breast cancer was oestrogen positive.

Goserelin was one of the first of this class to be discovered. It is a synthetic analogue of GnRH that has alteration of the amino acids in the sixth and tenth positions of the structure. These alterations make it bind more strongly to GnRH receptors, resulting in a sustained action compared to endogenous GnRH. Goserlin is given as subcutaneous implant, allowing it be given every 4 to 12 weeks. The side effects are similar to the androgen antagonists and resemble the symptoms of the menopause (e.g. hot flushes and sexual dysfunction). Leuprorelin, triptorelein, and buserelin have similar structures, mode of action, and side effects as goserelin. All except buserelin, which is given by nasal spray, are used as sustained-release depot injections every 4 to 12 weeks depending on the formulation.

Retinoids

Bexarotene is closely related to vitamin A (a retinoid) and activates retinoid X receptors (RXR). The RXRs are located in organs such as the liver and kidney, and exist in three forms (α, β, and γ). They are nuclear receptors that work by binding (dimerizing) to other nuclear receptors (e.g. thyroid receptors and peroxisome proliferator-activated receptor). When activated they cause a corepressor (a protein that suppresses gene expression) to dissociate and recruit a coactivator (a protein the increases gene transcription), which in turn promotes protein synthesis. Bexarotene is thought to activate the transcription of genes that influence cellular growth and differentiation. It has been shown to inhibit the growth of cancers of hematopoietic and squamous cell origin, and is used as a second-line agent, orally and topically, in the treatment of cutaneous T-cell lymphoma refractory to other treatments.

Interferons

Interferons are cell-signalling proteins involved in the immune system. There are two main types:

- type I attaches to interferon α receptors (e.g. interferon α and interferon β)
- type II attaches to interferon γ receptors (e.g. interferon γ).

The interferons have potent effects on cellular proliferation and work through what is called the JAK/ STAT signalling pathway (JAK = Janus kinase; STAT = signal transducers and activators of transcription). This involves phosphorylation of the interferon receptor, recruitment of the STAT, phosphorylation of the STAT, and homodimers (two connected molecules) of phosphorylated STAT entering the nucleus. Once in the nucleus, the STAT dimers bind to DNA and induce the transcription of genes. Interferon's effects in cancer cells is thought to be through a number of mechanisms, including inhibition of cellular growth and differentiation, induction of apoptosis by up-regulation of genes such as p53 and activation of capsases, and the recruitment of immune cells.

In cancer chemotherapy it is interferon α that is used. The marketed interferons used are α 2a and α 2b. They differ in the amino acid sequence, but no clinically significant difference has been found. Both are given by subcutaneous injection for a range of leukaemias and solid tumours. The side effects include flu-like symptoms, nausea, thyroid dysfunction, elevation of liver enzymes, and depression.

22.3.2 Chemotherapy targeted at the tumour RNA

The platinum compounds and fluoropyrimidines (e.g. cytarabine) affect RNA synthesis, but their main action is interfering with DNA synthesis. Dactinomycin (also called actinomycin D) is a cytotoxic antibiotic derived from *Streptomyces* spp. The main feature of dactinomycin is a central phenoxazone ring, which acts as a chromophore (gives the drug a red colour). Attached to this are two identical sets of cyclic polypeptides that include D-valine, L-threonine, and L-proline. The cross-linking between actinomycin and guanosine occurs as hydrogen bonds between the 2-amino group of each guanosine and the carbonyl oxygen of L-threonine on the actinomycin. At low doses it binds DNA at the transcription initiation complex and inhibits RNA polymerase, preventing chain elongation. However, at high doses it also stops DNA synthesis. Dactinomycin is given by intravenous injection, mainly to treat paediatric tumours (e.g. Wilms' tumour and Ewing's sarcoma). The main side effect is bone marrow depression, mainly affecting white cells and platelets.

New therapies in development are antisense oligonucleotides. Messenger RNA comprises a single chain of oligonucleotides. Production of proteins involves the binding of transfer RNA (tRNA) that has an antisense codon (a sequence of three oligonucleotides complementary to the mRNA). These new antisense oligonucleotides work by having a complementary chain of oligonucleotides that block the mRNA (for more details about mRNA see Box 21.1, Chapter 21). One such current therapy being investigated targets transforming growth factor-beta2 (TGF-β2), which is a potent promoter of tumour growth.

22.3.3 Chemotherapy targeted at the tumour proteins

This group of drugs can be further subdivided into those that target tumour membrane receptors (e.g. monoclonal antibodies against the protein CD20 and gefitinib) and those that work in the cytoplasm (e.g. imatinib and the vinca alkaloids). The drugs targeting the tumour membrane receptors are broadly divided into monoclonal antibodies and tyrosine kinase inhibitors, while those that work in the cytoplasm can be characterized as either tyrosine kinase inhibitors or tubulin inhibitors.

Table 22.5 Monoclonal antibodies used against tumour cells

Monoclonal antibody	Target
Rituxumab	CD20
Alemtuzumab	CD52
Cetuximab Penitumumab	EGFR (HER1)
Trastuzumab	HER2

CD20, cluster of differentiation 20; CD52, cluster of differentiation 52; EGFR, epidermal growth factor receptor; HER1, human epidermal growth factor receptor 1; HER2, human epidermal growth factor receptor 2.

Drugs targeting tumour membrane receptors: monoclonal antibodies

The monoclonal antibodies used against tumour membranes are summarized in Table 22.5.

Rituximab The first monoclonal antibodies developed for cancer therapy targeted lymphoid antigens (CD20 and CD52). CD20, which stands for cluster of differentiation 20 or cluster of designation 20, is a one of over 300 proteins that are expressed on the surface of leukocyte cells. It is a transmembrane protein that acts as a cation channel, probably transporting calcium, and is involved in cell activation and growth of B-lymphocytes. It is only found on pre-B-lymphocytes and mature lymphocytes, and is not found on stem cells, plasma cells, or other normal tissue. **Rituximab** is a chimeric (a fusion of human-derived and mouse-[murine]derived proteins) monoclonal antibody. When rituximab binds it produces a series of events that lead to cell death. First, it activates intracellular signalling (Box 22.2) through protein tyrosine kinases, which ultimately leads to the arrest of cellular cell division and possibly apoptosis. Another mechanism is through the activation of capsases, leading to apoptosis. The third mechanism that has been proposed involves complement activation. Attachment of rituximab results in activation of the complement cascade by the Fc portions on the rituximab binding with C1, finally resulting in the formation of a membrane attack complex. This causes lysis of the cell and is called complement-dependent cytotoxicity (CDC). The final proposed mechanism of action is through antibody dependent cellular cytotoxicity (ADCC). This involves activation of effector cells such as natural killer (NK) cells, monocytes, and eosinophils.

Rituximab is given by intravenous infusion for non-Hodgkin's lymphoma. It causes total depletion of both healthy and malignant B-cells, followed by regeneration of new, healthy B-cells over 6 months. Infusion-related reactions are common and include nausea, fever, chills, and rigors. A more severe form, associated with dyspnoea and hypoxia, called tumour lysis syndrome, can also occur 12–24 hours after the infusion. This is due to the rapid and large breakdown of cells, resulting in hyperkalaemia, hyperuricaemia, hyperphosphataemia, and hypocalcaemia. Premedication with antihistamines and paracetamol can be used to reduce the infusion-related reactions.

Alemtuzumab is similar to rituximab, but attaches to CD52 instead of CD20. The exact role of CD52 is still to be determined, but like CD20 it may be associated with cellular signalling, as well as cell adhesion. The exact mechanism of action of alemtuzumab is also being determined, but it is thought to induce tumour cytotoxicity through ADCC and CDC like rituximab. It is used for chronic lymphocytic leukaemia and is given intravenously. Like rituximab alemtuzumab is associated with infusion-reactions, and causes profound lymphopenia (extremely low lymphocytes) lasting up to 12 months.

Cetuximab and **panitumumab** are monoclonal antibodies that target epidermal growth factor receptor (EGFR). The EGFR, also known as human epidermal growth factor receptor 1 (HER1), is a membrane-based receptor involved in cellular growth. Activation of the EGFR results in intracellular signalling, resulting in cell differentiation and growth, and increased cell survival (Figure 22.15).

EGFR is one of four HERs (HER1, HER2, HER3, and HER4). The first step in the signal transduction by EGFR is the formation of homodimers (e.g. HER1-HER1) or hetrodimers (e.g. HER1-HER2) following activation by a ligand (e.g. epidermal growth factor, transforming growth factor alpha). This leads to activation of tyrosine kinase, resulting in auto-phosphorylation of the receptor on multiple tyrosine molecules. Adaptor proteins, such as growth factor receptor-bound protein 2 (Grb2), are then recruited. These starts a series of reactions leading to cell proliferation (e.g. through the Ras/MAPK pathway) and/or cell survival through anti-apoptosis signals (e.g. through the PI3K/Akt pathway).

Both cetuximab and panitumumab bind to the extracellular domain of the EGFR and prevent its activation. They may also work through ADCC, as rituximab does. Both are given intravenously and used for metastatic colon cancer expressing EGFR. Cetuximab is also used for advanced squamous cell cancer of the head and neck. Both can cause infusion-related reactions, similar to rituximab, which occur more often with cetuximab. Skin reactions occur in about 90% of patients, appearing as a papulopustular rash within the first few weeks of treatment.

Trastuzumab is a humanized monoclonal antibody targeted at another of the epidermal growth factor receptor family, HER2 (also called HER2/neu). The HER2, like HER1, is a membrane-bound receptor and is over-expressed in 20–30% of breast cancers. It is a tyrosine kinase receptor involved with cell signalling, with a similar pathway as outlined in Figure 22.15. Like HER1 it starts by forming homodimers or heterodimers. However, unlike HER1, it can adopt a conformation that resembles a ligand-activated state without the need for a ligand to attach. It can therefore produce homodimers in the absence of a ligand. Trastuzumab acts through several pathways. First, it attaches to HER2 and prevents it from dimerizing. Second, it activates effector cells such as natural killer (NK) cells and monocytes, leading to ADCC. Third, it causes down-regulation of the HER2 by promoting endocytosis of the receptor and degradation. Finally, HER2 has the capacity to 'shed' the external portion of the receptor, leaving the membrane-bound fraction intact to continue cell signalling. Trastuzumab prevents 'shedding' by inhibiting metaloproteinases that are involved in the cleavage of the external portion.

Trastuzumab is given by intravenous infusion for the treatment of local or metastatic HER2-positive breast cancer. Like the other monoclonal antibodies, it is associated with infusion-related reactions. It also produces cardiotoxicity and must be used with caution in patients with existing cardiac disease, particularly heart failure.

> Ngozi received trastuzumab as her breast cancer was found to be HER2 positive, as well as oestrogen positive. This is an unusual finding and the two receptors are often inversely related.

Drugs targeting tumour membrane receptors: tyrosine kinase inhibitors

Lapatinib, **gefitinib** and **erlotinib** are tyrosine kinase inhibitors and act on HER1 (lapatinib also inhibits HER2).

Box 22.2
Action of rituximab

Figure b

1. Binding of rituximab, particularly cross-linking of CD20, leads to activation of protein tyrosine kinases, which leads to activation of phospholipase C gamma (PLCγ). This further activates mitogen-activated protein kinase (MAPK). The PLCγ also cleaves phosphatidylinositol trisphosphate (PIP$_3$), which increases intracellular calcium. This leads to apoptosis.

2. The binding of rituximab causes inhibition if interferon 10. This then inhibits BCL-2, an anti-apoptotic gene. The result is activation of capases 9 and capsase 3, which induces apoptosis.

3. The Fc regions of two riuximab antibodies bind to and activate the complement system starting at C1. This then activates C$_2$ and C$_4$. The C$_1$, C$_2$, C$_4$ complex (called C3 convertase) activates C$_3$, causing it to split and leave a fraction on the cell membrane surface (C$_{3b}$). This activates C$_5$. The final step is the association of C$_{5b}$, C$_6$, C$_7$, C$_8$, and C$_9$ to produce a membrane attack complex (MAC). The MAC produces a 'pore' in the membrane, leading to lysis.

4. Receptors on natural killer (NK) cells interact with the bound rutiximab and results in the release of interferon gamma, granzymes (serine proteases). The granzymes cleave and activate capsases, leading to apoptosis. One granzyme released, perforin, attacks the cell wall, leading to lysis.

5. Monocytes are also activated by binding to the rutiximab-CD20 complex. This causes phagocytosis.

Fc region, fragment crystallizable region; PLCγ, phospholipase C gamma; IL-10, interleukin 10; INFγ, interferon gamma; NK, natural killer.

Adapted from: Smith, MR Rituximab (monoclonal anti-CD20 antibody): mechanism of action and resistance. *Oncogene* 2003; 22: 7359–68.

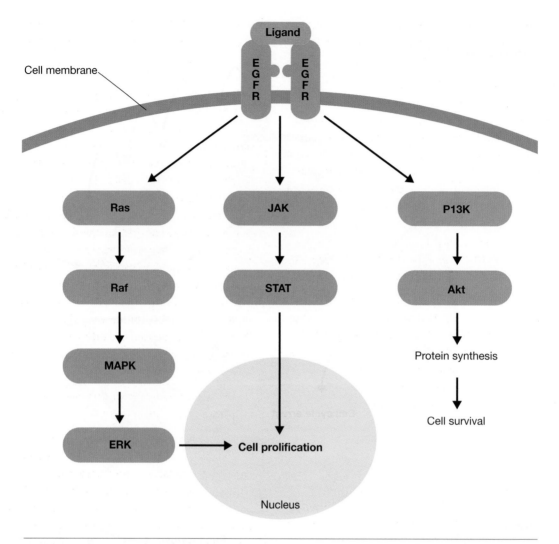

Figure 22.15 Cell signalling pathways promoted by EGFR. EGFR, epidermal growth factor receptor; Ras, rat sarcoma enzyme, a GTP binding protein; Raf, serine/thronine kinase; MAPK, mitogen-activated protein kinase; ERK, extracellular signal-regulated kinases; JAK, Janus kinases; STAT, signal transducers and activators of transcription; PI3K, phosphoinositide 3-kinase; Akt, Akt protein kinases (also called protein kinases B).

They all bind to the adenosine triphosphate (ATP) binding site on the HER, preventing the auto-phosphorylation of the dimers and hence the activation of their signalling pathways (see Figure 22.15). Gefitanib and erlotinib are used in the treatment of non-small-cell lung cancer and erlotinib in pancreatic cancer. Lapatinib is used for HER2 positive breast cancer. All are given orally and the common side effects are gastrointestinal. Erlotinib and gefitanib have been associated with interstitial lung disease and patients should be encouraged to report any breathing difficulties. An acne-like rash is reported to occur with erlotinib, and lapatinib can cause cardiotoxicity and hepatotoxicity.

Drugs targeting tumour intracellular pathways: tyrosine kinase inhibitors

Similar to the tyrosine kinase inhibitors that target membrane receptors, a number have been developed that target intracellular tyrosine kinases. These include **imatinib**, **dasatinib**, and **nilotinib**, and they bind to the ATP pocket on tyrosine kinase. The main target for these drugs is ABL–BCR fusion protein, which is formed through the Philadelphia chromosome. The Philadelphia chromosome is chromosomal defect where parts of two chromosomes (9 and 22) are translocated (swap places). Nearly all cases of chronic myeloid leukaemia (CML), approximately 30% of adult acute lymphoblastic leukaemia (ALL), about 5% of childhood ALL, and 2% of acute myeloid leukaemia (AML) are associated with the Philadelphia chromosome (called Ph positive).

The translocation results in a fusion between the breakpoint cluster region (BCR) gene and the Ableson (ABL) gene, resulting in the production of the ABL–BCR fusion protein. The ABL–BCR fusion protein is a constantly active tyrosine kinase that can bind effector proteins such as Grb2, leading to the promotion of cell differentiation and growth. This group of drugs also targets other tyrosine kinases, including c-KIT (a cell surface receptor expressed on blood cells) and platelet-derived growth factor receptor (PDGFR, a membrane-bound receptor). Both of these receptors, once activated, produce cell signalling through pathways similar to EGFR (see Figure 22.15).

Dasatinib, imatinib, and nilotinib are administered orally and are mostly used for leukaemias (e.g. CML and ALL). Imatinib is also indicated for stromal tumours of the gastrointestinal tract. The main side effects of concern are myelosuppression, including neutropenia, thrombocytopenia, and anaemia. They also cause gastrointestinal disturbance (nausea and diarrhoea) and liver dysfunction.

Drugs targeting tumour intracellular pathways: other kinase inhibitors

Temsirolimus is a drug that inhibits mammalian target of rapamycin (mTOR), a serine/threonine protein kinase that is involved in cell proliferation and survival. mTOR monitors cellular energy levels and nutrients, and coordinates inputs from sources such as the growth factors. Activation of mTOR leads to increased production of cell cycle proteins such as cyclin D and hypoxia-inducible factor-1a (HIF-1a), and VEGF. Blockage of mTOR leads to cell cycle arrest and inhibition of angiogenesis. It is particularly useful in renal cell carcinomas, as they often have a mutation that reduces the degradation of HIF-1a. Temsirolimus is given intravenously and the major side effects are injection related reactions, usually occurring on the first infusion (premedication with antihistamines recommended). Other adverse effects include hyperglycaemia, hypercholesterolaemia, hypertriglyceridaemia, and bone marrow suppression.

Drugs targeting tumour intracellular pathways – tubulin inhibitors

Tubulin is a globular protein that is the building block for the microtubules inside cells. The tubulin exists in two subunits, α-tubulin and β-tubulin. To produce microtubules the tubulin arranges in dimers, which then bind with guanosine triphosphate (GTP). The dimers are then assembled into the microtubules and the GTP is hydrolyzed to guanosine triphosphate. Microtubules start to be formed during G_2 phase and are essential for cell division (M phase). The M phase is divided into four main subphases. The first is prophase, where the two centromes form on either side of the cell and coordinate the production of the microtubules. The next phase is prometaphase, during which the microtubules from the centromes span across the cell and enter the nucleus. During this time some of the microtubules attach to the chromosomes through a protein called a kinetochore. Prometaphase is followed by metaphase, in which the duplicated chromosomes, attached to the kinetochore microtubules, align in the middle of the cell. This is followed by anaphase, during which the kinetochore microtubules shorten and 'pull' the chromosomes apart to each end of the cell. Once this is finished, the cell splits to form two new daughter cells.

The two main classes of drugs are targeted at tubulin are the vinca alkaloids and taxanes.

Vinca alkaloids The vinca alkaloids are among the oldest of the anticancer treatments. They were originally found in the Madagascar periwinkle plant (*Catharanthus roseus*), but are now synthetically produced. The common vinca alkaloids used as chemotherapy are **vincristine**, **vinblastine**, **vindesine**, and **vinorelbine**. They work by binding to tubulin and preventing its polymerization into the microtubules. This stops mitosis and arrests the cell in the M phase. They are used intravenously for a range of haematological and solid tumours, including leukaemia, sarcoma, and lung and breast cancer. The main side effect is myelosuppression with vinblastine, vindesine, and vinorelbine, while vincristine produces neurotoxicity, including peripheral and autonomic neuropathy. Extravasation of the vinca alkaloids leads to potential necrosis and patients must be monitored for signs such as pain at the injection site.

Taxanes Like the vinca alkaloids, the taxanes were originally discovered in extracts from plants. The first taxane, **paclitaxel** is derived from the bark of the Pacific yew tree (*Taxus brevifolia*). The other taxane, **docetaxel**, is a semi-synthetic derivative of paclitaxel. The taxanes work by binding to the β subunit of tubulin and stabilizing the microtubules. This prevents them from shortening (depolymerizing) or lengthening (polymerizing), stopping them from functioning inside the cell. The inability to depolymerize the microtubules leaves fragments in the cytoplasm that act as a trigger for apoptosis. Another trigger for apoptosis may come from taxanes binding to Bcl-2 (B-cell lymphoma 2), which is anti-apoptotic by suppressing the activation of capsases through inhibiting the release of cytochrome C from mitochondria. Both are given by intravenous injection and used to treat ovarian, breast, and non-small-cell lung cancer. Hypersensitivity reactions are common with both paclitaxel and docetaxel, and pre-medication with corticosteroids is recommended. The other side effects include peripheral neuropathies, cardiac arrhythmias, and myelosuppression. Docetaxel can also cause fluid retention.

22.3.4 Chemotherapy targeted at endothelium

As noted at the beginning of this chapter, an important feature of some solid tumours is angiogenesis, or the proliferation of blood vessels, to help maintain the growing tumour mass. A potent promoter of angiogenesis is vascular endothelial growth factor (VEGF). There are several subtypes of VEGF, of which VEGF-A is the most important, as it can attach to all three types of VEGF receptor. The VEGFRs are membrane-bound tyrosine kinase receptors that behave very similarly to the human epidermal growth factor receptors (HERs, see Figure 22.15). VEGFR1 (also called FLT1) and VEGFR2 (also called KDR or FLK1) are located on endothelial cells and are responsible for the promotion of angiogenesis. Suppression of angiogenesis has two effects on tumours. First, it 'starves' the tumour of nutrients and oxygen. Second, it reduces the ability of cancer cells to enter the bloodstream and metastasize.

Just like the treatments targeted against HER, the two main classes of drugs used to inhibit angiogenesis are either monoclonal antibodies or tyrosine kinase antagonists. **Thalidomide**, and its analogue lenolidamide, also has an effect on angiogenesis.

Monoclonal antibodies against VEGF

Bevacizumab is a recombinant humanized monoclonal antibody that attaches to VEGF (note it binds the ligand, not the receptor as the HER monoclonal antibodies do). It is given intravenously for the treatment of breast,

colorectal, renal, and small-cell lung cancer. Bevacizumab has some unusual side effects, including hypertension, thromboembolic disorders (e.g. myocardial infarction), and gastrointestinal perforation and obstruction.

Tyrosine kinase inhibitors against VEGFRs

Two tyrosine kinase inhibitors, **sorafenib** and **sunitinib**, target the VEGFRs. Sunitinib inhibits all three VEGFRs, while sorafenib inhibits VEGFR-2 and VEGFR-3, and serine/threonine kinases (see Figure 22.15). In addition, they both inhibit other cellular signalling receptors, including platelet-derived growth factor receptor (PDGFR) and stem cell factor receptor (c-Kit). They are used for renal cell carcinoma and gastrointestinal stromal tumours, and are administered orally. Sorafenib and sunitinib can cause what is called 'hand-foot' syndrome, where patients develop impairment in their sense of touch (dysaesthesia), which can progress to swelling, pain, erythema, and shedding of the outer skin (desquamation). They have both been associated with hypertension, and sunitinib with cardiac toxicity.

Thalidomide and lenolidamide

Thalidomide was first developed in the 1940s and promoted in the 1950s and 1960s as a safe and effective tranquillizer. It was also found to be an antiemetic and was used in pregnant women for morning sickness. Unfortunately, it turned out that thalidomide was teratogenic and it resulted in over 10,000 babies being born with deformities. The particular type of deformity is called phocomelia and presents as short or absent long bones in the legs and arms, and 'flipper-like' hands and feet. This deformity is thought to be caused by the effect thalidomide has on the blood vessels of the developing foetus. These effects are now used as anti-angiogenesis treatment in cancer.

Thalidomide, and its analogue **lenalidomide**, are potent immunomodulators. One of the most important effects is on tumour necrosis factor alpha (TNF-α). This pro-inflammatory cytokine plays an important role in host defences against microorganisms. Thalidomide has been shown to degrade the mRNA responsible for producing TNF-α, and hence reduce its activity. Although TNF-α is a potent inducer of angiogenesis, the effects on TNF-α are not thought to mediate thalidomide's anti-angiogenic action. Thalidomide reduces expression of VEGF and basic fibroblast growth factor (bFGF), which promote angiogenesis. It also suppresses interleukin-6 (IL-6), a factor that promotes cellular growth and survival in multiple myeloma. Thalidomide also has direct cytotoxic effects by increasing apoptosis through activating capsase 8, and down-regulating nuclear factor κB (NF-κB), which affects anti-apoptotic genes, especially those relating to the suppression of capsases. Other mechanisms related to its effects in multiple myeloma include modulation of the expression of surface adhesion molecules such as inter-cellular adhesion molecule 1 (ICAM-1) and vascular cell adhesion molecule-1 (VCAM-1), recruitment and activation of immune cells such as NK cells, increased production of interleukin-2 and interferon γ, and inhibition of the cycloxygenase 1 and 2 enzymes.

Thalidomide is non-enzymatically hydrolyzed in the plasma to several active metabolites. It may also undergo hepatic metabolism, and it is thought that it is metabolites, and not thalidomide, that have anti-tumour action. Lenalidomide does not require conversion and is up to 50,000 times more potent than thalidomide at inhibiting TNF-α *in vitro*. Both are given orally in the treatment of multiple myeloma. Thalidomide can cause drowsiness (hence given at bedtime) and peripheral neuropathy. Lenalidomide can cause thromboembolism and severe neutropenia.

Investigational drugs targeted at the endothelium and extracellular matrix

Combretastatins are a family of naturally occurring molecules with anti-angiogenesis properties that have been isolated from the bark of the African bush willow tree (*Combretum caffrum*). They have structural similarity to colchicine, a drug that affects the mitotic spindle, and one of the family (combretastatin A-4) has been investigated as a chemotherapy agent. Combretastatin A-4 binds to tubulin and prevents polymerization of the microtubules. Apart from their role in mitosis, microtubules are important for the internal organization and structure of the cell. When rapidly growing vascular endothelial cells are exposed to combretastatin it causes them to loose shape, resulting in vascular shut-down and increased vascular permeability.

Prinomastat (AG3340) is an inhibitor of matrix metalloproteinases (MMP), specifically MMP-2, -9, -13,

and -14. MMPs are zinc-dependent proteolytic enzymes involved with cleaving cell-surface receptors and activating/inactivating cytokines and chemokines. They play a role in tissue remodelling and are involved with angiogenesis and metastasis. Other MMP inhibitors include **marimastat** and **neovastat**.

22.3.5 Miscellaneous cancer chemotherapies

L-asparaginase

Asparagine is a non-essential amino acid used in protein synthesis. L-asparaginase is an enzyme that catalyses the conversion of asparagine to aspartic acid. In ALL the tumour cells are unable to synthesize asparagine and need to obtain it from the circulation. L-asparaginase depletes the asparagine, thus depriving the ALL cells of this amino acid. It is derived from several sources, but the most common source is from *Escherichia coli* (known as colaspase) or a closely related bacteria, *Erwinia chrysanthemi* (known as crisantaspase). Both are given by injection for ALL. The main side effects are allergic reactions, including possible anaphylaxis. Liver damage and clotting disorders are also possible.

Tretinoin

Tretinoin, also known as all-trans retinoic acid (ATRA), is used in the treatment of acute promyelocytic leukaemia (APML). It is also used in the treatment of severe acne (see Chapter 8). In APL there is translocation of chromosome 15 and 17, causing a fusion between the retinoic acid receptor alpha (RARα) gene and the promyelocytic leukemia gene (PML). The PML- RARα fusion causes arrest of maturation of leukocytes, resulting in the proliferation of immature cells. Tretinoin, which is structurally related to vitamin A, acts on the gene to promote the cells from immature into mature blood cells. It is given orally, as it is in acne, and the side effects are the same as seen when it is used for acne (e.g. dry skin and mucous membranes). However, there is also a more severe reaction seen only when it is used in APML, called retinoic acid syndrome. It occurs several days after starting treatment and presents as fever, dyspnoea, and respiratory distress. It can be life threatening and needs to be treated with corticosteroids.

22.4 Resistance to cancer chemotherapy

Just like microorganisms, cancer cells also develop ways of avoiding the effects of chemotherapy treatment. Broadly, resistance can be inherent (or innate) or acquired. Acquired resistance can develop due to adaptation from constant exposure to chemotherapy or more often by mutation given the unstable and erratic nature of cancer cells. The mechanisms of resistance can be classified as pharmacokinetic (e.g. related to the drug getting into or staying in the cells) or pharmacodynamic (e.g. modification of the drug's action once at its target).

> Out patient, Ngozi, was unfortunately found to develop resistance to her first chemotherapy regimen (anthracycline + cyclophosphamide + tamoxifen). She was then switched to trastuzmab + paclitaxel.

22.4.1 Pharmacokinetic resistance

Distribution of the drug within the tumour

Despite the potential for increased vascularization due angiogenesis, it is sometimes difficult for chemotherapy agents to reach their target tissue. A major barrier is changes in fluid dynamics in the interstitium (the space between cells). In tumour cells the interstitial fluid pressure gradient favours distribution to the peripheries and resists penetration of the chemotherapy into the tumour mass.

Drug efflux pumps

Just like with bacteria, some cancer cells have developed membrane transporters that push drug out of the cell. An example of this occurs with cisplatin. Some cells contain a plasma glycoprotein P-gp ('permeability glycoprotein') that can transport chemically unrelated compounds out of the cell. This leads to what is called 'multidrug resistance'.

Inactivation or metabolism

Some drugs can be metabolized within the cell. It has been observed that some cancer cells can express cytochrome P450 enzymes, which can metabolize chemotherapies. An example of this occurs with docetaxel. Platinum compounds have also been shown to be readily conjugated within some cancer cells. Another example is irinotecan, which requires conversion within the cell by human carboxy esterases. Resistance has been shown in cells with low carboxy esterase activity.

22.4.2 Pharmacodynamic resistance

Mutation of the p53 gene

The p53 gene is important in arresting cell division to allow repair to occur or if cellular insults are sufficient to initiate the process of apoptosis. If this gene becomes mutated a cell may loose p53 function. In this case cytotoxic agents that rely on this gene to initiate apoptosis after they cause intracellular damage may be ineffective. This is one of the possible sources of resistance to cisplatin-based chemotherapy.

Sensitivity to apoptosis

Some tumour cells over-express proteins that suppress apoptosis. Examples include the B-cell lymphoma 2 (Bcl-2) protein family, which suppress the activation of capsases by inhibiting the release of cytochrome C from mitochondria. Again, cisplatin resistance may be mediated, in part, by this mechanism.

Improved repair of DNA

The ability of a cell to repair DNA can influence the effectiveness of some chemotherapy agents. Cells that over-express proteins such as excision repair cross-complementing protein (ERCC1) have been shown to be resistant. This resistance mechanism is particularly important for the alkylating agents.

Changes to drug binding sites

Drug resistance can occur if the binding site of the chemotherapy is altered. This is a potential source of resistance to the topoisomerase inhibitors (e.g. irinotecan), due to mutations in topoisomerase I/II.

Adverse environment inside tumour cells

Rapidly dividing cells have a lower (more acidic) intracellular pH. As a consequence they often increase the expression of proton (H^+) pumps to maintain a healthy intracellular pH. The area surrounding the tumour will therefore tend to be slightly acidic. This means that weakly basic drugs (e.g. doxorubicin) would become ionized and therefore be less able to penetrate the cell membrane and enter the cancer cells. Another feature of tumour cells is hypoxia due to the high demands produced by rapidly dividing cells. This is important in producing resistance to bleomycin, which requires oxygen to induce strand breaks in DNA. Hypoxia also causes cells to try and survive by invoking survival responses that include increased expression of the multi-drug efflux pumps.

22.5 Combination chemotherapy regimens

It is rare today to see only a single agent used to treat a cancer. This is due largely to concerns about possible resistance to therapy. When choosing chemotherapies a number of questions are considered. These include:

- Do the drugs have different mechanisms of action? It is not logical to combine two drugs that target the exact same part of the cancer cell.
- Do the toxicities overlap? This is likely to increase the side effects and therefore limit the amount of either drug that can be given.

- Does the patient have the particular targets for the chemotherapy? For example it is may not be useful to include a HER2 blocker in a patient with breast cancer that is not HER2 positive.

Clearly, combinations are chosen largely on the evidence of effectiveness from clinical trials. However, there is still a significant amount of 'art' in combining chemotherapy regimens.

SUMMARY OF COMMON DRUGS USED FOR CANCER

Therapeutic class	Drug	Mechanism of action	Common clinical uses	Comments	Examples of adverse drug reactions
Alkylating agents	Busulfan Carmustine Chlorambucil Cyclophosphamide Estramustine Ifosfamide Lomustine Melphalan Tiotepa Treosulfan	Damage DNA by forming covalent bonds across the strands of DNA This is achieved through the formation of an unstable molecule called a carbonium ion, a carbon atom with a net positive charge. This carbonium ion then binds to the 7-nitrogen on the guanine molecule in DNA	Leukaemia Lymphomas Soft tissue sarcoma Solid tumours Myeloma Adenocarcinoma Breast cancer	Variable properties Chlorambucil, busulfan, lomustine, estramustine, and treosulfan are taken orally Thiotepa is administered into the bladder. The rest are generally administered intravenously A metabolite of cyclophosphamide called acrolein can cause haemorrhagic cystisis. This is prevented by administering mesna and hydration Cyclophosphamide is metabolized by hepatic enzymes CYP2B6 and CYP3A4, leading to interactions	Infertility Bone marrow suppresion Acute non-lymphocytic leukaemia Pneumonitis pulmonary fibrosis Stephen–Johnson's syndrome
Anthracyclines and other cytotoxic antibiotics	Bleomycin Dactinomycin Daunorubicin Doxorubicin Epirubicin Idarubicin Mitomycin mitoxantrone	1) The planar ring structure intercalates between DNA strands, causing structural distortion of the DNA stopping both DNA and RNA synthesis 2) Inhibit topoisomerase, the enzyme required for DNA replication	Leukaemia Lymphomas Squamous cell carcinoma Breast cancer	Daunorubicin and doxorubicin were the first drugs derived from bacteria streptomyces. Dactinomycin used for paediatric cancers Doxorubicin, eprirubicin and mitoxantrone in high cumulative doses can result in cardiomyopathy Liposomal formulations of doxorubicin are available to reduce cardiotoxicity Idarubicin is given by mouth and the rest intravenously	Bone marrow suppression Mucositis Nausea and vomiting Respiratory failure (bleomycin) Cardiomyopathy Hand foot syndrome (doxorubicin)

Therapeutic class	Drug	Mechanism of action	Common clinical uses	Comments	Examples of adverse drug reactions
Antimetabolites	Capecitabine Cladribine Clofarabine Cytarabine Fludarabine Fluorouracil Gemcitabine Mercaptopurine Methotrexate Nelarabine Pemetrexed Raltitrexed Tegafur with uracil Tioguanine	They act as 'false' versions of DNA and RNA building blocks and stop the synthesis of DNA/RNA precursors	Leukaemia Lymphomas Colorectal cancer Solid tumour Mesothelioma Non-small cell lung cancer	This class can be further subdivided in folate antagonists, purine analogues, and pyrimidine analogues Liposomal preparation of cytarabine is used intrathecal	Nausea Diarrhoea Bone marrow suppression
Platinum compounds	Carboplatin Cisplatin Oxaliplatin	Aquate DNA of molecules, during which water replaces a ligand In the case of cisplatin, the leaving group is chloride, for carboplatin it is dicarboxycyclobutane, and for oxaliplatin it is oxalate This results in a reactive intermediate that binds to the bases of DNA, in particular the 7-nitrogens of adenine and guanine The cross-linking causes bending of the DNA and denaturing, leading to apoptosis	Ovarian , head and neck cancer, testicular cancer, bladder cancer, lung and brain tumours, colorectal cancer	The platinum compounds are all given intravenously Cisplatin has the greatest toxicity of the platinum compounds and cannot be used in patients with impaired renal function Cisplatin and oxaliplatin are extensively bound to protein in the body, unlike carboplatin All of the platinum compounds undergo extensive renal elimination	Vomiting Renal toxicity Neuropathy Bone marrow suppression
Podophyllotoxins	Etoposide Teniposide	Bind to topoisomerase II enzymes involved in the relaxation and coiling of DNA	Leukaemia Neuroblastoma	Teniposide is primarily metabolized in the liver, whereas etoposide is both renally cleared unchanged and metabolized, with half-lives of 5 hours and 4–11 hours, respectively	Bone marrow suppression Allergic reactions
Topoisomerase I inhibitors	Irinotecan Topotecan Camptothecin	Stop DNA synthesis by inhibiting topoisomerase I and are specific for the S phase of cell replication	Colorectal cancer Metastatic ovarian cancer	Topotecan is newer and has fewer side effects than irinotecan	Bone marrow suppression Gastrointestinal Asthenia Alopecia Anorexia

Therapeutic class	Drug	Mechanism of action	Common clinical uses	Comments	Examples of adverse drug reactions
Hormone and anti-hormonal agents for breast cancer	Oestrogen receptor antagonists: tamoxifen toremifene fulvestrant Aromatase inhibitors: anastrozole exemestane letrozole	There are several approaches: 1) Hormones inhibit growth of tissues, e.g. oestrogens in prostatic tumours, which produce a negative feedback. resulting in decreased testosterone levels 2) Block the effect of the hormone on the tissue: hormone antagonists, e.g. anti-oestrogens used in hormone-dependent breast cancer 3) Reduce production of hormones, e.g. block aromatase hormone, which converts testosterone to oestradiol or gonadotropin-releasing hormone to reduce testosterone levels in prostate cancer	Breast cancer	Variable properties Breast cancer drugs ideally used in oestrogen receptor positive However, tamoxifen has some activity in receptor negative patients because of other mechanisms such as effects on protein kinase C, insulin-like growth factor 1 (IGF-1), and Ca(2+)-calmodulin-dependent cAMP phosphodiesterase Tamoxifen administered orally and extensively metabolized in the liver by cytochrome P450 into active metabolites, one of which is endoxifen which is 100 times more potent as an inhibitor of oestrogen receptors	Nausea Vomiting Diarrhoea Fatigue Dizziness Fluid retention Hot flushes Menstrual irregularities
Hormone and anti-hormonal agents for prostate cancer	Anti-androgens: cyproterone acetate bicalutamide flutamide nilutamide Gonadorelin analogues: buserelin goserelin leuprorelin triptorelin Others: estramustine		Prostate cancer	Cyproterone acetate is steroidal whilst the others are non-steroidal Estramustine contains a molecule of estrogen (oestradiol) and a molecule of nitrogen mustard (mechlorethamine, also called mustine) It is given orally for advanced prostate cancer and has the side effects of both alkylating agents, and oestrogens	Fluid retention Nausea Diarrhoea Gynecomastia Hot flushes
Other antineoplastic drugs	Dacarbazine	Following conversion in the liver it interacts with DNA to methylate the 6-oxygen and 7-nitrogen on guanine	Melanoma Sarcomas	Dacarbazine was the first agent in this class	

Therapeutic class	Drug	Mechanism of action	Common clinical uses	Comments	Examples of adverse drug reactions
	Bexarotene	Agonist at retinoid X receptor involved in regulation of cell differentiation and proliferation	T-cell lymphoma	Restricted for second-line use	Hyperlipidaemia Hypothyroidism Leucopenia Headache Rash Pruritus
	Hydroxycarbamide hydroxyurea	As an antimetabolites thought to involve interference with synthesis of DNA	Chronic myeloid leukaemia Cervical cancer polycythaemia		Myelosuppression Nausea Skin reactions
	Mitotane	Selectively inhibits activity of adrenal cortex	Adrenocortical carcinoma	Requires corticosteroid replacement	Anorexia Nausea Vomiting Hypogonadism Thyroid disorders
	L-asparaginase	An enzyme that catalyses the conversion of asparagine to aspartic acid, depleting the tumour cells of this amino acid which they are unable to synthesise and need to obtain it from the circulation	Acute lymphoblastic leukaemia	L-asparaginase is derived from several sources, but the most common is *Escherichia coli* Given by injection Test urine for glucose because could cause hyperglycaemia	Nausea Fever Allergic reactions Liver damage Clotting disorders
Monoclonal antibodies	Rituximab Alemtuzumab Cetuximab Trastuzamab Bevacizumab Panitumumab	Monoclonal antibodies against proteins that are expressed on the surface of leukocyte cells	Lymphoma Leukaemia Breast Colorectal Renal Small-cell lung cancer	Rituximab is a monoclonal antibody against CD20 and alemtuzumab against CD 52 Cetuximab and panitumumab are monoclonal antibodies that target epidermal growth factor receptor Trastuzumab is a humanized monoclonal antibody against HER2 Bevacizumab is a recombinant humanized monoclonal antibody that attaches to VEGF ligand It has unusual side effects, including hypertension, thromboembolic disorders (e.g. myocardial infarction), and gastrointestinal perforation and obstruction.	Infusion related (fever, chills, nausea, and vomiting, allergic reactions) Cytokine release syndrome

Therapeutic class	Drug	Mechanism of action	Common clinical uses	Comments	Examples of adverse drug reactions
				All are administered by intravenous infusion. Patients should be given premedication with analgesia and antihistamine before doses to reduce infusion related adverse drug reactions	
Tyrosine kinase inhibitors	Imatinib Dasatinib Nilotinib	Inhibit tyrosine kinase by binding to the ATP pocket on tyrosine kinase	Leukaemia Stromal tumours of the gastrointestinal tract	Given intravenously	Nausea Diarrhoea Liver dysfunction
Other kinase inhibitors	Temsirolimus	Inhibits mammalian target of rapamycin (mTOR), a serine/threonine protein kinase involved in cell proliferation and survival. mTOR monitors cellular energy levels and nutrients, and coordinates inputs from sources such as the growth factors. Activation of mTOR leads to increased production of cell cycle proteins such as cyclin D and hypoxia-inducible factor-1a (HIF-1a), and VEGF. Blockage of mTOR leads to cell cycle arrest and inhibition of angiogenesis	Renal cell carcinomas	Given intravenously. Patients should be given premedication before first dose	Hyperglycaemia Hypercholesterolaemia Hypertriglyceridaemia Bone marrow suppression
Tubulin inhibitors	Taxanes: docetaxel paclitaxel vinca alkaloids vincristine vindesine vinorelbine vinblastine	Inhibit tubulin, a globular protein that is the building block for the microtubules inside cells	Taxanes: ovarian, breast, and non-small cell lung cancer. Vinca alkaloids: leukaemia, sarcoma, lung and breast cancer	Hypersensitivity reactions are common with both paclitaxel and docetaxel, and pre-medication with corticosteroids is recommended	Peripheral neuropathies Cardiac arrhythmias Myelosuppression Neuropathy Extravasation, leading to necrosis

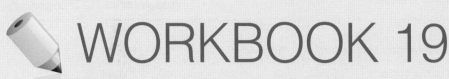

WORKBOOK 19
Cancer chemotherapy

Ngozi: a simplified case history

Today Ngozi is more nervous than usual because she will be told if the second chemotherapy regime has worked. She has given up trying to read her novel and has found her mind wondering back to the events leading to her diagnosis. Ngozi is a fourth-year medical student from Ibadan in Nigeria, and she still finds it incredible that her pharmacology modules in her degree could have saved her life. Ngozi can still vividly recall the particular pharmacology case study that made her decide she really ought to do a breast examination.

Thinking back, Ngozi now realizes that it was possible that her grandmother had died of breast cancer. Although the illness that lead to her death was never fully diagnosed, recalling the history of presenting complaint of her grandmother she wonders if it was metastatic breast cancer. The local doctor found three lumps in her grandmother's breast 3 weeks before she died, following symptoms of gradual weight loss, severe spinal pain, and breathlessness. The doctor said the lumps were just cysts and unrelated to the other symptoms. By the time her parents arrived to take her grandmother to a bigger hospital in town, her Nan was too weak to be moved.

Ngozi is initially unsure of how to carry out the self-examination because the pharmacology case study has no details. Luckily for her, she has internet access at home in Ibadan and so 'Googled' breast examination.

Ngozi was shocked when she actually found a lump on her left breast and possibly in her armpit. Ike, her husband, took her straight to the only oncologist they knew in the city, hoping to be seen on the same day. Unfortunately, the doctor was away on holiday and Ngozi was told to return in 3 weeks' time by the nurse in charge. After 3 weeks of no progress in Ibadan, they decided after much debate that Ngozi should fly to London for diagnosis and treatment. After arriving in London, Ngozi 's friend and former university flatmate, Rachel, who is now a pharmacist, insists on putting her up during her entire stay in the UK.

A table of clinical clerking abbreviations is given on page xi.

MEDICAL NOTES FOR NGOZI AT PRIVATE HOSPITAL

Age: 33 years

PC: Painless lump in the left breast

HPC: Breast lumps found whilst doing a self-examination 8 weeks earlier. Breast appears slightly distorted.

The early signs and symptoms of breast cancer include:

- *painless lump in the breast*
- *possible distortion of the breast*
- *nipple discharge (could be blood stained)*
- *lymphadenopathy (swelling and enlargement of lymph nodes).*

Ngozi's symptoms are indicative of a tumour in her breast. Other tests are required to confirm whether it is malignant or benign.

Sometimes the doctor will ask patients to come back in a couple of weeks for another physical examination of the breast because some breast tissue changes that are non-cancerous could disappear after a period.

PMH: Nil significant

DH: Microgynon 30 from the age of 17

Microgynon is an oral contraceptive containing oestrogen and progesterone.

SH: Married Nigerian medical student who lives in Ibadan. Has a 1-year-old son. BMI = 32 kg/m^2. Had first menstrual cycle at 10 years of age. Has two sisters—no history of breast cancer.

FH: Grandmother possibly had breast cancer

There are many risk factors for breast cancer. Confirmed risk factors include:

- *personal history of breast cancer = negative for Ngozi*
- *family history of breast cancer = possibly positive for Ngozi*
- *early menses (<15 years) and late menopause (>50 years) = positive for Ngozi*
- *late first pregnancy = positive for Ngozi*
- *age (>50 years) = negative for Ngozi.*

Other possible risk factors include:

- *diet high in fatty foods*
- *obesity = positive for Ngozi*
- *long-term use of oral contraceptives = positive for Ngozi*
- *alcohol.*

Ngozi has some of the above risk factors, which make it even more likely that the lump could be cancer.

O/E: Mass in upper quadrant of left breast. Lymphadenopathy in left axilla. No other findings.

After taking a medical history, a physical examination is undertaken at the clinic and the doctor checks for the presence of a lump in her breast, and swelling of the lymph nodes in the axilla (armpit) and supraclavicular area (neck). A lump is found in Ngozi's breast and the lymph nodes of her left armpit are swollen, signifying possible spread.

Diagnostic:

1) Breast ultrasound scan: 2.4 cm mass in upper outer quadrant

2) Needle biopsy: infiltrating ductal carcinoma

> *Initial diagnostic procedures for breast cancer include:*
>
> *1. Mammography*
>
> *This is an X-ray of the breast. It is usually not used in patients who are younger than 35 because their breasts are usually still dense and solid, and it could be difficult to make out a lump.*
>
> *2. Breast ultrasound*
>
> *Ultrasound waves are used to get pictures. This painless procedure takes just a few minutes. More commonly used in young women.*
>
> *3. Biopsy*
>
> *During this procedure, a small sample of cells or tissues of body parts (in this case the breast) are taken and examined under the microscope. The three main types of biopsy used are:*
>
> - *fine needle aspiration*
>
> - *needle biopsy: larger sample than fine needle aspiration*
>
> - *excision biopsy: gives the largest sample, but most invasive.*

A needle biopsy was chosen for Ngozi because it could be performed under local anaesthesia. It confirmed that the cancer was invasive and the mass in her axilla was probably a spread. However, more investigations were required.

Biochemistry and FBC:

Calcium: 2.8 mmol/L (reference 2.25–2.88)

Phosphorous: 1.22mmol/L (reference 0.81–1.45)

Liver function tests: normal

FBC: normal

> *Although diagnosis of solid tumours is usually made by biopsy, blood tests sometimes initially raise suspicion and prompt clinicians to do biopsies. They are also used to detect metastasis (spread). Blood tests are commonly used to diagnose haematological malignancies (e.g. leukaemia).*
>
> - *Examples of blood tests that are sometimes relevant are:*
>
> - *calcium: raised levels could indicate bone metastasis*
>
> - *haemoglobin: low levels could result from covert bleeding, which is present with some cancers, e.g. cancer of the colon*
>
> - *liver function tests: raised levels could indicate liver metastasis.*

Chest X-ray: Normal

Diagnosis: Invasive ductal carcinoma

Staging: T2N1M0

It is very important to diagnose and classify the tumour histologically (by the type of cells involved and their appearance) because this will influence the way in which it could progress and how it will respond to treatment. This is carried out by the pathologist after the tumour has been excised by a surgeon. Following this first step, further diagnostic tests/surgery could be required to help stage and remove the primary cancer.

Staging is an important process that works out how extensive the cancer is, plans treatment, and determines prognosis. If the cancer has not spread beyond her breast, surgery followed by radiation and or chemotherapy would be the common choice. However, if there is spread beyond the breast, surgery may not be performed and chemotherapy would be recommended.

Ngozi's T2N1M0 stage means she has a tumour size 2–3 cm, with lymph node involvement and no metastasis.

Plan 1 (following discussions with patient):

Lumpectomy

Mastectomy:	*breast removal surgery*
Radical mastectomy:	*removal of all the breast, axillary lymph nodes and pectoral muscles*
Lumpectomy:	*removal of the tumour tissue and only a small amount of surrounding tissue*

Results on tissue sample:

3) Oestrogen and progesterone receptors: positive

4) Human epidermal growth factor receptor (HER-2): positive

5) Lymph node involvement 5 out of 20

The results of above tests on the tissue sample of the tumour coupled with the size of the tumour are very important in predicting Ngozi's prognosis and the need for further treatment following surgery.

Oestrogen and progesterone receptors

These are mostly present in post-menopausal women. If receptors are positive, endocrine therapy is used. Unusually, Ngozi is pre-menopausal but has got positive receptors.

Human epidermal growth factor receptor (HER-2)

HER2 is a receptor found on the surface of certain cancer cells. When activated by human epidermal growth factor (HEGF) it can stimulate the cells to divide and grow. HER-2 positive tumours tend to grow faster than others and are more responsive to a HER-2 blocker.

Lymph node involvement

This will predict the possibility of the cancer recurring and the chances of the patient being cured by surgery alone.

Plan 2

1) Multidisciplinary team (MDT) to decide combination chemotherapy

2) Advised screening of first-degree relatives

3) Stop oral contraceptive

The questions that guide the MDT's choice of a regime include:

- *Do the agents have single-agent activity against the specific type of tumor?*

- *Do all the agents have different mechanisms of action that could complement each other?*

- *Do they have differing toxicities or if similar how can they be anticipated and minimized?*
- *What are other patient factors, e.g. what regime will least affect fertility in Ngozi, who wants to have more children?*

Plan following MDT:

Four cycles of anthracycline (doxorubicin) and cyclophosphamide regime plus tamoxifen

A Cyclophospahmide, methotrexate, and fluouracil (CMF) regime was considered and rejected because they have been shown to have a higher effect on fertility.

Although Ngozi was disappointed she would have to stay in England for longer than planned, she decided to focus on getting better so she could return to her family soon.

PART 1

The oncologist explained to Ngozi that she would have to come to the outpatient clinic every 3 weeks to receive intravenous doses (cycles) of the drugs in her regime. She had blood tests and ECG done before she could start chemotherapy.

Ngozi was given leaflets that explain everything about her cancer and treatment by the nurses and an appointment was made for her first appointment.

1a) What is cancer?

1b) Explain the difference between malignant tumours and benign tumours.

2) List two properties of cancer cells that make them different from normal cells.

3) What are oncogenes and what is their role in the aetiology of cancer?

4a) What is apoptosis?

4b) Name two signals that can initiate apoptosis.

5) What do the following terms mean?

a) Neoadjuvant chemotherapy

b) Adjuvant chemotherapy

6a) To what class does cyclophosphamide belong? What phase of cell growth is affected by this class of drugs?

6b) Describe the structure of alkylating agents and how this interacts with cancer cells to lead to apoptosis.

7a) What are other side effects of this class of drug?

7b) Why is it very important to hydrate patients receiving cyclophosphamide, and what drug is also given to help with this particular adverse effect?

8a) Describe the mechanism of action the main cytotoxic effect of doxorubicin.

8b) What is the adverse drug reaction that is most common with doxorubicin and associated only with the cytotoxic antibiotics?

> Hint: Ngozi had an ECG done before commencing treatment.

9) List two other cytotoxic antibiotics and briefly explain their mechanisms of action.

10a) What type of agent is tamoxixen and what is its mechanism of action?

10b) Discuss how fulvestrant and anatrozole's mechanisms of action differ from that of tamoxifin.

11) Describe two mechanisms of cancer chemotherapy resistance.

....

....

....

PART 2

The oncologist discusses two other possible options:

- CMF regime or
- herceptin-tax (trastuzumab and paclitaxel) regime

She explained that the herceptin-tax would be better because the drugs were two different classes and Ngozi was HER positive.

12) To what class does paclitaxel belong and what is its mechanism of action?

....

....

....

13) Explain how trastuzumab would destroy cancerous cells in Ngozi.

....

....

....

14) What is the action of fluorouracil on thymidylate synthesis?

....

....

....

The consultant also decides that Ngozi should discontinue the tamoxifen and take a combination of anastrozole and gosereln injection instead.

15) Describe the mechanism of action of goserelin in Ngozi's case.

Ngozi has made friends with a patient in clinic who was receiving the IFL (irinotecan, fluorouracil and leucovorin) regime for colorectal cancer.

16) What is the mechanism of action of irinotecan?

The doctor explains that the leucoverin is actually folinic acid, which is not really cytotoxic but is used to make the 5-fluorouracil more effective.

17a) What is the name of the cytotoxic agent that requires 'rescue' with folinic acid when high doses are used?

17b) What is the mechanism of action of this cytotoxic agent?

Ngozi has also met a few patients who suffer from haematological cancers. Several were receiving drugs called imatanib and rituximab.

18) List four common haematological malignancies.

19a) Describe the actions of imatinib.

19b) What is the particularly severe reaction called that can occur with rituximab and what is it caused by?

19c) Discuss two of the proposed mechanisms of action of rituximab.

> Ngozi has heard that they are now using thalidomide to treat cancers. She is aware of the controversy given the birth defects it produced in the 1960s. She wonders how it works in cancer.

20) What is the mechanism of action of thalidomide in cancers and how does lenolidamide compare?

21) How does angiogenesis occur and what is its importance in cancer?

22) What is the monoclonal antibody currently used to inhibit angiogenesis and how does it work?

Key references/suggested readings

General references

Australian Prescriber. http://www.australianprescriber.com.

National Institute for Health and Clinical Excellence (NICE). http://www.nice.org.uk/.

Rossi S. ed. *Australian Medicines Handbook*. Adelaide: Australian Medicines Handbook Pty Ltd, 2009.

British National Formulary. London: Pharmaceutical Press, 2008.

Lexi-COMP online. http://www.lexi.com/.

Rote Liste. https://www.rote-liste.de/.

med-news: Medizinische Informationen für Ärzte und Apotheker. http://www.gfi-online.de/.

Chapter 3: Pharmacokinetics

Birkett DJ. *Pharmacokinetics Made Easy*. Sydney: McGraw-Hill, 2002.

Chapter 4: Haemostasis and thromboembolic disorders

Osborne P, Dabin S, Rose P. A warfarin decision aid for patients on long-term therapy. *Prescriber* 2009; 20(13): 13–15.

Keeling D. Weighing up the risks and benefits of warfarin plus aspirin. *Prescriber* 2009; 20(4): 6–3.

Blann AD, Khoo CW. The prevention and treatment of venous thromboembolism with LMWHs and new anticoagulants. *Vasc Health Risk Manag* 2009; 5: 693–704.

Chapter 5: Hypertension

Ooi S-Y, Ball S. ACE inhibitors: their properties and current role in hypertension. *Prescriber* 2009; 20 (14): 15–28.

Chaplin S, McInnes G. ARBs: concise guide to properties and recommended use. *Prescriber* 2009; 20(7); 40–41.

Law M R, Morris J K, Wald N J. Use of blood pressure lowering drugs in the prevention of cardiovascular disease: meta-analysis of 147 randomised trials in the context of expectations from prospective epidemiological studies. *BMJ* 338: b1665.

Moser M, Setaro JF. Resistant or difficult-to-control hypertension. *New Eng J Med* 2006; 355: 385–392.

NICE. Hypertension: management of hypertension in adults in primary care. http://www.nice.org.uk/CG34.

Chapter 6: Atherosclerosis and ischaemic heart disease.

Abrams JMD. Chronic stable angina. *New Eng J Med* 2005; 352: 2524–2533.

Armitage J, Bowman L. Lipid-lowering treatment: today's recommended management. *Prescriber* 2009; 17 (10): 33–44.

Fox K, Ford I, Steg PG, Tendera M, Ferrari R. Ivabradine for patients with stable coronary artery disease and left-ventricular systolic dysfunction (BEAUTIFUL): a randomised, double-blind, placebo-controlled trial. *Lancet* 2008; 372: 807–816.

Chapter 7: Arrhythmias and heart failure

Taggar J, Lip G. Atrial fibrillation: current approaches to drug therapy. *Prescriber* 2008; 19(7): 48–59.

Mattson-DiCecca A-A, Reynolds E. Update: a 60-year-old woman with atrial fibrillation. *JAMA* 2009; 301: 1808.

Squire I. Evidence-based drug treatment of chronic heart failure. *Prescriber* 2009; 20(3); 22–36.

Chapter 8: Inflammation and the skin: dermatitis, acne, and psoriasis

Haider A, Shaw JC. Treatment of acne vulgaris. *JAMA* 2004; 292: 726.

Hengge UR, Ruzicka T, Schwartz RA, Cork MJ. Adverse effects of topical glucocorticosteroids. *J Am Acad Dermatol* 2006; 54: 1–15.

Management of atopic eczema in children from birth up to the age of 12 years: National Institute for Health and Clinical Excellence Clinical guidelines CG57, 2007. Available from http://guidance.nice.org.uk/CG57.

Winterfield LS, Menter A, Gordon K, Gottlieb A. Psoriasis treatment: current and emerging directed therapies. *Ann Rheum Diseases* 2005; 64: ii87–90.

Chapter 9: Rheumatoid arthritis

Chan ESL, Cronstein BN. Molecular action of methotrexate in inflammatory diseases. *Arthritis Res* 2002; 4(4): 266–273.

Kean WF, Kean IR. Clinical pharmacology of gold. *Inflammopharmacology* 2008; 16: 112–125.

Lee ATY, Pile K. Disease modifying drugs in adult rheumatoid arthritis. *Australian Prescriber* 2003; 26: 36–40. Available from http://www.australianprescriber.com/magazine/26/2/36/40/.

Nielsen OH, Ainsworth M, Csillag C, Rask-Madsen J. Systematic review: coxibs, non-steroidal anti-inflammatory drugs or no cyclooxygenase inhibitors in gastroenterological high-risk patients? *Aliment Pharmacol Therapeutics* 2006; 23: 27–33.

Olsen NJ, Stein CM. New drugs for rheumatoid arthritis. *New Engl J Med* 2004; 350: 2167–2179.

Rheumatoid arthritis: the management of rheumatoid arthritis in adults. National Institute for Health and Clinical Excellence Clinical guidelines CG79, 2009. Available from http://www.nice.org.uk/Guidance/CG79.

Saag KG, Teng GG, Patkar NM, Anuntiyo J, Finney C, Curtis JR, *et al.* American College of Rheumatology 2008 recommendations for the use of nonbiologic and biologic disease-modifying antirheumatic drugs in rheumatoid arthritis. *Arthritis and Rheumatism* 2008; 59: 762–784.

Chapter 10: Allergies and antihistamines: allergic rhinitis and urticaria

Barnes PJ. Molecular mechanisms of corticosteroids in allergic diseases. *Allergy* 2001; 56: 928–936.

Golightly LK, Greos LS. Second-generation antihistamines: actions and efficacy in the management of allergic disorders. *Drugs* 2005; 65: 341–384.

National Prescribing Centre. Common questions about hay fever. *MeReC Bulletin* 2004; 14(5): 17–20.

Ramey JT, Bailen E, Lockey RF. Rhinitis medicamentosa. *J Invest Allergol Clin Immunol* 2006; 16: 148–155.

Chapter 11: Respiratory disease: asthma and COPD

Global Initiative for Asthma. Global Strategy for Asthma Management and Prevention, 2008. Available from http://www.ginasthma.com/.

Guideline No. 101 British Guideline on the Management of Asthma: a national clinical guideline, 2009. Available from http://www.sign.ac.uk/guidelines/fulltext/101/index.html.

McKenzie DK, Abramson M, Crockett AJ, Glasgow N, Jenkins S, McDonald C, *et al.* The COPD-X Plan: Australian and New Zealand Guidelines for the management of Chronic Obstructive Pulmonary Disease, 2008. Available from http://www.copdx.org.au/guidelines/index.asp.

National Collaborating Centre for Chronic Conditions. Chronic obstructive pulmonary disease. National clinical guideline on management of chronic obstructive pulmonary disease in adults in primary and secondary care. *Thorax* 2004; 59 Suppl 1: 1–232.

Strunk RC, Bloomberg GR. Omalizumab for asthma. *New Engl J Med* 2006; 354: 2689–2695.

Chapter 12: Upper gastrointestinal tract disorders

Goyal RK, Hirano I. The enteric nervous system. *New Engl J Med* 1996; 334: 1106–1115.

Guideline No. 68 Dyspepsia: a national clinical guideline, 2003. Available from http://www.sign.ac.uk/guidelines/fulltext/68/index.html.

Hoyer D, Hannon JP, Martin GR. Molecular, pharmacological and functional diversity of 5-HT receptors. *Pharmacol Biochem Behav* 2002; 71: 533–554.

Huang JQ, Hunt RH. Pharmacological and pharmacodynamic essentials of H2-receptor antagonists and proton pump inhibitors for the practising physician. *Best Pract Res Clin Gastroenterol* 2001; 15: 355–370.

Montuschi P, Sala A, Dahlèn S-E, Folco G. Pharmacological modulation of the leukotriene pathway in allergic airway disease. *Drug Discovery Today* 2007; 12: 404–412.

Sachs G, Shin JM, Howden CW. The clinical pharmacology of proton pump inhibitors. *Aliment Pharmacol Therapeut* 2006; 23: 2–8.

Chapter 13: Disorders of the lower gastrointestinal tract

Kraft MD. Emerging pharmacologic options for treating postoperative ileus. *Am J Health-System Pharm* 2007; 64: S13–S20.

Mawe GM, Coates MD, Moses PL. Intestinal serotonin signalling in irritable bowel syndrome. *Aliment Pharmacol Therapeut* 2006; 23: 1067–1076.

Rome III Diagnostic Criteria for Functional Gastrointestinal Disorders. Rome Foundation. Available from http://www.romecriteria.org/edproducts/romeiii.cfm.

Schiller LRMD. Clinical pharmacology and use of laxatives and lavage solutions. *J Clin Gastroenterol* 1999; 28: 11–18.

Sentongo TA. The use of oral rehydration solutions in children and adults. *Curr Gastroenterol Rep* 2004; 6: 307–313.

Chapter 14: Diabetes mellitus and obesity

Australian Centre for Diabetes Strategies. National Evidence Based Guidelines for the Management of Type 2 Diabetes Mellitus. Canberra, National Health and Medical Research Council, 2005. Available from http://www.diabetesaustralia.com.au/.

Greenfield JR, Chisholm DJ. Thiazolidinediones-mechanisms of action. *Australian Prescriber* 2004; 27: 67–69. Available from http://www.australianprescriber.com/magazine/27/3/67/70/.

Harrold JA. Hypothalamic control of energy balance. *Curr Drug Targets* 2004; 5: 207–219.

Hiller-Sturmhfel S, Bartke A. The endocrine system. *Alcohol Health Res World* 1998; 22: 153–164.

Holst JJ. The physiology and pharmacology of incretins in type 2 diabetes mellitus. *Diabetes Obesity Metab* 2008; 10: 14–21.

The management of type 2 diabetes. National Institute for Health and Clinical Excellence Clinical Guidelines CG66, 2008. Available from http://www.nice.org.uk/CG66.

Vincent RP, Ashrafian H, le Roux CW. Mechanisms of disease: the role of gastrointestinal hormones in appetite and obesity. *Nature Clin Pract Gastroenterol Hepatol* 2008; 5: 268–277.

The prevention, identification, assessment and management of overweight and obesity in adults and children. National Institute for Health and Clinical Excellence Clinical Guidelines CG43, 2006. Available from http://www.nice.org.uk/CG043.

Chapter 15: The thyroid and contraception

Frye CA. An overview of oral contraceptives. Mechanism of action and clinical use. *Neurology* 2006; 66: 29–36.

Zhang J, Lazar MA. The mechanism of action of thyroid hormones. *Ann Rev Physiol* 2000; 62: 439–466.

Chapter 16: Epilepsy

Epilepsy in adults: quick reference guide. National Institute for Health and Clinical Excellence Clinical Guideline CG20, 2003. http://www.nice.org.uk/nicemedia/pdf/CG020adultsquickrefguide.pdf

Packham B. How to improve compliance with antiepileptic drugs. *Prescriber* 2009; 20: 12–20.

Chaplin S, Hart Y. Lacosamide: new adjunctive treatment for partial seizures. *Presciber* 2009; 20(10); 16–20.

Silver N, Cockerel C. Status epilepticus: features and appropriate management. *Prescriber* 2009; 20(6); 17–28.

Jon-Paul A. Manning, Douglas A. Richards, Norman G. Bowery. Pharmacology of absence epilepsy. *Trends Pharmacol Sci* 2003; 24(8): 428–433.

Chapter 17: Degeneration in the brain: Parkinson's disease and Alzheimer's disease

Metta V, Davidson C, Iqbal N. Treatment options for the management of parkinsonism. *Prescriber* 2009; 20(12): 32–45.

Lindvall O, Koaia Z. Prosepects of stem cell therapy fro replacing dopamine neurons in Parkinson's disease. *Trends Pharmacol Sci* 2009; 30(5): 260–267.

Gifford J, Jones R. Assessment and treatment of cognitive deficits in dementia. *Prescriber* 2009; 20(6): 45–49.

Andersen OM, Willnow TE. Lipoprotein receptors in Alzheimer's disease. *Trends Neurosci* 2006; 29(12): 687–694.

Brown D. Antipsychotics in dementia: use only if the risks are justified. *Prescriber* 2009; 20(8): 79.

Chapter 18: Schizophrenia

Laruelle M, Frankle WG, Narendran R, Kegeles LS, Abi-Dargham A. Mechanism of action of antipsychotic drugs: from dopamine D_2 receptor antagonism to glutamate NMDA facilitation. *Clin Therapeut* 2005; 27(Supple A): S16–S24.

Livingston M. Choosing an antipsychotic: an evidence-based approach. *Prescriber* 2009; 20(7): 7–9.

Lechner S. Glutamate-based therapeutic approaches: inhibitors of glycine transport. *Curr Opin Pharmacol* 2006; 6: 75–81.

Conn PJ, Lindsley CW, Jones CK. Activation of metabotropic glutamate receptors as a novel approach for the treatment of schizophrenia. *Trends Pharmacol Sci* 2009; 30(1): 25–31.

Chapter 19: Depression and anxiety

Anderson IM, Ferrier IN, Baldwin RC, Cowen PJ, Howard L, Lewis G, Matthews K, McAllister-Williams RH, Peveler RC, Scott J, Tylee A. Evidence-based guidelines for treating depressive disorders with antidepressants: A revision of the 2000 British Association for Psychopharmacology guidelines. *J Psychopharmacol* 2008; 22: 343–396.

Cowen P. Management of depression. *Prescriber* 2009; 20(7): 12–18.

Davies S, Nash J, Nutt D. Management of panic disorder in the primary-care setting. *Prescriber* 2009; 20(8): 17–26.

Chapter 20: Pain and its drug treatment

Campbell W. Current options in the treatment of mild-to-moderate pain. *Prescriber* 2009; 20(5): 31–45.

Zeppetella G. Effentora: fentanyl buccal tablet for breakthrough cancer pain. *Prescriber* 2009; 20(8): 28–33.

Chapter 21: The treatment of infections

Perea S, Patterson TF, Eliopoulos GM. Antifungal resistance in pathogenic fungi. *Clin Infect Diseases* 2002; 35: 1073–1080.

Hawkey PM. The origins and molecular basis of antibiotic resistance. BMJ 1998: 657–660.

Drlica K, Zhao X. DNA gyrase, topoisomerase IV, and the 4-quinolones. *Microbiol Molec Biol Rev* 1997; 61: 377–392.

Stratton CW. Dead bugs don't mutate: susceptibility issues in the emergence of bacterial resistance. *Emerging Infectious Diseases* 2003; 9: 10–16.

Back DJ, Burger DM, Flexner CW, Gerber JG. The pharmacology of antiretroviral nucleoside and nucleotide reverse transcriptase inhibitors: implications for once-daily dosing. *JAIDS* 2005; 39: S1–S23.

Clavel F, Hance AJ. HIV drug resistance. *New Engl J Med* 2004; 350: 1023–1035.

Antibiotics Expert Group. Therapeutic guidelines: Antibiotics. Version 13. Melbourne: Therapeutic Guidelines Ltd; 2006.

Chapter 22: Cancer chemotherapy

Clarke SJ, Sharma R, Mainwaring P. Angiogenesis inhibitors in cancer-mechanisms of action. *Australian Prescriber* 2006; 29: 9–12. Available from http://www.australianprescriber.com/magazine/29/1/9/12/.

Espinosa E, Zamora P, Feliu J, Gonz·lez BarÛn M. Classification of anticancer drugs: a new system based on therapeutic targets. *Cancer Treatment Rev* 2003; 29: 515–523.

Hesketh PJ. Chemotherapy-induced nausea and vomiting. *New Engl J Med* 2008; 358: 2482–2494.

Homsi J, Daud AI. Spectrum of activity and mechanism of action of VEGF/PDGF inhibitors. *Cancer Control* 2007; 14: 285–294.

Howell SJ, Johnston SRD, Howell A. The use of selective estrogen receptor modulators and selective estrogen receptor down-regulators in breast cancer. *Best Pract Res Clin Endocrinol Met* 2004; 18: 47–66.

Jordan MA, Wilson L. Microtubules as a target for anticancer drugs. *Nature Rev Cancer* 2004; 4: 253–265.

Mellor HR, Callaghan R. Resistance to chemotherapy in cancer: a complex and integrated cellular response. *Pharmacology* 2008; 81: 275–300.

Rawlings JS, Rosier KM, Harrison DA. The JAK/STAT signaling pathway. *J Cell Sci* 2004; 117: 1281–1283.

Smithy MR. Rituximab (monoclonal anti-CD 20 antibody): mechanisms of action and resistance. *Oncogene* (Basingstoke) 2003; 22: 7359–7368.

Wang JC. Cellular roles of DNA topoisomerases: a molecular perspective. *Nature Rev Molec Cell Biol* 2002; 3: 430–440.

Appendix
Summary of receptors

This summary of receptors is selective for the information relevant to the understanding of clinical pharmacology encountered in this book. For the most part only receptors known to be direct targets for clinical drugs are included, and receptor subtypes are shown only where they help understand the subject or are clinically significant. The main functions regulated by receptors are limited to those most relevant to clinical practice. Similarly, examples of agonists and antagonists are restricted. For a comprehensive pharmacological account of receptors and channels the reader is directed to Alexander *et al.* (2009), *Guide to Receptors and Channels*, 4th edn, published by the *British Journal of Pharmacology*. Many excellent reviews of the different types of receptors have also been published.

Abbreviations

PLC   phospholipase C

$[Ca^{2+}]_c$ cytosolic Ca^{2+} concentration

Acetylcholine receptors

There are two types of receptors for acetylcholine: the nicotinic acetylcholine receptor, which is a ligand-gated ion channel, and the muscarinic acetylcholine receptor, which is a G protein-coupled receptor (GPCR).

Nicotinic acetylcholine receptors (nAChR)

These are ligand-gated cation channels. All nAChR are made up of five subunits that cross the membrane and form a non-selective cation channel. These always include α-subunits, which contain the acetylcholine binding site.

> **Effects**   ↑ entry of Na^+, depolarizing the membrane (i.e. always excitatory). All sympathetic ganglia (fast responses). Widespread bodily effects. Also in brain.
>
> **Subtypes**   Multiple subtypes, three main groups: muscle (neuromuscular junction), ganglionic (at autonomic ganglia) and brain (widespread – one brain type is especially sensitive to nicotine). Their pharmacological profiles (agonist potencies and efficacies, and antagonist affinities) are not yet settled.
>
> **Agonists**   Acetycholine and (particularly at neuromuscular junction) suxamethonium.
>
> **Antagonists**   Non-depolarizing neuromuscular blocking drugs such as pancuronium and atracurium.
>
> **Desensitization**   Particularly with prolonged activation by the drug suxamethonium, resulting in a depolarizing neuromuscular blockade (i.e. the nAChR at the neuromuscular junction no longer responds, resulting in no muscle contraction).

Muscarinic acetylcholine receptors (mAChR)

These GPCRs couple through G_i and $G_{q/o}$ to increase phospholipase C activity (with elevated intracellular Ca^{2+} and protein kinase-C (PKC) activities) and reduce adenylyl cyclase (lower cyclic AMP levels).

Effects   Widespread – all effects of the parasympathetic nervous system. Clinically significant effects include salivary secretion, intestinal motility, bronchoconstriction, bradycardia, pupil constriction, brain function.

Subtypes M_1–M_5 receptors have been identified. Main clinically relevant knowledge focuses on M_1, M_2 and M_3:

M_1

Coupling   Mainly G_q: $\uparrow$ PLC, giving $\uparrow [Ca^{2+}]_c$ and $\uparrow$ PKC, with $\downarrow K^+$ channels.

Effects   Autonomic ganglia (slow excitatory response), $\uparrow$ salivary and gastric secretions, brain.

Agonists   Acetylcholine, carbachol.

Antagonists   Atropine, ipatropium, hyoscine, pirenzepine, dicycloverine.

M_2

Coupling $G_{i/o}$: $\downarrow$ cyclic AMP, $\uparrow K^+$ channels, $\downarrow Ca^{2+}$ channels.

Effects   Heart ($\downarrow$ rate, force and conduction). Brain.

Agonists   Aceylcholine, carbachol.

Antagonists   Atropine, ipatropium, dicycloverine.

M_3

Coupling G_q: $\uparrow$ PLC, giving $\uparrow [Ca^{2+}]_c$ and $\uparrow$ PKC.

Effects   Widespread. Glandular: $\uparrow$ gastric and salivary secretions. $\uparrow$ Smooth muscle contraction: airways, eye (iris, circular, ciliary muscle), gastrointestinal, bladder. Endothelium (vascular).

Agonists   Aceylcholine, carbachol, bethanechol, pilocarpine.

Antagonists   Atropine, dicycloverine, tiatropium.

Adenosine receptors

Also called P1 receptors, there are four types. Adenosine is a non-selective clinically used agonist, and theophylline (aminophylline) is a non-selective A_1/A_2 antagonist. Caffeine is also an agonist.

A_1

Coupling $G_{i/o}$: mainly $\downarrow$ cyclic AMP.

Effects   Widespread and diverse. Heart: $\downarrow$ pacemaker, $\downarrow$ atrioventricular conduction; increase (with A_{2A}) coronary vasodilatation; bronchoconstriction; $\downarrow$ neurotransmitter release (presynaptic); $\downarrow$ NMDA receptors.

A_{2A}

Coupling G_s: mainly $\uparrow$ cyclic AMP.

Effects   Coronary vasodilatation: widespread vasodilatation. Platelets: inhibits aggregation.

A_{2B}

Coupling G_s: mainly $\uparrow$ cyclic AMP.

Effects   Modulates mast cells degranulation, $\uparrow$ vasodilatation, $\uparrow$ cardiac fibroblast proliferation, $\uparrow$ intestinal epithelium Cl^- secretion, $\uparrow$ hepatic glucose production.

A_3

Coupling G_i/o

Effects $\uparrow$ Mast cell degranulation, cardioprotection.

Adrenoceptors

The main types of adrenoceptors, α-adrenoceptors and β-adrenoceptors, are further subdivide into α_1-, α_2-, β_1-, and β_2-adrenoceptors. Further subdivision of these subtypes can be made (e.g. α_1 may be divided into α_{1A}, α_{1B}, etc.) and other subtypes exist (e.g. β_3-adrenoceptors regulate lipolysis in fat tissue). Both adrenaline and noradrenaline are agonists at each of these receptor subtypes, but notably adrenaline has a relatively high potency at the β_2-adrenoceptors.

α_1-**adrenoceptors**

Coupling $G_{q/11}$: $\uparrow$ PLC, giving $\uparrow [Ca^{2+}]_c$ and $\uparrow$ PKC.

Effects $\uparrow$ Smooth muscle contraction: vascular, airways, gastrointestinal tract, uterus, vas deferens, bladder, iris (radial). Liver: $\uparrow$ glycogenolysis and gluconeogenesis. $\uparrow$ Sweat gland secretion. $\uparrow$ Salivary secretion.

Antagonists   Prazosin, doxazocin, indoramin, terazosin, labetalol (also β-adrenoceptor antagonist).

α_2-**adrenoceptors**

Coupling $G_{i/0}$: $\downarrow$ cyclic AMP, $\downarrow$ Ca^{2+} channels, $\uparrow$ K^+ channels.

Effects $\uparrow$ Gastrointestinal tract sphincter contraction. Pancreas: $\downarrow$ insulin, $\uparrow$ glucagon secretion. Presynaptic: $\downarrow$ neurotransmitter release. $\uparrow$ Platelet aggregation.

Agonists   Clonidine

β_1-**adrenoceptors**

Coupling G_s: $\uparrow$ cyclic AMP.

Effects $\uparrow$ cardiac output ($\uparrow$ heart rate, force, conduction). $\uparrow$ Renin secretion. $\uparrow$ amylase rich (viscous) saliva. Brain.

Agonists   Dobutamine.

Antagonists   Numerous β-blockers, e.g. propranolol, labetalol (also α_1-adrenoceptor blocker) and relatively β_1-adrenoceptor-selective (i.e. cardioselective) drugs, e.g. atenolol, bisoprolol.

β_2-**adrenoceptors**

Coupling G_s: $\uparrow$ cyclic AMP.

Effects $\uparrow$ Vasodilatation (particular skeletal and heart muscle vascular beds), bronchodilation, $\uparrow$ liver and muscle glycogenolysis, muscle tremor.

Agonists   Salbutamol, terbutaline, salmeterol, formoterol.

Angiotensin II receptors

Angiotensin II acts on AT_1 and AT_2 receptors, both of which have the 7-transmembrane structure characteristic of GPCRs. Clinically active drugs target the AT_1 receptor.

AT_1

Coupling $G_{q/11}$: $\uparrow$ PLC, giving $\uparrow [Ca^{2+}]_c$ and $\uparrow$ PKC.

Effects $\uparrow$ Vasoconstriction and vascular smooth muscle growth. $\uparrow$ Aldosterone secretion and kidney Na^+ reabsorption.

Antagonists   Losartan (and other 'sartans').

Dopamine receptors

The five dopamine receptor subtypes (D1–D5) are divided into two subfamilies, D1-like (D1 and D5) and D2-like (D2, D3, and D4). All are GPCRs. Further subdivisions (e.g. D_{1A} and D_{1B}) exist. Here we are concerned with dopamine receptors in the brain.

Antagonists Only show weak selectivity between receptor subtypes:

	D1	D2	D3	D4	D5
Chlorpromazine	+	+++	+++	+	+
Haloperidol	++	+++	+++	+++	+
Sulpiride	–	+++	++	–	–
Clozapine	+	+	+	++	+

D1

Coupling G_s: ↑ cyclic AMP.

Effects Widespread and abundant in dopamine projection areas, postsynaptic, modulating excitatory.

D2

Coupling $G_{i/o}$: ↓ cyclic AMP, ↓ Ca^{2+} channels, ↑ K^+ channels.

Effects Widespread and abundant in dopamine projection areas, presynaptic and postsynaptic inhibitory.

D3

Coupling $G_{i/o}$: ↓ cyclic AMP.

Effects Less abundant than D2, especially low in nigro-striatal areas, presynaptic and postsynaptic inhibitory.

D4

Coupling $G_{i/o}$: ↓ cyclic AMP.

Effects Low abundance, especially low in ni gro-striatal areas, presynaptic and postsynaptic inhibitory.

D5

Coupling G_s: ↑ cyclic AMP.

Effects Low abundance, especially low in nigro-striatal areas, presynaptic and postsynaptic modulating excitatory.

GABA receptors

There are two types of receptors for γ-aminobutyric acid (GABA): the $GABA_A$ receptor, which is a ligand-gated ion channel, and the $GABA_B$ receptor, which is a GPCR. $GABA_A$ and $GABA_B$ receptors can be further divided into subtypes (e.g. $GABA_{B1(a)}$, $GABA_{B1(b)}$ and $GABA_{B2}$).

$GABA_A$

Coupling Ligand-gated Cl^- channel inhibiting membrane depolarization.

Effects Widespread in brain: fast postsynaptic inhibition, slow presynaptic inhibition, suppressing uncontrolled excitation.

Agonists GABA, benzodiazepines (modulatory, at separate binding site).

Antagonists Flumazenil (at benzodiazepine binding site). Picrotoxin (blocks channel).

$GABA_B$

Coupling $G_{i/o}$: ↓ cyclic AMP.

Effects Pre- and post-synaptic inhibition in brain.

Agonists GABA, baclofen.

Antagonists Saclofen

Glucagon receptors

There are three members of the glucagon family of receptors (native agonists are glucagon and the glucagon-like peptides).

Glucagon R

Coupling G_s: ↑ cyclic AMP.

Effects ↑ Liver glycogenolysis and gluconeogenesis, ↓ glycogen synthase, lipolysis.

Glutamate receptors

Glutamate receptors fall into four types: three glutamate-gated receptors (NMDA, AMPA, and kainate receptors) and the GPCR metabotropic glutamate receptors. There are about eight metabotropic receptor subtypes.

NMDA receptors are notable for having a separate glycine binding site. Both the glutamate and the glycine binding sites must be occupied for activation. In addition we note that there are a number of clinically important channel blockers.

NMDA receptors
Coupling   Ligand-gated cation channel (Na^+ and Ca^{2+}).
Effects   Widespread in brain: postsynaptic excitatory. Also long-term modulatory (potentiation/depression).
Agonists   Glutamate, aspartate, and NMDA at glutamate site; glycine, D-serine, and cycloserine at glycine site.
Channel blockers   Dizolcipine, phencyclidine, ketamine, memantine, Mg^{2+}.

AMPA receptors
Coupling   Ligand-gated ion channel (fast Na^+, some variants with Ca^{2+} permeability).
Effects   Widespread in brain. Fast postsynaptic excitatory.
Agonists   Glutamate, AMPA, quisqualate.

Kainate receptors
Coupling   Ligand-gated cation channel (fast Na^+).
Effects   Pre- and post-synaptic, excitatory.

Metabotropic receptors
These are designated $mGluR_1$ to $mGluR_8$.

Coupling $mGluR_1$ and $mGluR_5$: $G_{q/11}$: $\uparrow$ PLC, giving $\uparrow [Ca^{2+}]_c$ and $\uparrow$ PKC.
$mGluR_2$ to $mGluR_4$, $mGluR_6$ to $mGluR_8$: $G_{i/0}$: $\downarrow$ cyclic AMP, $\downarrow Ca^{2+}$ channels, $\uparrow K^+$ channels.
Effects   Widespread in brain with diverse synaptic modulation effects.

Glycine receptors

The NMDA glutamate receptor (see above) has an obligatory binding site for glycine and so could be regarded as a glycine receptor. In fact it is always classed as a glutamate receptor. The dedicated glycine receptor of importance in the spinal cord is inhibitory, similar in function and role of the $GABA_A$ to the receptor in the brain. There are several variants of this glycine receptor.

Glycine receptor
Coupling   Ligand-gated Cl^- channel.
Effects   Widespread inhibitory function in spinal cord, suppressing uncontrolled excitation.
Antagonists   Strychnine.

Histamine receptors

There are four types of histamine receptor: H_1–H_4, all GPCRs. Clinical drug action is focussed on H_1 and H_2 receptors.

H$_1$

Coupling $G_{q/11}$: ↑PLC, giving ↑$[Ca^{2+}]_c$ and ↑PKC.

Effects   ↑Vasodilatation, ↑microvascular permeablility, giving local oedema, stimulation of local sensory nerves, giving itching.

Antagonists   Numerous 'antihistamines', including chlorpheniramine, loratidine, and cetirizine.

H$_2$

Coupling G_s: ↑cyclic AMP.

Effects   ↑Gastric acid secretion; cardiac stimulation.

Antagonists   Cimetidine, ranitidine, famotidine, nizatidine.

H$_3$

Coupling $G_{i/0}$: ↓cyclic AMP.

Effects   Presynaptic inhibition of neurotransmitter release.

5-hydroxytryptamine (serotonin) receptors

There are 14 to 15 types of 5-hydroxytryptamine (serotonin, 5-HT) receptors falling into seven classes: 5-HT$_1$ to 5-HT$_7$. Only some are mentioned here. They are all GPCRs with the exception of the 5-HT$_3$ receptors, which are intrinsic ion channel receptors. Their actions are widespread and complex because of the co-expression of different receptor subtypes in a single tissue regulating multiple and overlapping responses. Of particular clinical importance are the many receptor subtypes on the brain, and their increasingly recognized role in the gastrointestinal tract and the brain-gut axis. The clinical pharmacology of 5-HT receptors must be considered alongside the drugs which affect reuptake (e.g. the selective serotonin reuptake inhibitors).

5-HT$_{1A}$

Coupling $G_{i/0}$: ↓cyclic AMP.

Effects   Brain: presynaptic inhibition, affecting mood and behaviour, appetite, thormoregulation, sleep. Cardiovascular effects.

Agonists   Buspirone (partial agonist), aripiprazole, quetiapine, clozapine, ziprazidone.

Antagonists   Ergotamine, spiperone, propranolol.

5-HT$_{1B}$

Coupling $G_{i/0}$: ↓cyclic AMP.

Effects   Brain: presynaptic inhibition, affecting mood and behaviour, vasoconstriction.

Agonists   Ergotamine, sumatripan.

Antagonists   Pindolol, propranolol, meththiothpin.

5-HT$_{1D}$

Coupling $G_{i/0}$: ↓cyclic AMP.

Effects   Brain: cerebral vasoconstriction; behavioural.

Agonists   Sumatripan and related 'triptans', ergotamine.

Antagonists   Ketanserin.

5-HT$_{2A}$

Coupling $G_{q/11}$: ↑PLC, giving ↑$[Ca^{2+}]_c$ and ↑PKC.

Effects   Platelet aggregation, vasoconstriction, bronchiolar and gastrointestinal smooth muscle contraction. Brain: neuronal excitation giving diverse effects, e.g. mood and behaviour, sleep, thermoregulation.

Agonists   LSD, psilocybin.

Antagonists   Cyproheptadine, trazadone, aripiprazole, olanzapine, clozapine, risperidone, sertindole, ziprasidone.

5-HT$_{2B}$

Coupling   G$_{q/11}$: $\uparrow$ PLC, giving $\uparrow$ [Ca^{2+}]$_c$ and $\uparrow$ PKC.

Effects   Gastric contraction, vasoconstriction.

5-HT$_{2C}$

Coupling   G$_{q/11}$: $\uparrow$ PLC, giving $\uparrow$ [Ca^{2+}]$_c$ and $\uparrow$ PKC.

Effects   Brain: mood and behaviour; cerebrospinal fluid secretion. Gastrointestinal motility, vasoconstriction, erectile function.

Agonists   LSD, aripiprazole.

Antagonists   clozapine, cyproheptadine, fluoxetine, olanzapine, quetiapine, risperidone, trazodone.

5-HT$_3$

Coupling   Ligand-gated Na$^+$ and K$^+$ channel.

Effects   Neuronal depolarisation. Emesis, gastrointestinal motility. Anxiety.

Antagonists   Ondansetron and related 'setrons'.

5-HT$_4$

Coupling   G$_s$: $\uparrow$ cyclic AMP.

Effects   Brain: neuronal excitation; behaviour, mood and memory. Gastrointestinal motility.

Agonists   Metaclopramide.

Nicotinic acid receptors

High affinity nicotinic acid receptor (GPR109A)

Coupling   G$_{i/o}$: $\downarrow$ cyclic AMP.

Effects   Reduced adipocyte lipolysis.

Agonists   Nicotinic acid (low concentration).

Low affinity nicotinic acid receptor (GPR109A)

Coupling   G$_{i/o}$: $\downarrow$ cyclic AMP.

Effects   Putative reduced adipocyte lipolysis.

Agonists   Nicotinic acid (high concentration).

Opioid receptors

δ-opioid receptor

Coupling   G$_{i/o}$: $\downarrow$ cyclic AMP.

Effects $\uparrow$ Spinal analgesia, $\uparrow$ respiratory depression, $\downarrow$ gastrointestinal motility.

Agonists   β-endorphin and enkephalins. Etorphine. Morphine and codeine: weak agonists.

Antagonists   Naloxone and naltrexone (weak).

κ-opioid receptor

Coupling   G$_{i/o}$: $\downarrow$ cyclic AMP.

Effects $\uparrow$ Spinal and peripheral analgesia; sedation and confusion.

Agonists   β-endorphin and dynorphin. Etorphine. Morphine and codeine: weak agonists.

Antagonists   Naloxone and naltrexone (high affinity).

μ-opioid receptor

Coupling   G$_{i/o}$: $\downarrow$ cyclic AMP.

Effects $\uparrow$ Analgesia (all levels); $\uparrow$ respiratory depression; $\downarrow$ gastrointestinal motility; euphoria; sedation; addiction.

Agonists   Morphine and codeine; β-endorphin, dynorphin, and enkephalins; etorphine; methadone; meperidine, fentanyl.

Antagonists   Naloxone and naltrexone (high affinity).

Nucleotide receptors

Purinergic receptors are divided into the P1 receptors for adenosine (A_1–A_3: see above) and the P2 receptors for the purine and pyrimidine nucleotides. P2 receptors are further divided into two classes, P2X (ligand-gated ion channel receptors for ATP) and P2Y (GPCRs for ATP, ADP, UTP, UDP, and UDP-glucose), each class being divided further into a number of different receptors designated $P2X_1$–$P2X_7$ and $P2Y_1$, $P2Y_2$, $P2Y_4$, $P2Y_6$, $P2Y_{11}$, and $P2Y_{14}$. Only some are mentioned below.

$P2Y_1$
Coupling $G_{q/11}$: ↑PLC, giving ↑$[Ca^{2+}]_c$ and ↑PKC.
Effects   Widespread, e.g. vascular endothelium ↑prostacyclin release; platelet activation and aggregation; neuromodulation.
Agonists   ADP (ATP).

$P2Y_2$
Coupling $G_{i/0}$: ↓cyclic AMP and ↑PLC, giving ↑$[Ca^{2+}]_c$ and ↑PKC.
Effects   Widespread, e.g. vascular endothelium ↑prostacyclin release; regulation of hepatic glucose/glycogen metabolism; regulation of Cl⁻ fluxes in epithelia, e.g. in airways.
Agonists   ATP, UTP, diquafosol.

$P2Y_4$
Coupling   ↑PLC, giving ↑$[Ca^{2+}]_c$ and ↑PKC.
Effects   Placental and epithelial function.
Agonists   UTP.

$P2Y_6$
Coupling $G_{q/11}$: ↑PLC, giving ↑$[Ca^{2+}]_c$ and ↑PKC.
Effects   Widespread, including heart, blood vessels, and brain.
Agonists   UDP.

$P2Y_{11}$
Coupling G_s: ↑cyclic AMP and $G_{q/11}$.
Effects   Differentiation of immunocytes; vascular smooth muscle cells.
Agonists   ATP.

$P2Y_{12}$
Coupling $G_{i/0}$: ↓cyclic AMP.
Effects   Platelet aggregation and neuronal inhibition.
Agonists   ADP.
Antagonists   Clopidogrel (metabolite).

$P2Y_{13}$
Coupling $G_{i/0}$: ↓cyclic AMP.
Effects   Regulates immunocytes and neuronal cells.
Agonists   ADP.

$P2Y_{14}$
Coupling $G_{q/11}$: ↑PLC, giving ↑$[Ca^{2+}]_c$ and ↑PKC.
Effects   Widespread, role unclear.
Agonists   UDP-glucose.

P2X ligand-gated ion channel receptors for ATP
The ion channel of P2X receptors is permeable to Na^+ and K^+, and Cl⁻ in some cases (e.g. $P2X_5$). ATP is the native agonist in all cases; $P2X_1$ and $P2X_3$ have the highest affinity for ATP. The receptor family is broadly distributed across tissues, indicating a widespread role.

P2X$_1$

Platelets. Smooth muscle: vasculature, vas deferens, bladder, gastrointestinal tract.

P2X$_2$, P2X$_4$ and P2X$_6$

Synaptic modulation in brain and spinal cord – pain, memory, and learning, motor functions.

P2X$_3$

Brain and spinal cord – pain perception.

P2X$_5$

Differentiating and dividing tissues, some cancers.

P2X$_7$

Immunocytes, mediating immune responses, proliferation and apoptosis.

Prostanoid receptors

Placed into classes dependent on the most potent of the native prostanoids agonists: PGD$_2$–DP receptors, PGE$_2$–EP receptors, PGF$_{2\alpha}$–FP receptors, PGI$_2$ (prostacyclin)–IP receptors, thromboxane–TP receptors.

DP$_1$
Coupling   G$_s$: ↑ cyclic AMP.

DP$_2$
Coupling   G$_{i/o}$: ↓ cyclic AMP.

DP receptors
Effects   ↓ platelet aggregation, ↑ vasodilatation, ↑ smooth muscle relaxation (gastrointestinal and uterus), endocrine effects.

EP$_1$
Coupling   G$_{q/11}$: ↑ PLC, giving ↑ [Ca^{2+}]$_c$ and ↑ PKC.
Effects   ↑ smooth muscle contraction- bronchial and gastrointestinal.

EP$_2$
Coupling   G$_s$: ↑ cyclic AMP.
Effects   Gastrointestinal: ↑ smooth muscle relaxation and secretions. ↓ Bronchoconstriction, ↓ vasodilatation.

EP$_3$
Coupling   G$_{i/o}$: ↓ cyclic AMP.
Effects   ↓ Smooth muscle relaxation (gastrointestinal and uterus); ↑ gastric mucous, ↓ gastric acid secretion, presynaptic inhibition, ↑ uterine contractions (in pregnancy).

FP
Coupling   G$_{q/11}$: ↑ PLC, giving ↑ [Ca^{2+}]$_c$ and ↑ PKC.
Effects   Uterine contraction.

IP
Coupling   G$_s$: ↑ cyclic AMP.
Effects   ↓ Platelet aggregation, ↑ vasodilatation.

TP
Coupling   G$_{q/11}$: ↑ PLC, giving ↑ [Ca^{2+}]$_c$ and ↑ PKC.
Effects   ↑ Platelet aggregation, vasoconstriction, bronchoconstriction.

Index